Intracranial Pressure IV

Edited by
K. Shulman A. Marmarou J. D. Miller
D. P. Becker G. M. Hochwald M. Brock

With 235 Figures and 82 Tables

Springer-Verlag
Berlin Heidelberg New York 1980

Kenneth Shulman, M. D.
Anthony Marmarou, Ph.D.
Leo M. Davidoff Department of Neurological Surgery, Albert Einstein College of Medicine, Yeshiva University,
1300 Morris Park Avenue, Bronx, NY 10461 (USA)

J. Douglas Miller, M. D., Ph.D., FRCS
Donald P. Becker, M. D.
Virginia Commonwealth University, Medical College of Virginia, Division of Neurological Surgery, 1200 East Broad Street, Richmond, VA 23298 (USA)

Gerald M. Hochwald, M. D.
Department of Neurology, New York University Medical Center,
550 First Avenue, New York, NY 10016 (USA)

Prof. Dr. Mario Brock
Universitätsklinikum Steglitz, Neurochirurgische Klinik und Poliklinik, Freie Universität Berlin, Hindenburgdamm 30, D-1000 Berlin 45 (FRG)

ISBN-13: 978-3-642-67545-4 e-ISBN-13: 978-3-642-67543-0
DOI:10.1007/ 978-3-642-67543-0

Library of Congress Cataloging in Publication Data. International Symposium on Intracranial Pressure, 4th, Williamsburg, Va., 1979. Intracranial pressure IV. "Proceedings of the fourth International Symposium on Intracranial Pressure held in Williamsburg, Virginia, USA, June 10-14, 1979." Bibliography: p. Includes index. 1. Brain--Diseases--Congresses. 2. Intracranial pressure--Congresses. I. Shulman, Kenneth, 1928-. II. Title. [DNLM: 1. Intracranial pressure--Congresses. W3 IN995] RC386.I56 1979 616.8 79-29761

Softcover reprint of the hardcover 1st edition 1980

Offsetprinting: Beltz Offsetdruck, Hemsbach/Bergstr.

2127/3140-543210

Proceedings of the Fourth International Symposium on Intracranial Pressure
Held at Williamsburg, Virginia, USA, June 10–14, 1979

Organizing Committee

J. D. Miller, Richmond, Secretary
D. P. Becker, Richmond
G. M. Hochwald, New York
A. Marmarou, New York
K. Shulman, New York

Advisory Committee

T. W. Langfitt, Philadelphia, Chairman
J. W. F. Beks, Groningen
M. Brock, Berlin
P. Janny, Clermont-Ferrand
B. Jennett, Glasgow
N. Lundberg, Lund

Preface

This book contains the papers delivered at the Fourth International Symposium on Intracranial Pressure, held at Williamsburg, Virginia, USA, June 10–14, 1979. Divided into 12 sessions, they reflect the most recent developments in areas such as head injuries, pressure-volume studies, cerebrovascular complications, intracranial hemorrhage, brain edema, systemic factors and infectious processes, data recording and analysis, CSF formation and absorption, hydrocephalus, clinical aspects of ICP monitoring, anesthesia and intracranial pressure, treatment with barbiturates and steroids, and osmotherapy. The book concludes with a summary of the present state-of-the-art in the field as a whole by Dr. Langfitt.

There were two innovations at this Symposium. The first of these was poster sessions, the second, breakfast seminars. This volume contains all papers read plus all those presented as posters, and for this reason contains more pages than the three previous volumes.

The organizers wish to thank the Advisory Committee for the work done in paper selection and focus of the Conference. Appreciation is also given to the Chairmen and Co-chairmen of the sessions for the preparation of summary statements. Manuscript preparation was performed by Ms. Lucille Browne, and gratitude is expressed to her.

The next Symposium, the Fifth International Conference on ICP, will be held in Japan in 1982.

We also wish to acknowledge the technical help of Springer-Verlag and their celerity in producing this volume.

The Editors

Contents

Session I. Head Injury

Chairman: D. P. BECKER; *Co-chairman:* I. PAPO

Session II. Pressure-Volume Studies

Chairman: A. MARMAROU; *Co-chairman:* A. L. BENABID

Session III. Cerebrovascular Aspects

Chairman: J. D. MILLER; *Co-chairman:* N. N. ZWETNOW

Session VI. Systemic Factors and Infectious Processes

Chairman: J. W. F. BEKS; *Co-chairman:* A. CROCKARD

Session VII. Data Recording and Analysis

Chairman: J. O. ROWAN; *Co-chairman:* R. L. GRIFFITH

Session X. Clinical Aspects of ICP Monitoring

Chairman: T. W. LANGFITT; *Co-chairman:* N. LUNDBERG

Session XI. Anesthesia and Intracranial Pressure

Chairman: M. S. ALBIN; *Co-chairman:* C. ALEXANDER

Session XII. Barbiturate, Steroid, and Osmotherapy

Chairman: J. T. HOFF; *Co-chairman:* W. GOBIET

Session I
HEAD INJURY

Chairman: D.P.Becker
Co-chairman: I.Papo

SUMMARY

It is now clear that ICP monitoring in patients with severe head injury is an invaluable adjunct to patient management. Clinics with large trauma services are reporting reduced mortality figures, and they relate this, in major part, to ICP monitoring and control of ICP. (BYRNES and DRUCKER). The evidence is mounting that elevated ICP itself may increase morbidity and mortality, and it is now recommended that in head injury ICP be kept below 20-25 mmHg. High levels of ICP do not always reflect degree and extent of irreversible brain damage, and therefore elevated ICP should be treated vigorously. ICP monitoring can be particularly helpful in patients harboring intracranial hematomas or contusions where the surgeon is not sure decompression is needed. TEASDALE and co-workers showed that such patients who have ICP >20 mmHg are likely to deteriorate soon. Finally, prognostic power in head injury can be improved by adding the ICP level to information on the neurological exam. PITTS and co-workers suggest ICP level at 24 hours carries the greatest correlation with outcome.

An important observation regarding ICP in experimental head injury was made by GENNARELLI et al from Philadelphia. Marked ICP rises were seen in the seconds and minutes following mild and moderate acceleration injuries. ICP went as high as 80-90 mmHg for a number of minutes before declining, even in surviving animals. The authors postulate marked cerebrovascular dilation as the cause. A number of discussants suggested that the primary culprit is the marked systemic arterial blood pressure elevation that comes on immediately following the concussive injury. This can cause cerebrovascular dilation and even damage the vascular endothelium (possibly from local prostaglandin release). A presentation by CORALES and colleagues in a later session confirmed the early ICP elevation, and they also showed there was no evidence of brain edema accumulation, further strengthening the vascular etiology hypothesis.

Is external decompression a worthwhile maneuver for control of elevated ICP in head injury? NAKATANI and co-workers from Osaka measured brain tissue pressure in brain underlying an external decompression. The operation did not decrease the brain tissue pressure and appeared to increase the hydrostatic edema propagation. Several discussors supported this position, and suggested it is generally desirable to replace the bone flap and control elevated ICP my medical means (after evacuation of large intracranial masses).

ICP AND OUTCOME IN PATIENTS WITH SEVERE HEAD INJURY

L.H.PITTS, J.V.KAKTIS, R.JUSTER, AND D.HEILBRON

Introduction

The measurement of intracranial pressure (ICP) is important in directing therapy for intracranial hypertenison; it may also improve our ability to predict outcome following coma-producing craniocerebral trauma. Although prognostic schemes exist, they include physical examination data primarily and cannot confidently predict outcome in as many as 35% of patients (3).

We have examined ICP data from our head injured population to determine the relationship between ICP and outcome and to evaluate ICP as a prognostic factor.

Patient Population and Methods of Analysis

Data from ICP monitoring, physical examination, results of surgery, and outcome at 3 months (2) were sequentially collected and subsequently analyzed in an IBM 370 computer. Data for 88 patients with severe head injury who were in traumatic coma (no eye opening, no verbal response, not following commands) for six hours or more and who had continuing monitoring of ICP for at least 12 hours were examined.

ICP monitoring by subdural or intraventricular catheter began within 6 hours of onset of coma in 80% of patients and within 18 hours in all patients. ICP elevations above 25 torr in all patients were treated using hyperventilation and osmotherapy. Monitoring continued until ICP values remained below 20 torr for 24 hours or the patient died. Data were analyzed using both 6 hour mean ICP values and a weighted ICP (ICP_{wt}) derived from values recorded during the first 24 hours of monitoring and weighted using a PASCAL distribution (Figure 1).

We estimated the effect of ICP_{wt} when taken in combination with a variety of other prognostic factors, using a linear logistic regression analysis to develop predictors of outcome using all these variables. Tests for mean differences and linearity were performed using the Breakdown Procedure in the Statistical Package for the Social Sciences (SPSS).

Results

Figure 2 shows the 6 hour mean ICP values for patients in 5 outcome categories determined 3 months after injury. P-values for group differences in mean ICP values and p-values for the linear relationship of group mean ICP to outcome are shown. After an initial 6 hour period of stabilization of ICP, there is a significant linear relationship between ICP and outcome between 6-24 hours. After 24 hours there is no linear relationship between ICP and outcome; some patients died, or monitoring was discontinued after normalization of ICP during the first day.

ICP_{wt} was calculated for various outcome groups (Table I). There were significant differences in mean ICP_{wt} for various groupings of outcome categories. ICP_{wt} was significantly linearly related to outcome for 5 outcome categories (death-D; vegetative state-VS; severe disability-SD; moderate disability-MD; good recovery-GR) and 3 outcome categories (D, VS-SD, MD-GR).

The linear logistic analysis indicates that increasing ICP_{wt} by 1 torr lowers the odds of a "good" outcome (GR, MD) by a multiplicative factor of 0.964; e.g., a 5 torr increase lowers the odds by $(0.964)^5 = 0.73$. ICP_{wt} increases of 1 torr lowers the odds of survival by 0.94; a 5 torr increase lowers the odds by $(0.94)^5 = 0.73$. Our patient study population is not large and the results of this type of analysis vary depending on which prognostic factors are considered and the grouping of outcome categories in a given analysis. Nonetheless, ICP_{wt} compared favorably with age, motor response, eye opening, pupillary response and extraocular movement as a predictor of outcome.

Discussion

Since LUNDBERG'S (5) description in 1964 of ventricular fluid pressure monitoring in head injured patients, ICP determination and control of intracranial hypertension have been mainstays in the treatment of

Table I

	Outcome vs. ICP_{wt}	
DEATH	21 ± 3	
VS	15 ± 4	
SD	16 ± 2	$p < 0.025$
MD	13 ± 3	$p_{lin} < 0.001$
GR	11 ± 1	
DEATH, VS, SD	19 ± 2	$p < 0.01$
MD, GR	12 ± 1	
DEAD	21 ± 2	$p < 0.002$
ALIVE	14 ± 1	
DEATH	20 ± 2	$p < 0.02$
VS, SD	16 ± 2	$p_{lin} < .004$
MD, GR	12 ± 1	

ICP_{wt} given as group mean in torr ±s.e.

See text for abbreviations.

craniocerebral trauma (6, 7). Although elevated ICP is acknowledged to be prejudicial against a good outcome following severe head injury, LANGFITT (4) has pointed out that there is little agreement as to what ICP level is "bad," and notes also that there are major variations in descriptions of outcome categories. In most publications, ICP is reported as normal-elevated or normal-moderate elevation-severe elevation (2, 6, 7). Few data are available regarding mean ICP's in different outcome categories and no data are available regarding a specific ICP value and its relation to outcome.

Our data demonstrate a significant linear relationship between ICP and outcome, and show that the differences in ICP among outcome groups are most pronounced between 6-24 hours after injury. Before 6 hours, there is some ICP instability, perhaps due to resuscitation or postoperative intracranial changes. After 24 hours, given that some patients have died with overwhelming brain damage and uncontrollable ICP elevation and no longer contribute to group mean ICP's, the differences in ICP among groups are not linearly related.

We have defined a weighted ICP value that takes advantage of the group differences between 6-24 hours. Although other improved ICP derivations may be developed, our choice demonstrates statistically significant ICP differences among outcome groups. It further shows that surprisingly low ICP values (i.e., ICP_{wt} 15-21 torr) are associated with death, vegetative state, or severe disability. This suggests that even more aggressive management of intracranial hypertension, i.e., treating ICP greater than 20 torr, might be indicated in head injury.

Our analysis indicates that ICP may be as important a prognostic factor as pupillary or motor responses, or eye movement; only age consistently provided more prognostic information than ICP values. Since JENNETT(3) has shown that outcome cannot confidently be predicted in as many as one-third of severely head injured patients using physical examination features alone, we feel ICP data should be collected and analyzed routinely in an attempt to define more accurately its role in outcome prediction.

Summary

ICP values collected between 6-24 hours after severe head injury are linearly related to outcome. A weighted ICP value is described that shows significant differences among outcome groups. Weighted ICP values for poor outcome groups are surprisingly low, between 15-21 torr, suggesting that more aggressive ICP management may be indicated in the future. Analysis of our data suggests that ICP may be an important prognostic factor and should be included in any data collection scheme for traumatic coma.

References

1. Collice M, Rossanda M. Beduschi A, Porta M (1976) Management of head injury by means of ventricular fluid pressure monitoring. In: Beks JWF, Bosch DA, Brock M (eds) Intracranial Pressure III. Springer, Berlin Heidelberg New York, p 101

2. Jennett B, Bond M (1975) Assessment of outcome after severe brain damage. A practical scale. Lancet I:480-484

3. Jennett B, Teasdale G, Braakman R, Minderhoud J, Knill-Jones R (1975) Predicting outcome in individual patients after severe head injury. Lancet I:1031-1034

4. Langfitt TW (1976) The incidence and importance of intracranial hypertension in head-injured patients. In: Beks JWF, Bosch DA, Brock M (eds) Intracranial Pressure III. Springer, Berlin Heidelberg New York, p 67

5. Lundberg N, Troupp H, Lorin H (1964) Continuous recording of the ventricular fluid pressure in patients with severe acute traumatic brain injury. J Neurosurg 22:581-590

6. Marshall LF, Smith RW, Shapiro HM (1979) The outcome with aggressive treatment in severe head injuries. Part I: The significance of ICP monitoring. J Neurosurg 50:20-25

7. Miller JD, Becker DP, Ward JD, Sullivan HG, Adams WE, Rosner MJ (1977) Significance of intracranial hypertension in severe head injury. J Neurosurg 47:503-516

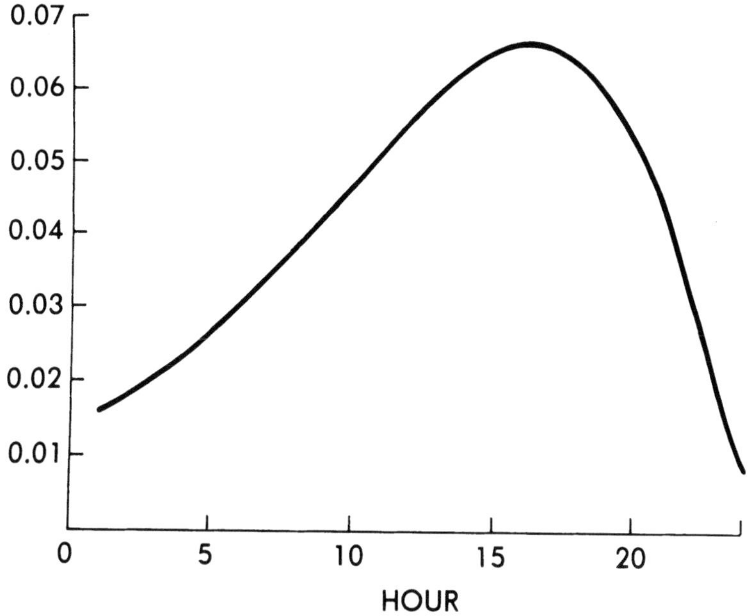

Fig. 1. The PASCAL distribution weighting factors applied to ICP values during the first 24 hours of monitoring, used to produce ICP_{wt}

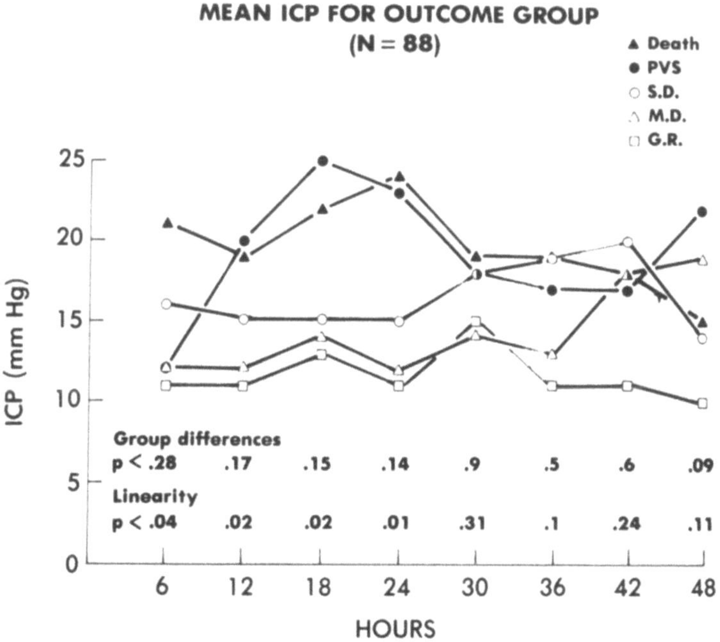

Fig. 2. Six hour ICP mean values for 5 outcome groups. ICP is linearly related to outcome only during the first 24 hours after injury

PROGNOSTIC SIGNIFICANCE OF INTRACRANIAL PRESSURE AND NEUROLOGICAL CONDITION IN ACUTE BRAIN LESIONS

K.E.Richard and R.A.Frowein

Introduction

The significance of intracranial pressure increase in regard to the prognosis of the patients with acute brain lesions until now was not unanimously assessed (1 - 6). Therefore in the present analysis the question which has to be examined is which position the intracranial pressure takes within prognostic factors, especially the age of the patients and the degree of neurologic disorders.

Materials

In 267 patients with an acute intracranial pressure increase before and after surgery of brain tumors (N=145), after head injuries (N=35) and in non tumorous hydrocephali (N=87) the mean ventricular fluid pressure ($VFP\bar{x}$) was calculated from a continuous pressure curve of one day. These values were correlated with the daily checked neurological state. The following states were differentiated:

A. Full consciousness
- I. without neurological disorders,
- II. with moderate neurological disorders,
- III. with severe neurological disorders.

B. Clouded consciousness
- I. without neurological disorders,
- II. with moderate neurological disorders,
- III. with severe neurological disorders.

C. Coma
- I. without neurological disorders,
- II. with paresis/unilateral pupillary dilatation,
- III. with spontaneous extensor rigidity
- IV. with hypotonic musculature/bilateral pupillary dilatation.

These parameters as well as the age of the patients - children as well as teenagers 0-19 yrs; young adults 20-39 yrs; older adults over 40 yrs- were correlated to the outcome: surviving patients; patients who died early, i.e., up to the 14th day; patients who died later, i.e., after the 14th day.

Results

In Fig. 1 for each patient within the first postoperative/posttraumatic week the day of the highest VFPx as well as of the severest neurologic disturbance was taken.

1. Age

In the range of non pathologically elevated pressure values (VFPx 0-20 mmHg) 84% of the children and teenagers, 70% of the young adults, and 52% of the older adults survived. In the higher range of $VFP\bar{x}$ the survival rate decreased and in the older adults with very high pressures over 40 mmHg the survival rate dropped to 30%.

2. Neurological state

Adding to age the neurologic state, the prognostic significance of this parameter becomes apparent. All patients without a disorder of consciousness survived, independently of the VFP level and the age. If the patients were clouded, the outcome was favorable in all instances in which the $VFP\bar{x}$ did not exceed the level of 20 mmHg and the neurologic state did not show any disorder beyond clouded consciousness or a minimal disorder such as a hemiparesis. With pressures over 20 mmHg the survival rate dropped to 71%, respectively to 55% in cases with severe neurologic disturbances.

If the patients were unconscious, the survival rate dropped further with increasing depth of coma and increasing $VFP\bar{x}$. Only 6 children and one young adult postoperatively survived a shortlasting coma grade IV, but only one child had a $VFP\bar{x}$ higher than 20 mmHg.

3. Time factor

In Fig. 2 mean pressures are plotted in relation both to the degree of neurological disturbances and to the postoperative or the posttraumatic periods of time.

Patients after surgery of brain tumor, who were clear or clouded, generally survived mean pressures up to 40 mmHg. Patients with severe hemiparesis survived pressures above 20 mmHg less frequently. The course of the unconscious patients always was unfavorable, if the $VFP\bar{x}$ after the third postoperative day continued to exceed 20 mmHg.

In patients with head injury (Fig. 3) VFP monitoring was not undertaken in slight injuries with undisturbed consciousness. It was only practiced in severe injuries with coma. Patients in coma grades I and II frequently survived pressures up to 40 mmHg. However, none of the patients with coma grades III and IV survived pressures over 20 mmHg. In pressures below 20 mmHg transitory improvements up to apallic syndrome were achieved. All these patients ultimately expired.

Patients with a non-tumorous hydrocephalus rather seldom showed severe disturbances of consciousness (Fig. 4). The course was overwhelmingly favorable even for patients with considerable increases of $VFP\bar{x}$.

Conclusion

In summary it follows that the degree and the duration of disturbed consciousness, the age of the patients and the associated neurologic disorders are the essential prognostic parameters.

The intracranial pressure level and its behavior under treatment, however, gain increasing significance in the course of the patients with severe disturbances of brain function, recognizable by depth and duration of coma.

References

1. Bruce DC, Schut L, Bruno LA, Wood JH, Sutton LM (1978) Outcome following severe head injuries in children. J Neurosurg 48: 679-688

2. Jennet B, Johnston JH (1972) Continuous monitoring of intracranial pressure in patients with head injury. Proc Roy Soc Med 65:885-886

3. Miller JD, Becker DP, Ward JD, Sullivan HG, Adams WE, Rosner MJ (1977) Significance of intracranial hypertension in severe head injury. J Neurosurg 47:503-516

4. Papo I, Caruselli G (1977) Intracranial pressure monitoring in intensive care patients suffering from acute head injuries. Long term intracranial pressure monitoring on comatose patients suffering from head injury. A critical survey. Acta Neurochir (Wien) 39:187-200

5. Richard KE, Frowein RA (1978) The relationship between intracranial pressure disturbances of brain function and prognosis. Neurosurg Rev 1 - 2:25-36

6. Vapalahti M (1970) Intracranial pressure, acid-base status of blood and cerebrospinal fluid and pulmonary function in the prognosis of severe brain injury. Thesis, Helsinki

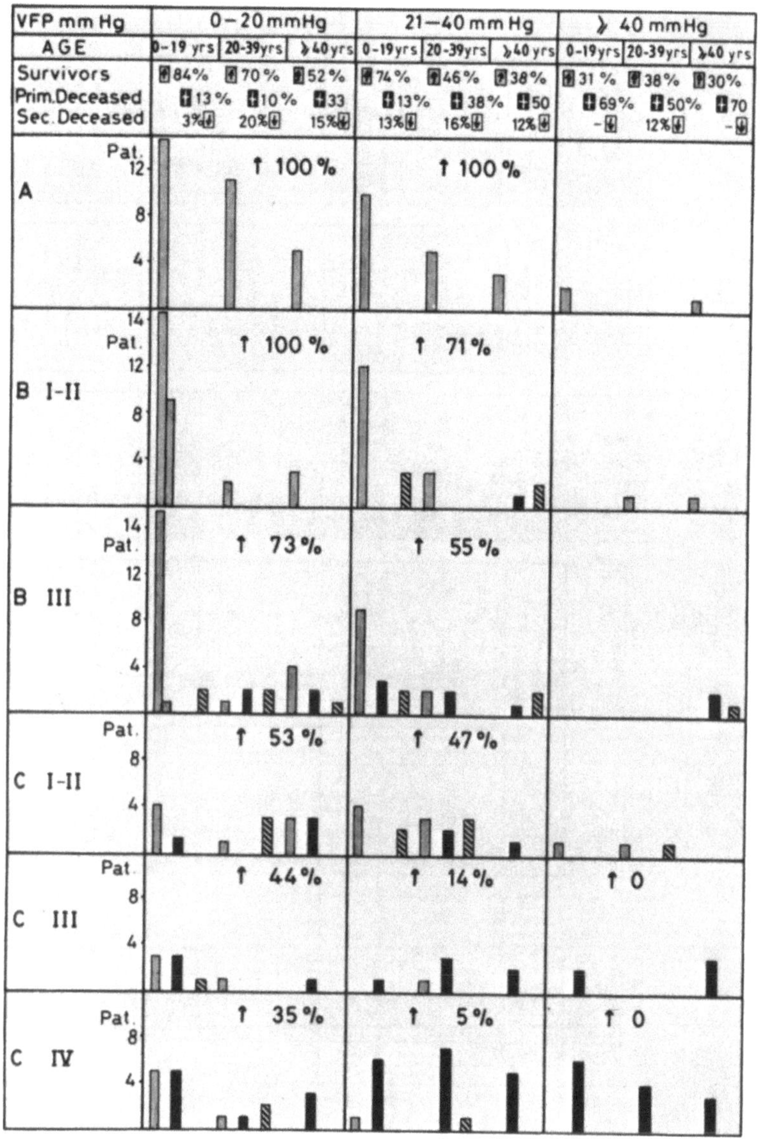

Fig I. Intracranial pressure, age of patients, neurological state and outcome. (For the VFPx and neurological state the worst values of the first post postoperative resp. posttraumatic week were taken).

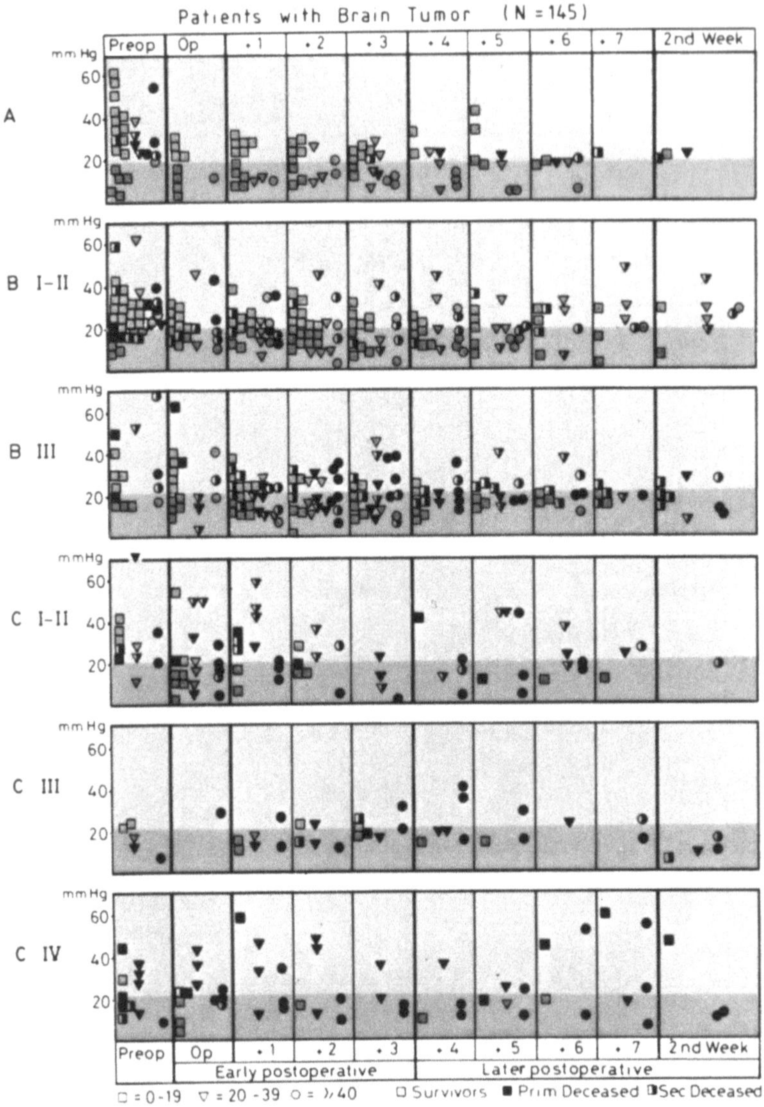

Fig 2. Intracranial pressure and neurological state in the first 2 postoperative weeks after brain tumor surgery.

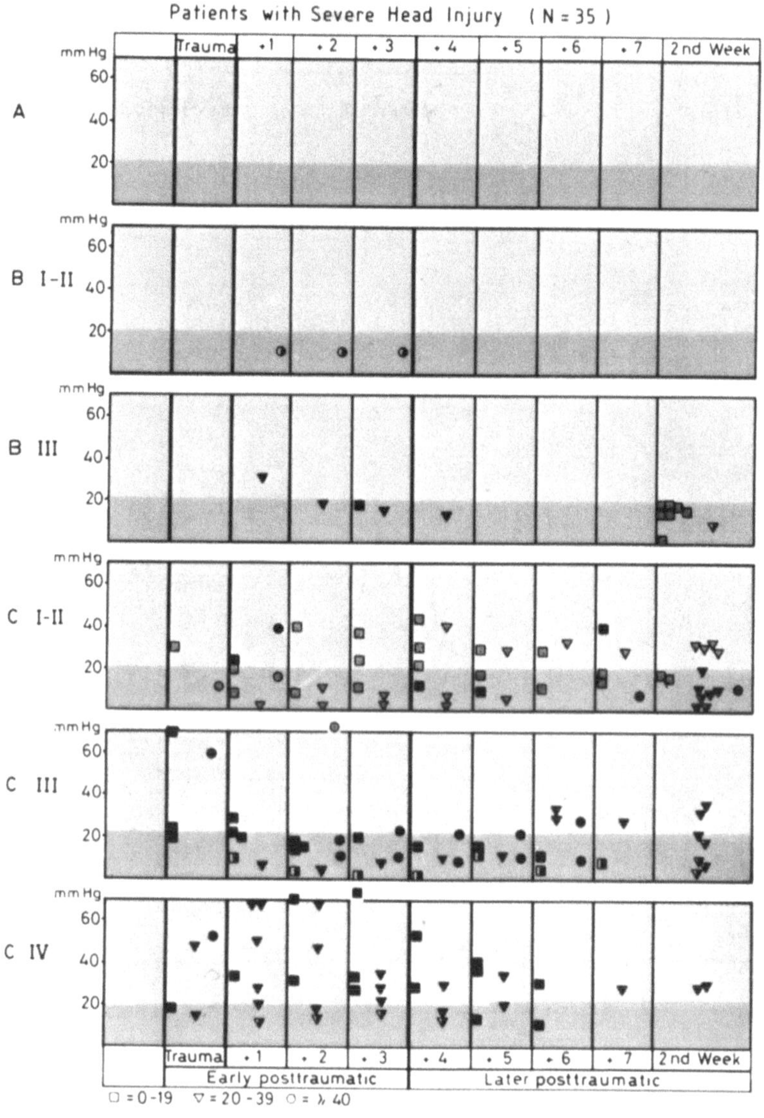

Fig 3. Intracranial pressure and neurological state in the first two posttraumatic weeks after severe head injury.

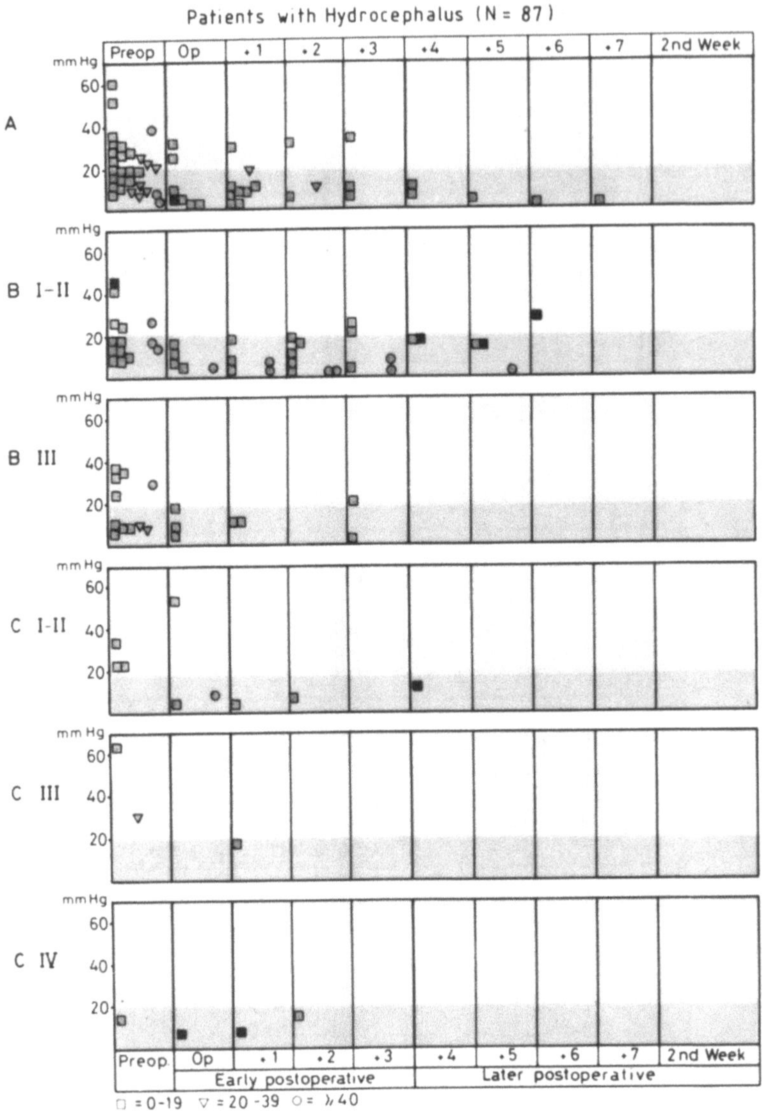

Fig 4. Intracranial pressure and neurological state in the first two weeks in patients with non-tumorous hydrocephali.

ROLE OF ICP MONITORING IN PATIENTS SUFFERING FROM SEVERE BRAIN INJURIES

M.COLLICE, P.VERSARI, G.VECCHI, A.SCORNAJENGHI, AND V.D'ANGELO

Introduction

In order to further evaluate the role of intracranial pressure (ICP) monitoring in brain injured, comatose patients, in terms of both prognostic significance and usefulness for treatment, our total series of monitored patients has been reviewed.

Materials and Methods

The Neurosurgical Department was opened in the Ospedale Maggiore Niguarda in May 1970. Since then 106 comatose patients with severe brain injuries have been studied by ventricular fluid pressure (VFP) continuous monitoring. During the first two years, however, ICP monitoring was used only occasionally, but since then, the indications for VFP monitoring have been standardized and the technique used more frequently.

Of the 106 patients 37 underwent surgery for different types of mass lesions. At admission time or before surgery all were comatose: 68 did not show any signs of midbrain dysfunction (MBD) (purposeful or decorticate motor response); 38 showed some signs of MBD (usually bilateral decerebrate response and/or abnormal or absent oculocephalic reflex). VFP monitoring started within the first 24-48 hours from the onset of coma or soon after surgery. Recording was continued for 5-8 days when coma persisted. Standard treatment consisted of early and hyperoxic hyperventilation, i.v. dexamethasone, and in addition, osmotic diuretics and barbiturates. CSF drainage was given when there was a sustained rise of ICP above 20 mmHg.

Results

The results of the whole series are reported in Table I. Of the 106 patients, 40 (or 37.7%) died and 26 of these showed a high intracranial pressure (HICP), that is, an ICP more than 15 mmHg. The overall mortality rate in patients with HICP was 58.6%, while it was 21.6% in those with normal ICP (significant difference, x^2:10.9). If mortality rates in patients with normal ICP, moderate HICP (15-45 mmHg) and severe HICP (more than 45 mmHg) are considered separately, a significant difference is found only between patients with normal ICP and severe HICP (x^2:29). Also, in this group of patients with severe HICP 3 out of 5 survivors were under 8 years. When the patients are divided in two categories according to clinical presentation (with and without MBD) mortality in HICP group is significantly higher than in normal ICP group only for patients with MBD (x^2:6.635).

Table 1. ICP and final outcome in 106 patients with severe brain injury according to clinical presentation and presence or absence of mass lesion. (Number of dead in brackets.) In patients with mass lesion only postoperative recordings have been considered
MBD: Midbrain dysfunction

		ICP CLASSES (mmHg)			
		0 - 15	16 - 45	45	TOTAL
COMA WITHOUT MBD	MASS	17 (3)	2 (0)	1 (0)	20 (3)
	NO MASS	29 (4)	12 (2)	7 (4)*	48 (10)
COMA WITH MBD	MASS	6 (2)	7 (5)	4 (4)	17 (11)
	NO MASS	8 (4)	5 (5)	8 (7)**	21 (16)
TOTAL		60 (13)	26 (12)	20 (15)	106 (40)

* Two of 3 survivors were under 8 years.
** The only survivor is 4 years.

Table 2. Mortality rate in severe brain injury patients without MBD and without mass lesion in ICP monitored series and in non-monitored series

	Cases No.	Mortality
Monitored series	48	20.8%
Non-monitored series	62	37.0% (No s.d.)

Conclusions

ICP and prognosis
The relationship between ICP and outcome is confirmed in this series, i.e., intracranial hypertension has a definite negative influence on clinical results. Obviously, this is particularly true for patients with severe intracranial hypertension and/or for those showing MBD signs and for patients over 8 years.

As LANGFITT (1) pointed out at the last meeting in Groningen, there is no general agreement regarding the prognostic value of ICP monitoring in patients with brain injury. We would like to stress that among other factors, the type of treatment used might have a role in determining the different results reported. In other words, early hyperventilation and sedation may avoid intracranial hypertension due to acute post-traumatic hyperemia; thus, in these circumstances, HICP may reflect a more severe diffuse injury.

ICP as a guide for treatment
Because of the relatively low incidence of HICP in postoperative course of patients presenting without MBD signs before surgery (3 out of 20 patients) and due to the very high mortality rate in all patients with MBD (21 out of 23 patients), despite intensive therapy,

it seems to us that ICP monitoring could be of particular value in patients presenting without MBD and without mass lesion. In fact, in this group of patients HICP incidence was approximately 40% and overall mortality relatively low (20%).

In an attempt to confirm this hypothesis we tried to compare outcome in this group of monitored patients with outcome in a previous group of non-monitored patients presenting with similar clinical features. Survival seems to be better in the monitored series although statistical significance was not reached and the comparison between the series may be open to criticism. (Table 2)

In summary, in brain injured patients, ICP monitoring may give some useful information on prognosis in cases with MBD and help to improve the management of patients with less severe brain damage.

Reference

1. Langfitt TW (1976) The incidence and importance of intracranial hypertension in head-injured patients. In: Beks JWF, Bosch DA, Brock M (eds) Intracranial Pressure III. Springer, Berlin Heidelberg New York, p 67

BRAIN DAMAGE IN FATAL NON-MISSILE HEAD INJURY WITHOUT NEUROPATHOLOGICAL EVIDENCE OF HIGH ICP

D.I.GRAHAM, J.H.ADAMS, AND D.DOYLE

Introduction

If a high intracranial pressure (ICP) is sustained after head injury then the outcome is less good than in patients with a normal ICP (11,6). On the other hand some patients in whom the monitored ICP has not been raised die or remain vegetative (5,6). These clinical reports, which reflect uncertainty about the relationship between ICP and outcome, do not include pathological data.

We report here the types of brain damage that are found in fatal non-missile head injuries in which there is no neuropathological evidence of the ICP having been high during life.

Material and methods

In a comprehensive neuropathological analysis of 280 patients, all of whom had been managed in the Department of Neurosurgery, Institute of Neurological Sciences, Glasgow, there were 48 without evidence of raised ICP.

The brains and spinal cords were fixed in 10% formal saline for at least 3 weeks before dissection. After transecting the midbrain, the cerebral hemispheres were cut in the coronal plane into slices 1.0 cm thick. Representative blocks of cerebrum, cerebellum and brain stem were stained by NISSL'S method using cresyl violet and by WOELKES' modification of HEIDENHAIN'S technique for myelin, and by various other techniques when they were considered appropriate.

Results

Using criteria established previously (1), these 48 (17%) patients had no neuropathological evidence of a significantly high ICP during life: furthermore none had evidence of secondary brain stem damage. There were 37 males and 11 females. The age range was from 3 months to 78 years, and the length of survival after injury ranged from 2 hours to 20 months. There was a fracture of the skull in 30 (62%) and multiple injuries in 13 (27%). In the great majority death was due to "medical" complications that included bronchopneumonia, pulmonary embolism, sepsis and renal failure.

Ischaemic brain damage of the types defined preiously (3) was present in 34 (71%) cases; of the 20 cases with lesions in the cerebral cortex there were 7 with diffuse necrosis, 8 in which the ischaemic damage was centered on the boundary zones between the major arterial territories, 4 in which the ischaemic damage was centered on the anterior or middle cerebral arterial territories or both, and 1 in whom there was multiple foci of necrosis. There was ischaemic damage in the hippocampus in 28, in the basal ganglia in 22 and in the cerebellum in 22.

TABLE

	n	Talked	Ischaemic brain damage	Supratentorial haematoma	Acute meningitis	Cerebral fat embolism	Diffuse brain swelling
Cases with severe impact injury (not avoidable)*	17	0	11	1	1	0	2
Cases without severe impact injury (avoidable)	31	19	23	11	4	3	5
	48	19	34	12	5	3	7

*Includes cases in which the principal neuropathological findings were diffuse injury to white matter (13), primary haemorrhages in brain stem (2), a large depressed fracture of the skull (1) and severe cerebral contusions (1).

Ischaemic brain damage was severe in 9 (26%), moderately severe in 11 (32%) and mild in 14 (42%).

There was diffuse damage to white matter of immediate impact type in 13 (27%) cases (2).

In 5 cases there was acute meningitis, in 7 diffuse brain swelling, in 3 massive cerebral fat embolism, in 2 multiple small hemorrhages in the brain stem of the type described by TOMLINSON (10) and in 1 a large depressed fracture of the skull with severe underlying cerebral contusions. There were 12 cases in which more than one type of major brain damage was present. Contusions were absent or slight in 42, moderately severe in 4 and extensive in 2; there were 6 cases in which damage to the cerebral hemispheres was restricted to contusions. In 6 cases there was minimal brain damage, death being due to extracerebral complications.

Nineteen (40%) of the 48 patients "talked and died" (8), and in 12 (25%) a supratentorial haematoma had been evacuated (see Table). None of the 17 patients with severe impact damage (not avoidable) "talked", whereas 19 of the 31 (61%) cases without severe impact damage (avoidable) "talked" before death.

Discussion

In none of these cases was there neuropathological evidence of the ICP having been high in life (1) and yet 17 (35%) had sustained severe brain damage (not avoidable) at impact. In the remaining 31 (65%) cases without evidence of severe impact damage, it is reasonable to assume that much of the brain damage must have been secondary. That 19 (61%) of these 31 cases "talked" before dying (8) is further evidence that severe brain damage had not been sustained at impact. This raises the possibility that death might have been avoided, either by preventing or by treating complications more effectively (9,4,7).

Ischaemic brain damage was identified in 34 (71%) of the cases and is therefore the most common type of potentially avoidable injury. Even though we have previously shown (3) that there is a statistically significant association between ischaemic brain damage and raised intracranial pressure, the present study shows a remarkably high incidence of ischaemic brain damage in cases without evidence that ICP was high in life. Ischaemic brain damage therefore appears to be a major factor contributing to the mortality and persisting morbidity associated with severe head injury whether or not the ICP has been raised.

A common avoidable factor contributing to death after head injury is delay in the treatment of an intracranial haematoma (9). It is therefore of interest to note that in 12 patients there was no neuropathological evidence of a high ICP even though a supratentorial haematoma had been successfully evacuated; in 7 of these 12 cases however, there was another major type of brain damage. Other important but less common secondary complications include diffuse brain swelling, meningitis and massive cerebral fat embolism.

Whilst a sustained rise of ICP may be harmful to the brain, or may be evidence of severe damage already sustained, the corollary is not true. Severe impact damage and serious secondary brain damage are compatible with normal ICP, and avoidable factors were judged to have contributed to death in more than half of the cases reported here without evidence that ICP had been high in life. Whilst measures to control increasing ICP are sometimes important, they should not become the sole objective of clinical management. Neither should a normal ICP be regarded as necessarily indicative of a favorable outcome.

Conclusion

A detailed neurohistological analysis of 280 fatal head injuries showed that there were 48 in which there was no neuropathological evidence of a high ICP. In 17 severe brain damage (not avoidable) was sustained at impact, whereas in 25 of the remaining 31 cases there were potentially avoidable and/or treatable complications contributing to the brain damage (sometimes severe) after the head injury. The absence of a high ICP cannot therefore be equated with a good outcome.

References

1. Adams JH, Graham DI (1976) The relationship between ventricular fluid pressure and the neuropathology of raised intracranial pressure. Neuropath Appl Neurobiol 2:323-332

2. Adams JH, Michell DE, Graham DI, Doyle D (1977) Diffuse brain damage of immediate impact type. Its relationship to "primary brain stem damage" in head injury. Brain 89:489-502

3. Graham DI, Adams JH, Doyle D (1978) Ischaemic brain damage in fatal non-missile head injuries. J Neurol Sci 39:213-234

4. Jennett B, Carlin J (1978) Preventable mortality and morbidity after head injury. Injury 10:31-39

5. Johnston IH, Jennett B (1973) The place of continuous intracranial pressure monitoring in neurosurgical practice. Acta Neurochir 29:53-63

6. Miller JD, Becker DP, Ward JD, Sullivan HG, Adams WE, Rosner MJ (1977) J Neurosurg 47:503-516

7 Miller JD, Sweet RC, Narayan R, Becker DP (1978) Early insults to the injured brain. J Amer Med Assoc 240:439-442

8 Reilly PL, Graham DI, Adams JH, Jennett B (1975) Patients with head injury who talk and die. Lancet II:375-377

9. Rose J, Valtonen S, Jennett B (1977) Avoidable factors contributing to death after head injury. Br Med J 2:615-618

10. Tomlinson BE (1970) Brain-stem lesions after head injury. J Clin Path 23 Suppl (Roy Coll Path)4:154-165

11. Valpalahti M, Troupp H (1971) Prognosis for patients with severe brain injuries. Br Med J 3:404-407

RELATIONS OF CEREBRAL PERFUSION PRESSURE AND HEMATOCRIT WITH HEMISPHERIC CEREBRAL BLOOD FLOW DURING POST – TRAUMATIC COMA

F. ARTRU, B. PHILIPPON, M. BERGER, AND R. DELEUZE

Introduction

In head-injured patients, previous reports on correlations between cerebral blood flow (CBF) and cerebral perfusion pressure (CPP), intracranial pressure (ICP) and arterial blood pressure were discordant (4,1,5,3). In this study, we examined these relations after a correction of CBF values was made for changes due to variations of $PaCO_2$.

Materials and methods

We studied 10 patients with severe brain injuries. All were in deep coma and under controlled ventilation. The epidural pressure was monitored with the technique of de ROUGEMONT et al. (2). Hemispheric CBF measurements were performed bilaterally 16 times, using a modification of OBRIST ^{133}Xenon method. Patients were divided in 2 groups: the symmetrical (sym.) group where the CBF on the two hemispheres differed by less than 5 ml/100g/min and the asymmetrical (asym.) group where the difference was larger. From computerized tomograms (CT), we evaluated also the symmetry or asymmetry of hemispheric lesions in every patient. $PaCO_2$, systolic arterial blood pressure (BP) and hematocrit were measured during each CBF study. We determined the relation between variations of $PaCO_2$ ($\Delta PaCO_2$) and variations of HCBF (ΔHCBF) in 6 patients who were studied twice. All HCBF were then corrected, using this relation, to their theoretical values for an arbitrary $paCO_2$ of 30 mmHg (HCBF').

Results

Average values of HCBF, HCBF', $PaCO_2$, CPP and BP are shown on Table 1. We found a linear relation between ΔHCBF and $\Delta PaCO_2$: $\Delta HCBF = 0.8\ \Delta PaCO_2 + 0.3$ ($r = 0.88$; $p < 0.01$). No significant correlations of HCBF' with CPP, ICP or BP appeared in the series as a whole. The sym. group, however, showed a positive correlation of HCBF' with CPP ($r = 0.45$; $p - 0.07$) and BP ($r = 0.59$; $p < 0.02$; see Fig. 1) but no correlation with ICP (Table 2). In the asym. group, HCBF' on the less perfused side correlated negatively with CPP ($r = -0.68$; $p < 0.05$) and BP ($r = -0.63$; $p = 0.07$), and positively with ICP ($r = 0.84$; $p < 0.01$; see Fig. 2). The better perfused hemisphere did not show significant correlations.

Hematocrit and HCBF' correlated negatively in the whole series ($r = -0.40$; $n = 32$; $p < 0.05$) and in the sym. group ($r = -0.78$; $p < 0.02$). The relation was still significant ($r = -0.70$; $p < 0.05$) when the mean Xenon partition coefficient used in HCBF calculation was assigned a standard value (=1.3), instead of varying with hematocrit.

Examination of CT revealed that patients in the sym. group had inapparent or symmetrical hemispheric lesions, while, in the asym. group,

Table 1. Average values of HCBF, HCBF', PaCO2, ICP and BP in the symmetrical and asymmetrical groups and in the whole series of patients

	SYMMETRICAL GROUP (n=6)	ASYMMETRICAL GROUP (n= 4)		TOTAL (n=10)
		HCBF'+*	HCBF' -*	
HCBF** (ml/100g/min)	33.5 ± 4.3	39.0 ± 3.7	30.3 ± 5.4	34.6 ± 5.4
HCBF' (ml/100g/min)	32.1 6.9	38.7 7.7	21.9 7.6	33.9 8.2
PaCO2 (mmHg)	32 ± 8	30.5 ± 8.1		31 ± 8
CPP (mmHg)	126 ± 17	104 ± 22		114 ± 21
ICP (mmHg)	21 ± 10	17 ± 6		19 ± 9
BP (mmHg)	146 ± 16	121 ± 16		133 ± 20

* + = more perfused hemisphere;
  - = less perfused hemisphere.

** normal value = 47.6 ± 5.0.

Table 2. Correlations of HCBF' with CPP, ICP and BP in the symmetrical and asymmetrical groups and in the whole series of patients

	SYMMETRICAL GROUP	ASYMMETRICAL GROUP HCBF' +	HCBF -	TOTAL
HCBF' and CPP	r = + 0.45 n = 16 p = 0.07	n.s.	r = - 0.68 n = 8 $p < 0.05$	n.s.
HCBF' and ICP	n.s.	n.s.	r = + 0.84 n = 8 $p < 0.01$	n.s.
HCBF' and BP	r = + 0.59 n = 16 $p < 0.02$	n.s.	r = - 0.63 n = 8 p = 0.07	n.s.

the lesions were always very asymmetrical. Furthermore, the hemisphere where the lesions predominated had always the lower CBF value.

Discussion

Correlations of HCBF with other parameters (except hematocrit) were not readily apparent in this series. It was first necessary to eliminate artificially the effect of PaCO2 variations on the CBF results. The existence of a linear Pa CO2/CBF relationship facilitated this correction. Secondly, the patients had to be divided in 2 groups.

In the sym. group, the positive correlations of HCBF' with BP and CPP are in agreement with the results of GOBIET et al. (5), and point to an impairment of CBF autoregulation. In this group, ICP bore no relation with HCBF'.

In the asym. group, on the side of the less perfused hemisphere, ICP appeared to be a function of CBF and not a flow limiting factor. This was previously reported in similar patients with asymmetrical hemispheric lesions (4,1). In these cases, the apparent flow dependence of ICP could be due to an increase of intracranial blood volume caused by the mass displacement of the hemisphere and the consecutive obstruction of venous return. We have no explanation for the paradoxical (negative) relation of HCBF' with CPP and BP. Hematocrit changes noted in this series may have influenced HCBF by modifying blood viscosity.

Summary

Patients with head injuries were divided in 2 groups according to whether the CBF was symmetrical on the two hemispheres or asymmetrical. The former group showed a positive relation of HCBF with BP. In the latter group, the ICP was a function of the HCBF. Hematocrit and HCBF were negatively correlated.

References

1. Bruce DR, Langfitt TW, Miller JD, Schutz H, Valpalahti MP, Stanek A, Goldberg HI (1973) Regional cerebral blood flow, intracranial pressure and brain metabolism in comatose patients. J Neurosurg 38:131-144

2. de Rougemont J, Barge M, BenabidAL(1971) Un nouveau capteur pour mesure de la pression intracranienne. Valeur de la dure-mere en tant que membrane susceptible de transmettre les pressions. Neuro-chir 17:579-580

3. Enevoldsen EM, Jensen FT (1976) The relation between intracranial pressure and regional cerebral blood flow in the acute phase of severe head injury. In: Beks JWF, Bosch DA, Brock M (eds) Intracranial Pressure III. Springer, Berlin Heidelberg New York p 127

4. Fieschi C, Beduschi A, Agnoli A, Battistini N, Collice M, Prencipe M, Rixxo M (1972) Regional cerebral blood flow and intraventricular pressure in acute brain injuries. Europ Neurol 8: 192-199

5. Gobiet W, Bock WJ, Grote W, Bettag M (1975) Cerebral blood flow in patients with traumatic cerebral edema. In: Lundberg N, Ponten U, Brock M (eds) Intracranial Pressure II. Springer, Berlin Heidelberg New York p 508

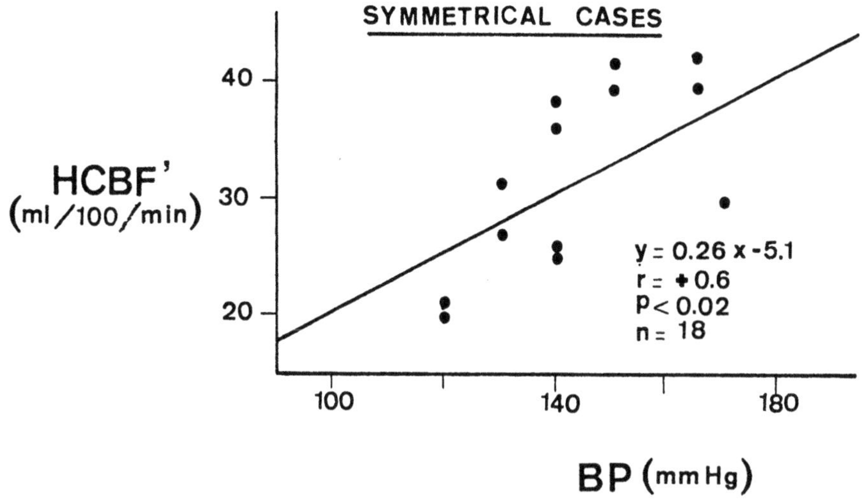

Figure I. Relationship, in the symmetrical group, between hemispheric cerebral blood flow corrected for PaCO2 changes (HCBF') and systolic arterial blood pressure (BP). Regression line and equation are shown.

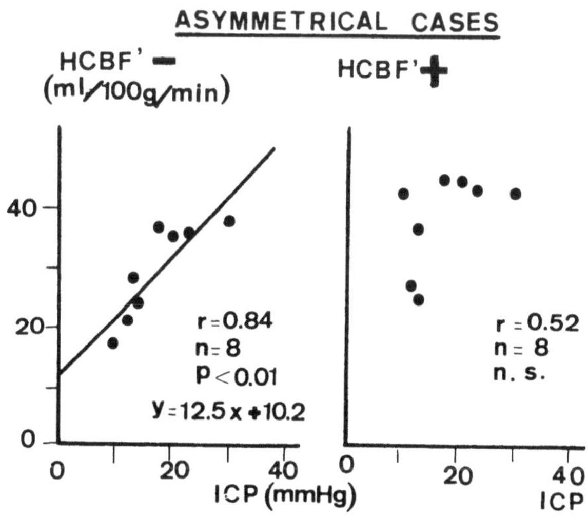

Fig. 2. Relationship, in the asymmetrical group, between hemispheric cerebral blood flow corrected for PaCO2 changes (HCBF') and intracranial pressure (ICP). On the left diagram, in ordinate, CBF of the less perfused hemisphere (HCBF'−).

ICP IN EXPERIMENTAL HEAD INJURY

T.A.Gennarelli, Z.Czernicki, H.Segawa, R.Wiser, K.Marsh, U.Wald, H.Adams, and D.Graham

Introduction

Changes in intracranial pressure (ICP) immediately after acceleration head injury are virtually unknown. Although ICP during acceleration may rise to high levels for several milliseconds, ICP measured by cisternal or lumbar subarachnoid pressure reportedly remains normal immediately after cerebral concussion unless an intracranial hematoma is present (1,2). This report demonstrates that there are profound increases in intracranial pressure in the first few minutes after acceleration injury. These appear to be a function of injury severity and normalize quickly unless acute subdural hematomas occur.

Materials and Methods

Thirty-four supine Macaque monkeys were subjected to a single angular acceleration of the head by an acceleration apparatus capable of producing graded injuries from subconsussive to instantaneously lethal (3). Resulting injuries fell into several groups and were graded by an experimental trauma severity (ETS) system. This report deals with ICP measurements in mild reversible traumatic unconsciousness (ETS 3), severe but recoverable unconsciousness (ETS 4), and animals which did not survive the insult (ETS 5). Intracranial pressure was measured by a modified right angle subarachnoid bolt which was screwed into the right frontal area. The dura was punctured and a hollow subarachnoid bolt was attached to a fluid filled teflon tube attached to a Hewlett-Packard manometrically calibrated pressure transducer. Because of transducer saturation during the acceleration, the transducer was temporarily disconnected for 30 seconds before and for 10 seconds after acceleration injury. Systemic arterial pressure (SAP) was simultaneously recorded from a femoral artery catheter and the cerebral perfusion pressure (CPP) was obtained by the difference between the mean SAP and the mean intracranial pressures. These pressures were recorded for at least two hours following injury. Non-surviving animals were sacrificed on the day of the experiment while surviving animals were sacrificed one week later. Sacrifice by perfusion fixation with Formalin-Acid-Methanol (FAM) was performed, after which the head was immersion fixed for 24 hours before the brain was removed. After removal, the brain was immersion fixed for 24 hours in FAM and then placed in 70% methanol. Whole coronal sections were fixed in paraffin and colloidin and stained with hematoxylin-eosin, cresyl violet, and luxol-fast blue. Care was taken to describe any ischemic brain damage in all serial sections.

Results

Figure 1, A through C depicts the ICP values in individual animals as a function of time after injury in each of the three grades of injury severity. The degree of variability within each grade can be noted.

Figure ID shows the mean values of ICP for each of the three injury grades. The mildly concussed animals (ETS 3) demonstrate moderate elevations of intracranial pressure which are maximal 30 seconds after injury (mean 42 mmHg) and progressively diminish such that by 5 to 10 minutes after injury they have normalized. Animals in ETS grade 4 are those that suffered severe but reversible cerebral concussion and demonstrate a slightly wider variation of ICP values. Maximum ICP is not reached until 1 to 2 minutes after injury (mean of 72 mmHg) but again, like that of ETS 3 the ICP progressively diminishes and normalizes by 10 minutes. The mean value of ICP at 30 and 60 seconds is somewhat skewed to the high side by two animals who exhibited extremely high values of 90 to 130 mmHg. Animals in ETS grade 5 did not survive the impact and all died a neurological death within six hours after the injury. Almost all of these animals died because of extremely large subdural hematomas. Of the three groups this one has the greatest variability of ICP. Two patterns are present however, Several animals have the same initial ICP-time history as those of grades 3 and 4 but then a secondary ICP rise occurs 5 to 10 minutes after injury as the subdural hematoma accumulates. Others exhibit a high ICP which never decreases to normal until terminally when the blood pressure falls.

Figure 2 demonstrates the changes in CPP in the same groups. In all groups arterial pressure increased transiently after injury. The minimal change in CPP of ETS 3 suggests that the blood pressure change was the same as the intracranial pressure change. In group 4 there was a marked decrease in perfusion pressure which recovered as the intracranial pressure recovers. This suggested that any rise in blood pressure was not quite as great as the rise in the intracranial pressure. In ETS 5 marked decrease in perfusion pressure occurs and this does not recover. Thus despite a rise in blood pressure the rise in intracranial pressure was overwhelming. It should be noted also that during the secondary ICP elevation 5-15 minutes after injury the perfusion pressure did not change whatsoever, suggesting a completely passive role of the intracranial pressure at this time.

Microscopic examination of the brains of 22 of these animals showed ischemic changes in one or both Ammon's horn in 8 of the 15 animals of the ETS 3 and 4 groups but only in two of the 7 animals of the ETS 5 group. The paucity of pathological evidence of ischemia in Ammon's horn in the non-survivors (ETS 5) may be attributed to the short survival period (mean 3 hours). However the presence of ischemic change in the surviving animals is unexpected since the intracranial pressure was never lower than the expected threshold for brain ischemia.

Discussion

It is clear that rather impressive rises in intracranial pressure can accompany completely reversible mild cerebral concussion (ETS 3). More severe traumatic unconsciousness (ETS 4) is associated with an even larger and slightly longer rise in intracranial pressure and also is accompanied by a significant but temporary drop in the CPP. Animals with subdural hematomas (ETS 5) develop massive intracranial hypertension such that the CPP drops to ischemic levels and these animals die from lack of cerebral perfusion. The finding of Ammon's horn ischemic changes in 53% of animals in grades 3 and 4 is unexpected and suggests that Ammon's horn ischemia need not be associated with prolonged elevation of ICP or with markedly decreased CPP.

Transient, marked cerebrovascular dilatation best explains the initial

ICP rise. Other possible causes, such as abrupt and temporary changes in CSF formation or absorption, in brain bulk, or in interstitial or intracelluar water seem unlikely. In these animals, the ICP changes are always accompanied by parallel changes in the SAP. Two explanations are possible. First, if the rise in SAP is the primary change then the ICP passively follows the blood pressure because of impaired cerebrovascular autoregulation (4). However, under similar conditions GRUBB and co-workers have reported high ICP in absence of elevated SAP so this explanation cannot be entirely valid (5). The alternative explanation is that vasodilatation increases ICP by the rapid addition of a small volume of intravascular blood to the intracranial space. Because of the rapidity of the change, a CUSHING response is elicited causing the SAP to increase (4,6). Restitution of the ICP to normal occurs as a result of spatial compensation taking place over the next few minutes and also because of recovery of normal vasomotor control of the cerebral blood vessels. The authors favor the latter hypothesis.

Summary

Acceleration induced head injury in the monkey was produced and ICP, SAP and CPP measured. Conclusions are as follows:

1. Elevation of ICP to as high as 100 mmHg occurs after cerebral concussion.
2. If subdural hematoma does not occur, then ICP becomes normal by 5-10 minutes after injury.
3. If subdural hematoma occurs, a secondary rise of ICP occurs and CPP becomes zero.
4. The magnitude of the initial ICP rise is related to injury severity.

The data best fit the concept that the temporary increase of ICP results from abrupt vasodilatation.

References

1. Gurdjian ES, Lissner HR (1944) Mechanism of head injury as studied by the cathode oscilloscope. J Neurosurg 1:393-399

2. Ommaya AK (1966) Experimental head injury in the monkey. In: Caveness W (ed) Head Injury. Lippincott, Philadelphia p260

3. Abel J, Gennarelli TA & Segawa H(1978) Incidence and severity of cerebral concussion in the rhesus monkey following sagittal plane angular acceleration. In 22nd Stapp Car Crash Conference Proceedings, SAE, New York, p 33

4. Langfitt TW, Kassel N, Weinstein J (1968) Cerebral vasomotor paralysis produced by intracranial hypertension. Neurol 15:622-641

5. Grubb RL, Naumann RA, Ommaya AK (1970) Respiration and the cerebrospinal fluid in experimental cerebral concussion. J Neurosurg 32:320-329

6. Nakatani S, Ommaya AK (1972) A critical rate of cerebral compression. In: Brock M and Dietz H (eds) Intracranial Pressure. Springer, Berlin Heidelberg New York, p 144

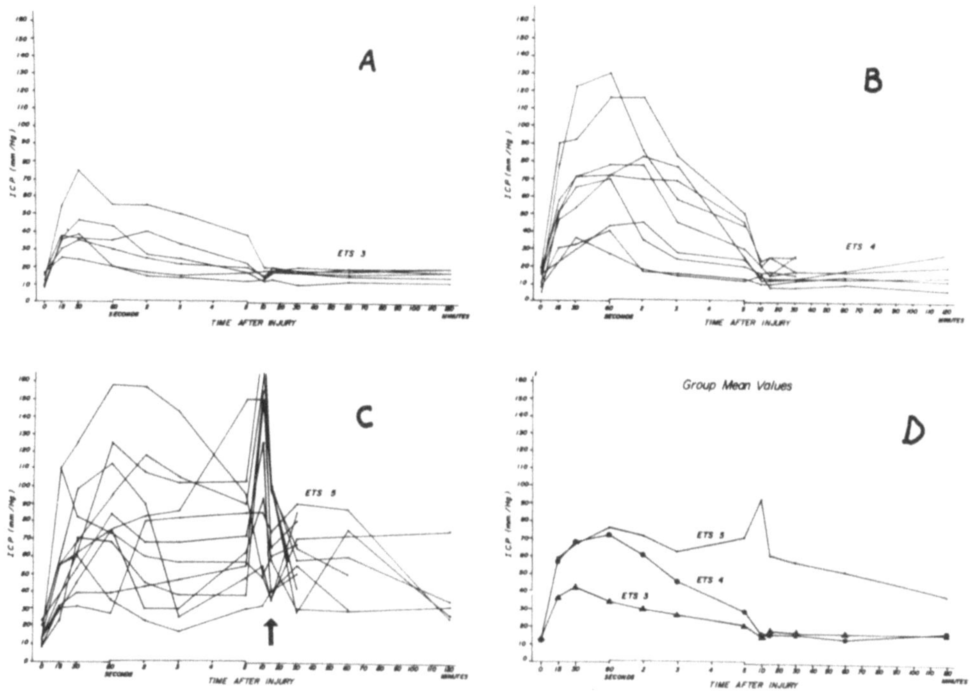

Figure 1. A-C: ICP-time histories of individual animals in ETS grades 3, 4, and 5 respectively. Arrow in C notes the secondary ICP rise due to the expanding subdural hematoma.

D: Mean ICP values of all animals in each severity classification

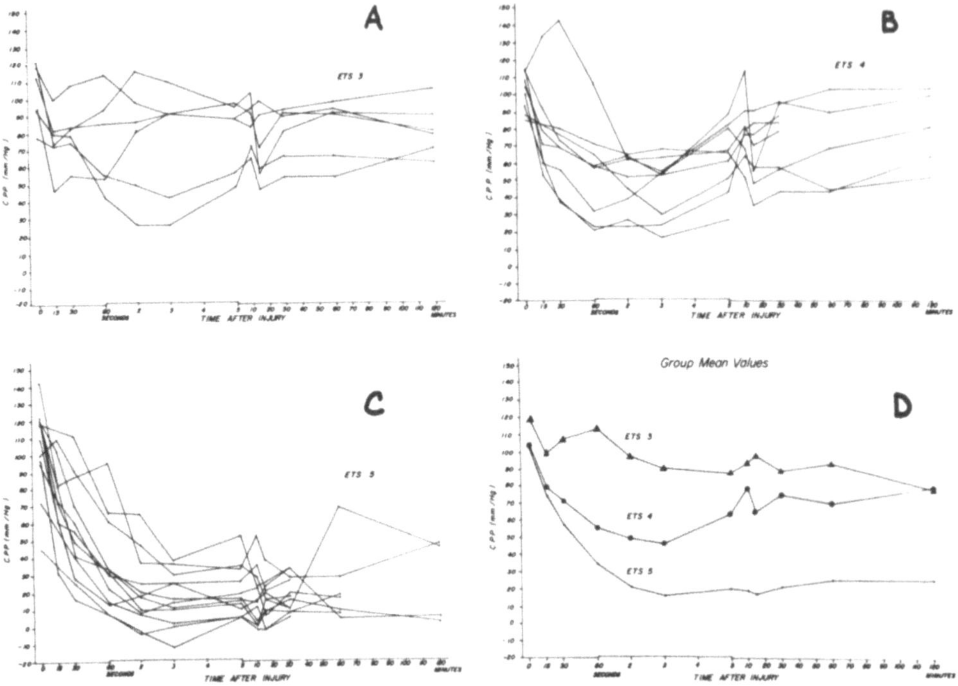

Figure 2. A-C: CPP-time histories of individual animals in ETS grades 3, 4 and 5 respectively.
D: Mean CPP values of all animals in each severity classification.

TIME COURSE IN INTRACEREBRAL TRAUMATIC HEMATOMAS

I. PAPO, G. CARUSELLI, AND M. SCARPELLI

Introduction

According to the neurosurgical experience of the past three decades the prognosis of traumatic intracerebral hematomas and/or brain lacerations, whether surgically or conservatively treated, seems to depend to a great extent on the state of consciousness of the patients. Thus, the mortality rate is extremely high in patients who are already in deep coma within 12 hours of the injury, while it is minimal in cases exhibiting only minor disturbances of consciousness. So far only little attention has been paid to ICP behavior in such lesions. As a matter of fact, in all series reported in literature, mass lesions, whatever their type, are compared with diffuse lesions, and therefore intracerebral hematomas are never taken into account as an homogeneous group.

Methods

ICP was recorded continuously by LUNDBERG'S intraventricular technique in 17 patients for whom the diagnosis of traumatic intracerebral hematomas and/or brain laceration was made by CT scan. Altogether 13 patients were operated upon: in 4 cases well defined hematomas were removed through a small craniotomy or a craniectomy. In 7 patients with extensive lacerations the lesion was cleaned out and a subtemporal decompression performed as well, while in the last 2 patients only a decompression was carried out.

The patients were classified in three groups: 1) patients in deep coma scoring 4 to 5 points on Glasgow Coma Scale; 2) patients with intermediate disturbances of consciousness scoring 6 to 10 points; 3) patients with minor disturbances of consciousness scoring more than 10 points.

Results

Group 1 (Table 1): All patients exhibited high ICP, with baseline ranging between 40 and 60 mmHg. In 3 patients after early operation ICP dropped definitely to 20-30 mmHg and never rose again. In 1 patient ICP fell postoperatively onto to rise again with vasoparalytic tracing. In none of these patients noticeable clinical improvement occurred; all of them died within a few days. In the last patient, harboring a deep located hematoma, only a bone decompression was performed. ICP was reduced but no clinical advantage ensued.

Group 2 (Table 2 a): 3 patients underwent delayed operation (4 to 6 days after injury). Intracranial hypertension was not significantly reduced after surgery and began to subside after several days. However all patients improved slowly making a satisfactory recovery. The last patient, with a bilateral frontal laceration and moderately elevated ICP was not operated on.He died of sepsis 23 days after injury.

Group 3 (Table 2b): In 3 patients with temporal hematomas and severe intracranial hypertension, ICP dropped immediately after delayed surgery; all patients improved quickly. In another patient, with a large temporal laceration, a subtemporal decompression was sufficient to normalize ICP and relieve clinical condition. One patient with a temporal hematoma improved clinically but ICP was normalized only after several days of continuous ventricular drainage. Finally, 3 patients were not operated upon. ICP decreased slowly (after a ventricular drainage in one patient). All patients recovered quite well.

Discussion

In the patients of the first group even if ICP was significantly reduced by surgery outcome was not influenced. It may be inferred, therefore, that irreversible lesions were associated to high levels of intracranial hypertension.

In the patients of Group 2 the reduction of intracranial hypertension and clinical improvement took place very slowly after surgery. As regards Group 3, it is worth noting that in some patients with localized lesions severe intracranial hypertension was tolerated suprisingly well. After surgery, ICP in patients with traumatic hematomas behaved quite differently from most patients underoing delayed operation for primary intracerebral hemorrhage; in trauma cases raised ICP fell definitely and did not rise again, while in "vasculopathic" patients ICP dropped only for a few hours. Routine CT scan in head injuries has clearly demonstrated that traumatic intracerebral hematomas and/or brain laceration with mild symptomatology are extraordinarily common. In a majority of such patients fairly raised ICP declines spontaneously and a satisfactory recovery takes place. Nevertheless, in some cases intracranial hypertension may persist for a long time and justify delayed surgery. It must be stressed as well the role played by CSF dynamics disturbances in the pathogenesis of sustained intracranial hypertension. From the practical standpoint, the most valuable indications for long-term ICP monitoring seem to be huge lesions on CT scan with mild symptomatology and subacute lesions with stagnant symptomatology. In both circumstances ICP monitoring may prove of real use in making surgical decisions.

Table I: Group I: deeply comatose patients (4 to 5 on G.C.S.) No lucid interval, early surgery (within 48 hours).

N.	Sex	Age	Lesion	ICP (mmHg)	Postop ICP (mmHg)	Outcome
1	M	17	T.BL.	60	30	died 10th day
2	M	73	F.BL	60	15*	died 6th day
3	M	40	B G.H.	40**	20	died 3 months
4	M	42	T.BL.	60	25	died 7th day
5	M	20	T.BL.	60	30	died 5th day

Abbreviations: T = temporal; F - frontal; BG - basal ganglia; BL = brain laceration; H = hematoma.

* ICP rose to its preoperative level after 18 hours.
** Pressure wave to 80 mmHg before decompression.

Table 2. A) Patients with intermediate disturbances of consciousness
B) Patients with minor disturbances of consciousness

(A)

N.	Sex	Age	Lesion	ICP (mmHg)	Treatment	PostopICP (mmHg)	Outcome
1	M	17	T.BL.	35	op.6th day	30	recovered
2	F	16	T.BL.	40	op.4th day	35	recovered
3	F	23	T.BL.	40	op.4th day	40	recovered
4	M	31	bil.F.BL.	25	medical	--	died(sepsis) 23rd day

(B)

N.	Sex	Age	Lesion	ICP (mmHg)	Treatment	PostopICP (mmHg)	Outcome
1	M	48	T.H.	45	op.12th day	20	recovered
2	M	47	T.H.	45	op. 3rd day	15	recovered
3	M	64	T.H.	60	op. 5th day	15	recovered
4	M	64	T.BL.	45	op. 7th day[0]	10	recovered
5	M	40	T.H.	35	op. 9th day	35(VD)	recovered
6	M	33	F.BL.	40	medical	- -	recovered
7	M	40	F.BL.	50	VD	- -	recovered
8	F	17	T.BL.	25	medical	- -	recovered

[0]Only subtemporal decompression.

Abbreviations: T = temporal; F = frontal; H = hematoma; BL=brain laceration; VD=ventricular continuous.

OPERATE OR OBSERVE?
ICP AND THE MANAGEMENT OF THE 'SILENT' TRAUMATIC INTRACRANIAL HAEMATOMA

G. TEASDALE, S. GALBRAITH, AND B. JENNETT

Introduction

Since the introduction of CT scanning it has become apparent that an intracranial haematoma can be present in a head injured patient who is not, as yet, deteriorating. Some of these haematomas will resolve spontaneously but others, because of progressive cerebral compression, have to be removed. We have studied 21 patients to determine the value of continuous monitoring of intracranial pressure in the management of these patients, particularly in identifying soon after the discovery of a haematoma, the likelihood of spontaneous resolution.

Patients and Methods

There were 21 patients who had an acute traumatic intracranial haematoma diagnosed by CT scanning 1-13 days after injury; in each, the clinician in charge decided that there was a good prospect of recovery without operation because of a lack of deterioration in conscious level or of the development of focal signs since injury. Each patient had some impairment of consciousness but only 3 were in coma (no eye opening, no comprehensible verbal response, not obeying commands). Eight haematomas were frontal, 6 temporal and the remainder fronto-temporal or diffuse. Management consisted of careful observation of clinical responsiveness and continuous monitoring of intracranial pressure by intraventricular catheter; steroids and artificial ventilation were not used and osmotics rarely. It became necessary to evacuate the haematoma in 8 cases, in 7 because of deteriorating responsiveness and in 1 because of persisting failure to improve. The interval from the start of monitoring to operation varied from 12 hours to 7 days. In the remaining patients responsiveness improved and intracranial pressure remained or returned to normal levels (<15mmHg).

Results

1) Comparison of operated and non-operated patients

The age of the two groups was similar, and there were no characteristic clinical or radiological features which distinguised them. The level of intracranial pressure during the first one or two hours of monitoring was however different (Table 1). No patient whose intracranial pressure remained below 20 mmHg in this period deteriorated within the next few days; the one patient with initially normal ICP who required operation did not deteriorate until 7 days later, at which time his intracranial pressure was high. By contrast, the majority of patients whose basal intracranial pressure level was above 20 mmHg deteriorated and required operation within the next 1-3 days. This event was usually associated with a further rise in intracranial pressure, and B waves were frequent in this group. Two of 4 patients managed conservatively despite an initially high intracranial pressure also temporarily deteriorated before recovering.

Table 1. Initial Features and Subsequent Management

		Conservative	Operative
Age (years + SD)		51 ± 16	42 ± 17
Coma	Absent	12	6
	Present	1	2
Shift	Absent	4	2
	Present	9	6
ICP	<20 mmHg	9	1
	>20 mmHg	4	7

Table 2. Outcome after Trial of Conservative Management

Final Management	Dead	Severe Disability	Moderate/ Good Recovery
Conservative	1	1	11
Operation	2	2	4

2) Outcome (Table 2)
Bad outcomes were commoner in the patients who required operation, but the deaths were due to delayed complications and not to irreversible brainstem compression.

Discussion

The patients considered for a trial of conservative management are only a small proportion of traumatic intracranial haematomas seen in our Institute. What is the best management of such patients with clinically silent haematomas remains uncertain and controversial. We have confirmed that some patients can be successfully managed wihtout operation (2); all but one patient in this group made good recoveries. Some patients, however, will deteriorate. A prophylactic operation (1) would decrease the risk of secondary brain damage in the latter cases, but this would result in some patients being operated upon unnecessarily, unless the patients who can be successfully managed without surgery could be identified at an early stage. Reliable criteria have not yet emerged but the level of intracranial pressure during a period of continuous monitoring does provide some indication of the likelihood of success of conservative management; in the rest it may be a valuable indication of when operation is needed.

Summary

In 21 patients with an acute traumatic intracranial haematoma, ICP monitoring helped to distinguish between patients requiring operation and those managed conservatively.

References

1. Weigel K, Ostertag B, Mundinger F (1978) CT follow-up control of traumatic intracerebral hemorrhage. In: Frowein RA, Wilcke O, Karimi-Nejad A, Brock M, Klinger M (eds) Advances in Neurosurgery5. Springer, Berlin Heidelberg New York,p 62

2. Becker DP, Miller JD, Ward JD, Greenberg RP, Young HF, Sakalas R (1977) The outcome from severe head injury with early diagnosis and intensive management. J Neurosur 47:491-502

BRAIN INTERSTITIAL FLUID PRESSURE MEASUREMENT IN HEAD INJURY PATIENTS

S. NAKATANI, K. KOSHINO, H. MOGAMI, Y. SAWADA, AND T. SUGIMOTO

Introduction

The wick catheter was applied successfully to the measurement of the brain interstitial fluid pressure (BIFP) (1). BIFP is high within the edema fluid territory as compared to that of CSF and of normal brain tissue (6). This pressure gradient induces a propagation of the edema fluid into the surrounding extracellular space (7). The decrease in Hounsefield number in CT scan is directly proportional to the increased water content of the brain tissue and in turn reflects the intracompartmental pressure gradients (4). These recent developments led us to try the simultaneous monitoring of CSF pressure and the BIFP within the brain parenchyma of acute head injury patients, to compare with the printed-out Housefield numbers in CT scan. This study proposed to find out which of the internal or external decompression is more rational treatment in the early management of head injury.

Material and Methods

The wick catheter was made, utilizing the polyethylene tube (an inner diameter 1 mm) with multiple side holes at the tip filled with 10-0 non-filament nylon threads. Dynamic property of the wick catheter was tested in thirty cats anesthetized with pentobarbital sodium (30 mg/kg bw). Wick catheters were left in situ during operation at one or two sites of the white matter of the brain of the head injured patients who were admitted to the Emergency Service, Traumatology ICU of the Osaka University Hospital in coma or semicoma and subjected to surgery. In patients who underwent decompressive craniectomy, one of the wick catheters was left in the subcutaneous space on the cortical surface. The intraventricular CSF pressure was measured from a cannula inserted into the anterior horn of the lateral ventricles. The catheter was connected to the Statham and Nihon-Kohden strain gauge pressure transducers. Systemic arterial and intracranial pressure, EKG, heart rate, respiratory rate and EEG were recorded with Nihon-Kohden polygraph. Proper arterial pO_2, pCO_2 and pH were maintained, being checked frequently by IL meter. Water and electrolyte balances were kept properly. Pre- and postoperative CT scans were taken and the mean Hounsefield numbers at the regions of interest were calculated from the printed-out numbers.

Results

Using the wick catheter devised by us, the pressures were recorded simultaneously from the cisterna magna, the supratentorial subdural space and the white matter of the cerebral hemisphere of the cats. Arterial pulsation and respiratory oscillation were recorded satisfactorily from the brain tissue as compared with that from other compartments. A positive BIFP of 6 mmHg was obtained. Tracheal occlusion in the spontaneously breathing tracheostomized cats caused a large increase in BIFP associated with a marked elevation of arterial blood pressure. Intravenous injection of noradrenalin in the artificailly ventilated normocapnic cats induced a large increase in BIFP. These responses are the same as BROCK et al reported (2).

Fifteen severe head injury patients subjected to this study were categorized into three groups. In patients who developed low density edema region in the brain on CT, pressure gradients were obtained between CSF, non-edematous brain tissue and edematous brain tissue. These pressure gradients became larger firstly and then smaller with a propagation of edema into a generalized uncontrollable increased ICP (Fig. 1). In patient who underwent decompressive craniectomy, an initial subcutaneous pressure was very low, whereas BIFP deep in the edematous brain tissue was high. The pressure gradients decreased with increasing scalp tension and with increasing general ICP (Fig.2). In patients with brain stem lesion and normal density white matter, no pressure gradient was observed between CSF pressure and BIFP(Fig.3).

Discussion

BRUCE et al reported that ICP does not correlate well with the severity measured by clinical criteria except at extremely high levels (1). NAKATANI and OMMAYA have demonstrated that slowly increasing volume may reach the lethal level with only a slight increase in ICP and that the level of ICP depends not only on that volume but also on its rate of accumulation (2). The lack of significant correlation between prognosis and/or regional blood flow may well be due to the lack of correlated data on tissue pressure and the rate of such volumetric changes. BIFP is more important than a general ICP in evaluating the pathological condition of the brain. POLL et al suggested a useful clinical application of brain tissue pressure measurement (5). However, no report on the clinical measurement of BIFP in neurosurgical patients has been followed. We have tried and succeeded in continuous BIFP recording in severe head injury patients using the wick catheter devised by us, which responded in the same way described by BROCK et al. (1). Only preliminary data were obtained on the correlation between BIFP and Hounsefield number of CT scan. It is, however, important that a higher BIFP was recorded in low density area of the brain of clinical patients, which confirmed the experimental data. Much more data are necessary before we can discuss a significance of the intracranial pressure gradients in relation to the general ICP.

From the BIFP data obtained we inferred the better surgical management of head injured patients. We have tried a theoretical reasoning on the movement of the fluid in the brain during increased ICP and after decompression (3) using SHULMAN'S simplified equation: $FM = k(Pc - Pif - 25\ \text{mmHg})$ (8), which serves enough for our present purpose. Pc is the mean capillary hydrostatic pressure. Pif is the pressure in the interstitial compartment. Difference of the colloid osmotic pressure of the blood and interstitial fluid is the critical effective capillary filtration pressure (CECFP, 25 mmHg). In increased ICP, Pc increases. However, Pc - Pif decreased and becomes less than CECFP. Fluid movement is supposed to be from the brain tissue to the blood stream. Even if it actually is not so, we at least can say that an increased ICP per se would neither induce nor aggravate brain edema in the closed cavity. On the contrary, it will counterbalance an increase in Pc and prevent an edema development. Decompressive craniectomy disrupts the normal physical condition of cerebrovascular hemodynamics. An increase in cerebral blood flow, whether caused by arterial hypertension or high pCO_2 will increase cerebral blood volume and vascular transmural pressure unopposed by the corresponding increase in CSF pressure. Pc increases by vasodilation and arterial hypertension. Pif decreases to become greater than the CECFP. Then, the movement of fluid must be from the blood stream to the brain tissue and an extensive hydrostatic edema will be induced. It is well known that by increased transmural pressure, arterial hypertension aggravates brain edema (9). Increased BIFP gradient developed will enhance an edema propagation. Intracerebral hemorrhage and intraventricular bleeding may be induced on some occasions. On the other hand, the internal decompression, i.e., removal of intracranial mass and of the source of edema propagation prevents deleterious secondary insults to the brain maintaining the homeostatic mechanism of the closed calvarium by replacement of the bone flap. Thus, intensive medical treatment being carried out, generous internal decompression is a choice surgical policy in the management of head injury patients.

Summary

BIFP recorded continuously in acute head injury patients was found higher in the lower density edematous area than in normal density area of CT scan. In patients who underwent decompressive craniectomy, an initial subcutaneous pressure was low, whereas BIFP deep in the edematous brain tissue was high. Pressure gradients decreased with increasing general ICP. It is concluded that the generous internal decompression is a choice of surgical policy in the early management of head injury patients.

References

1. Brock M, Winkelmüller W, Pöll W, Markakis E, Dietz H (1972) Measurement of brain-tissue pressure. Lancet II:595-596

2. Nakatani S, Ommaya AK (1972) A critical rate of cerebral compression. In: Brock M, Dietz H (eds) Intracranial Pressure. Springer, Berlin Heidelberg New York, p 144

3. Nakatani S, Ommaya AK (1977) Fluid movement in the brain: Is decompressive craniectomy rational in the management of head trauma? Excerpta Medica Internat Congr Series 418:230

4. Penn RD, Kurts D (1977) Cerebral edema, mass effects and regional blood volume in man. J Neurosurg 46:181-189

5. Pöll w, Brock M, Markakis W, Winkelmüller W, Dietz H (1972) Brain tissue pressure. In: Brock M, Dietz H (eds) Intracranial Pressure. Springer, Berlin Heidelberg New York,p 188

6. Reulen HJ, Kreysch HG (1973) Measurement of brain tissue pressure in cold induced cerebral edema. Acta neurochir 29:29-40

7. Reulen HF, Graham R, Spats M, Klatzo I (1977) Role of pressure gradients and bulk flow in dynamics of vasogenic brain edema. J Neurosurg 46:24-35

8. Shulman K (1965) Small artery and vein pressures in the subarachnoid space of the dog. J Surg Res 5:56-61

9. Shutta HS, Kassel NF, Langfitt TW (1968) Brain swelling produced by injury aggravated by arterial hypertension. Brain 91:281-294

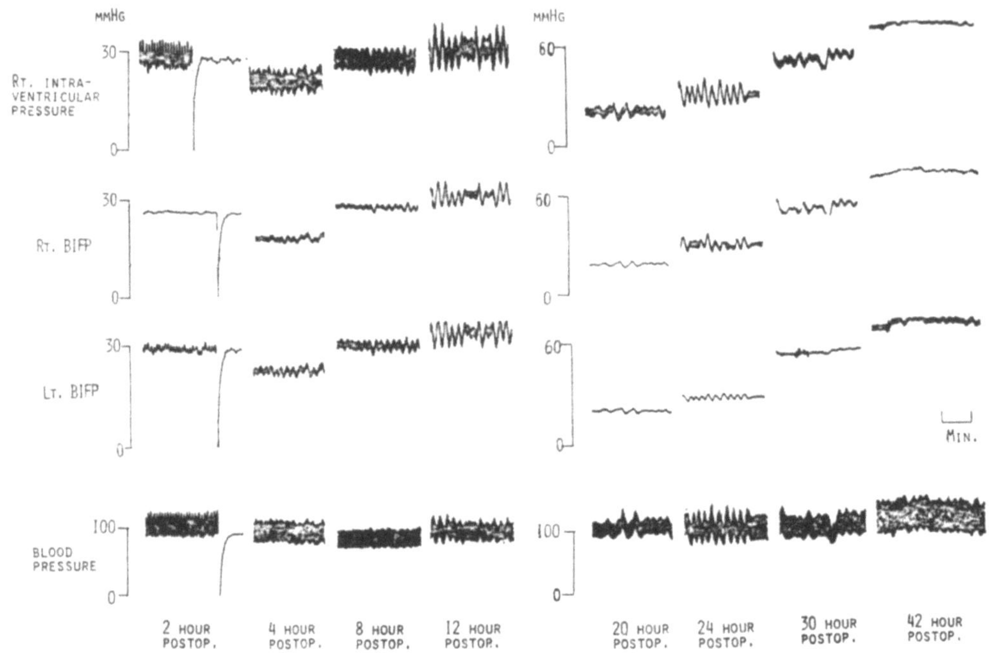

Figure 1. Record from 20 year old male with traumatic hematoma in right basal ganglia. The wick catheters were placed in the non-edematous white matter of the right frontal lobe and in the edematous brain tissue adjacent to the hematoma cavity. For twelve postoperative hours the left BIFP is higher than the right BIFP and right ventricular CSF pressure. Then, pressure gradients decreased and ICP increased uncontrollably to over 70 mmHg. Mean Hounsefield numbers at the regions of BIFP measurement were 28 on the left and 40 on the right, calculated from the printed-out CT of the 3rd postoperative hour.

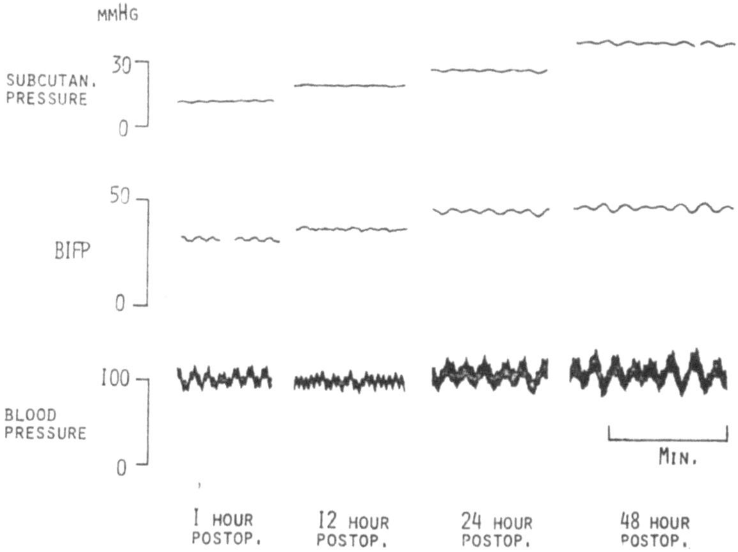

Figure 2. Record from 43 year old male with multiple skull fractures and diffuse brain contusion. Subcutaneous pressure was obtained from the wick catheter placed over the right cerebral convexity. BIFP was recorded from the wick catheter left in situ deep in the white matter of the left frontal lobe. Note the pressure gradient between them. At the start of the record BIFP was as high as 30 mmHg, whereas the subcutaneous pressure was only 10 mmHg. By the time of the cerebral death, BIFP rose to 50 mmHg when the latter pressure reached 40 mmHg with an increased scalp tension. Mean Hounsefield number at the region of BIFP measurement was 36 at the twelfth postoperative hour.

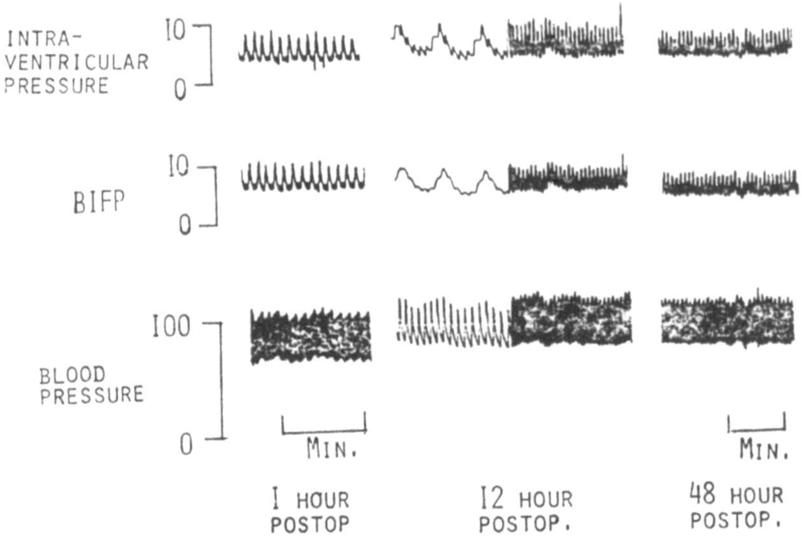

Figure 3. Record from 65 year old male with basal skull fracture,BIFP was recorded from the wick catheter placed in the white matter of the right frontal lobe through the burr hole for the ventricular tap. No pressure gradient. Continuous low pressure throughout the record. Mean Hounsefield number at the BIFP measurement was 42, in normal range.

RELEVANCE OF CAT-SCAN FOR THE LEVEL OF ICP IN PATIENTS WITH SEVERE HEAD INJURY

L. AUER, R. OBERBAUER, H. TRITTHART, W.D. SAGER, AND G. CLARICI

Introduction

The knowledge of intracranial pressure (ICP) is a matter of predominant interest in patients with severe head injury. An outstanding improvement in the diagnosis of posttraumatic mass lesions was the introduction of CAT-scanning (4-6,8,9). This new method gives a picture of morphological changes intracranially, hence of compartmental volume changes. Thus, brain edema can be diagnosed (7): a typical consequence of tissue-mass increase in narrowing of the ventricular system. This morphological observation can lead to plausible but unproven conclusions on "increased ICP' when CAT-scan shows brain swelling and narrowing of the ventricular system.

Methods

Intraventricular pressure was measured during CAT-scanning in 8 patients with severe head injury. Pressure measurement was performed similar to LUNDBERG'S method by tapping a lateral ventricle and connecting the drainage to a Statham transducer and a Datascope-monitor. Twelve scans were made in an EMI-1010 tomograph; ventricular volume was calculated and correlated with intraventricular pressure.

Results

Our present experience covers 3 main groups of pathological pictures:

1. Narrow or even closed ventricles with normal ICP (Fig.2).
2. Unilateral acute hydrocephalus with increased ICP and contralateral mass lesion.
3. Normal or enlarged ventricles with increased ICP. (Fig.1).

There was no correlation to observe between the level of ICP and the size of the ventricular system (Fig.3).

Discussion

Out of our present data it appears most critical to draw conclusions on the level of ICP from CAT-scan pictures of the supratentorial compartment. There is no reliable relation between morphological pictures and level of ICP.

It becomes evident from the recent literature (8,9), that a considerable number of severely head injured have normal CAT or slightly altered density and ventricular volume, although they are in a deeply comatose state. CAT in such cases is not contraindicative for any surgery, since there is no information regarding the level of ICP. It appears, therefore, as an advantage to measure ICP continuously through a ventricular drainage and, if necessary, withdraw CSF to lower ICP. Following the pressure-volume relationship, the CSF-volume, necessary to effectively lower ICP, is the smaller, the higher ICP is. Therefore, a withdrawal of a few milliliters of CSF can be enough. We have utilized this system in more than 100 patients with a very low incidence of complications (2). If ICP remains increased despite drainage, medical treatment and all intensive care measures, bitemporal decompression can be performed successfully (1-3).

Summary

Intracranial pressure was monitored via ventricular catheter during CAT-scanning in patients with severe head injury. Ventricular volume was calculated and plotted against intracranial pressure: there was no correlation at all. This observation does not allow determination of the level of intracranial pressure by the CT picture of the supratentorial ventricular system.

References

1. Auer L (1977) Therapeutical consequences of simultaneous ICP and blood pressure monitoring in patients with severe head injury. Proc 6th Int Congr Neurosurg, Exc Med 418:115-116

2. Auer R (1979) Long-term monitoring of ventricular fluid pressure in patients with head injury - problems and indications. Neurosurg Rev In press

3. Heppner F (1972) Für und wider die subtemporale Entlastungstrepanation. Schw Arch Neurol Neurochir Psych 111:275-283

4. Huk W, Schiefer W (1976) Computerized axial tomography in craniocerebral trauma. In: Lanksch W, Kazner E (eds) Cranial Computerized Tomography. Springer, Berlin Heidelberg New York, p 310

5. Jennet B, Teasdale G, Galbraith S, Steven LJ (1977) The role of T.A.C. in the diagnosis of traumatic intracranial haematoma. In: DuBoulay GH, Moseley IF (eds) Cranial Computerized Axial Tomography in clinical practice. Springer, Berlin Heidelberg New York, p 62

6. Kruger J, Becker H, Rub H, Hacker H (1976) Concerning the influence of CTT in the treatment of cerebral trauma. In: Lanksch W, Kazner E (eds) Cranial Computerized Tomography. Springer, Berlin Heidelberg New York, p 329

7. Lanksch W, Kazner E (1976) CT findings in brain edema. In: Lanksch W, Kazner E (eds) Cranial Computerized Tomography. Springer, Berlin Heidelberg New York, p 344

8. Perini S, Mashio CA, Beltramello A, Benati A, Bricolo A (1978) The role of computed tomography in the diagnosis and management of head injuries. J Neurol Sci 22:51-62

9. Zimmermann RA, Bilaniuk LT, Gennarelli T, Bruce D, Dolinskas C, Uzzell B(1978) Cranial computed tomography in diagnosis and management of acute head trauma. Am J Roentgenol 131:27-34

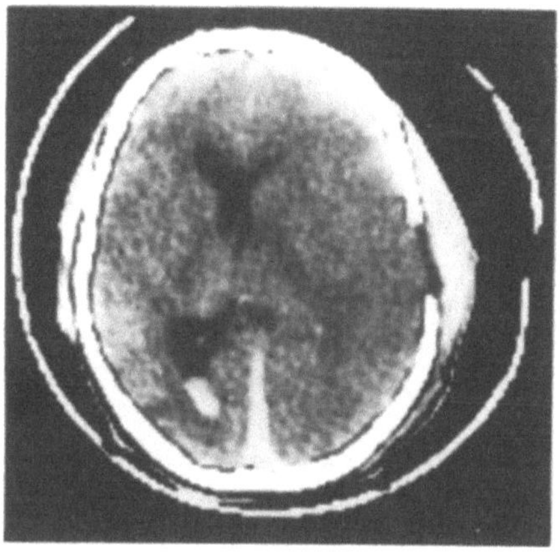

Figure 1. CAT-scan of a 17 year old man two days after severe head injury and evacuation of an acute subdural hematoma. During scanning, intraventricular pressure was 74 mmHg. The patient had fixed dilated pupils and was unreactive to pain. CAT-scan showed an open ventricular system, somewhat displaced to the left, even enlarged on the left.

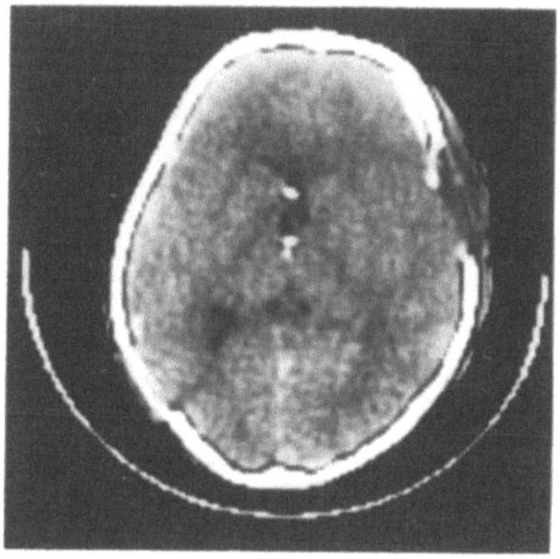

Figure 2. Considerably narrowed ventricular system in a 4 year old girl four days after head injury with a right temporal and a left occipital depressed fracture. During this CAT-scan, intraventricular pressure was normal at a level of 8 mmHg.

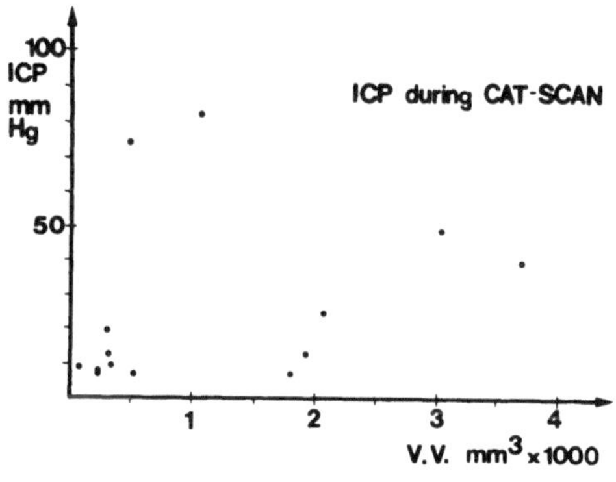

Figure 3. Intraventricular pressure (ICP) plotted against ventricular volume (VV). There is no relation between the two parameters.

CAN CT SCAN FINDINGS PREDICT INTRACRANIAL PRESSURE IN CLOSED HEAD INJURY PATIENTS?

F.L.HAAR, V.K.SADHU, R.S.PINTO, P.L.GILDENBERG, AND J.M.SAMPSON

Introduction

The current study attempts to determine if the CT scan can be used to help predict whether the intracranial pressure (ICP) is normal or significantly elevated in a common group of head injured patients who would require no early surgery other than the placement of the ICP measuring device itself.

Methods

Two consecutive series of patients with closed head injury and a Glasgow Coma Score of 8 or less was studied to determine whether intracranial hypertension could be predicted from CT scans. A total of 65 scans on 42 patients were examined. Patients with missile injuries or intracranial hematomas requiring early surgical evacuation were excluded.

In the first series, 39 CT scans on 24 patients were reviewed by a neuroradiologist who had no prior knowledge of each patient's ICP or clinical status. The indices observed were ventricular size, assymmetrical ventricular compression, midline shift, obliterated cisterns and/or sulci, and temporal horn dilatation on the side which the third ventricle was shifted. Each of these CT features was evaluated, and a composite subjective predictive value of 0 (ICP < 12 mmHg) to 4 (ICP > 40 mmHg) was assigned and subsequently compared to measured ICP's.

In most cases, initial ICP was measured by ventriculostomy or Richmond bolt within 90 minutes of the CT scan obtained on admission. If the CT scan was repeated on a later day, it was correlated with the ICP measured just after the patient returned to the Intensive Care Unit from the CT scan room

Results

Of the 11 scans predicted to depict a normal or borderline ICP, the measured ICP was less than 20 mmHg in all 11 (100%) (Fig.1). However, only three (11%) of the remaining 28 scans predicted to demonstrate elevated ICP had a measured ICP of greater than 20 mmHg (Fig.2). ICP was normal despite slit-like ventricles or mild ventricular shift in most cases (Fig.3). Marked ventricular shift with temporal horn dilatation on the side to which the shift was directed correlated most consistently with elevated ICP (Fig.2).

On the basis of this initial study, the criteria for prediction were modified in a subsequent series of 26 scans on 18 closed head injury patients reviewed by the same neuroradiologist. In this series, less emphasis was placed on the presence of small ventricles and mild to moderate ventricular compression and shift, and greater emphasis on dilatation of a portion of the ventricular system opposite the side of the greater mass effect, as well as marked ventricular shift. Of the 18 scans predicted to show normal or near normal ICP, measured ICP was actually 20 mmHg or less for 17 (94%). The one exception is seen in Figure 4. In only 2 (25%) of the 8 remaining scans thought to demonstrate elevated ICP was the ICP actually elevated.

Discussion

ICP may be within normal range in patients with severe, non-penetrating closed head injuries but no intracranial hematoma (1,2), an incidence of 65% being reported in one series (3). Normal or near normal CT scans on admission have been reported in 38 - 41% of patients with severe, non-penetrating head injuries (4,5). None of our patients with a CT scan of this description had an early ICP of greater than 20 mmHg. Although narrowed or "slit" ventricles have been described as the most frequent single abnormality in this group of patients (5) it did not indicate intracranial hypertension.

The most reliable CT scan finding to suggest an increase in ICP is dilatation of the temporal horn on the side opposite the hemisphere with the greater mass effect. Possible mechanisms for this finding include uncal herniation, compression of the aqueduct against the opposite tentorial edge, direct compression of the ipsilateral ventricular system by the mass effect and protection from direct compression of the contralateral temporal horn by the anterior and posterior clinoid and clinotentorial ligaments(6).

A marked unilateral ventricular compression associated with shift of the ventricular system to the opposite side also correlated well with the presence of intracranial hypertension, although the same findings to a lesser degree may exist with no elevation of intracranial pressure.

It should be emphasized that, even after a preliminary study suggesting which CT scan findings correlated with increased ICP, only 2 of 8 patients meeting those criteria actually had increased ICP.

We conclude that the prediction of an elevated ICP on the basis of an abnormal CT scan is far less accurate than the prediction of normal ICP on the basis of a normal or near normal CT scan.

Summary

In our series of 65 CT scans on 42 patients, a normal or near normal initial CT scan signified normal intracranial pressure (ICP). A dramatically abnormal CT scan did not necessarily signify elevation of the ICP. Significant unilateral ventricular compression with marked shift to the opposite side, and dilatation of the temporal horn on the side opposite the greater mass effect, were the most reliable predictors of intracranial hypertension. Narrow or "slit" ventricles and milder degrees of ventricular shift and compression were not reliable predictors.

References

1. Fleischer AS, Payne NS, Tindall GT (1976) Continuous monitoring of intracranial pressure in severe closed head injury without mass lesions. Surg Neurol 6:31-34

2. Hahn FJY, Schapiro RL (1976) The excessively small ventricle on computed axial tomography of the brain. Neuroradiol 12:137-139

3. Jennett B, Johnston IH (1972) The uses of intracranial pressure monitoring in clinical management. In: Brock M, Deitz H (eds) Intracranial Pressure. Springer, Berlin Heidelberg New York, p353

4. Johnston IH, Jennett B (1970) Intracranial pressure changes following head injury. Jancet II:433-436

5. Snoek J, Jennett B, Adams JH, et al(1979) Computerized tomography after recent severe head injury in patients without acute intra-cranial haematoma. J Neurol Neurosurg & Psych 42:215-225

6. Zimmerman RA, Bilaniuk LT, Gennarelli T, et al (1978) Cranial computed tomography in diagnosis and management of acute head trauma. Am J Roentgenol 131:27-34

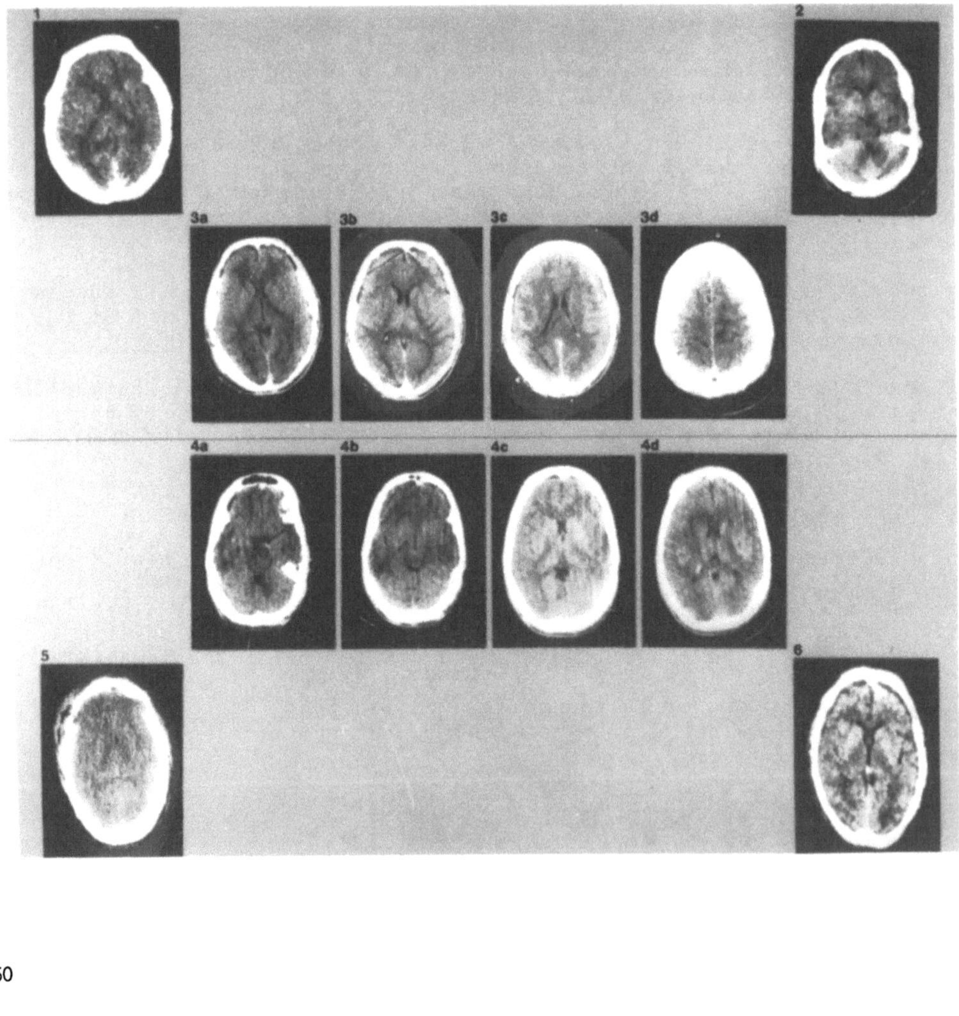

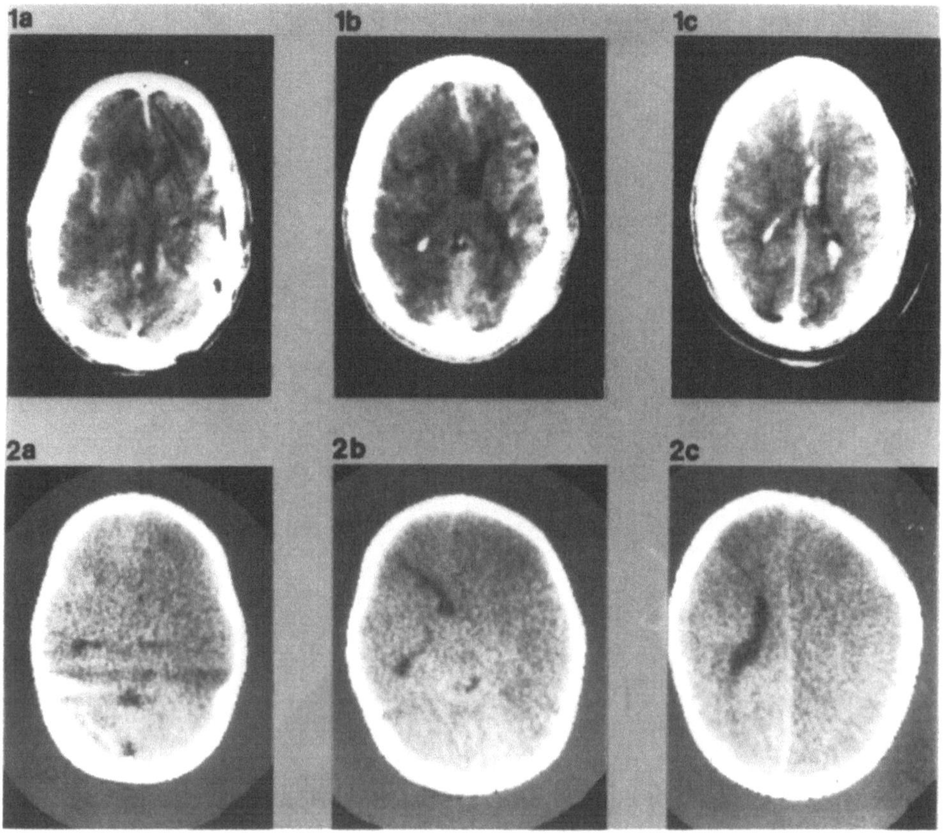

Fig. 2. Examples of CT scans thought to reflect significantly elevated ICP in patients whose ICP measured 20 - 70 mmHg. Note the temporal horn dilatation in 2a and 2b.

For each illustration, a new number represents a new patient and small letters represent various CT sections for a given patient.

◁ Fig. 1. Examples of CT scans thought to reflect normal or mildly elevated ICP in patients with ICP measured < 20 mmHg.

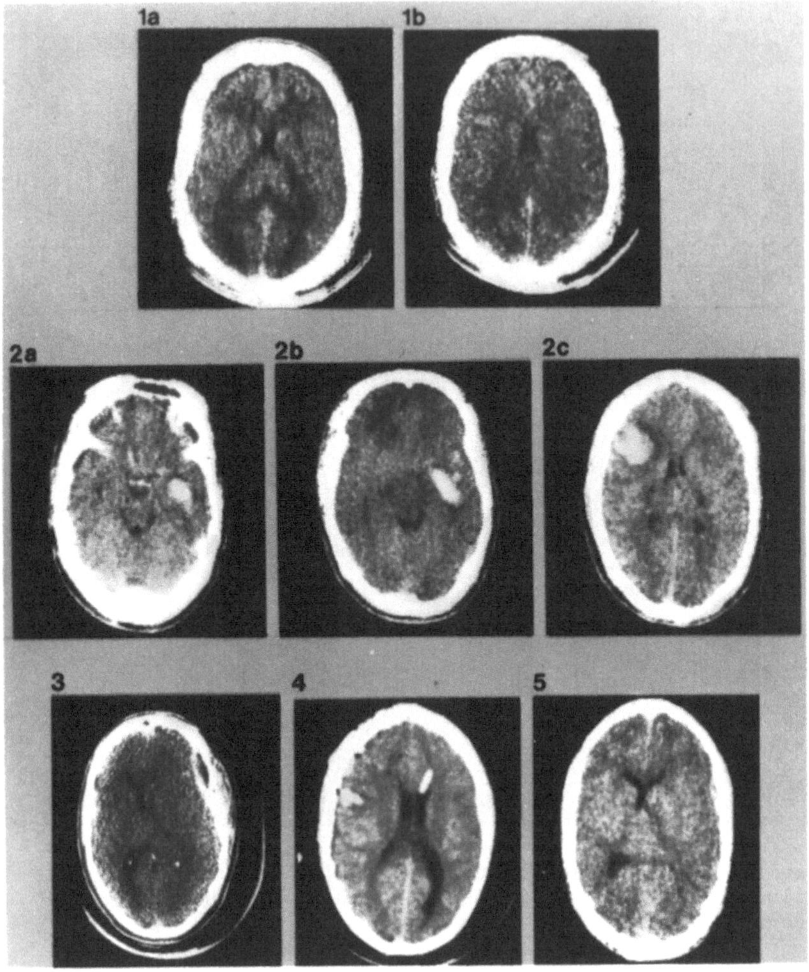

Fig. 3. Examples of CT scans thought to reflect significantly elevated ICP in patients whose ICP measured < 20 mmHg ("false positive").

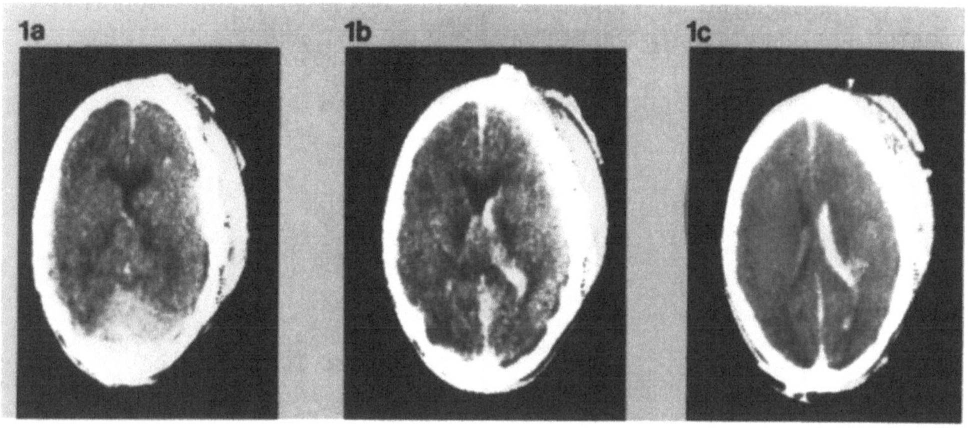

Fig. 4. CT scan thought to reflect normal ICP in patients whose ICP measured 60 mmHg (the only "false negative" in 42 patients).

FACTORS INFLUENCING SURVIVAL AND QUALITY OF SURVIVAL IN PATIENTS TREATED FOR ELEVATED INTRACRANIAL PRESSURE

C.P.McGRAW AND G.HOWARD

Introduction

Does controlling intracranial pressure (ICP) have an effect on mortality or recovery for patients with increased ICP? Can other information be valuable in predicting the ICP and, in combination with the ICP, be valuable in predicting outcome? This study was done in an attempt to answer those questions.

Matherial and Methods

In 300 monitored patients, three classes of variables were examined:

1) Factors determined at the onset of monitoring (age, race, sex, Glasgow coma level, delay before monitoring was initiated and initial ICP).

2) Measures of ICP (average ICP, highest hourly average ICP)

3) Measures of outcome (Glasgow recovery scale and survival to discharge).

Since the ability to predict is the ultimate test of understanding, regression analysis was employed to predict:

1) ICP during hospital stay, using the factors determined at onset of monitoring.

2) Patient outcome, using both factors determined at onset of monitoring and ICP factors.

The analysis was done for all patients with intracranial lesions and the data were then grouped into categories; all cases, closed head injuries, all head injuries, infarctions, hemorrhages, hemorrhages and infarctions, and inflammations.

Results

Initial ICP. 1) In patients with head injury, age, the level of coma and the delay in monitoring were predictive of initial ICP. The younger the patient, the milder the coma; the shorter the delay before monitoring, the lower the initial ICP. 2) In stroke, initial ICP was not predictive. 3) In all cases combined, age and coma level were the major predictors of initial ICP.

Average ICP. Except in the inflammation group, level of coma and ICP (most of the explanation) accounted for 37% to 44% of variation in average ICP. Initial ICP was affected by a delay in monitoring in closed head injuries only.

Highest Hourly Average ICP. In predicting the highest hourly average ICP, the initial ICP proved to be the primary predictor. Coma proved to be a predictor only in the all-cases and in the all-head-injuries groups (accounting for 16% to 66% of variation).

Survival. The overall average ICP was important to survival in head injuries, while the highest hourly average ICP was of predictive value in hemorrhages and strokes. Age was a factor in the head injury group but not in the hemorrhage group. The level of coma was a factor in all cases, all head injuries and strokes. When outcome was plotted against average and highest ICP, it could be seen that patients with an average ICP higher than 31 mmHg did not live, nor did patients with a highest ICP greater than 100 mmHg. For stroke, the highest hourly average ICP was more detrimental, while the overall average ICP was more detrimental for head injuries.

Glasgow Recovery Scale. The primary predictors were average ICP and highest hourly average ICP. Age was a factor except in intracranial hemorrhage; the level of coma was a factor in head injuries. Individual factors that significantly ($p < 0.05$) affected the Glasgow recovery scale were coma (15%), highest hourly average ICP (13%), and average ICP (6%). Initial ICP (2%) was not a predictor($p > 0.05$).

Although significant predictions in Glasgow recovery scale and dis-change status could be made in respect to the hemorrhage group, such predictions accounted for less variation (10% to 18%) than for other diagnoses (27% to 59%).

Conclusions

1) In patients with head injuries, the level of coma was the major predictor of initial ICP, followed by age of patient and delay until monitoring, the three together accounting for 6% to 16% of the variance.

2) Initial ICP was the major predictor of both average and highest ICP.

3) For patients with head injuries, age was a factor in predicting outcome, but not in stroke patients. The level of coma was a factor in predicting outcome only in all patients combined, in the head injuries group and in the stroke group.

4) In strokes, the highest ICP was important in predicting outcome, while in head injuries, the average ICP was more important.

5) No patient lived to be discharged in any group with an overall average ICP above 31 mmHg. No head injury patient lived to be dis-changed with a highest hourly average ICP above 100 mmHg, while no stroke patient lived to be discharged with a highest hourly average ICP above 60 mmHg.

6) The Glasgow recovery scale was improved for patients who did not have as high a highest hourly average ICP.

THE PROGNOSTIC VALUE OF INTRACRANIAL PRESSURE (ICP) MEASUREMENT IN RELATION TO THE DIFFERENT FACTORS THAT CAN AFFECT ICP

E.B.BONGARTZ, H.E.NAU, L.GERHARD, J.LIESGANG, AND W.J.BOCK

Introduction

To predict the patient's outcome after a severe head injury, neurological findings, the posttraumatic course and other clinical data have been analyzed including the results of different treatments(1-6). This retrospective study correlates ICP with outcome and with other factors. We tried to analyze the possible differences between a group of survivors and compared them with the same number of patients who died.

Material and Methods

We investigated 120 patients with a minimum unconsciousness of 24 hours. Follow-up of diagnostic measurements (CT, EEG), neurological investigations, control of ICP and in those who died a detailed postmortem examination were done by means of a standardized list of questions. Nearly 80 factors were distinguished and divided into pretraumatic, traumatic and posttraumatic factors (Table 1). Epidural ICP was measured in patients with midline shift, intracranial mass lesions or with CT-visible brain damage. All patients were treated in a half-sitting position under moderate controlled hyperventilation and with high dose dexamethasone therapy. The percentage of autopsies among the deceased was 78%. Among our patients 70% were male; 17% of the patients were under the age of 10. In the survivors' group 30% were under the age of 10 in contrast to 2% of the non-survivors. The average age of the non-survivors was 41, of the survivors 22.

Results

Pretraumatic diseases did not influence the posttraumatic ICP with the possible exception of chronic alcoholism. Among the pedestrians (20%) and bicycle riders (8%) there was no difference in regard to increased ICP (20%), but there was a better survival rate among the younger patients (30%) which indirectly influenced the correlation between pedestrians and survival and ICP.

The fact that more patients with late admission after trauma (16%) have shown an increased ICP (63%) may be correlated not so much directly to the time of admission and ICP, but to a couple of other factors such as age (82% above 50 years), time of day of the accident (25% between 6:00 and 18:00 o'clock), localization of the accident (35% in big cities, 65% in villages), etc.

It is remarkable that those patients who developed raised ICP showed minor and fewer neurological symptoms, but these patients had a higher incidence of extensive diffuse brain damage in CT (38%).

Table I. Extract of the investigated factors in severe head injury

PRETRAUMATIC FACTORS	
age	sex
preexisting diseases	place of accident
TRAUMATIC FACTORS	
kind of accident	time between accident and admission
state of consciousness	pain reaction
respiration	shock
pupils / light reaction	reflex/ moror disturbance
extension mechanisms	additional injuries
instrumental skull investigations	intracranial space occupying lesions
morphological findings	
POSTTRAUMATIC FACTORS	
kind of operation	state of consciousness
pain reaction	extension mechanisms
pupils / light reaction	reflex / motor disturbance
blood chemistry	infections
vegetative disorders	seizures
instrumental skull investigations	patho-morphological findings

Among the non-survivors there were many more patients with the combination: vegetative disregulation and raised ICP (42%). Raised ICP was found in 30% of the non-survivors, in the survivors only in 5%. An extract of the other results is shown in Table 2.

Discussion

The multifactorial problem in the evaluation of influences upon ICP could be demonstrated in a couple of examples, such as the correlation between age, ICP and type of accident or the correlation between pedestrians, survival and increased ICP. To establish the importance of two different factors influencing ICP it is necessary to prove the interaction of those 2 factors with each other. For example: extension rigidity was found in 80% of the patients without increased ICP and only in 45% of those with increased ICP. The results are in contrast to the common opinion that extension rigidity has a negative prognostic value. Such a contrast suggests the influence of another

Table 2. Extract of the results after evaluation of the standardized list of questions (see also text)

	survivors 60 patients	non-survivors 60 patients
Kind of accident: pedestrians	15 patients	9 patients
bicycle riders	5	5
car drivers	8	7
fall	10	20
Reason for admission		
primary unconsciousness	36 patients	49 patients
secondary unconsciousness	6	5
lateralization of symptoms	4	2
Average time before admission	10 hours	11 hours
Average hours of unconsciousness	198	235
Signs of shock at admission	13 patients	21 patients
Intubated at admission	22 patients	32 patients
Skull fracture	22 patients	30 patients
CT: midline shift (edema)	16 patients	10 patients
midline shift (hematoma)	11	23
diffuse brain damage	8	10
Extension rigidity after 24 hours	19 patients	19 patients
Osmotherapy (sorbitol/mannitol)	3 patients	15 patients
Temperature/blood pressure disorders after 48 hours (10 +)	6 patients	21 patients
Infections after 48 hours (10 +)	20 patients	20 patients
Post-mortem investigations:		
Heart diseases (coronary sclerosis, hypertrophy, scars)		27 patients
Lung diseases (pulmonary sclerosis, emphysems, scars)		21 patients
Diseases of other organs (except liver/kidney) (aorta and brain vessel sclerosis, stomach, etc)		34 patients
Fractures (fractures of the skull base: 41 patients)		53 patients
Signs of infections (tracheobronchitis, pneumonia, etc)		48 patients
Diseases of vessels (laceration, thrombosis, embolism)		18 patients
Brain: cortical lesions		44 patients
diffuse internal lesions		24
circumscribed internal lesions		38
midbrain lesions		13
signs of local brain pressure		48

unknown factor. This factor can easily be demonstrated in the CT results where extension rigidity is combined with a high percentage (66%) with more localized brain damage. Important is the correlation of raised ICP and vegetative disregulation. The connecting mechanism is not known. It may be that vegetative temperature and blood pressure disregulation causes blood brain barrier damage and therefore causes increased ICP. It may also be that raised ICP evokes hypothalamic disfunction and by this way temperature and blood pressure disregulation.

By interconnecting loops it is possible that ICP can be influenced more by pathophysiological factors than by physiological factors, and therefore it is shown that a correlation of different factors to brain pressure only makes sense if brain pressure is a part of this complex control system.

Summary

120 patients with severe head injury were studied. 60 patients had a favorable outcome. 60 died and underwent an extensive post-mortem investigation. By a standardized list of questions we analyzed nearly 80 factors of each patient by which it could perhaps be possible to predict a patient's outcome and their possible influence upon ICP. These factors were differentiated in pretraumatic, traumatic and posttraumatic factors. No significant correlation between pretraumatic or traumatic factors and posttraumatic ICP was found. Only posttraumatic factors like vegetative disorders and raised ICP were significantly increased in the group of the non-survivors. Other factors had a possible influence upon outcome, like time of admission (a traumatic factor), but to be sure of this, bigger groups of patients have to be investigated.

References

1. Becker DP, Miller JD, Ward JD, Greenberg RP, Young HF, Sakalas R (1977) The outcome from severe head injury with early diagnosis. J Neurosurg 47:491-502

2. Bricolo A, Turazzi A, Alexandre A, Rizzuto N (1977) Decerebrate rigidity in acute head injury. J Neurosurg 47:680698

3. James HE, Madauss WC, Tibes PA, McCloskey JJ, Bean JR (1977) The effect of high dose dexamethasone in children. Acta Neurochir 48:225-236

4. Lundberg N, Kjallquist A, Bien C (1959) Reduction of increased ICP by hyperventilation. Acta psych neurol Scand Suppl 139:5-64

5. Marshall LF, Smith RW, Shapiro HM (1979) The outcome with aggressive treatment in severe head injuries. J Neurosurg 50:20-30

6. Nau HE, Bongartz EB, Bock WJ, Weichert C (1979) Computerized tomography, electroencephalography and clinical symptoms in severe head injuries. Acta neurosurg 45:209-216

DOES THE PRESSURE-VOLUME RELATIONSHIP EXIST?

A.L.BENABID, J.DE ROUGEMONT, J.P.CHIROSSEL, AND M.BARGE

Introduction

The pressure-volume relationship (PVR), since described in 1966 by LANGFITT, has become the best known feature in the literature concerning intracranial pressure (ICP). Much work has been done, many curves have been published, and authors try to explain all aspects of ICP in terms of PVR; however, in some instances, the shapes of the curves are different, and the physiopathological statements lack mathematical basis.

Critical Review of Literature: a non-exhaustive review of the literaturs is sufficient to demonstrate the discrepancies between the experimental data. If plotted using the same coordinates, the curves of the ICP increases above the normal pressure Po, with respect to the volume V injected, are all different (Fig 1): some are exponential-like shaped, others linear, and others reach a plateau; MARMAROU (1973) demonstrated that the PVR he obtained was exactly exponential. All these differences can be related to technological features: the animal may be the monkey (5), the cat (4,7,8) or the dog (3,6); the new intracranial volume is performed either by a bolus injection(3); by a steady state infusion (4,5,6,8) or by repetitive bolus equivalent to steady state infusion (7), using either a balloon (5,8) or an injection in CSF space (3,4,6,7). The injection rates also are different: 0.017 ml/mn (5) 0.023 ml/mn (8) 0.5 ml/mn (4) 0.6 ml/mn (7) and 15ml/mn (6). So it could be that what is always reported under the term PVR corresponds in fact to different phenomena, and not to the cerebral vascular compliance alone.

Theoretical Aspects: Any injection of a new volume into a system induces a change in ICP, the pattern of which depends on the internal structure of this system. In the case of a closed system, the pressure increase is directly related to the compliance S of the internal contents so that $\Delta V/\Delta P = S$, which is a constant or a function of the pressure; in this case only, the PVR directly reflects the compliance S. In the case of an open system, the ratio $\Delta V/\Delta P$ dependant on the compliance S, the CSF pathways conductance K and the rate of infusion r, is given in our model (3) by the relation: $\Delta V/\Delta P = S.r / (r - K\{P-Po\})$. Therefore the PVR curve no longer reflects the compliance S alone, but also other characteristics of the system (like K) and the conditions to which it is submitted (like the rate r and the pressure P). This ratio is reduced to the compliance S only when the rate of infusion r is infinite, (which corresponds to a bolus injection and the pressure must be measured at the peak level) or when the CSF conductance K is equal to zero,(which corresponds either to a theoretically perfect hydrocephalus, or to the decompensated stage of intracranial hypertension). This has been achieved experimentally by LANGFITT with a balloon (5): while the CSF volume has not been completely evacuated, ICP remains low because r is low; when the whole CSF is replaced by the balloon, or if CSF resorption is no longer possible because of the brain shift, the system appears to be closed and then ICP increases according to the brain compliance. Therefore the PVR of LANGFITT is the only one which describes the changes of intracranial compliance, the experimental situation reproducing fairly well the pathological conditions; but this PVR curve is theoretically unable to describe the physical laws ruling out the behavior of the system in lower or normal ICP ranges. For this purpose, the pressure volume response of the system must be studied by bolus injections (3) where the ratio of $\Delta V/\Delta P$ at the peak is equal to the compliance S. In cases of steady state infusion, the PVR pattern reflects the parameters S, K and r, and the analysis of the experimental data contained in this curve can be only done according to a detailed mathematical model, the vascular compliance being not the sole characteristic of the system determining and changing the shape of the curve. So, the determination of the so-called PVR curve in patients or in animals may not be used as a tool for studying the intracranial compliance. When an amount of fluid ΔVi is injected, however fast the rate may be, a part ΔVs is stored in the system by way of a vascular compression dependent on the vascular compliance S and another part ΔVa is absorbed by the CSF pathways depending on the conductance K. Therefore, the equation $\Delta Vi = \Delta Vs + \Delta Va$ can be written: $r.\Delta t = S.\Delta P + K.(P-Po)\Delta t$; this differential equation is the general mathematical model of the system, the solution of which depends on the assumptions concerning the mathematical structure of S and K. Nevertheless, in all cases, the ratio $\Delta Vs/\Delta P$ represents the compliance S which is to be measured; but in all experiments reported, this has been assessed experimentally by measuring the only data accessible $\Delta Vi/\Delta P$, without mathematical interpretation of the curve according to a model. This explains, in our opinoin, why the results are so different, and the interpretations in this field so varied.

Results and Discussion

Previously (1,3) we have developed a mathematical model of CSF dynamics. From the same experiments on 53 dogs, there is an hyperbolic relationship between conductance K and ICP, and the compliance S has been found statistically constant with respect to pressure, before any vasomotor response occurs. The mean statistical data of S and K have been reintroduced into this model and the computer calculation of the equations gives a series of pressure-volume curve highly dependent on the rate of infusion r (Fig. 2). When r increases, the initial part of the curve tends asymptotically to a straight line, the slope of which is 1/S. The last part of the curve is always a plateau, the height of which depends only on K and r. Therefore, a very large amount of fluid can be injected without significant ICP increase, if the rate is sufficiently low and the CSF pathways not disturbed by a brain shift, as induced by an inflating balloon. These curves may be compared to those reported in the literature (Fig. 1). Excepting the ones from balloon inflation (the mechanism of which is different, as we say), the other curves (on considering their initial part) fall in the same area as ours. FURUSE'S curves are similar to ours, reaching a plateau depending on the degree of obstruction of the CSF pathways during experimental hydrocephalus by soot dispersion; the MARMAROU'S curve is in the same ICP range as ours, but the volume range is narrower, and we believe that, for larger volumes, a plateau would have been obtained. The question of exponential-like shape of some curves is now raised; in our experience this shape is not often observed, the most common exhibiting a continuously decreasing slope; but in some cases, the initial part is curved upwards. Following cerebral blood volume measurements using an impedance technique (2), it can be shown that a vasodilatation response occurs when ICP is increased, its rate degree dependent on the ICP increase rate (Fig. 3). This delayed vasodilatation, which is probably achieved to keep constant the cerebral blood flow, is responsible for the initially exponential-like shape of some curves.

Conclusions

Changes in vasomotor tone obviously occur when ICP increases, as is shown by the increase in ICP pulse height. Therefore the consecutive changes in vascular compliance represent one of the most important functional features of CSF dynamics and their assessment is of great interest. However, owing to the open nature of the system, the brain compliance can be assessed only by careful mathematical analysis of the CSF system response to a given disturbance, obtained by volume injections. This can be achieved by computer calculation according to a strict mathematical model, leading to valuable information concerning vascular compliance and CSF conductance, which can never be separated.

Summary

The experimental evidence of ICP changes induced by volume injection have been widely published by several authors using various techniques. In many cases,physiopathological interpretations do not take into account the role of CSF absorption. Only a mathematical approach involving a strict model permits analysis of the data and the characterization of the basic system response to a disturbance. It is shown that the shape of the so-called Pressure Volume curve is determined by both the compliance and the CSF conductance; the curve reaches an equilibrium plateau dependent on the infusion rate, and the exponential-like shape of the initial part of the curve is of vasomotor origin. The basic behavioral law of the system is in fact ruled out by a pressure-infusion rate relationship.

References

1. Benabid AL, Rougemont j de, Barge M (1975) CSF dynamics: a mathematical approach. In: Lundberg N, Ponten U, Brock M (eds) Intracranial Pressure II. Springer, Berlin Heidelberg New York, p 54

2. Benabid AL, Persat JC, Piquard JF, et al (1976) Rheographic assessment of CBV and correlations with changes in ICP. Acta Neurochir (Wien) 34:287-294

3. Benabid AL (1978) Modelisation et caracterisation d'un phenomene biologique: la pression intracranienne. D Sc Physics Thesis, Grenoble University

4. Furuse M, Hasuo M, Brock M, Dietz H (1976) The role of CSF resorption on the intracranial pressure volume relationship. In: Beks JWF, Bosch DA, Brock M (eds) Intracranial Pressure III. Springer, Berlin Heidelberg New York, p 20

5. Langfitt TW, Weinstein JD, Kassell NF (1966) Vascular factors in head injury: contribution to brain swelling and intracranial hypertension. In: Caveness WF, Walker AE (eds) Head Injury Conference Proceedings. Lippincott, Philadelphia Toronto, p 172

6. Lofgren J, von Essen C, Zwetnow NN (1973) The pressure volume curve of the cerebrospinal fluid space of dogs. Acta Neurol Scand 49:557-574

7. Marmarou A (1973) A theoretical and experimental evaluation of the cerebrospinal fluid system. PhD Thesis, Drexel University

8 Sullivan HG, Miller JD Becker DP et al (1977) The physiological basis of ICP change with progressive epidural brain compression: an experimental evaluation in cats. J Neurosurg 47:532-550

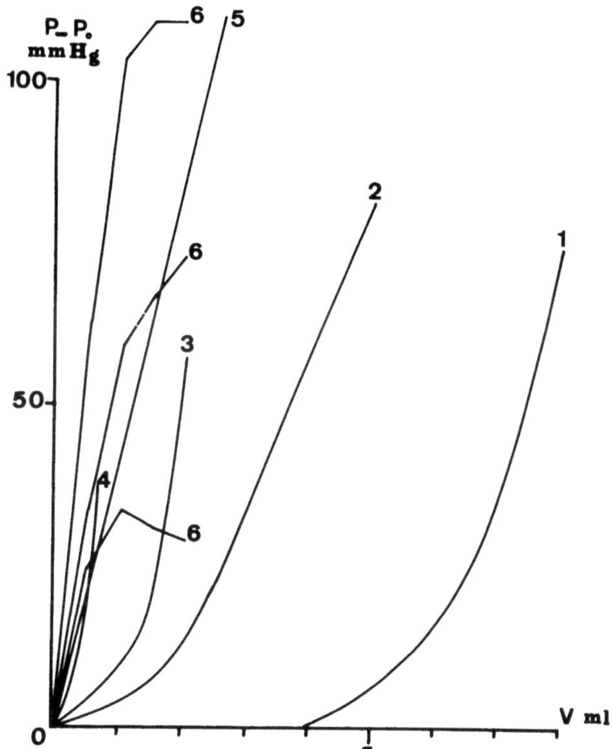

Fig. 1. Literature aspects of pressure volume relationships: Curves have been replotted from the literature data; ICP changes are related to normal pressure Po.
1 -LANGFITT (monkey, balloon, steady state infusion, 0.017 ml/mn)
2 -LOFGREN (dog, cisterna magna, steady state infusion, 15 ml/mn)
3 -SULLIVAN (cat, balloon, steady state infusion, 0.023 ml/mn)
4 -MARMAROU (cat, ventricle, repetitive bolus, 0.6 ml/mn)
5 -BENABID (dog, cisterna magna, bolus injection)
6 -FURUSE (cat, cisterna magna, steady state infusion, 0.5 ml/mn)

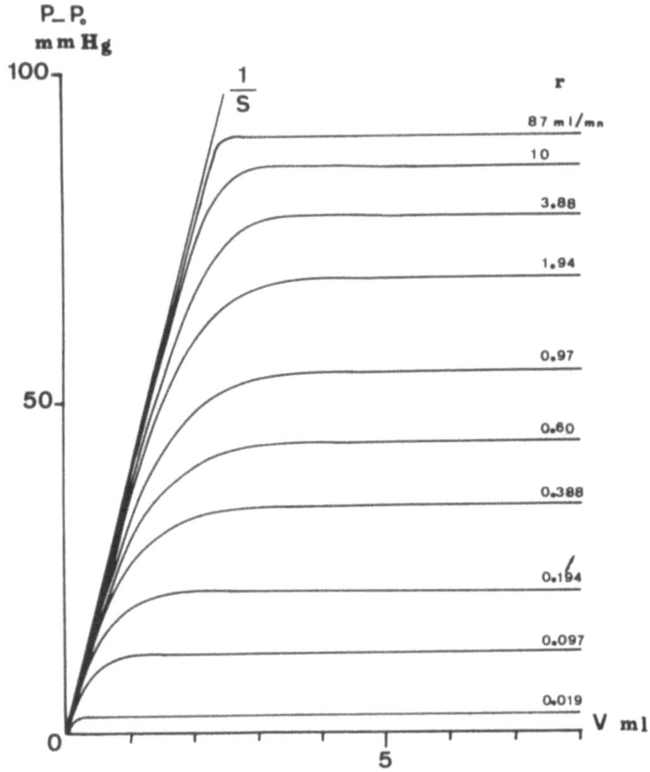

Fig. 2. Pressure volume relationships according to infusion rate r: The data have been computed by reintroducing into the model the experimental values of compliance S and conductance K determined on 53 dogs.

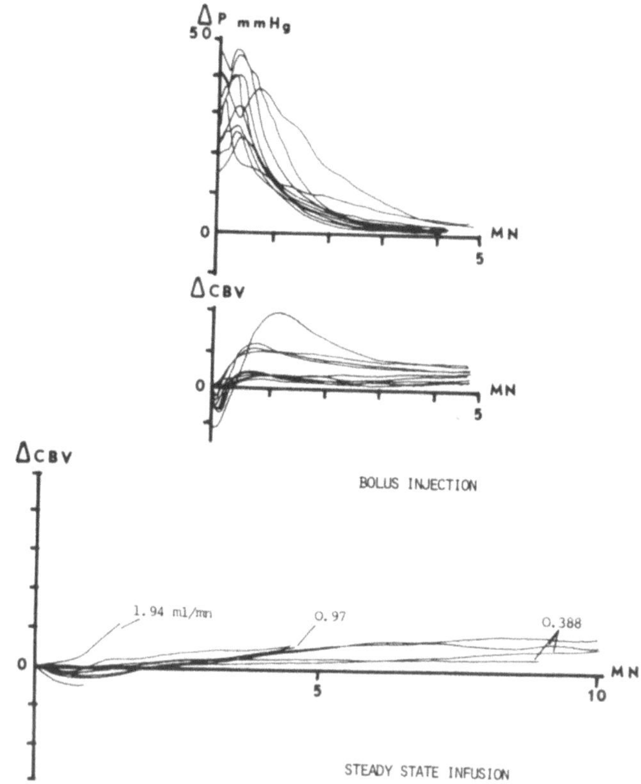

Fig. 3. Cerebral blood volume changes relation to injection rate. In case of bolus injection, a rebound of ICP is shown to be due to an active vasodilatation. In case of steady state infusion, the vaso-dilation speed depends on the injection rate.

EXPERIMENTAL BRAIN INJURY IN THE DOG: PATHOPHYSIOLOGICAL CORRELATION

R.J.CLUBB, R.MAXWELL, AND S.CHOU

Introduction

Despite the utilization of standardized brain injury created by the inflation and subsequent deflation of an epidural balloon, two general response patterns were observed: 1. Absence of significant postdeflation intracranial hypertension and prolonged survival. 2. Postdeflation intracranial pressure (ICP) rise exceeding 40 torr, plateau waves, and brain death within several hours of deflation. This paper aims to provide insight into the causes of the variability in responses to a standardized injury by correlating physiological behavior with autopsy findings.

Material and methods

In dogs anesthetized with nitrous oxide, hyperventilation and gallamine, end-expiratory CO_2, blood pressure (SAP), electrocardiogram, blood gases, temperature, ICP, electroencephalogram (EEG) were recorded. An epidural balloon was placed over the temporal lobe through a burr hole. Balloon inflation continued until the EEG became isoelectric. Static balloon inflation (constant volume) was then maintained for 3, 15 and 30 minutes in Groups I,III, and II, respectively. The balloon was then removed. After expiration or sacrifice, autopsy evaluation was performed.

Group I included ten dogs (inflation rate: 0.4cc/5 min) observed for six hours after deflation. Five received one 30 mg/kg injection of pentobarbital. Group II included eight dogs (inflation rate: 1.0cc/5 min) observed for six hours after deflation. Three received pentobarbital and one received nitroprusside. Group III included 41 dogs (inflation rate:1.0cc/5 min). Animals of Group III in which ICP did not exceed 40 torr within three hours of inflation were sacrificed or observed until death several days later. Animals in which ICP exceeded 40 torr within three hours were observed five additional hours. These were divided into control, pentobarbital, and nitroprusside treatment groups.

Results

In three dogs of Group I, ICP exceeded 40 torr within 80 minutes of balloon removal. They exhibited plateau waves of ICP alone or of ICP and SAP. All expired within several hours of deflation. Autopsies revealed midbrain hemorrhages in all three but no mass lesions. ICP did not exceed 40 torr in seven dogs of Group I. One expired after barbiturate injection while six survived several days after termination of anesthesia. These dogs exhibited neither midbrain hemorrhages nor mass lesions.

In every Group II animal, ICP exceeded 40 torr within 38 minutes of deflation. Four untreated animals exhibited plateau waves of ICP and SAP exceeding 200 torr. Pentobarbital or nitroprusside prevented systemic hypertension and discrete pressure waves but ICP still increased to within 30 torr of SAP. Brain death was evident within five hours of deflation in all eight dogs. Autopsies revealed transtentorial herniation and posterior thalamic hemorrhages ipsilateral to the balloon site in all animals and midbrain hemorrhages in all but one. Mass lesions were absent.

In 23 dogs of Group III (Subgroup A), ICP exceeded 40 torr within three hours of deflation while, in 18, (Subgroup B), ICP did not exceed this level. All but three dogs in Subgroup A were brain dead at the end of observation. All animals of Subgroup B which were not sacrificed at three hours after deflation survived several additional days. All but one non-barbiturate treated animal of Subgroup A exhibited plateau waves of ICP alone or of ICP and SAP (exceeding 200 torr). Most animals in Subgroup A exhibited transtentorial herniation (Figure 1) and midbrain and thalamic hemorrhages (Figure 2). These lesions were absent in most animals of Subgroup B. Intergroup differences were highly significant (midbrain: $p < .01$, thalamus: $p < .025$, herniation: $p < .005$), but not absolute. Mass lesions were absent in Group III dogs.

Increased time of static inflation resulted in a significant increase in incidence of post-deflation intracranial hypertension, herniation and midbrain and thalamic hemorrhages.

Discussion

Despite standardized brain injury, significant post-deflation intracranial hypertension and plateau waves were present in some dogs and absent in others. Global ischemia was the same in dogs with both behavioral patterns and probably does not account for the observed brain swelling and plateau waves. Significant autopsy findings were confined to the midbrain-thalamic junction and tentorium. Mass lesions and significant areas of contusion or necrosis were absent. Superficial and deep venous obstruction resulting from mass expansion were probably similar in all animals. Thus, the marked differences between the two patterns of post-deflation behavior were unlikely due to relatively minor and inconsistent differences in magnitude of ischemia, vasogenic edema, masses, or venous obstruction. There is indirect evidence that plateau waves, especially of ICP and SAP, are related to transtentorial herniation and are caused by cerebral vasoparalysis (1,2,3,4). Since dogs with similar plateau waves and intracranial hypertension exhibited a much higher incidence of herniation and midbrain hemorrhages than those without these lesions, we postulate that brain swelling and plateau waves may be related to midbrain dysfunction which probably interrupts rostral control over caudal centers for cerebral vasoparalysis.

Summary

Dogs which sustained standardized brain injury by the inflation of an epidural balloon exhibited two general response patterns: 1. Those with significant brain swelling and plateau waves. 2. Those without these phenomena. Dogs with the first pattern had a significantly higher incidence of transtentorial herniation and midbrain hemorrhages.

Based on these data, brain swelling may be related to midbrain dysfunction.

References

1. Beks J, ter Weeme CL (1967) The influence of urea and mannitol on increased intraventricular pressure in cold-induced cerebral edema. Acta Neurochir (Wien) 16:97-107

2. Langfitt T, Kassell N, Weinstein J (1965) Cerebral blood flow with intracranial hypertension. Neurol 15:761-73

3. Langfitt T, Winstein J, Kassell N (1965) Cerebral vasomotor Paralysis produced by intracranial hypertension. Neurol 15:622-41

4. Weinstein J, Langfitt T, Kassell N (1964) Vasopressor response to increased intracranial pressure. Neurol 14:1118-31

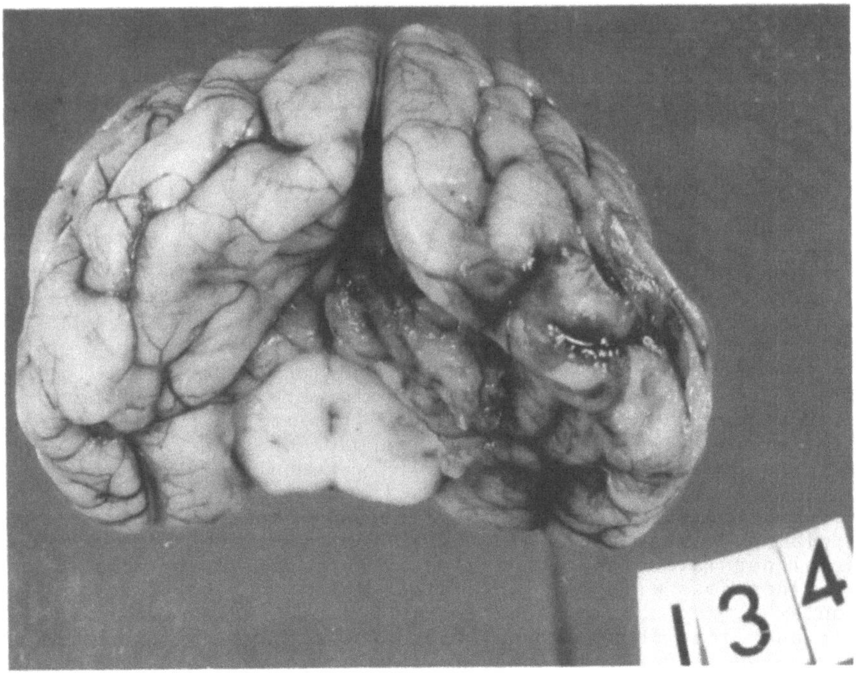

Figure 1. Transtentorial herniation on the right producing midbrain distortion.

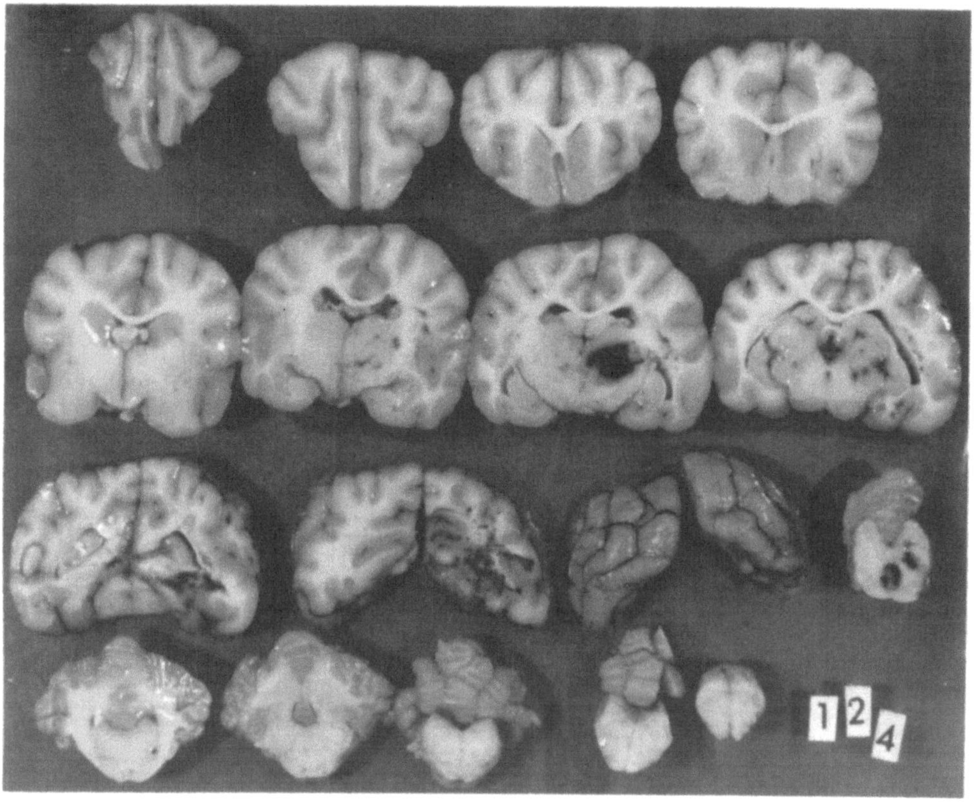

Figure 2. Typical cross sections of the cerebral hemispheres and brain stem in animals with significant post-deflation brain swelling. Significant lesions confined to the posterior thalamus and midbrain. Note medial temporal lobe infarction in region of herniation and in distribution of posterior cerebral artery.

CORRELATIONS BETWEEN INTRACRANIAL PRESSURE, NEUROLOGIC DEFICIT AND COMPUTER TOMOGRAPHIC FINDINGS IN PATIENTS WITH ACUTE SEVERE HEAD INJURY
A CLINICAL STUDY

P.FASOL, H.BINDER, T.REISNER, R.SCHEDL, L.SCHMID, AND M.STRICKNER

Introduction

The aim of the present paper was to investigate interrelations between ICP, neurologic status and data of computerized axial tomography during the acute stage after admission of patients with acute severe head injury.

Clinical material and methods

In 47 patients with severe head injury ICP monitoring was started as soon as possible after admission. Table I shows the distribution of neurosurgical diagnosis and mean ICP levels within the first 24 hours. ICP was measured in the epidural space using the Ladd monitor equipment (Ladd Research Industries, Inc.). Neurological status was investigated immediately after admission, if possible always by the same neurologist. These examinations were repeated twice or three times within 24 hours. Neurologic deficits have been classified in 4 stages of midbrain dysfunction syndrome and bulbar brain syndrome. The particular symptoms of midbrain syndromes I-4, and bulbar brain syndrome as well are seen as follows (I):

Midbrain syndrome (MBS) I: sudden or delayed adversive reaction, mass movements, rotary motion, normal tonus, normal bulbus position, pendulans bulbus movement, pupils narrow with normal light reaction.

MBS 2: delayed reaction, absence of adversive movement, mass movements of arms, extension synergisms of legs, hypertonus in legs, bulbus position normal but movement disconjugated, pupils small, light reaction delayed.

MBS 3: flexion synergisms of arms, extension synergisms of legs, hypertonus in all extremities, bulbus position divergent and movement absent, pupils small, sluggish light reaction.

MBS 4: extension synergisms of arms and legs, extension posture of all extremities, bulbus position divergent and movement absent, pupils narrow, light reaction sluggish.

Bulbar brain syndrome (BBS): motor reaction and movement absent, atonic posture, bulbi divergent, pupils maximally enlarged, light reaction absent.

In computerized axial tomography we distinguished three different stages of ICP level:
Stage I: no signs of ICP elevation

Stage 2: incipient herniation of one temporal lobe, subfalcial herniation, eventual enlargement of contralateral and compression of homolateral ventricular system.

Table 1. 47 patients with severe head injury: neurosurgical diagnosis, mean ICP level for the first 24 hours
(brackets: number of deaths)

	ICP		
	I 0 - 20	II 21 - 50	III > 50
Cerebral contusion	8(3)	13(6)	7(7)
Acute subdural hematoma	3(2)	3(3)	4(4)
Acute epidural hematoma	2(0)	-	-
Frontobasal fracture	1(0)	4(2)	-
Missile injury	-	2(2)	-

Table 2. Interrelations between ICP level and stage of midbrain disfunction (MBD)

Number of patients	Deaths	ICP	MBD	Interrelation
8	2	I	1,2	excellent
8	7	III	1 4	excellent
8	8	III	4	good
13	6	II	1,2	good
3	0	I	3 1	good
2	1	I	1 4	not clear
2	1	I	3	not clear
1	1	III	1	not clear

Table 3. Interrelations between ICP monitored and evidence of ICP elevation in CAT. 21 investigations

	CAT		
ICP	I	II	III
I	1	4	1
II	-	6	3
III	-	2	4

Stage 3: compression of basic cisterns, ventricular system subtotal or total compressed.

CAT examinations were performed in 21 cases, in some of those ICP monitoring has been continued during CAP recording.

Results

Considering interrelations between ICP level and neurologicl deficit we can distribute our patients to several groups showing no marked differences (See Table 2). There are 8 patients with normal ICP and moderate neurologic disfunction and further 8 patients with severe neurologic damage and ICP exceeding 50 mmHg. In altogether 11 cases there was seen a short time discrepance between ICP and neurologic status disappearing after a few hours. However, in 5 of our patients interrelations between ICP and neurologic stage are not clear and interpretations rather speculative.

Estimating the correlations between ICP and CAT recordings we can point out that all cases with ICP elevation had CAT evidence of increased pressure. There are still 5 cases with signs of ICP elevation in CAT with normal ICP monitored (Table 3).

Conclusions

Within the first 24 hours in the acute stage of cerebral trauma there are near interrelations between mean ICP and neurologic deficit. For successful treatment knowledge of ICP level is necessary. Short time changes in ICP are not discernable by neurologic investigation and CAT examination as well. However, exact knowledge of actual neurologic status and CAT examinations for identifying of intracranial mass lesions are unalterable requirements for the management of head injured patients.

Reference

1. Gerstenbrand F, Lucking CH (1970) Die akuten traumatischen Hirnschaden. Arch Psychiat Nervenkr 213:264-281

CONTINUOUS MEASUREMENT OF INTRACRANIAL PRESSURE IN 127 SEVERE HEAD INJURIES

D.P.BYRNES AND T.B.DUCKER

Introduction

In the United States the commonest cause of death between the ages of 1 and 40 is trauma. Some 70% of these deaths are due to head injuries. The conventional methods of head injury care are resuscitation, operation if needed, and observation. The latter is mainly to check for signs of rising intracranial pressure which may signal hematoma, cerebral edema, or hydrocephalus.

Unfortunately the physical signs of rising intracranial pressure (ICP) are not always consistent or reliable. This is particularly so if the patient has suffered multiple injuries. Such a patient often requires many hours of anesthesia. and ventilation in the intensive care unit (ICU) for his other injuries. This situation makes the ongoing repeated clinical neurological examination invalid or indeed impossible. So some other method of monitoring is needed. Logically that method is the direct measurement of intracranial pressure continuously. As well as providing a continuous qualitative measurement of ICP the visco-elastic state of the brain can be assessed, i.e., the patient's position on the pressure volume compliance curve can be charted; additionally with the ventricular catheter system CSF can be removed at any time to allow reduction in intracranial pressure.

We now have the apparatus and expertise to do that on a practical and routine basis. The Maryland Institute for Emergency Medical Services Systems is a 50 bedded unit within the University of Maryland Hospital. This unit handles approximately 1200 acutely ill patients per year. The vast majority are victims of trauma. In the years 1977-78, 245 (non-penetrating) severe head injuries were admitted to the Institute. Severity was, among other criteria, defined as a level of consciousness below 7 on the Glasgow Coma Scale (1) for six hours. Twenty-six of these patients died within a very short time. Ninety-two others showed rapid improvement when resuscitation and care of other injuries was completed. This improvement precluded the need for measuring ICP.

Onehundred twenty-seven patients underwent continuous intracranial pressure monitoring. Thirty-two percent (75) of these patients required craniotomy for hematoma - epidural, subdural or intracerebral. The vast majority of these procedures were done within hours of injury. Prior to ICP being measured several required craniotomy at a later time from 1 to 7 days after injury. The need for surgery in these was usually made known by the very effective combination of ICP measurement and the CT scan. In those operated on early the ICP was measured after surgery.

Seventy-two percent of these injuries was due to road traffic accidents. There were 96 males and 31 females. Multiplicity of injuries in terms of non-CNS was a common feature. Sixty percent had another major system injury in addition to cranio-cerebral one. Twenty-five percent had two additional system injuries. These extra cranial problems were: penetrating chest, lung contusions, liver and spleen lacerations, and major limb fractures. Approximately 6% had a cervical spine injury also. There was an overall mortality of 39%.

Methods

Intracranial pressure was measured by ventricular catheterization. This was done by means of a small diameter infant feeding tube (No.5 Argyle Sherwood Medical Company) attached to a Statham P 37 or P 50 transducer fixed to the patient's head. A wall mounted multi-channel digital readout and oscilloscope system is used with variably set six built-in alarms. This allows simultaneous recording of blood pressure (systolic, diastolic, and mean); venous pressure on pulmonary artery pressure; heart rate and temperature. The catheter is inserted in the operating room under full sterile conditions. It is done here for infection prevention measures. The multiple injured patient is a notorious infection risk.

A small twist drill burr hole is made to the right of the midline frontally behind the hairline. The dura is opened usually with a large diameter needle. The feeding tube with a trocar of steel wire inside it is inserted into the front horn of the right lateral ventricle. The failure rate in this maneuver is less than 5% with practice. Approximately 1-1/2 ml CSF is removed for cell count, culture and various biochemical tests. The proximal end of the tube is led in the subgaleal plane for approximately 4-5 cm and out through a separate stab wound. By means of the 3-way stopcock it is attached to the transducer. The 3rd port of the stopcock has a self-sealing rubber diaphragm which allows later withdrawal of CSF without opening the system to the atmosphere.

The patient is transferred back to the ICU and the wall hook-up completed. The catheter is usually removed in 72-96 hours unless needed for CSF drainage. The overall infection rate was approximately 5%, infection being defined as positive culture from either ventricular or lumbar CSF. Occasionally if ventricular catheterization could not be achieved a subarachnoid screw was inserted. These, however, are not included in the following results.

Patients who had intracranial pressure greater than 20 mmHg for 10 minutes were treated. The methods used were routine endotrachial intubation, hyperventilation (pCO_2 approximately 25 mmHg), steroids, and sedation to prevent movement. Mannitol, CSF venting either continuously or intermittently, decompressive surgery and occasionally barbiturates were used as the need to combat rising ICP occurred.

In patients whose ICP did not exceed 24 mmHg for more than 10 minutes, 62 or 74% survived and 22 or 26% died. In patients whose sustained ICP is greater than 10 minutes over 25 mmHg in spite of vigorous therapy, only 7 or 16% survived and 36 (84%) died. The latter group of patients who have ICP of over 25 mmHg for 10 minutes can be further subdivided. In those whole pressures did not exceed 35 mmHg for greater than 10 minutes 35% survived and 65% died. In patients who had sustained ICP greater than 35 mmHg, often greater than 40 mmHg, none survived.

Figure 1 summarizes our results of our 127 patients. Those patients who, in spite of therapy, had sustained ICP recording after craniocerebral trauma are subdivided into less than 25 mmHg, 30 - 35 mmHg, and greater than 35 mmHg, had survival rates of 75%, 35%, and 0% respectively.

Figure 1. Sustained High ICP in Head Trauma with Active Treatment.

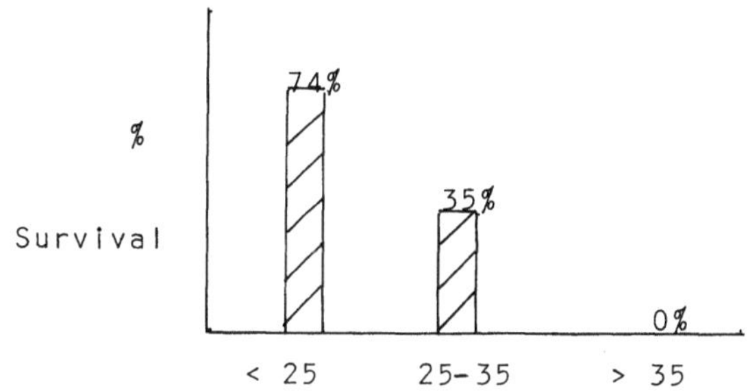

Conclusion

We concluded from this that: (a) routine measurement of ICP in some head injuries is practical; (b) it allows better continuous neurologic assessment of patients whose other injuries require continuous sedation or anesthesia; (c) intraventricular catheterization allows CSF venting and is therefore the only potentially therapeutic method; and (d) failure to control intracranial pressure markedly increases mortality.

Reference

1. Teasdale G, Jennet B (1974) Assessment of coma and impaired consciousness. A practical scale. Lancet 2:81-84

Session II

PRESSURE-VOLUME STUDIES

Chairman: A. Marmarou
Co-chairman: A. L. Benabid

SUMMARY

SKLAR et al investigated pressure volume relationships in a variety of disease states, including pseudotumor cerebri, hydrocephalus and brain atrophy, by rapidly changing ICP from one constant pressure plateau to another using infusion technique. They reported that the elasticity slope $\{(dP/dV)/ICP\}$ is directly proportional to ventricular size. Shapiro et al studied normal children and adults to obtain normal reference values for the Pressure Volume Index (PVI). They reported that compliance as measured by PVI is proportional to neural axis volume with children having lower compliance solely as a function of smaller neural axis volume. During the discussion, SHAPIRO stated ventricular size in hydrocephalic children did not necessarily correlate with compliance. He suggested that pressure volume studies should be performed in patients with similar disease states in order to make valid comparisons.

The underlying theory of pressure volume relationships was challenged in the report by BENABID. He viewed brain compliance as a theoretical concept based on vasomotor tone and expressed that perhaps it would be better to study vasomotor tone as an index of brain stiffness. On the basis of findings reported by SULLIVAN, who studied $P/\Delta V$ relationships before and after cardiac arrest, arteriole and hydraulic pressures do make a significant contribution to the CSF $P/\Delta V$ curve. In discussion, ZWETNOW cited the earlier work by LOFGREN and ZWETNOW where effects of blood pressure upon elastance were clearly demonstrated. The issue, however, was not resolved and SULLIVAN'S findings could not be explained on the basis of current concepts.

The analysis of PV studies conducted in man by FRIDEN and EKSTEDT showed that elastance was not proportional to the CSFP as would be expected in an exponential relationship between pressure and volume. The elastance pressure curve was found to be complex and they suggested that errors in estimation of compliance and outflow conductance may be introduced by linear approximations of the elastance curve, particularly if the elastance pressure curve is assumed to equal zero at zero pressure.

Methods for describing brain visoelastic properties were presented by WALSH and SCHETTINI. These workers used a pressure displacement transducer for calculation of elastic response parameters obtained from brain surface depth insertion tests conducted in vivo. Using similar principles, MARMAROU and co-workers used an electrodynamometer, capable of more precise dynamic control, to measure force-deformation curves of brain tissue. Both groups found non-linear visoelastic response characteristics. The need for further investigation in basic tissue properties to complement the pressure volume studies was clearly emphasized by the results of experiments by YONEDA et al who found that it is possible for considerable shearing stresses to develop within brain tissue in the absence of a detectable rise in the ICP.

THE PRESSURE-VOLUME FUNCTION OF BRAIN ELASTICITY AND ITS RELATIONSHIP WITH VENTRICULAR SIZE

F.H.SKLAR, C.W.BEYER,JR., H.HAGLER, M.RAMANATHAN, AND W.K.CLARK

Introduction

The exponential nature of the pressure-volume function of brain elastance has been well documented in animals (10) and man (7). It follows mathematically that the slope relating the natural logarithm of pressure to volume is equivalent to the slope relating elastance (dP/dV) to pressure (10). This slope parameter will be referred to as the elasticity slope.

Whether or not the elasticity pressure-volume function is influenced by ventricular size has not received attention in the literature. MILLER et al could demonstrate a linear relationship between elastance and pressure only in patients with normal sized ventricles, but not in patients with hydrocephalus (4). SHULMAN and MARMAROU could show no correlation between the pressure-volume elasticity relationship and head circumference measurements in hydrocephalic children (7). In the present study, the pressure-volume function of brain elasticity as indicated by the elasticity slope is examined as a possible function of ventricular volume in patients with diverse clinical disorders.

Methods

The slope of the semi-logarithmic pressure-volume elasticity function was measured with a rapid rate infusion/withdrawal technique (10) in 12 patients with active communicating hydrocephalus, compensated hydrocephalus, brain atrophy, and pseudotumor cerebri. Ages ranged from 6 months to 68 years. Pressure-volume measurements were made as the patients were studied with servo-controlled lumbar infusions to determine CSF dynamics as a function of intracranial pressure (ICP) (9). Elasticity pressure-volume measurements were made as ICP was rapidly changed from one constant pressure plateau to another (Fig. 1A and B).

A calibrated syringe plunger position detector was used to monitor the volume changes. The infusion apparatus had reciprocally arranged syringes and a solenoid valve switching device to make unnecessary interruption of the procedure to refill a syringe. The volume data along with mean CSF pressure were sampled at one second intervals with a PDP 11/34 computer. The elasticity slope relating the natural logarithm of pressure versus volume infused (or withdrawn) was calculated with simple linear regression techniques. Four to twenty-four (average 12) elasticity determinations were done in each patient, and these results were averaged. From CT scans, ventricular volumes were digitized and calculated as a percent of total intracranial volume with a PDP 11/05 computer.

Results

The pressure-volume data fit an exponential model with statistical significance for each rapid rate infusion/withdrawal elasticity determination, without exception. The original computer display of the data for a single patient with enlarged ventricles after meningitis is shown in Figures 1A and B. The elasticity slope showed no correlation with age, net CSF absorptive capacity, or resting pressure as determined from the measurements of CSF dynamics. However, the elasticity slope showed a directly proportional relationship with ventricular volume considered as a percentage of total intracranial volume with statistical significance ($p < 0.005$) (Figure 2).

Discussion

The clinical significance of the elasticity function remains obscure. The results of the present study suggest that at a given ICP, patients with ventriculomegaly show a greater pressure response to a given volume change such as with respiratory and cardiac fluctuations than do patients with small or normal sized ventricles. Increased amplitude of the intracranial pulse pressure has been reported in patients with normal pressure communicating hydrocephalus (3,6). The serial measurements of SATO et al. indicate that despite the maintenance of constant ICP, pulse amplitudes progressively increase as hydrocephalus develops after intracranial hemorrhage and trauma (6). An increased elasticity slope related to ventricular dilatation could account for these observations.

BERING has emphasized the importance of the choroidal pulse wave in the pathophysiology of the ventricular enlargement in hydrocephalus (1). He found that unilateral choroid plexectomy resulted in asymmetrical hydrocephalus in dogs treated with intracisternal kaolin; the ventricle without a choroid plexus failed to enlarge. WILSON and BERTAN similarly produced communicating hydrocephalus with intracisternal lampblack (11). Of 13 hydrocephalic dogs, 10 had a smaller lateral ventricle on the side that the anterior choroidal artery had been surgically divided. The pulse amplitude was reduced on the side of the interrupted artery. CSF pulse pressure differences between the two lateral ventricles were accentuated by changing the CSF pressure (11). This observation suggests that in a single animal there were differing elasticity relationships for the two cerebral hemispheres.

Hydrocephalus has been induced in lambs by mechanically increasing the intraventricular pulse pressure with a pulsating ventricular balloon synchronized to the cardiac cycle (5). Asymmetrical ventricular enlargement occurred, the larger ventricle on the side of the pulsating balloon. The brains of these animals showed pathologic features characteristic of obstructive hydrocephalus (2).

It is therefore apparent that the elasticity pressure-volume function may indeed be of etiologic importance in diseases of the CSF compartment. For instance, in the present series, patients with pseudotumor cerebri had lower elasticity slopes than did the patients with active hydrocephalus. These pseudotumor patients had CSF absorptive defects (8), yet they had small ventricles on CT scan. Perhaps the elasticity relationship accounts for why the ventricles fail to enlarge in pseutotumor cerebri. In hydrocephalus, it remains to be clarified whether these elasticity changes are the result or the cause of the ventricular enlargement.

Summary

The elasticity slope relating elastance to ICP is directly proportional to ventricular size. This relationship results in an increased ICP pulse amplitude in hydrocephalic patients. The pressure-volume function of brain elasticity may be of etiologic importance in diseases of the CSF system.

References

1. Bering EA Jr (1962) Circulation of the cerebrospinal fluid. Demonstration of the choroid plexuses as the generation of the force for flow of fluid and ventricular enlargement. J Neurosurg 19:405-413

2. Di Rocco C, Di Trapani G, Pettorossi VE, Caldarelli M (1979) On the pathology of experimental hydrocephalus induced by artificial increase in endoventricular CSF pulse pressure. Child's Brain 5:81-95

3. Maira G, Rossi GF, Vignati A (1975) Intracranial pressure and pathogenesis of "normotensive" hydrocephalus. In: Lundberg N, Ponten U, Brock M (eds) Intracranial Pressure II. Springer, Berlin Heidelberg New York,p 128

4. Miller JD, Leech PJ, Pickard JD (1975) Volume-pressure response in various experimental and clinical conditions. In: Lundberg N, Ponten U, Brock M (eds) Intracranial Pressure II. Springer, Berlin Heidelberg New York, p 97

5 Pettorossi VE, DiRocco C, Mancinelli R, Caldarelli M, Velardi F (1978) Communicating hydrocephalus induced by mechanically increased amplitude of the intraventricular cerebrospinal fluid pulse pressure: Rationale and method. Exp Neurol 59:30-39

6. Sato K, Fuchinove T, Yahagi Y (1975) CSF pulse wave changes in cases with normal pressure hydrocephalus. In: Lundberg N, Ponten U, Brock M (eds) Intracranial Pressure II. Springer, Berlin, Heidelberg New York, p 133

7. Shulman K, Marmarou A (1971) Pressure-volume considerations in infantile hydrocephalus. Dev Med Child Neurol 13(Suppl 25): 90-95

8 Sklar FH, Beyer CW Jr, Ramanathan M, Cooper PR, Clark WK (to be published) Cerebrospinal fluid dynamics in patients with pseudotumor cerebri. Neurosurg

9. Sklar FH, Beyer CW Jr, Ramanathan M, Elashvili I, Cooper PR, Clark WK (1978) Servo-controlled lumbar infusions: A clinical tool for the determination of CSF dynamics as a function of pressure. Neurosurg 3:170-175

10. Sklar FH, Elashvili I (1977) The pressure-volume function of brain elasticity. Physiological considerations and clinical applications. J Neurosurg 47:670-679

11. Wilson CB, Bertan V (1967) Interruption of the anterior choroidal artery in experimental hydrocephalus. Arch Neurol 17:614-619

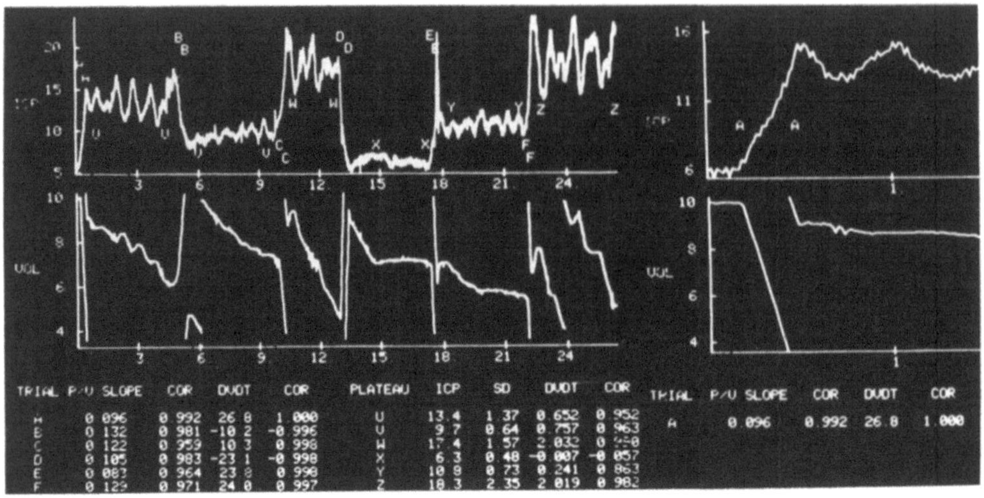

A **B**

Figure 1A. Original computer display of 26 minutes of a servo-controlled lumbar infusion protocol in a 12 month old black female with enlarged ventricles and developmental delay after meningitis. Upper, ICP (mmHg) vs. time (min); lower, volume (cc) vs. time (min). Elasticity determinations indicated by Trials A to F; P/V SLOPE represents the elasticity slope. Constant pressure plateaus to determine CSF dynamics as a function of ICP are indicated by letters U to Z.
COR, coefficient of correlation; DVDT, pump rate calculated from linear regression; SD, standard deviation.
From the constant pressure plateau data, the calculations indicate a normal net CSF absorptive capacity at 0.18 cc/min/mmHg ($p < 0.01$) with a resting pressure of 7.3 mmHg.

Figure 1B. Original computer display of data for single elasticity determination (from 1A). With linear regression techniques, the computer calculates the elasticity slope (P/V SLOPE) relating the natural logarithm of pressure to volume infused.

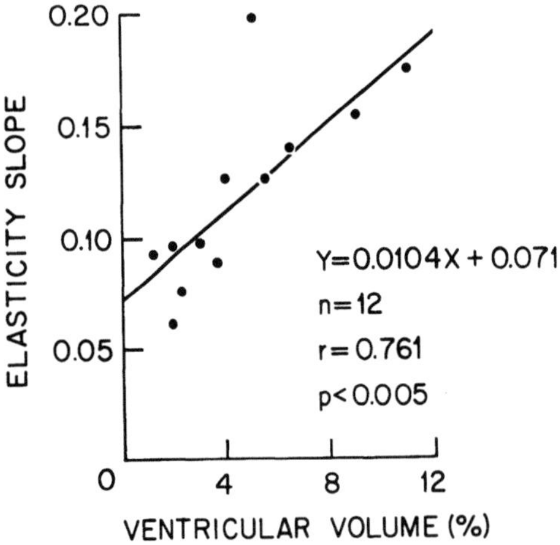

Figure 2. Elasticity slope vs ventricular volume expressed as a percentage of total intracranial volume.

A METHOD FOR PREDICTING PVI IN NORMAL PATIENTS

K. SHAPIRO, A. MARMAROU, AND K. SHULMAN

Introduction

The description of the Pressure-Volume Index (PVI) by MARMAROU (3) provides a simple bolus technique for measuring neural axis pressure-volume relationships and characterizing CSF hydrodynamics. The present study was undertaken to define normal values in humans using these techniques.

Methods

Twenty-three children, ages 3 months to 14 years, and 7 adults, ages 19 through 55 years, without intracranial mass pathology were studied using the PVI technique. Adults were studied awake using 18-gauge spinal needles placed in the lumbar subarachnoid space (5), or with indwelling ventricular cannulae (2). All children were anesthetized (Halothane 0.75%) for air myelograms; the cisterna magna was cannulated with a 20-gauge spinal needle. All cannulae were connected to low-volume displacement electrical transducers whose output was monitored on strip chart recorders. All pressures were referenced to the right atrium. Bolus manipulation of CSF was performed as previously reported (4). Equations used for calculating PVI, as well as CSF formation rate (I_f) and the outflow resistance (R_O) were previously reported (3).

Results

One-hundred sixty-three bolus manipulations were performed in 30 subjects of this report. Mean CSF pressure for the entire group was 13.2 mmHg. Although the mean PVI for the 7 adults was 25.6 ± 3.7 ml, the PVI in children ranged from 8.2 to 30.6 ml.

We attempted to explain the variation in the pediatric PVI determinations by relating PVI to neural axis volume. Since the previous work from this laboratory showed that in the cat, 68% of total PVI is contributed by the intracranial compartment and the remaining 32% by the spinal compartment (2), we used the ratio of each child's intracranial and spinal volumes to those of the normal adult, to estimate the relative contribution of each compartment to total PVI. These volumes were estimated from external measurements (5). This data is incorporated in the nomogram (Figure 1) which enables one to predict the relative contribution of each compartment using external measurements. With this nomogram, we attempted to predict PVI for the pediatric patients of this study. The actual PVI for the entire series was measured with a correlation coefficient between predicted PVI and measured PVI of r = .93.

Using bolus withdrawal to measure CSF formation rates in all patients, the mean I_f for the entire series was 0.36 ± 8 ml/min, with a range of 0.29 - 0.58 ml/min.

Using bolus injections to calculate resistance to the absorption of CSF (R_o), the mean R_o determined for the children was 2.9 ± 0.8 mmHg/ml/min; the mean R_o for the adults was 2.4 ± 0.7 mmHg/ml/min. Bolus injection was carried out to raise CSFP from 5 mmHg to 25 mmHg above baseline; there were no statistically significant differences between R_o determined at higher CSFP as compared to those determined at relatively low CSFP.

Discussion

The PVI for one normal patient may differ markedly from the next. Two variables were identified which accounted for this difference,namely, intracranial and spinal volumes. From the study it appears that the major determinant of neural axis compliance is the intracranial volume. Bolus manipulation was used to alter CSFP within a range of 5 - 40 mmHg. PVI determinations performed at low CSFP were similar to those at higher CSFP in each subject. We conclude that within this CSFP envelope, P-V relationships are constant.

If one used compliance (C = .4343 PVI/CSFP) as an index of the relative elasticity of the neural axis, the infants studied had lower compliance at similar CSFP than the older children and adults. Whether these differences are purely a function of smaller neural axis volumes or related to different biomechanical properties of the immature brains is not clear.

The rate of CSF formation determined by the PVI method of bolus manipulation is comparable to that determined by other techniques. The mean I_f for this entire series was 0.36 ± 0.8 ml/min, similar to that obtained by perfusion techniques.

Although R_o determinations were consistent throughout this study, our results differed from previous studies utilizing infusion techniques. By extrapolating data from others (1), the normal R_o obtained by infusion is 4.5 - 12 mmHg/ml/min as compared to our mean R_o of 2.8 ± .8 mmHg/ml/min, using bolus injection. Since our normal R_o values were of the same order of magnitude as those extrapolated from infusion techniques, we believe that the bolus technique provides a valid estimate of R_o. However, normative values of R_o may depend on the technique employed to measure this hydrodynamic parameter.

This study provides normative data for evaluating PVI determinations performed in clinical settings. In addition to providing normal values of I_f and R_o determined by the PVI technique, it also shows that P-V relationships depend upon the neural axis volume of the individual studied.

References

1. Ekstedt J (1978) CSF hydrodynamic studies in man. Normal hydrodynamic variables related to CSF pressure and flow. J Neurol Neurosurg & Psychiat 41:345-353

2. Marmarou A, Shulman K, LaMorgest J (1976) Compartmental analysis of compliance and outflow resistance of the cerebrospinal fluid system. J Neurosurg 43:523-534

3. Marmarou A, Shulman K, Rosende R (1978) A nonlinear analysis of the cerebrospinal fluid system and intracranial pressure dynamics. J Neurosurg 48:332-344

4. Shapiro K, Marmarou A, Shulman K (1976) Clinical applications of the Pressure Volume Index. Presented at the 44th Annual Meeting of the American Association of Neurological Surgeons, San Francisco (Paper No. 75)

5. Shapiro K, Marmarou A, Shulman K (to be published) Characterization of clinical CSF dynamics and neural axis compliance using the Pressure Volume Index: I. The normal Pressure Volume Index. Ann Neurol

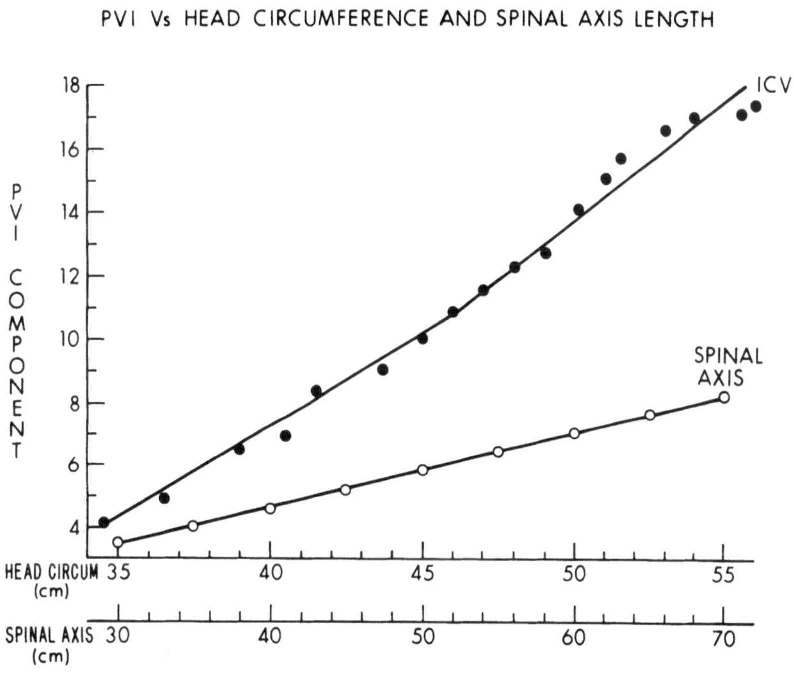

Figure 1. Nomogram used to derive predicted PVI based on contributions of cranial and spinal compartments. Head circumference and spinal length (foramen magnum to S_2) are measured. Plotting the measurement on the appropriate abscissa, a vertical line is drawn to the corresponding portion of the graph and the PVI contribution of that compartment taken from the ordinate. The predicted PVI is obtained by adding the cranial and spinal contributions.

DRASTIC DEHYDRATION AS A TREATMENT OF INTRACRANIAL HYPERTENSION IN SEVERE HEAD INJURIES

A.L.BENABID, A.BAUD, J.DE ROUGEMONT, F.FACCIOLI, M.BARGE, AND J.P.CHIROSSEL

Introduction

As long ago as 1955, the analysis of metabolic changes in head injuries (hyponatremia by water retention) and of their causes (hypersecretion of A.D.H. and rise of cortisol) led the French school (5) to put forward the idea of water restriction. Today some neurosurgeons (4) advise a daily amount of 1000 ml of water. In order to fight against a secondary brain edema we have sought a negative water balance by reducing the water intake to 250-500 ml per day.

Materials and methods

Forty-five severe head injuries were selected for this study; 23 of them were operated on for expansive hematomas (12 subdurals, 5 epidurals, 1 subepidural, 5 intracerebrals). 22 were diffuse brain damage (13 of them with posturing reaction). The water intake was limited to 250-500 ml glucose without Na and with a small amount of K per day intravenously for 3 to 5 days. All the patients were subjected to artificial ventilation (PCO_2 = 30-35 mmHg) and ACTH therapy. The water balance was checked each day by comparing assessable values only (perfusion intake and urinary, gastric, CSF output). Blood gases, electrolytes, urea, creatinine were checked twice a day; electrolytes and urea were measured in the urinary output.

In 24 patients continuous monitoring of intracranial pressure (ICP) and arterial blood pressure (ABP) was carried out for calculating ICP/ABP which we call the brain vasomotor index (BVMI) (3).

As soon as the patient came under our control, water intake was strictly limited to 250 ml/day.

Subsequent adjustments were made according to the urinary output, level of urea and creatinine, BVMI, clinical status; usually step by step rehydration begins on the third or fourth day.

Results

1 Biological results - See Figure 1

a) The water balance remained negative and the loss of water amounted to an average of 2 liters; this result represents a minimal estimation because we did not take into account unassessable water loss.

b) There was always a rise of urea and to lesser degree of creatinine and Na, while the urinary output remained almost stable. These changes disappeared when rehydration began. We observed three renal failures in patients who had had renal troubles previously.

c) On average the ratio of ICP/ABP remained almost normal (< 0.2); nevertheless a few rose into the area between 0.2 and 0.5 which can be dangerous. Figure 2 shows that there was a connection between positive or negative water intake and the change of the ratio ICP/ABP monitored 2 days after water intake. A statistical relationship exists between changes in the ICP/ABP ratio and water movement, the slope of which is dependent upon the intensity of brain damage. The slope is near zero for a normal brain and, in brain injury, the greater the damage, the greater the slope.

Clinical results can be summarized as follows:
--16 deaths out of 45 patients (cerebral causes 5, extracerebral causes 11, gastric hemorrhages 5, cardiac failure 2, pulmonary infection 2, renal failure 1, septicemia 1).

--Complications: pulmonary infection 13, venous thrombosis 2, renal failure 3

--The late outcome of the 29 surviving patients according to the JENNETT and BOND (2) scale is: grade 1-2 (professional life) 16; grade 3 (family life) 7; grade 4 (severe psychiatric disability) 4; grade 5 (prolonged coma) 2.

Conclusions

The tolerance of this drastic dehydration looks good. Renal functions have to be checked carefully; they can be used as a guide for adjustment of the water intake. There is a connection between ICP and water intake. Dehydration prevents the ICP from rising to a dangerous level in the majority of cases. Clinical results in severe head injuries compare favorably with other results (5) as regards mortality (35%) as well as late outcome.

Summary

A drastic dehydration in the order of 250 ml/day without Na has been applied to 45 severe head injuries. This dehydration is well tolerated but renal functions must be checked closely. This treatment allows us to control ICP in the majority of cases and seems to improve the prognosis.

References

1 Becker DP, Miller JD, Ward JD, Greenberg RP, Youn HF, Sakalas R (1977) The outcome from severe head injury with early diagnosis and intensive management. J Neurosurg 47:491-502

2. Jennett B, Bond M (1975)Assessment of outcome after severe brain damage. A practical scale. Lancet 1:480-484

3. Rougemont J de, Benabid AL, Chirossel JP, Barge M (1976) The brain vasomotor tone index as a prognosis leader in severe head injuries. In: Beks JWF, Bosch DA, Brock M (eds) Intracranial Pressure III. Springer, Berlin Heidelberg New York, p 119

4. Shenkin HA, Bezier HS, Bouzarth WF (1976) Restricted fluid intake: rational management of the neurosurgical patient. J Neurosurg 45:432-436

5. Wertheimer P, Descotes J (1955) Les perturbations humorales dans les traumatismes craniens recents. Memoires de l'Academia de Chirurgie 81:6190627

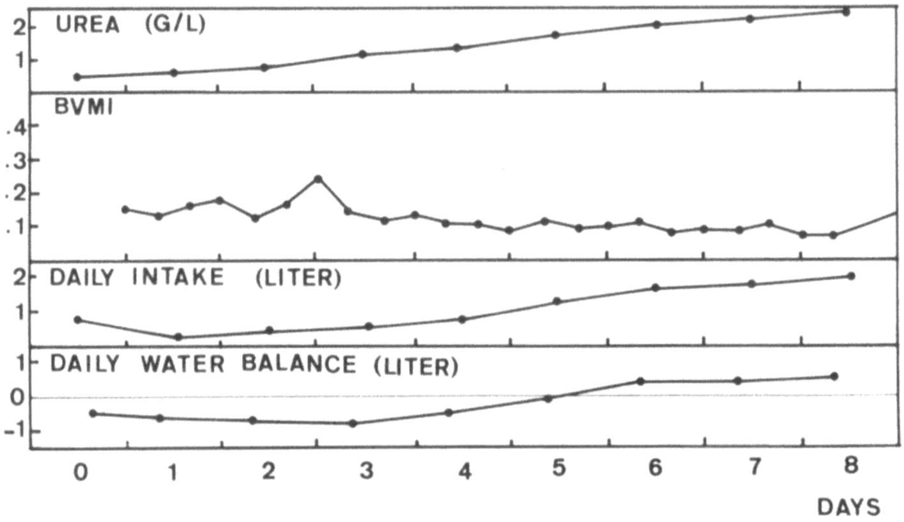

Figure 1. Changes in the water balance, urea and ratio ICP/ABP (BVMI) during restriction of the water intake (average values).

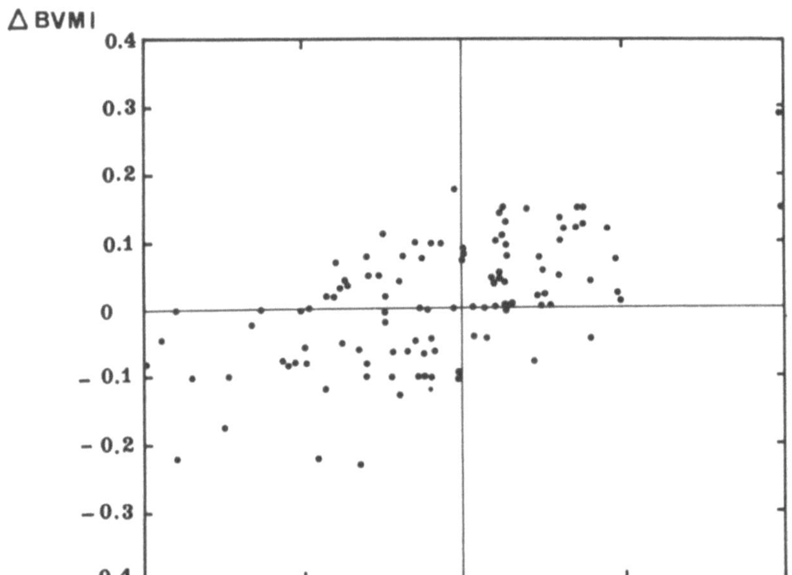

Figure 2. Changes in the ratio ICP/ABP (BVMI) checked 48 hours after modification of the water balance.

THE CSF PRESSURE-VOLUME RELATIONSHIP BEFORE AND AFTER CARDIAC ARREST

H.G.SULLIVAN, J.D.MILLER, AND R.L.GRIFFITH

Introduction

This study evaluates the significance of intra-arterial and capillary hydrostatic pressures in determining the shape of the CSF P/ΔV curve. We report CSF P/ΔV curves determined before and after cardiac arrest in the cat.

Material and Methods

Fifteen cats were anesthetized with i.v. methohexital sodium, paralyzed with a continuous i.v. infusion of succinylcholine chloride, and maintained on controlled ventilation. A 21 G needle was placed stereotaxically into both the right and left frontal horns of the lateral ventricles. One needle was used for recording CSF pressure and the other was connected to a normal saline reservoir of variable height.

In each animal two sets of three, 0.3 ml, bolus intraventricular injections were made and for each injection a value of the parameter b was calculated from the equation

$$b = \frac{\ln\{P_p/P_o\}}{\Delta V}.$$

This is the standard exponential known to define, for normal physiological conditions, the relationship between ΔV and P_{csf} (1,2). b is thought to be constant for a given animal under stable physiological conditions. P_{eq} was obtained before and after each set of three intraventricular injections. For each animal the mean values of b and P_{eq} were used to plot the CSF P/ΔV curve over a ΔV range of from zero to 0.4 ml (10% of total CSF volume) and over a pressure range of up to 50 mmHg.

After determining the CSF P/ΔV curve for normal physiological conditions each animal received 200 units of heparin i.v. and ten minutes later cardiac arrest was induced by i.v. KCl solution. After cardiac arrest, P_{csf} fell to zero, and infusion of normal saline from the reservoir was used to return P_{csf} to the pre-cardiac arrest level of P_{eq}. Beginning at this level of P_{csf} sixteen bolus intraventricular injections, consisting of four sets of 0.1, 0.2, 0.3 and 0.4 ml, were made. Each injection was initiated from a P_{csf} approximating the pre-cardiac arrest P_{eq}. To define the CSF P/ΔV curve after cardiac arrest, peak pressure after injection was plotted as a function of ΔV. This curve was compared with the relationship derived from the pre-cardiac arrest data.

Results

For 8 animals the CSF P/ΔV relationship after cardiac arrest was not different from the pre-cardiac arrest relationship. The remaining 7 animals demonstrated a statistically significant difference (linear model analysis and t test) between the pre- and post-cardiac arrest CSF P/ΔV curves. However, the physiological importance of this difference is open to question since in all of these animals P_{csf} remained an exponential function of ΔV and with one exception the parameter b was within the normal range of 2.0 ml^{-1} to 5.7 ml^{-1} for 48 normal animals previously studied in our laboratory. The one animal with statistically different pre- and post-arrest curves, where b was outside the normal range, had a b value of 6.0 ml^{-1} as compared to the 5.7 ml^{-1} upper limit of normal.

Discussion

The shape of the CSF P/ΔV curve is a reflection of how readily tissues around the CSF space tolerate distortion by changes in CSF volume. Since brain is one of the major tissues surrounding the CSF space, it is logical to ask whether hydraulic pressures in cerebral arterioles and capillaries make any contribution to the ability of the brain to resist deformation by CSF volume change. In the experiments reported here, the arteriole and capillary hydraulic pressures were reduced to zero by cardiac arrest. Animals were heparinized so that venous blood could still be squeezed out of the brain by CSF volume change. Pre- and post-arrest curves were compared with respect to the same baseline P_{csf}. We conclude that if the exit pathway for venous blood remains open, parameters such as arterial and capillary hydrostatic pressures do not make a significant contribution to the shape of the CSF P/ΔV curve. The shape of the CSF P/ΔV curve would seem to be more a mechanical than a biological property of the craniospinal system. It seems unlikely that total CSF volume at P_{eq} before cardiac arrest would correspond to total CSF volume at P_{eq} after cardiac arrest. If the pre- and post-cardiac arrest pressures were plotted against the total CSF volume instead of ΔV, one would very likely have two curves of similar shape, but separated from one another on the V_{csf} axis. The primary effect of biological changes in the craniospinal system may be to shift the CSF P/V curve along the V_{csf} axis while the shape of this curve is dictated by mechanical properties of brain tissue, dura, and venous exit channels.

References

1. Marmarou A, Shulman K, Rosende R (1978) A non-linear analysis of the cerebrospinal fluid system and intracranial pressure dynamics. J Neurosurg 48:332-344

2. Sullivan HG, Miller JD, Griffith RL, Carter W, and Rucker S (1979) Bolus vs steady-state infusion for determination of CSF outflow resistance. Ann Neurol 5:228-238

This work was supported by NIH grants #1 R01 NS 14309-01 and #7 R01 NS 15995-01

CSF PRESSURE-VOLUME RELATION AND PULSE RELATED CSF PRESSURE VARIATIONS IN MAN

H. FRIDÉN AND J. EKSTEDT

Introduction

The intracranial volume/pressure (V/P) relationship (1,2,4,5,6) has been studied by many investigators. Most experiments have been made on animals and very little is known about the quantitative aspects in man. The present paper deals mainly with the reference values for the different V/P variables and the deviations from normal found in some pathological states.

Methods

With the patient in the supine position and by means of continuous lumbar CSF drainage at constant pressure, the ICP of the patient was decreased to 0.5-0.1 kPa below the pressure at which the pulse related ICP-variations had their minimum. The CSF formation rate was determined at this pressure level. Then, with a constant flow rate of 50 mm^3/s, artificial CSF was infused until the pressure reached 5-6 kPa. When the highest level was reached the pressure was regulated and reduced in steps of 1.0 kPa. The resulting steady state flow was measured at each level. From these values the conductance of the CSF outflow pathways was calculated. The elastance/pressure (E/P) relationship was calculated from the constant flow rate infusion part of the recording. The pressure recording of this part was divided into small increments and the volume infused during the time of the increment measured. The CSF formed and the total volume of fluid eliminated during the same time was compensated for. The pulse-related pressure variations at different pressure levels were measured from the recording. The equipment used has been described in detail (3).

Results

Figure 1 - The E/P curve passed a minimum and then increased with rising pressure in a way somewhat between linear and exponential. It was characterized by its value at CSF resting pressure, E_r, its minimum value, E_{min}, the pressure at this point $p_c(E_{min})$, and a linear regression line of its ascending part.

The V/P relationship was best described as having a straightened-out sigmoid form with its maximum inclination at the pressure of minimum elastance, then levelling-off to an almost asymptotic value as the pressure increased. Two volume values were chosen to characterize the curve; the volume difference between that of minimum elastance and the levelling-off level, here called the "buffer volume", V_{buff}. The pulse-related pressure-variations/pressure ($\Delta P/P$) curve was characterized in the same way as the E/P curve: by its value at CSF resting pressure, Δp_{cpr}, its minimum value Δp_{cpmin}, the pressure at this point $p_c(\Delta p_{cpmin})$, and a linear regression line of its ascending part. The fit of this line was usually very good. From the total group of

Table I. Averaged "reference values" of the CSF pressure/volume variables in man, obtained from 18 patients selected as "normals" from a material of 105 patients

ELASTANCE		n	Mean value	S.D.	Dimension
Value at resting pressure	(E_r)	15	59.2×10^{-6}	24.4×10^{-6}	[kPa· mm^{-3}]
Minimum value	(Emin)	15	16.8×10^{-6}	6.1×10^{-6}	[kPa· mm^{-3}]
CSFP at minimum value	[Pc(Emin)]	15	0.96	0.24	[kPa]
Slope of linear fit	(AE)	16	212.2×10^{-6}	89.0×10^{-6}	[mm^{-3}]
Pressure axis intercept of linear fit	(BE)	16	1.24	0.31	[kPa]
PULSE RELATED VARIATIONS					
Value at resting pressure	(Δ pcpr)	18	0.22	0.11	[kPa]
Minimum value	(Δ pcpmin)	8	0.06	0.03	[kPa]
CSFP at minimum value	[pc(Δ pcpmin)]	9	0.95	0.16	[kPa]
Slope of linear fit	(AD)	16	0.47	0.06	-
Pressure axis intercept of linear fit	(BD)	16	1.18	0.42	[kPa]
VOLUME					
"Level off volume"	(V lo)	13	34.5	8.5	$\times 10^3$[mm^3]
"Buffer volume"	(V buff)	15	15.3	4.5	$\times 10^3$[mm^3]

patients it was possible from clinical history and investigations to select 18 patients as probably "normal". The averaged values for these patients are shown in Table I.

In the typical hydrocephalus syndrome cases the recorded relationships were essentially unaffected compared with those of the normal material. The CSFP resting point had deviated to the right along the pressure axis, towards a higher elastance, higher pulse related CSFP variations and lesser buffer volume.

A different picture was seen in the patients with sinus thrombosis. Here the whole set of curves and the resting point were off-set to the right. The resting point remained essentially unchanged relative to the curves, thus maintaining normal elastance, pulse related CSFP variations and buffer volume.

In patients with a sinus thrombosis also affecting the CSF outflow pathways a mixed picture of both above-described findings were found.

Discussion

The pressure of minimum elastance corresponds to a pressure at which volume variations have their least effects on the CSFP, which probably means that there are blood vessels that at this pressure are maximally compressible. This should be the case when the pressure inside the vessel equals that of outside, i.e., the intracerebral venous pressure.

A theory (2,4,5,6,7) supported by many authors is that the elastance is directly proportional to the CSFP. From our material it seems very unlikely that there is such a relationship behind the E/P curve. Furthermore, using that concept for calculating the results of a bolus injection test can give underestimation of the elastance as well as overestimation of the conductance of the CSF outflow pathways; an overestimation which increases with decreasing conductance. Yet a straight line was fitted, but then only to the ascending part of the

E/P curve. This was done mainly in order to make comparisons from patient to patient.

The pulse-related CSFP variations at each CSFP level are thought to be the product of a constant net blood volume change per cardiac cycle and the elastance at that pressure level. This was, in general, the case but there were also significant exceptions.

Summary

The pressure effects caused by CSF volume changes were studied in 105 patients. The effects were quantified and reference values from 18 patients, considered as normal, are presented as well as some pathological deviations.

1. Avezaat CJJ. Van Eijndhoven JHM, De Jong DA, Moolenaar WCJ (1976) A new method of monitoring intracranial volume/pressure relationship. In: Beks JWF, Bosch DA, Brock M (eds) Intracranial Pressure III. Springer, Berlin Heidelberg New York, p308

2. Cohadon P, Castel JP, Nouillant A, Vandendriessche M (1975) Volume pressure relationship in clinical and experimental conditions of raised ICP. In: Lundberg N, Ponten U, Brock M (eds) Intracranial Pressure II. Springer, Berlin Heidelberg N Y, p 107

3. Ekstedt J (1977) CSF hydrodynamic studies in man. I. Method of constant pressure CSF infusion. J Neurol Neurosurg, Psych 40:105-119

4. Lofgren J, Von Essen C, Zwetnow NN (1973) The pressure-volume curve of the cerebrospinal fluid space in dogs. Acta Neurol Scand 49:557-574

5. Marmarou A, Shulman K, Rosende RM (1978) A non-linear analysis of the cerebrospinal fluid system and intracranial pressure dynamics. J Neurosurg 48:332-344

6. Sklar FH, Elashvili I (1977) The pressure-volume function of brain elasticity. J Neurosurg 47:670-679

7. Sullivan HG, Miller JD, Griffith RL, Carter W Jr, Rucker S (1978) Bolus versus steady-state infusion for determination of CSF outflow resistance. Ann Neurol 5:228-238

Supported by grant No. B79-04X-04125-06 from the Swedish Medical Research Council.

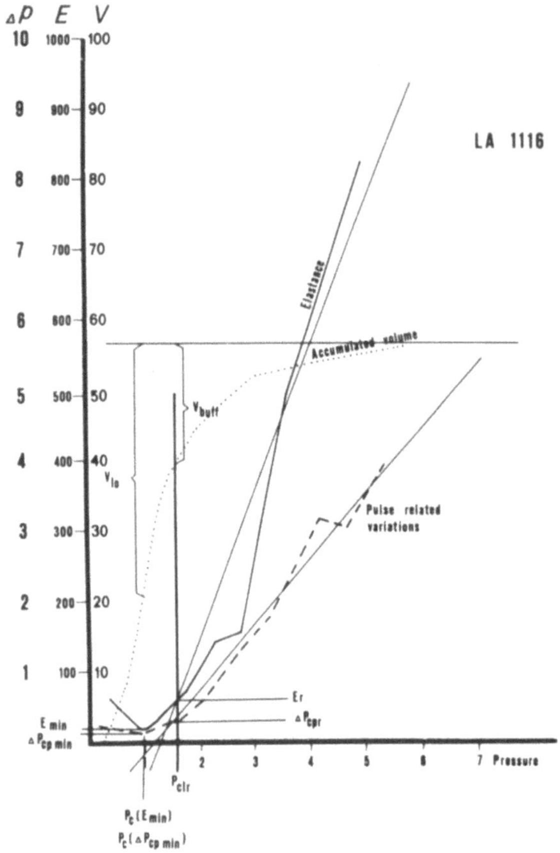

Figure I. Elastance, accumulated volume and pulse related CSF pressure variations in the normal man as functions of the CSF pressure. Points used to characterize the relationship are marked out as well as linear regression lines.

EFFECTS OF CEREBRAL EDEMA UPON VISCOELASTIC PROPERTIES OF BRAIN TISSUE

A. MARMAROU, H. TAKAGI, C.W. HARGENS, AND K. SHULMAN

Introduction

The intracranial pressure/volume curve from which parameters such as the PVI and VPR are derived is obtained from manipulations of CSF volume and describes the bulk compliance of the craniospinal axis. Although these parameters reflect the combined visoelastic properties of the brain, other techniques are more suitable for measurement of individual viscous and elastic components. The objective of this study was to examine the viscoelastic properties of cat brain by measuring the deformation in response to a known force applied to the surface of the tissue.

Methods

The instrument used for the viscoelastic measurements consisted of an electrodynamometer with a gas suspended armature which oscillated in response to a changing magnetic field (Figure 1). The magnetic field variation induced by a surrounding coil on the device was controlled in frequency and amplitude by a conventional function generator which operated in a sinusoidal mode. The force was directly proportional to the electrical current applied to the coil. The displacement of a probe connected to the armature was monitored by a linear variable differential transformer (LVDT). The outputs of the coil (force) and displacement (LVDT) were recorded on a storage oscilloscope with force displayed on the vertical axis and deformation on the horizontal axis. Application of force in a sinusoidal mode produced a pattern in the form of a hysterisis loop from which viscoelastic parameters were derived. The slope of the major axis of the loop (y/x) is a measure of the dynamic spring rate (DSR) in gm/mm. The dynamic spring rate is the summation vector of two parameters: the elastic spring rate (ERS) which represents the purely elastic or "Hookean" component and the loss rate (LR) which is a measure of the viscous component and reflects the amount of energy converted to heat and lost within the tissue per cycle. The phase lag between applied force and resulting deformation is a measure of the loss angle (θ) which defines the phase angle between the dynamic spring rate (DSR) and elastic spring rate (ESR). The loss angle (θ) can be obtained from the ratio of loop opening to displacement of the sample (1). From measure of DSR and θ, the LR and ESR components can be calculated (Sin θ=LR/DSR, Cos θ=ESF/DSR(Fig.2).

The white matter of the left frontal lobe of adult cats (n = 5) maintained under nitrous oxide anesthesia was made edematous by an infusion technique described in another report in this volume. For in-vivo tests, a 1 cm O.D. burr hole was trephined in the left frontal pole and the electrodynamometer probe positioned directly over the site of the infusion. The dura was left intact. A similar site was prepared in the opposite control hemisphere. The probe tip manipulated by a stereotaxic apparatus was carefully lowered on the brain surface and the amount of pre-load (gms) or pre-strain (mm) was noted. Pre-load, amplitude, and frequency of force application were independently controlled and could be easily changed during the test. In addition to in-vivo measurements viscoelastic tests of dead brain were conducted on animals with infusion edema of the left hemisphere and sacrificed at 6 hours and 7 days. Brains were removed rapidly and kept chilled until time of test. The right hemisphere served as control for each brain tested.

Results

Viscoelastic response tests conducted on the surface of dead brain with dura intact yielded an exponential force-deformation curve. The amount of force necessary to compress the brain increased with deformation indicating a stiffening of the tissue. The exponential form of the curve was more clearly evident when deformations exceeded 2.0 mm. For deformations less than 2.0 mm the compressive phase of the force cycle was more linear. When force was reduced the tissue did not recover as rapidly producing a phase lag (θ) between force and deformation. This delay between force and deformation was observed in all tests indicating the presence of a viscous component within the tissue. The amount of delay increased as the forcing frequency was increased from 0.5 to 4.0 Hz. The dynamic spring rate (DSR) at 0.5 Hz equalled 5.7 gm/mm and increased to 9.0 gm/mm when forcing frequency was increased to 4 Hz indicating a stiffening of the tissue with increasing rate of force application. The values of DSR obtained from the major axis of the loop at higher frequencies represent the average of approximately 8 cycles, and differences between cycles were not evident at the higher rates of force application. The purely elastic component (ESR) under these conditions averaged 70 to 80% of the dynamic spring rate. When dura was removed from the surface of the dead brain the DSR decreased by 8% at 0.5 Hz (Table I). The decrease of DSR with dura removed was greater with increasing frequency (13.0%). Changes in ESR and LR paralleled the decrease in DSR when dura was removed.

The DSR in areas of edema decreased by 4% in the acute experiment where the animal was sacrificed 6 hours after the start of infusion (Test 17A vs 18A). This softening of the tissue was accompanied by an increased LR and θ demonstrating an increase in the viscous component. The brain edema in the animal sacrificed 7 days after infusion had a more pronounced effect on the viscoelastic response. The DSR decreased by 33% compared to control levels in this series of tests (Test 9 VSR). Similar reductions of DSR were observed in verified edema areas of sectioned brain.

Surface viscoelastic response tests conduced in-vivo with dura intact showed a similar exponential force-deformation curve for compressions exceeding 1.0 mm. Below the level, the initial compressive force cycle was fairly linear with a pronounced hysterisis effect on the return phase. The DSR measured on the surface of a region previously infused with fluid showed a marked reduction (C13 vs C9 Table I).

Upon sacrifice, the DSR decreased compared to control followed by a gradual increase to twice normal level within 15 minutes. Values of ESR and LR paralleled the changes in dynamic spring rate.

Discussion

The application of the electrodynamometer test apparatus described provides an effective and versatile means of evaluating the viscoelas-

Table I. Viscoelastic response of brain tissue

Test	Condition	FREQ (Hz)	DSR	ESR rm/mm	LR	θ DEG
Acute Experiment (6 hours after infusion) - In Vitro						
Control Area						
17A	Dura Intact	0.5	5.70	5.59	1.09	11.1
19A	Dura Removed	0.5	5.25	5.14	1.10	12.1
17B	Dura Intact	4.0	9.00	8.54	2.83	18.3
19B	Dura Removed	4.0	7.89	7.59	2.18	16.0
Edematous Area						
18A	Dura Intact	0.5	5.49	5.30	1.43	15.1
20A	Dura Removed	0.5	5.04	4.87	1.28	14.8
18B	Dura Intact	4.0	7.89	7.59	2.18	16.0
20B	Dura Removed	4.0	7.00	6.74	1.86	15.4
Chronic Experiment (7 days after infusion) - In Vitro						
Control Area						
9	Dura Intact	0.5	7.14	6.85	2.02	16.4
-	Dura Removed	0.5	-	-	-	-
Edematous Area						
12	Dura Intact	0.5	4.76	4.63	1.12	13.6
12	Dura Removed	0.5	3.90	3.76	1.35	15.4
Chronic Experiment (7 days after infusion) - In Vivo						
C13	Dura Intact Normal	0.5	11.19	10.88	2.63	0.80
C9	Dura Intact Edema	0.5	7.23	6.95	1.99	0.64

tic properties of brain tissue. The technique has the advantage of rapid assessment of viscous and elastic tissue components which can be studied under control of amplitude and pattern of force application. Effects of pre-load and initial compression must be taken into consideration.

We preferred to select a test frequency range in the relatively low end of the scale and well within the spectrum of cardiovascular pulsations (<100 Hz).

KOENEMAN (3) has evaluated the tissue properties in the frequency range of 100-500 Hz and found the storage modulus to be relatively constant with frequency. The differences found in the very low range, where other data is not available, could be due to the variation of the dynamic properties with frequency which is usually found in most viscoelastic materials.

An increase in elastic modulus after death was reported by METZ et al who evaluated elasticity of brain tissue using a miniaturized inflation probe (4). These results are consistent with our studies; however we observed a transient decrease (softening) of tissue followed by a gradual increase in stiffness.

This initial softening of the tissue may be due to the loss of pressure at sacrifice. Further tests at multiple sites must be conducted to resolve this issue.

The exponential force-deformation curve supports the findings of SCHETTINI and WALSH (5) and problems arise in the analysis of the viscoelastic response using conventional linear techniques. For this reason, deformations must be maintained at low levels. The findings of decreased stiffness with increased viscous loss in edematous tissue is in agreement with increased compliance values measured by other techniques (6). The changes in viscoelasticity observed in dead brain emphasizes the need for apparatus capable of determining brain material properties in-vivo.

References

1. Christensen MS, Hargens CW, Nacht S, Gans EH (1977) Viscoelastic properties of intact human skin: instrumentation, hydration effects and the contribution of the statum corneum. J Invest Dermatol 69:282-286

2. Galford JE, McElhaney JH (1970) A viscoelastic study of scalp, brain and dura. J Biomech 3:211-221

3. Keoneman JB (1966) Viscoelastic properties of brain tissue. Masters Thesis, Case Institute of Technology

4. Metz H, McElhaney J, Ommaya AK (1970) A comparison of the elasticity of live, dead, and fixed brain tissue. J Biomech 3:453-458

5. Schettini A, Walsh EG (1974) Experimental identification of the subarachnoid and subpial compartments by intracranial pressure measurements. J Neurosurg 40:609-616

6. Walstra G. et al (this book) Tissue compliance.

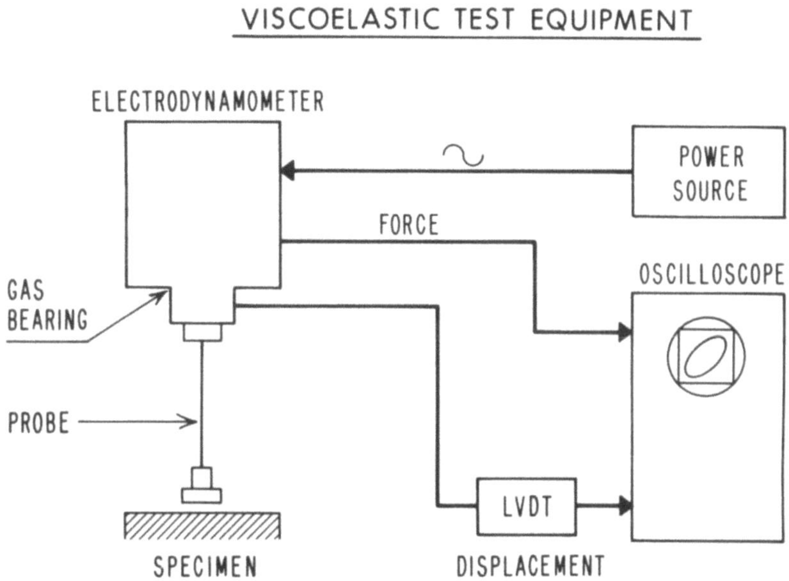

Figure 1. Schematic diagram of the test configuration. A power source (function generator) controlled the current to the electrodynamometer and was proportional to force (y-axis). Displacement was increased by an LVDT (x-axis). A gas bearing virtually eliminated friction of the armature normal to the brain surface.

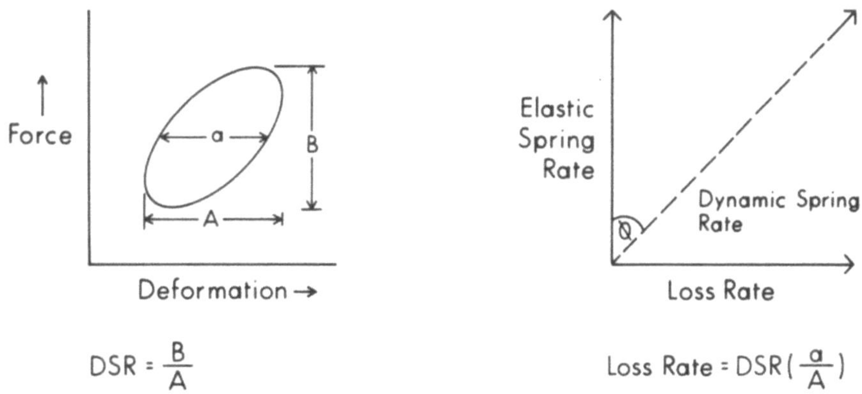

Figure 2. Analysis of the force-displacement loop. Dynamic spring rate is defined as the resultant vector of the ESR (elastic spring rate) and LR (loss rate).

PARAMETERS FOR IDENTIFYING BRAIN RESPONSE PROPERTIES IN VIVO

E.K.WALSH AND A.SCHETTINI

Introduction

Under normal conditions brain tissue exhibits viscoelastic response which can be characterized by viscoelastic parameters including the instantaneous (short-time) and equilibrium (long-time) elastic response, relaxation behavior, and creep behavior. To measure the material coefficients associated with these types of response it is necessary to perform experiments which, for brain tissue, must be done in-vitro. Nevertheless, certain experiments can be performed on brain tissue in-vivo in which case (i) the measured parameters, e.g. pressure, displacement, can be used in the solution to the mechanics problem, which best simulates the experimental configuration, to calculate the actual material coefficients (cf. 1,3), or (ii) the measured parameters can be considered as pseudo response coefficients and used directly to monitor and identify controlled changes in the system (cf. 1,2). Here we consider the latter point of view and describe several pseudo response parameters which are directly measurable in-vivo and which are analogous to material response coefficients used to characterize nonlinear viscoelastic materials.

Materials and methods

Figure 1a shows a schematic diagram of the pressure-displacement transducer with the coplanar pressure sensor mounted at the base of the center shaft and the core of a displacement transducer (LVDT) mounted at the upper part of the shaft. Figure 1 b is an expanded schematic of the transducer base indenting the brain substance through the intact dura membrane. As the transducer shaft is depressed, the pressure sensor causes a compression of the subpial brain substance resulting in an increase in pressure, while the depth of insertion is measured simultaneously by the LVDT.

Results

Here we will concentrate on the results of two response tests which we identify as the elastic response test and the pressure test. The differences between the tests are in the rate of insertion and in the control of the insertion depth following maximum insertion.

Elastic response test: For the elastic response test the insertion rate is relatively rapid so that the 0.5-1.0 mm subpial insertion occurs in approximately one second. At maximum insertion the system is held fixed for 3-4 sec and then withdrawn. The solid trace shown in Fig. 2 is the pressure-insertion depth response for this test as measured directly on an X-Y graphic recorder. The change in slope identified as δ_S indicates the depth such that subsequent insertion results in subpial compaction. Thus the curve beyond δ_S represents the pressure-depth response of the in-vivo brain substance. The nonlinear character of the response is clear from the curvature of the trace. We can identify two response parameters. The first, designated simply as the pressure-depth ratio, G_o, is the slope of the tangent line to the response trace at δ_s and is exactly analgous to the "instantaneous" elastic tangent modulus in nonlinear viscoelasticity. The second, called the secant pressure-depth ratio, G_s, is determined as the slope of the line connecting the points (p_s, δ_s) and (p^*, δ^*) where p^* is a nominal pressure near the maximum pressure of the test. Clearly the difference between G_o and G_s is a measure of the nonlinearity of the response.

Pressure test: The transducer insertion rate for the pressure test is considerably less than for the elastic response test with subpial insertion requiring about twenty seconds. Insertion is carried out at a uniform rate to a depth corresponding to approximately 40 mmHg following which the system is immediately withdrawn at the same uniform rate. Figure 3 shows the results of a pressure test recorded directly on an X-Y graphic recorder. Essentially, the loading phase of the pressure test is the same as that of the elastic response test with the exception of the loading rate. The fact that the subpial insertion rate is greater than the characteristic relaxation time for in-vivo brain tissue means that the measured pressure can be considered to be an equilibrium response. Clearly, both an equilibrium tangent modulus and an equilibrium secant modulus can be constructed. Figure 3 shows only the equilibrium tangent modulus designated as G_e. The difference between G_o and G_e for a given animal is a measure of the anelastic behavior of the material.

Discussion

Some numerical values for G_o, G_s, and G_e and a discussion of the use of these parameters to monitor changes in the system is given in these Proceedings (2).

Summary

In-vivo parameters analogous to the instantaneous and equilibrium tangent and secant moduli of nonlinear viscoelastic materials can be directly measured with the pressure-displacement transducer and used to monitor changes in the intracranial system.

References

1. Metz H, McElhaney J, Ommaya AK (1970) A comparison of live, dead and fixed brain tissue. J Biomech 3:453-458

2. Schettini A, Walsh EK. Influence of large doses of steroids on brain compression, epidurally. These Proceedings.

3. Walsh EK, Schettini A (1976) Elastic behavior of brain tissue in-vivo. Am J Phycical 230:1058-1062

Work supported by V.A.Medical Research & Merck Research Institute.

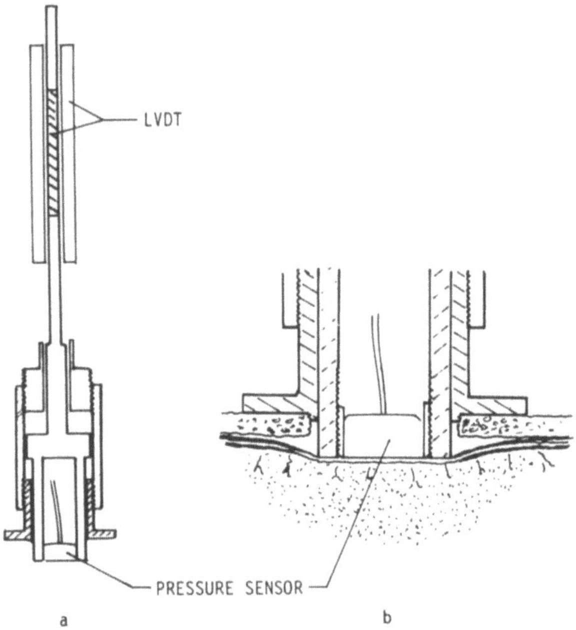

Figure 1. Pressure displacement transducer. 1a is an overall schematic showing the LVDT and the pressure sensor. 1b shows the base of the transducer with the sensor indenting the brain substance.

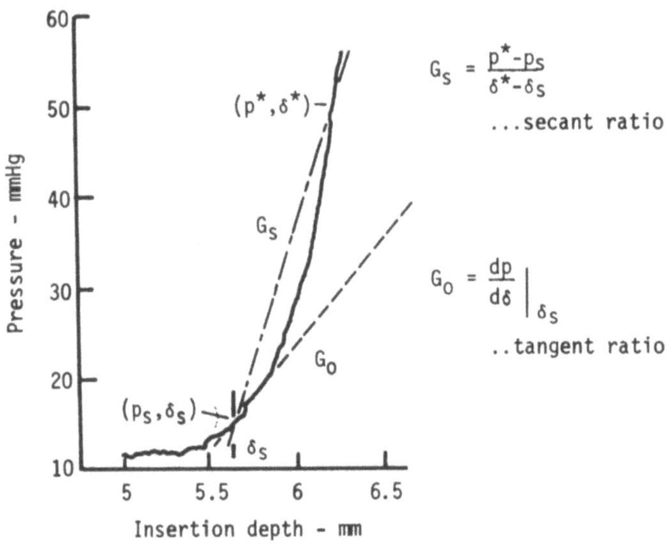

Figure 2. Elastic response test. The solid trace is the pressure-depth response. The broken line labelled G_o represents the tangent pressure-depth ratio; the line G_s represents the secant pressure-depth ratio. δ_s indicates the position of the subpial region.

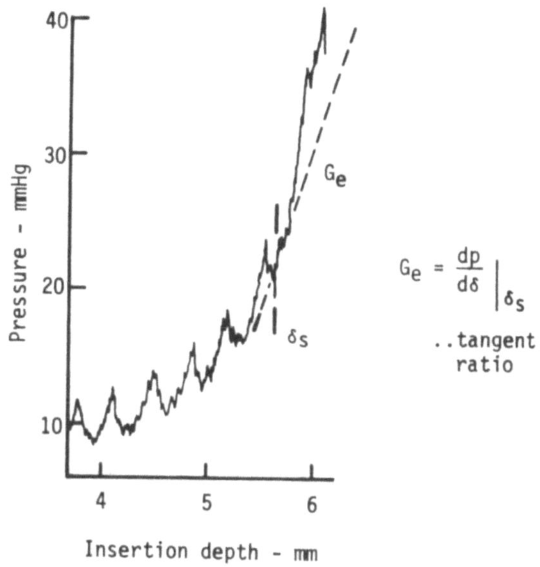

Figure 3. Pressure test. The solid trace is the pressure-depth response. The broken line labelled G_e represents the equilibrium tangent pressure-depth ratio. δ_s indicates the position of the subpial region.

DYNAMICS OF TRANSTENTORIAL HERNIATION

S. YONEDA, M. MATSUDA, H. HANDA, H. GOTOH, AND E. TSUDA

Introduction

Increased intracranial pressure with supratentorial mass lesion causes a pressure difference between the supratentorial and infratentorial compartments, which eventually causes transtentorial herniation(2). Since the brain tissue is a kind of viscoelastic substance, the distorted brain develops the shearing stress. The present experiment was undertaken in an attempt to measure the shearing stress which develops in the herniated brain at the edge of the tentorium.

Material and methods

Experiments were performed in 23 monkeys weighing 4.1 to 8.6 kg. The animals were anesthetized with intravenous injection of sodium pentobarbital[1], 20 to 25 mg/kg. After tracheostomy and cannulation for intravenous administration of fluid and drug, and for measurement of systemic blood pressure, the animals were placed prone on the stereotaxic apparatus, and right temporo-occipital craniotomy was performed. A small balloon was placed extradurally in the temporal region to raise the intracranial pressure (ICP). A miniature device[2] was attached to the tentorial edge in order to measure the force per unit area which was given to the herniated brain at the edge of the tentorium. This force was regarded as the shearing stress. The animals were x-rayed at intervals so that the descent of the tentorium was measured. Epidural pressure (EDP) was measured by means of an SFT transducer (5) attached directly to the dural surface through a burr hole in the left parietal and suboccipital regions. The dural defect was closed with teflon patch and the cranial defect with resin. The extradural balloon was continuously inflated by infusing the contrast material at the rate of 1.1 to 4.4 ml/hr. The shearing stress, respiration, systemic blood pressure, supratentorial EDP and infratentorial EDP were all recorded simultaneously. All the procedures were performed under spontaneous respiration. Arterial blood gases analyzed at intervals were within normal range except in the terminal stage.

At the end of experiment, the supratentorial portion of the brain was removed and calibration of the sensing device attached to the tentorial edge was done with the use of a load transducer[3]. The force given to the herniated brain was calculated by comparing the actually recorded curve with the calibrated one, and the sensing area of the device was measured with the use of a universal tool microscopic measuring[4]. Then, the force per unit area (gm/mm^2) was figured out and converted

---

[1] Nembutal®
[2] KFC-C11 strain gauge, Kyowa Electric Co., Ltd., Tokyo
[3] 20T-10B, Kyowa Electric Co., Ltd., Tokyo
[4] Type TUM 200, Tokyo Kogaku Co., Ltd., Tokyo

to the terms of mmHg, so that the shearing stress was easily compared with ICP.

Results

The supratentorial EDP was always higher than the infratentorial EDP. The shearing stress at the edge of the tentorium began to develop as soon as the balloon was inflated, and increased progressively even in the initial stage of inflation when the increase of ICP was minimal and the pressure difference was not apparent between the supratentorial and infratentorial compartments (Fig. 1). The difference between the shearing stress and ICP (supratentorial EDP) became remarkable after ICP exceeded 30 mmHg.

The extent of the descent of the tentorium accompanying the increase of supratentorial EDP varied from animal to animal. When the supratentorial EDP was increased to 50 to 70 mmHg, the tentorium ceased to descend. The shearing stress reached 80 to 140 mmHg when the descent of the tentorium came to the maximum (Fig. 2). Table 1 shows the values of the shearing stress and infratentorial EDP in relation to the increase of supratentorial EDP.

Table 1. Shearing stress and infratentorial EDP in relation to the increase of supratentorial EDP. The shearing stress at the tentorial edge is far greater than ICP (supratentorial EDP)

mmHg

Supratentorial EDP	10	20	30	40	50	60	70	80	90	100	110	120
Shearing Stress	11 ±9	23 ±26	37 ±28	57 ±28	87 ±22	122 ±24	142 ±20	155 ±24	169 ±20	179 ±40	193 ±47	202 ±52
Infratentorial EDP	10 ±2	16 ±4	22 ±7	31 ±7	39 ±12	45 ±9	56 ±10	65 ±10	74 ±10	83 ±11	91 ±10	97 ±12

mean±SD

DISCUSSION

When a mass expands within the intracranial space, the volume of the mass is accommodated to some extent by displacement of cerebrospinal fluid and expression of blood from the brain (3,4), so that the ICP increase is absent or kept minimal. In addition, the descent of the tentorium and transtentorial herniation are working in the manner to reduce the supratentorial ICP. Therefore, the tolerance to increased ICP might be greater in the monkeys which have fibrous tentorium than in other experimental animals such as the dogs and cats which have bony tentorium. The wide variation of the values of the shearing stress when the tentorium ceased to descend will be due to anatomical variation of the tentorial incisura and partly due to the position of the sensing device.

The pressure is not uniformly transmitted throughout the brain when the ICP is increased by an intracranial mass lesion (1,3). The pressure difference develops within the brain. This is because the brain contains elastic material such as arteries that resist distortion and displacement (1). Strictly speaking, the term "pressure" should be used only in a hydrostatic system, not in the system where the pressure differences develop (4). We use the term "shearing stress" for the force given to the herniated brain at the edge of the tentorium.

It is clear from the present experiment that the shearing stress at the tentorial edge begins to develop even in the initial stage when the supratentorial mass is small and there is no significant increase of ICP or no significant pressure difference between the supratentorial and infratentorial compartments. The shearing stress at the tentorial edge is always greater than ICP (supratentorial EDP), and the former is extremely high compared with the latter in the later stage of intracranial hypertension. As the ICP increases, the characteristics of the brain substance changes from elastic to plastic. So does the tentorial edge as it is displaced downwards and stretched. The tissue damage caused by the strained edge of the tentorium is supposed to be tremendously extensive. The functional significance of the shearing stress should be elucidated by studying the morphological and neurophysiological changes.

Summary

The present data shows that the shearing stress given to the herniated brain at the edge of the tentorium develops in the very early stage of intracranial mass lesion when ICP is not significantly increased. The shearing stress is extremely high compared with the ICP. It is this shearing stress rather than the ICP itself that is of prime importance in the pathophysiological manifestations of the transtentorial herniation.

References

1. Cairns H (1939) Raised intracranial pressure: hydrocephalic and vascular factors. Br J Surg 27:275-294

2. Langfitt TW, Weinstein JD, Kassell NF, Simeone FA (1964) Transmission of increased intracranial pressure. I. Within the craniospinal axis. J Neurosurg 21:989-997

3. Langfitt TW, Weinstein JD, Kassell NF, Gagliardi LJ (1964) Transmission of increased intracranial pressure. II. Within the supratentorial space. J Neurosurg 21:998-1005

4. Weinstein JD, Langfitt TW, Bruno L, Zaren HA, Jackson JLF (1968) Experimental study of patterns of brain distortion and ischemia produced by an intracranial mass. J Neurosurg 28:513-521

5. Yoneda S, Matsuda M, Shimizu Y, Handa J, Handa H, Oda F, Matsuo K, Taguchi N (1973) SFT - A new device for continuous measurements of intracranial pressure. Surg Neurol 1:13-15

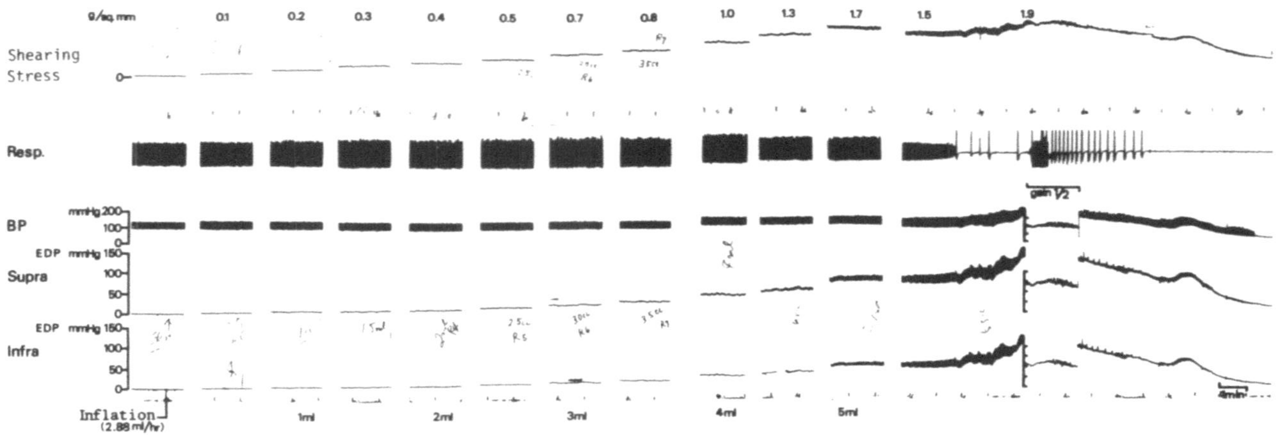

Fig. 1. Simultaneous recording of the shearing stress, respiration, systemic blood pressure, supratentorial EDP and infratentorial EDP. Infusion of the extradural balloon is started at an arrow at the rate of 2.88 ml/hr. The shearing stress at the edge of the tentorium develops in the very early stage of balloon inflation when ICP is not yet significantly increased.

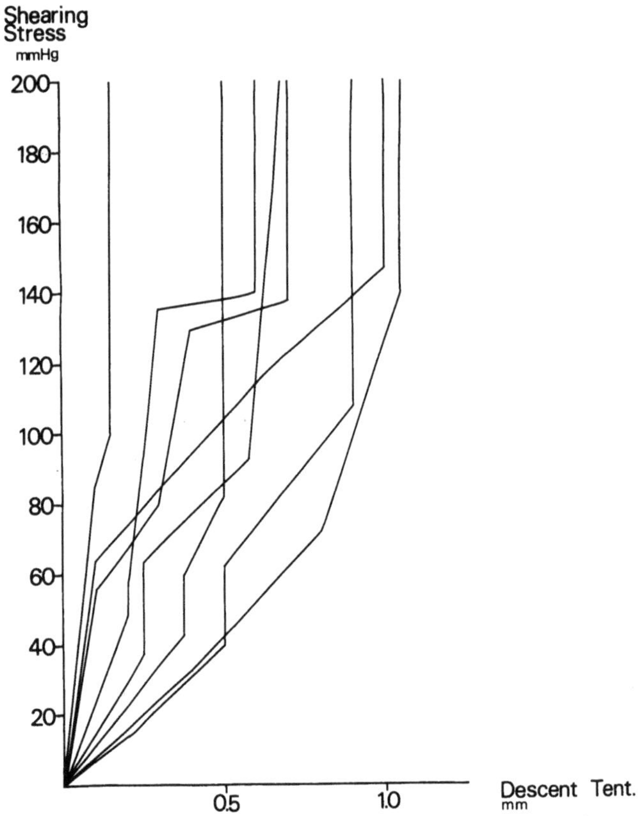

Figure 2. When the descent of the tentorium comes to the maximum with increasing ICP, the shearing stress reaches 80 to 140 mmHg. Thereafter, the shearing stress continues to increase as ICP is increased.

INTRABRAIN PRESSURE, CEREBROSPINAL FLUID PRESSURE AND THE PV FUNCTION OF CRANIOSPINAL SYSTEM ELASTICITY IN PATIENTS AFTER THE EXTRACTION OF TUMORS FROM THE BASAL REGION AND POSTERIOR FOSSA

E.I.PALTSEV AND E.B.SIROVSKY

Introduction

In order to determine the mechanical parameters of the craniospinal system in neurosurgical patients, we have studied the effects of changes in the volume of the fluid in the ventricular system of the brain on the ventricular CSF pressure and on the intrabrain interstitial fluid (ISF) pressure. We supposed that these effects in patients with increased CSF pressure, after the extraction of tumors from the posterior fossa would be noticeably different from those in patients with decreased or normal CSF pressure, after the extraction of tumors from the basal region. We have also studied in these patients the time constants of the relaxation in the craniospinal system with increase in the fluid volume in this system, and of the recovery of the CSF pressure to its initial value after rapid decrease of the fluid volume.

Materials and methods

Measurements of intrabrain ISF pressure and CSF pressure were made by methods which we have described earlier (1). Local ISF pressure was measured by means of a perforated catheter 1.5 mm(O.D.) with very small holes at the end. This catheter was introduced into the right premotor zone to a depth of about 2.0-2.5 cm. CSF pressure was measured by a catheter 2.0 mm(O.D.). The catheter was inserted into the lateral ventricle (as described by LUNDBERG). This catheter also served for injecting or withdrawing fluid. The compliance (or the elasticity) of the craniospinal system was studied by injecting saline through a 3-way tap. The velocity of flow was from 4 to 10 ml/min. In our investigations the CSF Pressure at the end of the injection of saline never exceeded 60 torr. In all, 15 patients were investigated during the first three to four days after the operation.

Results

In Fig. 1a is shown a typical example of the changes in ventricular pressure and local ISF pressure caused by withdrawing or introducing fluid. It is clear that the CSF pressure during withdrawal of fluid decreased, but during the introduction fluid into the ventricle increased more abruptly (a type of hysteresis is apparent). A study of the relationship between CSF pressure and the volume introduced shows that this dependence may be approximated by the exponential function $P(v)=(Po+b/a)\exp(av)-b/a$. Here P(v) is the intraventricle pressure, v is volume of the injected fluid, Po is the initial CSF pressure. Po and P(v) in this approximation are average pressure (without taking into account pressure pulsations). From this approximation for P(v) it follows that $dp/dv=E(p)=a.p+b$. Thus, a, b and p are constants characterizing the elastance or compliance of the craniospinal system. We have determined approximately (Fig. 1b) the constants a, b in

Table 1. The average values of CSF pressure, ISF pressure $\bar{a}$, $\bar{b}$ and elastance $\bar{E}(=\bar{a} \cdot \bar{p} + \bar{b})$ in the first group of patients after the extraction of tumors from the basal region, and in the second group of patients after the extraction of tumors from the basal region, and in the second group of patients after the extraction of tumors from the posterior fossa

1st group	$\bar{P}$csf,torr	$\bar{P}$isf,torr	$\bar{a}$, ml^{-1}	$\bar{b}$,torr/ml	$\bar{E}$,torr/ml
1st day	+11.9	-3.5	+0.070	+0.85	1.68
2nd day	+12.8	-0.2	+0.080	+0.70	1.74
3-4 days	+14.0	-4.3	+0.068	+0.80	1.75
2nd group					
1st day	+22.0	+0.0	+0.142	-1.20	1.92
2nd day	+23.4	-4.4	+0.108	-0.60	1.93
3rd day	+29.8	-3.6	+0.112	-0.15	2.19

patients for all PV dependences. In Fig. 1c are shown the approximated relationships between E and P in patients after the extraction of tumors from the basal region and in patients after the extraction of posterior fossa tumors. It is clear that the relationships are different for these two groups of patients. An analysis of the results allowed us to determine the distribution of observed values of CSF pressure, ISF pressure, a and b. Histograms of these values are nonsymmetrical. Their boundary values and average values were determined. The average values are given in Table 1. The changes of ISF pressure are not always simply connected with the volume alterations in the ventricular system. During withdrawal of cerebrospinal fluid the ISF pressure usually decreases together with the CSF pressure, but a slight increase in the ISF pressure may occur towards the end of the phase of removal of liquid. In patients with posterior fossa tumors, an initial fall and subsequent rise in the pressure of the interstitial liquid may be seen during the introduction of liquid (Fig. 1d).

Fig. 1a) A typical response of the ventricular CSF pressure and tissue ▷ ISF pressure to the slow withdrawal of CSF and subsequent injection of saline into the ventricle. Downward pointing arrows indicate the beginning of these procedures, and upward arrows, the end. The reduction of the CSF pressure is seen clearly, and also a wave of ISF pressure.

1b) A graphical construction of the approximate relationships between CSF pressure (P) and volume (V) and between elastance (E) and pressure (P).

Figure 1c) The approximate elastance pressure relationships in patients after the extraction of tumors from the basal region (solid lines) and after the extraction of tumors from the posterior fossa (dotted lines).

1d) Difference in the response of the CSF pressure and the local ISF pressure to the introduction of saline into the lateral ventricle. Downward pointing arrows indicate the beginning of the injection. After the end of the introduction the reduction in the CSF pressure and a wave of the ISF pressure are clearly seen. Horizontal arrows indicate the initial pressure levels.

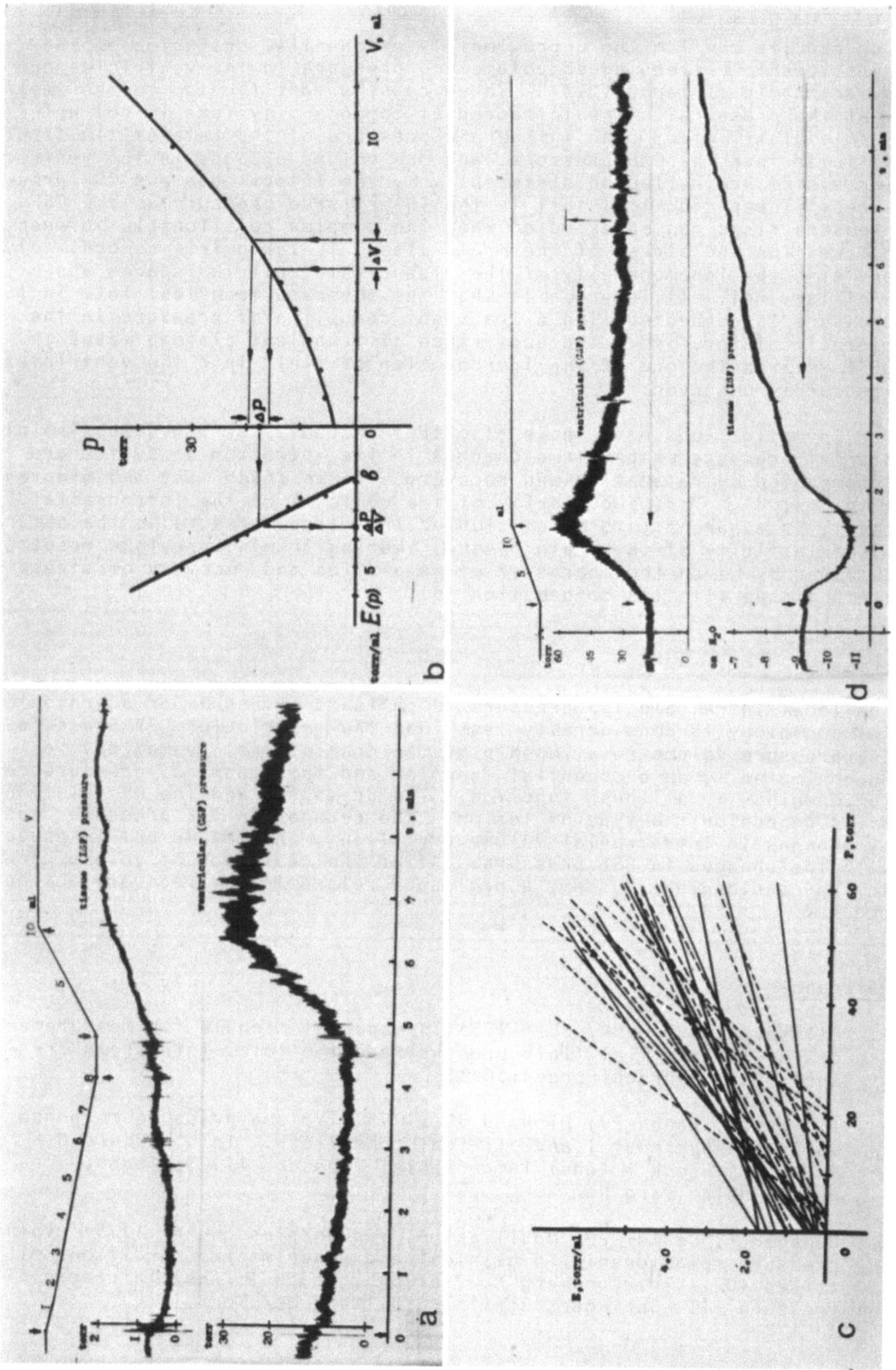
a
b
c
d
tissue (ISF) pressure
ventricular (CSF) pressure
torr
torr/ml
V, ml
E(p)
ΔP
ΔV
E, torr/ml
P, torr
cm H2O

Discussion

Our results confirm the approximately exponential character of the relationship between added volume and pressure in the ventricles and subarachnoid cisterns (2-4). These results testify also to the fact that the pressure in the intracranial component systems is not uniformly distributed; the intrabrain pressure of the interstitial fluid is lower than the CSF pressure, and the volume changes in the ventricular system are reflected differently by the intertissue and CSF pressures. The paradoxical fall in the intertissue pressure as the CSF pressure rises can be expected when the complex relationship between deformation and stress of the brain tissue is taken into account (5), and also the inhomogeneity of the tissue-intercellular spaces and capillary net. It is probable that the observed transient fall in ISF pressure is connected with a transient reduction of pressure in the microcirculatory bed. The appearance of transient plateau waves in CSFP towards the end of the introduction of fluid into the ventricles was rarely observed.

Our investigations have shown also that increases or decreases in intracranial pressure with volume changes in the intracranial system are accompanied by relaxation and recovery effects which last 3-5 minutes (Fig. 1a, d). This peculiarity of the contents of the intracranial cavity is apparently to be attributed in a large measure to the natural viscoelasticity of the brain tissue, bearing in mind previous results obtained by us on the character of relaxation and recovery of stress in brain tissue with its deformation (6).

Summary

The local intrabrain ISF pressure in patients with sub- or supratentorial pathology is considerably less than the ventricular CSF pressure. The pressure volume relationship of the craniospinal system may be approximated by an exponential function and the elastance pressure relationship - by a linear function. The pressures and the PV relationships depend on the type of lesion. The changes in ISF pressure caused by changes in intracranial volume are slight, and may be not in phase with the changes in CSF pressure. After the cessation of volume changes in the craniospinal system, a prolonged relaxation or recovery action occurs.

References

1. Paltsev EI, Sirovsky EB (1975) The special cannula for measurement of the interstitial fluid pressure and the total intrabrain pressure. Vopr Neurochirurg 4:56-58

2. Miller JD, Leech PJ, Pickard JD (1975) Volume pressure response in various experimental and clinical conditions. In: Lundberg N, Ponten U, Brock M (eds) Intracranial Pressure II. Springer, Berlin Heidelberg New York, p97

3 Cohadon F, Castel JP, Nouillant A, Vandendriessche M (1975) Volume pressure relationship in clinical and experimental conditions of raised ICP. In: Lundberg N, Ponten U, Brock M (eds) Intracranial Pressure II. Springer, Berlin Heidelberg New York, p107

4. Sklar FH, Elashvili I (1977) The pressure-volume function of brain elasticity (physiological consideration and clinical application). J Neurosurg 47:670-679

5. Hakim S, Venegas J G, Burton JD (1976) The physics of cranial cavity, hydrocephalus and normal pressure hydrocephalus: mechanical interpretation and mathematical model. Surg Neurol 5:187-210

6. Paltsev EI, Sirovsky EB (1975)The viscoelasticity and the plasticity of the brain. Biomekhanika 13:16-23 Riga :Ed.RNIIOT

CLINICAL EXPERIENCES WITH INTRACRANIAL VOLUME-PRESSURE RESPONSE

I. NYARY, J. VAJDA, AND E. PASZTOR

Introduction

On the basis of recent investigations (1,2) the subject of intracranial pressure-volume relationships has become clarified. However, despite the few but promising clinical reports gathered to validate the theory that had been established in animal studies, many important areas need to be explored by human investigations. The aim of this study was to adapt and test the model proposed in patients presenting with presumably decreased intracranial compliance.

Materials and Methods

A total of 37 patients were investigated. This group was further divided according to the etiology of their intracranial pathology: 16 cases of axial tumors with concomitant hydrocephalus; 15 cases of non-tumoral hydrocephalus; 3 cases of supratentorial tumors with dilated ventricles and 3 cases of post-traumatic hydrocephalus. ICP was assessed by measurement of ventricular fluid pressure (VFP) via a catheter placed into the lateral ventricle. The bolus technique was used to investigate brain stiffness. After sufficient time was allotted to reach baseline conditions, increasing volumes of 1-4ml mock CSF were injected into the CSF space through the same catheter and elicited VFP responses were recorded. The last diastolic value of VFP at the inspiratory nadir before the volume-injection was designated as P_o, the corresponding value immediately after injection as P_t. In many patients with decreased intracranial compliance, there occurred subsequent to the immediate pressure increase due to volume load, a further, prolonged ICP elevation topped by induced secondary waves, P_{max}. Volume-pressure response (VPR) and pressure volume index (PVI) were calculated for both P_t and P_{max} using standard equations (1). Investigations were carried out in awake, conscious patients, and no complications were encountered during and subsequent to the studies.

Results

Figure 1 (panel A) shows original recordings obtained from a patient with cerebellar astrocytoma. It can be seen that on volume load an immediate step-like pressure increase occurred without any tendency to decrease. On the contrary, further increases could be registered, especially after greater volumes, that very often precipitated a regular B wave. The pattern demonstrated on Figure 1 (panel A) was almost unexceptionally uniform and reflected so well the patients' clinical state that we have considered it as an unequivocal sign of decreased intracranial compliance. After removal of the tumor measurements were repeated and considerably smaller reactions to the same volume load were monitored (Figure 1, panel B). Induced secondary waves as registered preoperatively were never encountered after removal of space occupying mass.

Table I. Resting ICP(mmHg; P_r), VPR(mmHg/ml; VPR_t, VPR_{max}) and PVI ml; PVI_{max} in patients with history of axial tumor and concomitant hydrocephalus

No.	P_r	VPR_t	VPR_{max}	PVI_{max}
1	1.1	2.3	5.3	2.2
2	3.7	1.5	5.2	7.1
3	4.0	2.6	9.0	3.5
4	5.7	5.1	19.3	3.2
5	6.1	2.9	4.8	8.2
6	6.2	4.5	14.6	3.6
7	6.1	4.6	5.0	11.2
8	11.3	3.8	14.7	3.3
9	17.3	3.9	6.9	9.9
10	17.8	2.7	16.0	6.3
11	18.8	1.8	8.1	10.3
12	25.5	5.4	15.0	6.2
13	30.7	3.8	10.8	9.0
14	35.7	7.4	11.3	11.9
15	36.0	1.8	4.2	25.3
16	40.0	6.1	13.1	7.9
MEAN		3.8	10.2	8.1
SD		1.7	4.8	5.5
SE		0.42	1.2	1.4

To demonstrate our experiences regarding numerical analysis, results obtained in a homogenous group of 16 patients with history of axial tumor are presented in Table I. Since elicited VFP responses did not tend to decrease toward pre-response levels, we were unable to determine PVI by plotting volume changes against log pressure changes. Instead, PVI was determined from each pressure response and VPR was also calculated for different volume loads. We have analyzed the relationship between VPR_t, VPR_{max}, PVI_t, PVI_{max} and P_o as well as ΔV. No correlation could be found between VPR and increasing P_o, therefore, individual values were averaged. Calculated values of PVI_t have shown an increase with increasing volume load while corresponding estimates of PVI_{max} were similar within reasonable limits, and were also averaged for each patient.

In Table I patients were aligned according to their registered resting ICP (P_r). It can be seen that only some patients had ICP values indicating intracranial hypertension, some others presented with quite normal ICP. Calculated VPR and PVI do not show any correlation with the resting level of ICP. Mean VPR_{max} was significantly higher ($p<0.001$) than VPR_t. The mean value of PVI_{max} (8.1 $\pm$ 1.4ml falls very close to the corresponding figure of 8.4 $\pm$ 1.3ml found in the hydrocephalus group, discussed in detail elsewhere (5). Mean values of VPR and PVI presented in Table I can be compared with corresponding data obtained from three patients of the hydrocephalus group who were considered normotensive and ineligible for shunt operation (VPF: 1.2 $\pm$ 0.32mmHg/ml, PVI: 22.4 $\pm$ 6.4 ml).

Discussion

In this series of patients we were unable to reproduce volume-pressure responses similar to that of MARMAROU (1) obtained in healthy, normal cats. The different pattern of responses, inconsistency between calculated VPR and PVI, the occurrence of high VPR along with high PVI, might indicate that different mechanisms are operative in cases of decreased intracranial compliance due to space occupying mass. This assumption can be confirmed indirectly by the fact that in patients considered normal or in the same patient after tumor removal the pattern was substantially different and PVI resembled more or less that presented by MARMAROU et al. On the other hand, analysis of volume-pressure responses provided a sensitive and reliable indicator of brain stiffness even in quantitative terms when VPR or PVI were calculated using P_{max} instead of P_t.

References

1. Marmarou A, Shulman K, LaMorgese J (1975) Compartmental analysis of compliance and outflow resistance of the cerebrospinal system. J Neurosurg 43:523-534

2. Miller JD, Garibi J, Pickard JD (1973) Induced changes of cerebrospinal fluid volume: Effects during continuous monitoring of ventricular fluid pressure. Arch Neurol 28:265-269

3. Miller JD, Leech PJ (1975) Assessing the effects of mannitol and steroid therapy on intracranial volume pressure relationships in patients. J Neurosurg 42:274-281

4. Sullivan HG, Miller JD, Griffith RL, Becker DP (1978) CSP pressure-volume dynamics in neurosurgical patients: a preliminary evaluation in six patients. Surg Neurol 9:47-54

5. Vajda J, Horvath M, Nyary I (1979) Ventriculo-lymphatic shunt and decompensated intracranial volume-pressure relationship. Acta Neurochir Suppl 28:521-525

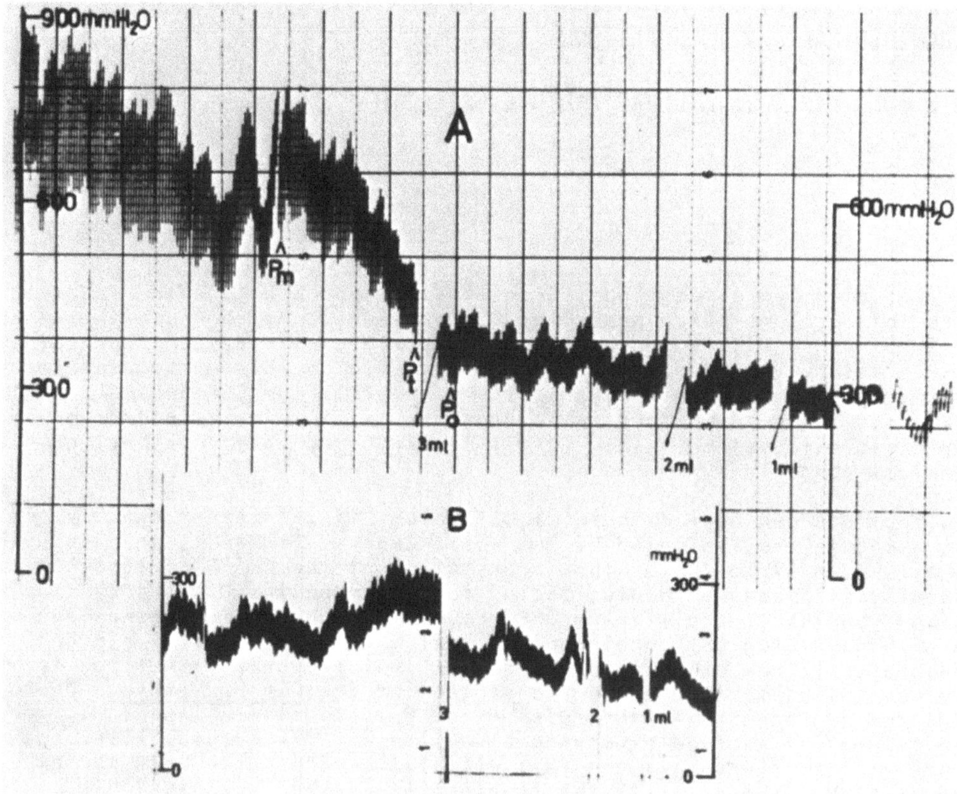

Figure 1. VFP tracings and volume-pressure responses of a patient presented with cerebellar astrocytoma prior to (panel A) and after (panel B) tumor removal.

A DIAGRAMMATIC, TWO-DIMENSIONAL MODEL FOR INTERPRETATION OF CRANIOSPINAL P/V INTERACTIONS

H.G.SULLIVAN, J.D.MILLER, AND R.L.GRIFFITH

We report a two-dimensional, diagrammatic approach to help visualize the interactions which may alter CSF pressure. As shown by the dashed axes of Figure 1, we begin with the experimentally determined plot of CSF pressure vs CSF volume change. In defining this curve experimentally, volume loading always begins at equilibrium CSF pressure (P_{eq}) which is taken to be the stable pressure level which results when the craniospinal system is left totally unperturbed under constant physiological conditions.

So that one can deal with total CSF volume (V_{csf}) rather than ΔV, we have chosen, as indicated by the solid axes in Figure 1, to change the X axis from ΔV to V_{csf}. This translation of the CSF P/ΔV function is permissible because volume loading to determine the P_{csf} vs ΔV plot always begins at equilibrium CSF volume (V_{eq}) which is constant under stable physiological conditions so that $V_{csf} = Veq + \Delta V$. In order to separate it from other craniospinal P/V relationships, we refer to the curve obtained by the above translation as the CSF P/V curve. When P_{eq} and V_{eq} are stable the response of P_{csf} to alterations in V_{csf} may be thought of as a point moving along the CSF P/V curve. After such a volume alteration, P_{csf} and V_{csf} will follow the curve back to the original P_{eq} and V_{eq}. If the craniospinal system (C/S-syst) is altered so that either or both P_{eq} or V_{eq} are changed, the CSF P/V curve will be moved to a new location with respect to the P_{csf} and V_{csf} axes. If the craniospinal system is altered so that it is more or less tolerant of CSF volume change, the CSF P/V curve will become more or less steep. The above alterations of the CSF P/V curve are indicated by the arrows in Figure 1.

In order to analyze the ways in which the CSF P/V curve may be altered by changes in the C/S-syst we divide the C/S-syst into two subsystems: 1) the hydraulic subsystem (HS), and 2) the viscoelastic subsystem (VES). The HS is the CSF space including the mechanisms for inflow and outflow of CSF while the VES is all tissues around the CSF space. Under a given set of physiological conditions a stable P_{eq} requires that V_{eq} may be non-changing. If V_{eq} is constant then CSF influx must equal CSF efflux. At any particular CSF pressure CSF absorption depends on CSF outflow resistance (R) and sagittal sinus pressure (P_{ss}). Thus, the level of P_{eq} is set by the magnitude of R, P_{ss}, and CSF formation, all of which are parameters of the HS. The level of P_{eq} is set only by parameters of the hydraulic system and P_{eq} moves up or down on the P_{csf} axis only in response to a change in HS. Changes in the VES may cause transient changes in P_{csf} but the level of P_{eq} will remain stable. V_{eq} is the volume which must fill up the CSF space in order to generate the pressure, P_{eq}. Thus, the magnitude of V_{eq} depends upon the level of P_{eq} and upon how readily the tissues around the CSF space tolerate distortion by CSF volume changes. For a given P_{eq}, if the VES is not easily deformed by CSF volume change, V_{eq} will be small, while, if the VES is not so stiff, V_{eq} will be large. Changes in V_{eq}, therefore, may reflect changes in the HS, the VES, or both. The shape of the CSF P/V curve is a reflection of how readily the tissues around the CSF space accept distortion by changes in CSF volume and, thus, the shape of the CSF P/V curve changes only in response to changes in properties of the VES. The above relationships are summarized within the parentheses on Figure 1.

Figure 2 shows how the diagrammatic approach advocated here may be applied in evaluating a plateau wave. Since the patient is not at steady state beginning CSF pressure (*) is not P_{eq}. In segment 1 of Figure 2a assume that CBF and CBV are measured and are stable. P_{csf} must, therefore, be ascending a CSF P/V curve toward P_{eq}. If P_{csf} is elevated P_{eq} must also be elevated and the pathological processes at work in the C/S-syst must have altered one of the parameters of the HS. In segment 2 of Figure 2, cerebral vasodilatation occurs, making the VES less readily deformed by V_{csf} and causing a sudden shift from CSF P/V curve #1 to curve #2. The shift to the new CSF P/V curve results in the dramatic increase in P_{csf}. The peak pressure now declines slowly while CBV remains elevated. This decline is due to movement down CSF P/V curve #2 toward the new P_{eq}. In segment 4, Figure 2, P_{csf} suddenly declines as CBV is rapidly diminished giving the VES improved tolerance for distortion by CSF volume and resulting in a shift back to CSF P/V curve #1. Since CSF volume is now below V_{eq}, P_{csf} increases again toward P_{eq}.

The authors hope that the diagrammatic approach presented here will be useful in dealing with C/S-syst P/V interationns. We emphasize that it is probably not correct to employ a single P/V curve to relate P_{csf} to all volume alterations (blood, mass, edema, or CSF) within the craniospinal system. Only CSF volume change alters P_{csf} by movement of a point along a single P/V curve (the CSF P/V curve). Volume changes in all other C/S compartments alter P_{csf} by changing P_{eq}, V_{eq}, or the shape of the CSF P/V curve. After such a change the total CSF volume is related to a new CSF P/V curve to generate a new level of P_{csf}. If the C/S-syst remains stable in the new state, P_{csf} and V_{csf} will follow the new curve and come to rest at the new P_{eq} and V_{eq}.

This work was supported by NIH grants #1 R01 NS 14309-01 and #7 R01 NS 15995-01.

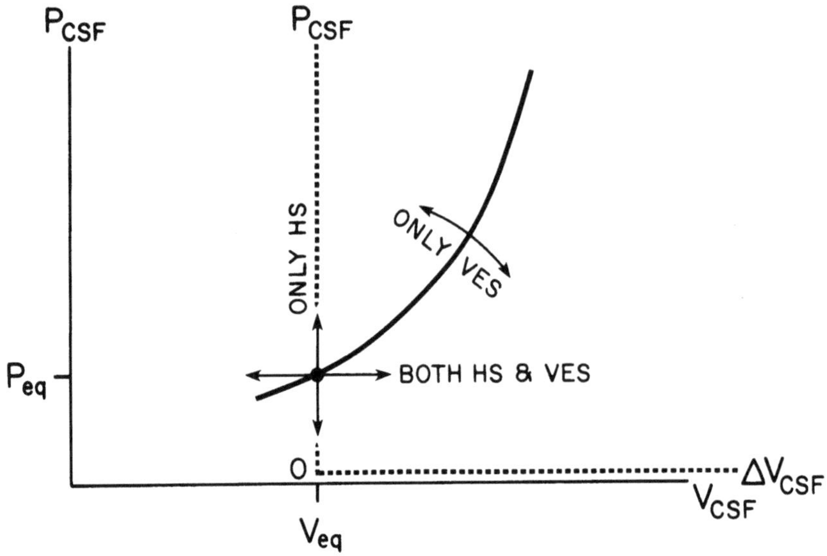

Figure 1. Translation of P_{csf} vs ΔV to P_{csf} vs total csf volume (V_{csf}) This translation is allowed because $V_{csf} = V_{eq} + \Delta V$.

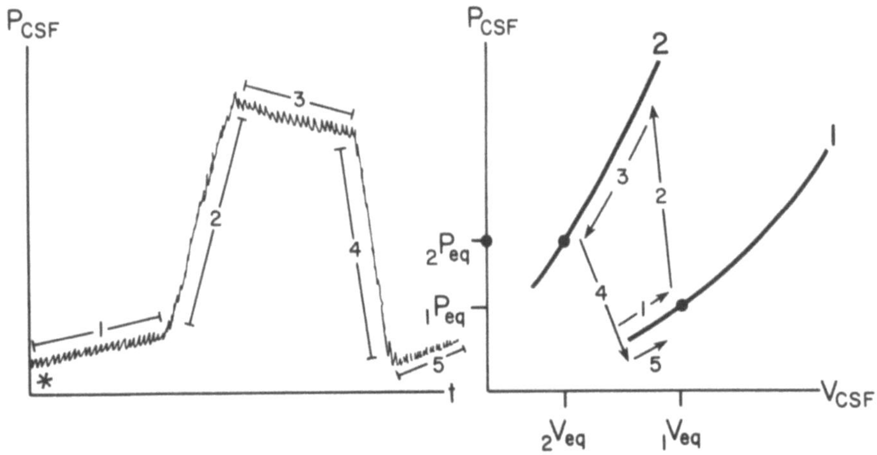

Figure 2. Two dimensional diagrammatic approach applied to hypothetical plateau wave.

ETIOLOGY OF B-WAVES

S.C.SØRENSEN, F.GJERRIS, AND S.E.BØRGESEN

Introduction

B-waves are observed in pressure recordings from the glaucomatous eye and the hydrocephalic brain. These pressure variations must be the result of changes in vascular volume. It is not known whether B-waves are the consequence of exaggerated alterations in the volume of the vascular bed or an exaggerated pressure response to alterations in vascular volume. We have tested the latter hypothesis by examining whether the presence of B-waves could be related to conductance to outflow of cerebrospinal fluid (C_{out}) and/or compliance of the craniospinal space (C_{css}).

Material and Methods

Twenty-four patients were studied because of suspicion of normal pressure hydrocephalus. They all fulfilled the following criteria: Progressing dementia, gait disturbances, increased ventricular size on CT-scan and abnormal isotope cisternography. Intraventricular pressure was recorded continuously for 24 hours. The pressure recording was analyzed for duration of periods with B-waves. B-waves were defined as pressure fluctuations occurring with a frequency of 1-2/min during periods lasting more than ten minutes. Following pressure monitoring the bolus-injection test described by MARMAROU et al (3)was performed. During steady state 6 ml of Ringer lactate solution was injected into the subarachnoid space through a lumbar cannula within 2-4 seconds. C_{css} was calculated from the pressure recording (2). Subsequently, the lumbo-ventricular perfusion test for measuring C_{out}(1) was performed.

Results

In none of the patients did the mean ventricular pressure exceed 12 mmHg. The duration of periods with B-waves varied between 0-75% of the recording time. The C_{css} values varied between 0.29-0.98 ml/mmHg, and the C_{out} values varied between 0.019-0.511 ml/min x mmHg.The total durations of periods with B-waves as percentage of total recording time were plotted against C_{out} values and C_{css} values respectively. The best power fits showed a poor correlation for both plots,i.e. correlation coefficients of 0.42 and 0.51 respectively. However, when C_{out} and C_{css} values for each patient were simply added, the plot of C_{out} + C_{css} versus duration of B-waves could be fitted by an exponential curve with a correlation coefficient of 0.84. It should be noted, that the ratio between the highest and the lowest C_{css} values were only 3 compared with a ratio of 27 for the C_{out} values.

Discussion

We are assuming that B-waves are the result of changes in cerebral vascular volume, because oscillations in blood flow to different organs are well known (4). They are probably due to cyclic variations in vascular resistance, the so-called Traube-Hering waves. The pressure response to a change in cerebral vascular volume depends both on C_{css} and C_{out}. Therefore, we have tested whether the duration of periods with B-waves could be correlated to either of these two variables. Low correlation coefficients were observed. If C_{out} and C_{css} were simply added this sum was inversely related to duration of periods with B-waves with a correlation coefficient of 0.84. This relationship suggests that an increase in duration of B-waves reflects an exaggerated response to volume changes. However, B-waves are an on-off phenomenon and cannot be explained by this relationship only, but a low C_{css} and/or a low C_{out} may be one prerequisite for the occurrence of B-waves.

Summary

In 24 patients with suspicion of normal pressure hydrocephalus conductance to outflow of CSF (C_{out}) was studied with a lumbo-ventricular perfusion technique, and compliance of the craniospinal space (C_{css}) was measured with a bolus injection technique. IVP was measured continuously for 24 hours and duration of periods with B-waves were calculated. Duration of periods with B-waves did not correlate with either C_{out} or C_{css}, but was inversely related to the sum $C_{out} + C_{css}$ with a correlation coefficient of 0.84, suggesting that an increase in duration of B-waves reflects an exaggerated response to vascular volume changes.

References

1. Borgensen SE, Gjerris F, Sorensen SC (1978) The resistance to CSF-absorption in humans. Acta Neurol Scand 57:88-96

2. Borgesen SE, Gjerris F, Sorensen SC (to be published) Cerebrospinal fluid conductance and compliance in normal pressure hydrocephalus. J Neurosurg 51

3. Marmarou A, Shulman K, LaMorgese J (1975) Compartmental analysis of compliance and outflow resistance of the cerebrospinal fluid system. J Neurosurg 43:523-534

4. Thorburn W (1972) Recordings of applanation force at constant intraocular pressure. Acta Ophthalmol 51:270-285

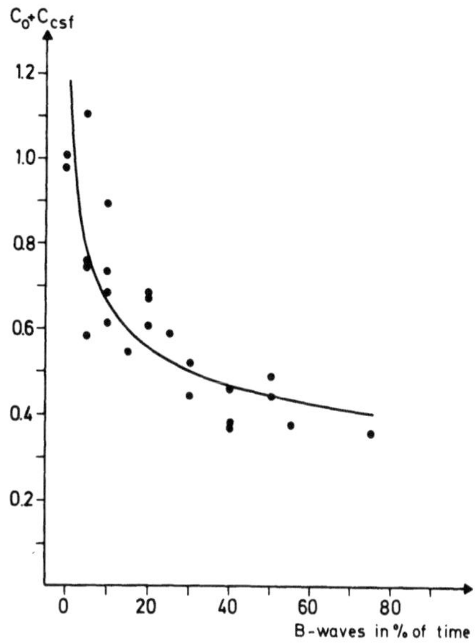

Fig. 1. Sum of C_{css} and C_{out} in relation to duration of periods with B-waves with a correlation coefficient of 0.84 (From (2), published with permission)

Session III

CEREBROVASCULAR ASPECTS

Chairman: J.D.Miller
Co-chairman: N.N.Zwetnow

SUMMARY

One of the most encouraging features of this session was the progress reported in the interpretation of changes in the amplitude and configuration of the pulse pressure waves of continuous recordings of ICP. Until recently, there has been little data by which one can compare changes in the pulse pressure which would be related to changes in blood volume with precisely measured bolus changes in CSF volume. The contributions of AVEZAAT and EIJNDHOVEN, STEVENAART, PORTNOY and CASTELL have gone a long way to filling this important gap in our information. Although much work remains to be done, the challenge for the next ICP meeting is clear. It is to define changes in intracranial pulse pressure waves in terms of their origins in changes in cerebrovascular volume, in brain stiffness or in CSF dynamics.

Difficulties remain in the resolution of the precise effects of changes in arterial pressure and arterial PCO_2 on CSF dynamics in pressure volume relationships. In noting that increases in arterial blood pressure in the absence of autoregulation produced stiffening of the brain and an increase in elastance, MARMAROU and his colleagues have ascribed this to an increase in intravascular pressure and cerebral blood volume. If this were the case, then it would be expected that increases in arterial PCO_2 would have the same effect. This is not the case, however, and it is likely that the distribution between the arterial and venous portions of the cerebrovascular bed and the intravascular pressure gradient from the arterial to the venous ends play a crucial factor in determining the effects of these physiological changes. Until it becomes possible to measure not only blood volume intracranially, but its distribution and to measure the intravascular pressure at precise loci along the cerebrovascular bed, difficulties will remain in predicting the effects of vascular changes on intracranial pressure volume relationships.

Elevations of intracranial pressure which accompany rises of arterial blood pressure are another example of the same problem. While on some occasions, the change in ICP may be a precise mirror of the changes in arterial pressure, often this is not the case. ICP rises progressively only after maximum arterial hypertension has been attained for some time and ICP may again decrease prior to any fall in arterial pressure. Again, there are many factors at work including changes in cerebral blood volume intravascular pressure and in cerebral edema.

The work of ALBIN and his colleagues presented in this session raised an interesting issue in discussion which was also referred to in a later session by MARMAROU. This was the production of widespread reduction in cerebral blood flow by a localized distortion of one cerebral hemisphere,produced in ALBIN'S experiments by the application of a brain retractor, and in other studies by focal brain edema. Drowsiness and lethargy which are seen in some patients with focal brain lesions may be due, not to distortion of the reticular formation, but to generalized depression of cerebral blood flow produced by a focal lesion.

INTRACRANIAL PRESSURE AND REGIONAL CEREBRAL BLOOD FLOW RESPONSES TO EXPERIMENTAL BRAIN RETRACTION PRESSURE

M.S.ALBIN, L.BUNEGIN, P.HELSEL, A.MARLIN, AND M.BABINSKI

During the past four years we have been delineating the physiopathological responses of brain to forces developed on it by graded retraction pressure (1,2,3,4). We have noted that the pressure threshold for the development of histological changes after one hour of retraction at normotensive levels was greater than 20 torr and at induced hypotensive levels greater than 10 torr (2,3). We have shown the correlation of somatosensory cortically evoked responses (SER) to the development of lesions and to cerebral perfusion pressures (CPP) - with a higher CPP showing a smaller decrease in SER and greater resistance to histopathological changes (4,5). We have evaluated brain retraction pressure (BRP) changes during intracranial procedures in the human and indicated that high BRP can be generated (3) (>125 torr). Finally, we have developed a counter pressure BRP monitoring unit that is sensitive and reliable.

During intracranial procedures with brain retraction localized to one hemisphere or to the posterior fossa, we were interested in determining:

1. whether there was a concomitant distribution of this focal pressure,
2. how cortical blood flow was affected by BRP and changes in mean arterial blood pressure levels since induced hypotension is frequently used in neurosurgical procedures on vascular tumors, aneurysms, and A-V malformations.

This will be the subject of this report.

Materials and methods

Using light pentobarbital, endotracheal anesthesia in acclimated mongrel canines, a craniectomy was performed over the right temporal-parietal cortex. Each animal was monitored for ECG, mean arterial blood pressure (MAP), central venous pressure (CVP), pulmonary artery pressure (PAP), pulmonary capillary wedge pressure (PCWP), discontinuous blood gases and electrolytes obtained through previously inserted catheters, monitoring leads and discontinuous arterial blood samples. An epidural counter pressure sensor for ICP was introduced through a burr hole over the contralateral (left) hemisphere (area of somatosensory cortex) and a cisterna magna catheter also inserted for ICP monitoring. The animals were divided into a normotensive and hypotensive group with induced hypotension produced by lowering the MAP to 55 torr using intravenous sodium nitroprusside.

After craniectomy, the dura was incised and reflected exposing an area at the level of the somatosensory cortex. A 12.00 mm De Martel retractor fitted with a pressure-sensitive sleeve was fixed onto a micromanipulator and 20 torr of BRP was applied to the area of the somatosensory cortex for one hour. Regional cerebral blood flow (6) was quantified in brain sections 1.0 cm^2 and 0.5 cm in thickness in 10 normotensive and 10 hypotensive animals using I_{125}, Ce_{141}, Sr_{85} and

Sc_{46} labelled microspheres. The 15 μm spheres were injected via a catheter located in the left ventricle prior to retraction, at 15 and 60 minutes during retraction and 5 minutes after removal of the retractor blade. In a special control group, hemispheric and local cortical flows were calculated in 3 normotensive and 3 hypotensive animals where only craniectomies were performed and the animals not subjected to retraction.

Results

ICP. The application of 20 torr of BRP produced an immediate rise of epidural ICP to 19.0 ± 1 torr on the contralateral side as well as a rise in Cisterna Magna pressure to 14.5 ± 3 torr. The ICP rise was sustained for as long as brain retraction was carried out.

Mean Arterial Blood Pressure at Normotension - Ranged between 90 and 125 torr.

Mean Hemispheric Blood Flows. As noted in Table 1, a significant change in flow occurred in both the retracted and contralateral hemisphere under normotensive and hypotensive conditions. Flow returned to near normal limits five minutes after termination of retraction in the normotensive animals. The hypotensive group showed a significant decrease in flow in the control as compared to the normotensive group and a marked decrease during retraction in both retracted and contralateral hemispheres. Unlike the normotensive group, hemispheric flows in the hypotensive group did not return to normal five minutes after termination of retraction.

Local Cortical Flow (Fig. 1). Indicates the same order of magnitude of changes as found in the hemispheric blood flows (Table 1). The local cortical flow corresponds to the cortical area directly beneath the retractor blade and the equivalent area on the contralateral cortex. Again, under induced hypotension, there was a marked decrease in flow in both retracted and contralateral cortex after removal of the retractor.

Discussion

It is not surprising that there would be transmission of retraction forces to the other portions of brain as manifested by the contralateral ICP as well as the responses in CM pressure. We have noted a sequence of events related to retraction of the viscoelastic mass that characterizes the brain, regardless of location of retraction. When constant fixed retraction is initially applied to brain, a compensation can occur as the brain bulk adjusts by moving away from the retractor into the available space in the adjacent areas. This compensatory movement may not occur if the brain is already occupying all available intracranial space because of a mass lesion and/or accompanying cerebral edema. In this initial phase, the fixed BRP may even decrease slightly as the brain falls away from the retractor. After this period of adjustment, BRP and contralateral ICP may even increase as brain mass now moves against the retractor. This may have serious repercussions in terms of potential injury and might explain the appearance of intracerebral hemorrhage or ischemia distant from the retracted area after retractor release. The danger of retraction under induced hypotension became more obvious when it is noted that autoregulation was lost (Table 1, Fig. 1) under nitroprusside in the hypotensive controls. Local cortical flow under the retractor as

Table I. Mean Hemispheric Flow (ml/min/100gm. - retraction time 60min)

Retracted	Time (min)	Contralateral
Normotensive (n=10)		
25.0±3.4	Control	26.0±5.1
19.4±3.6 p<.005	15	19.7±4.1 p<.005
20.1±3.5 p<.005	60	20.6±3.7 p<.005
22.6 3.5 p<.05	65	22.9 ±3.4 p<.220
Hypotension (n=10)		
15.2±4.3	Control	21.0±6.3
4.0±1.6 p<.001	15	6.0±2.2 p<.001
3.1±1.2 p<.001	60	4.4±1.0 p<.001
6.7±1.6 p<.001	65	9.0±2.2 p<.001

well as corresponding contralateral area was reduced by 20% in the normotensive group, while 80% reduction in flow was measured in both the retracted and contralateral cortical sections of the hypotensive group.

In a previous paper we demonstrated the effects of graded BRP on cortical somatosensory evoked responses (SER), a reduction in SER amplitude greater than 50% for more than 15 minutes indicated the possibility of lesion formation. In Figure 2 we have superimposed SER amplitude changes for 20 torr BRP under normotensive and hypotensive conditions on local cortical flow and we can appreciate the correlation between these two parameters. This indicates the possibility of using the SER as both an indication of changes in rCBF and a means of monitoring critical BRP changes during neurosurgical procedures. Since ICP/BRP increased and rCBF decreased similarly on both retracted and non-retracted contralateral cortex, an explanation for some of the histopathological findings reported in our earlier studies have to be considered due to the factor of excessive mechanical shear stresses generated by the edge pressures of the retractor blade. This is especially important in the face of a low perfusion pressure and loss of autoregulation. While we realize the necessity of brain retraction, it becomes important not to use ridged and deformed retractors with sharp edges; to attenuate edge pressure by use of an energy absorbing material and better retractor design; to monitor retractor pressures and to release retractor periodically; and to employ induced hypotension as sparingly as possible. A study might be designed to see if any correlation exists between the depth and duration of induced hypotension to the incidence of postoperative vasospasm after aneurysm surgery. Our aim should be to always encourage as adequate a cerebral perfusion pressure that is compatible with surgical reality and hemostasis.

Summary

20 torr of brain retraction pressure for a period of one hour on the right somatosensory cortex in 10 normotensive and 10 hypotensive animals revealed a rise in epidural ICP to 19.0 ± 1 torr on contralateral cortex and rise in CM pressure to 14.5 ± 3 torr; a decrease in

mean hemispheric and local cortical blood flow in retracted and contralateral areas which was considerably greater under induced hypotension than in the normotensive animals; and loss of autoregulation in the hypotensive group.

References

1. Albin MS, Bunegin L, Dujovny M, Bennett MH, Janetta PJ, Wisotskey HM (1975) Brain retraction pressure during intracranial procedures. Surg Forum 26:199-200

2. Albin MS, Bunegin L, Dujovny M, Bennett MH, Dujovny M, JannettaPJ (1976) Physiopathological responses to graded brain retraction pressure under induced hypotension. Proc. AANS Meeting, San Francisco, Paper No. 23

3. Albin MS, Bunegin L, Bennett MH, Dujovny M, Jannetta PJ (1977) Clinical and experimental brain retraction pressure monitoring. Acta Neurolog Scand Suppl 64, 56:522-523

4. Bennett MH, Bunegin L, Albin MS, Dujovny M, Hellstrom H,Jannetta PJ (1977) Evoked potential correlates of graded brain retraction pressure. Stroke 8:487-492

5. Laha RK, Dujovny M, Rao S, Barrionuevo PS, Bunegin L, Hellstrom HR Albin MS, Taylor FH (1979 to be published) Cerebellar retraction: Significance and Sequelae. Surg Neurol

6. Marcus ML, Heistad DD, Ehrhardt JD, Abboud FM (1976) Total and regional cerebral blood flow measurement with 7-10-, 15-, 25-, and 50 µm microspheres. J Appl Physiol 40:501-507

Supported in part by NINCDS Grant No. 1531601.

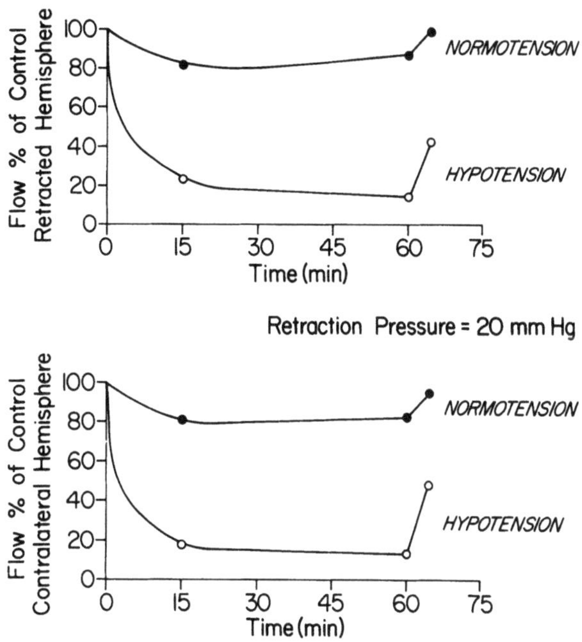

Fig. 1. Local cortical flow (cortical area directly beneath retractor blade and similar geography on non-retracted contralateral cortex). BRP at 20 torr for 60 min. under normotension (90-125 torr) and induced hypotension (55 torr using sodium nitroprusside).

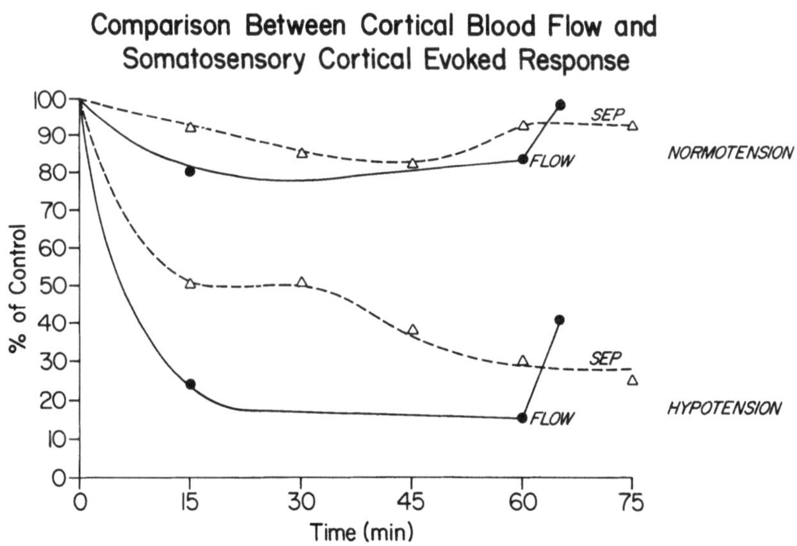

Fig. 2. Somatosensory evoked potential and local cortical flow compared as percentage of control against time. BRP of 20 torr for 60 min under normotension and induced hypotension.

ELECTROPHYSIOLOGICAL CHANGES ASSOCIATED WITH LOCAL BRAIN COMPRESSION

S. FUJIMOTO, H. KUYAMA, K. NISHIMOTO, T. AKIOKA, S. NAGAO, AND A. NISHIMOTO

Introduction

Brain retraction is a mandatory neurosurgical maneuver. However its electrophysiological studies are scanty. Changes in somatosensory evoked potential (SEP) with median nerve stimulation and cortical blood flow (CoBF) measured by hydrogen clearance method following brain retraction with graded local compression pressure (LCP), were studied in dogs.

Material and method

Under light ketamine anesthesia, animals were paralyzed with succinylcholine chloride. Ventilation was controlled to maintain arterial blood gas and pH at normal levels. As the first step, changes in SEP CoBF and pathological findings following reduction of cerebral perfusion pressure (CPP) were studied. CPP was reduced by three different methods, namely, exsanguination (n=9), cisterna magna infusion of saline (n=11) and continuous local brain compression (n=11). CPP was decreased by 10 mmHg every 30 minutes. As the second step, intermittent local brain compression was performed. LCP at 20 mmHg (n=5) for 30 minute duration was consequently applied four times with five minute intermission periods during which time the pressure was completely released. In the same way, the procedures were done at varying levels of LCP, namely 40 (n=8), 60 (n=6) and 80 (n=6) mmHg respectively. Local brain compression with a brain spatula was applied at the primary somatosensory area after right frontotemporal craniectomy and opening of the dura. LCP was monitored by a polyethylene microballoon attached to the tip of the brain spatula.

Results

In the exsanguination group, N_1 amplitude abruptly began to decrease when CPP decreased to 40-50 mmHg (CoBF decreased to 65%) and was suppressed to 50% at 30-40 mmHg, and it was finally abolished when CPP became 20-30 mmHg (CoBF decreased to 45%). In contrast to exsanguination, cisterna magna infusion showed a decrease of N_1 amplitude when cisterna magna pressure (CMP) rose to 30-50 mmHg while CoBF remained actually unchanged. N_1 amplitude decreased to 50% when CMP rose to 70 mmHg (CPP, 70-80 mmHg), and became flat when CMP went beyond 110 mmHg (CPP, below 30 mmHg). Local compression decreased markedly both N_1 amplitude and CoBF, more than in the other two groups. N_1 amplitude decreased as soon as local compression was started, and was suppressed to 50% at 50 mmHg of LCP (CPP, 90-100 mmHg) (Figure 1). In these animals, there was a shift of midline structures and distortion of brain tissue adjacent to the compression site. Disruption of nerve fibres were also demonstrated histologically at the compression site. During intermittent compression at the levels of 40, 60 and 80 mmHg of LCP, the more the number of repetitive compressions were increased at each pressure level or the more LCP was raised, the more both N_1 amplitude and CoBF decreased. At 60 and 80 mmHg of LCP, N_1 amplitude decreased to 35 and 11% during compression and remained reduced to 70 and 35% respectively at two hours after compression ceased (Figure 2). When N_1 amplitude was reduced by less than 50% of control during compression (n=12), it recovered to 101% at two hours after compression was released. However when N_1 amplitude was reduced more than 50% (n=11), it remained reduced to 55%. In these dogs, the compression area showed histologically, cortical microhemorrhage and edema.

Discussion

In the exsanguination group, as reported in middle cerebral artery occlusion (1), there was a threshold type relationship between N_1 amplitude of SEP and CoBF. This suggests that neuronal suppression is mainly attributed to a reduction of cerebral blood flow. In the continuous compression group, both N_1 amplitude and CoBF decreased more markedly than the other two groups. It is presumed that immediate occurrence of severe neuronal suppression is due to a disturbance of cerebral circulation and brain distortion secondary to mechanical compression. In the intermittent compressed group where LCP was more than 40 mmHg and/or N_1 amplitude decreased by more than 50% during compression, SEP did not recover for two hours after compression ceased.

Summary

Local compression decreased N_1 amplitude and CoBF more markedly than in the other two groups. And the more the number of repetitive compressions were increased at each pressure or the more LCP raised, the more both N_1 amplitude and CoBF decreased. It is concluded that LCP over 40 mmHg and/or reduction of N_1 amplitude by greater than 50% during brain retraction produce postoperative neuronal dysfunction and histological changes.

Reference

1. Branston NM, Symon L, Crockard HA, Pasztor E (1974) Relationship between the cortical evoked potential and local cortical blood flow following acute middle cerebral artery occlusion in baboon. Exp Neurol 45:195-208

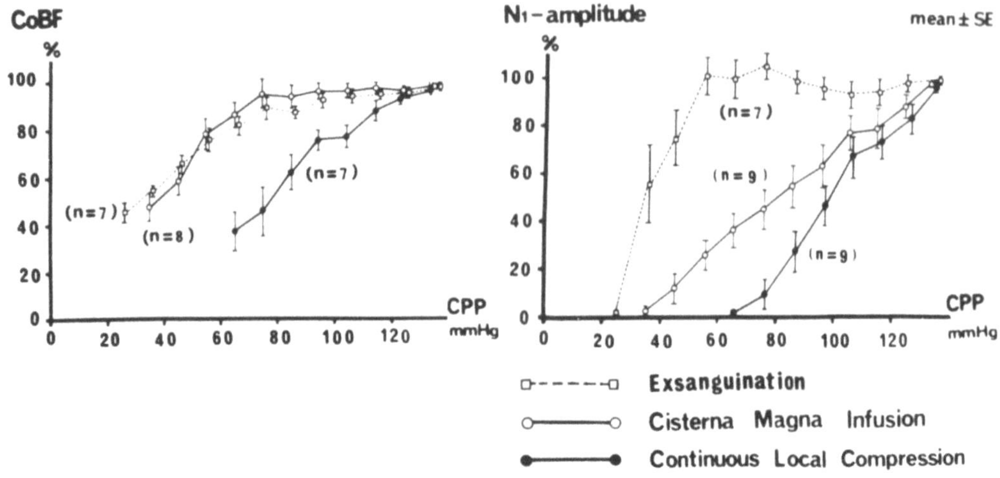

Fig. 1. Changes in SEP and CoBF following reduction of cerebral perfusion pressure. See text for discussion of results.

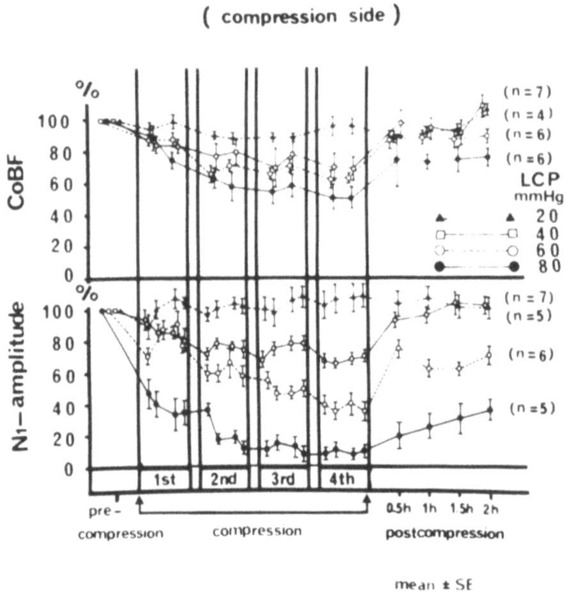

Fig. 2. Changes of SEP and CoBF following intermittent local compression. See text for discussion of results.

INFLUENCE OF MILD HYPERCAPNIA ON INTRACRANIAL PRESSURE IN ISCHEMIC, NON-INFARCTED BRAIN TISSUES

Y. NAKAGAWA, Y. L. YAMAMOTO, W. FEINDEL, E. MEYER, AND M. TSURU

Introduction

The authors clarified that mild hypercapnia between 43 and 55 mmHg is beneficial in enhancement of perfusion flow in the area of experimental "pure ischemia" without infarcted portion (Figure 1) (2,3,4). These results were obtained in experiments done on cats with closed cranium as well as dogs with open cranium. It is well known that elevation of arterial carbon dioxide pressure ($PaCO_2$) tends to induce an additional increase of ICP (1,5). Therefore, this study was designed to clarify how much ICP is increased under mild hypercapnia.

Methods

Six cats were anesthetized with intraperitoneal and intravenous pentobarbital and the ventilation was controlled by a respirator. In four cats, the trunk of the left middle cerebral artery was occluded by transorbital approach and the bone defect was sealed tightly. Two cats were subjected to control study without arterial occlusion. A flexible rubber tube with an inside diameter of 2 mm was placed in the subdural space of the left parietal area and connected to a pressure transducer. The hypercapnic state was maintained by regulation of the respiratory rate and volume with gas containing CO_2 of 5, 10 or 25%. The ICP monitoring was performed during six hours after occlusion of the middle cerebral artery.

Results

Maximum rise of ICP was 0.19 ± 0.03 mmHg (N=7) in control and 0.15 ± 0.03 mmHg (N=10) with arterial clipping, respectively, in response to 1 mmHg elevation of $PaCO_2$ (Figure 2). Therefore, the maximum rise of ICP to elevation of $PaCO_2$, for example, from 37 to 52 mmHg, was calculated only as 2.25 mmHg. After ICP reached the maximum, there was a gradual decline in pressure in all cases regardless of whether the artery was occluded or not. The ICP level, immediately before Co_2 inhalation was initiated, or after CO_2 with higher concentration was added, was at low level. There was no evidence of infaraction in all specimens at postmortem examination.

Discussion

Since the increase of ICP under hypercapnia of 43 to 55mmHg range was found to be minimum, an early increase of cortical blood flow measured with ^{85}Kr (hatched area in Figure 1) was judged to be the accepted result. The cause of the prolongation of the time interval to a maximum rise of ICP in the group with arterial occlusion appeared to be due to leakage of cerebrospinal fluid at the time of surgical procedure to the middle cerebral arteries.

Summary

The influence of mild hypercapnia on intracranial pressure in ischemic non-infarcted brain tissues was studied. The increase of ICP was slight in degree under hypercapnia between 43 and 55 mmHg, as far as the resting ICP remained at low level.

References

1. Kindt GW, Gosch HH (1972) Arterial PCO_2 effect at various levels of intracranial pressure. In: Brock M, Dietz H (eds) Intracranial Pressure. Springer, Berlin Heildelberg New York, p 210

2. Nakagawa Y, Yamamoto YL, Meyer E, Hodge CP, Feindel W (1978) A study of method for enhancement of perfusion flow in experimental cerebral ischemia - Part I: Effects of Hypercapnia. Neurol Med Chir (Tokyo) 18:Part II:713-723; - Part 2: Hypercapnia with mannitol. Neurol Med Chir (Tokyo 18:Part II:725-732

3. Nakagawa Y, Tsuru M, Yamamoto YL, Feindel W (1979) Enhancement of perfusion flow in an ischemic, non-infarcted brain tissue by mild hypercapnia. In: Gotoh F, Nagai H, Tazaki Y (eds) Cerebral Blood Flow and Metabolism. Munksgaard, Copenhagen, p 278

4. Nakagawa Y, Yamamoto YL, Meyer E, Hodge CP, Feindel W (to be published) Stroke

5. Teasdale GM, Lennox G, Lubcke H, Harper AM (1974) Intracranial pressure and intracerebral steal. In: Lundberg N, Ponten U, Brock M (eds) Intracranial Pressure II. Springer, Berlin Heidelberg New York, p 276

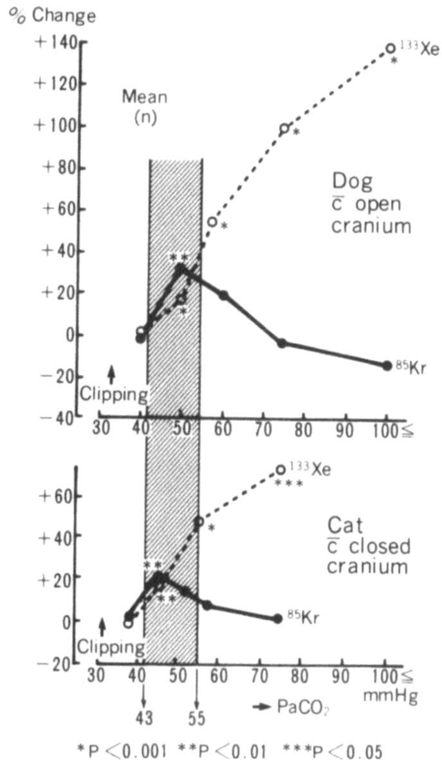

Figure 1. Changes of cortical blood flow measured with ^{85}Kr and regional cerebral blood flow measured with ^{133}Xe, under hypercapnia following occlusion of the left middle cerebral artery. This figure clearly indicates that hypercapnia between 43 and 55 mmHg (hatched area) is beneficial in enhancement of perfusion flow in the area of ischemia (3)

	Control N = 7	With Clipping N = 10	t-Test
Increase of ICP (mmHg) / Increase of $PaCO_2$ (mmHg)	0.19 ± 0.03	0.15 ± 0.03	ns
Time Interval up to Maximum Rise of ICP (Minutes)	7.7 ± 0.8	13.0 ± 1.0	$p < 0.001$
ICP before CO_2 Inhalation (mmHg)	9.7 ± 1.0	7.8 ± 0.8	ns

Figure 2. Degree of increase of intracranial pressure (ICP) following CO_2 inhalation.

SIMULTANEOUS SUBACUTE MEASUREMENT OF ICP AND BRAIN O_2 AVAILABILITY

R.B.MORAWETZ, H.L.MITCHEM, E.R.STRONG, J.G.GALBRAITH, AND J.H.HALSEY

Introduction

Inadequate oxygen delivery to brain tissue represents an important component of the deleterious effect of raised intracranial pressure (ICP). In an effort to develop techniques for direct assessment of brain tissue oxygenation, a ventricular catheter has been constructed which allows simultaneous continuous measurement of ICP and focal oxygen availability. A description of the device and initial experience with it are presented.

Materials and methods

A standard, commercially available ventricular catheter has been modified by the addition of four platinum electrodes along its shaft so that when the tip of the catheter lies within the lumen of a lateral ventricle the electrodes are in contact with brain tissue along its shaft, chiefly white matter. The electrodes are constructed of .003 inch bare platinum wire (90% platinum, 10% iridium), and each electrode can be monitored independently. O_2 availability (O_2a) is measured (1,2) continuously at the four electrodes using a polarographic technique, while ICP is measured (4) using a standard pressure transducer. Introduction and use of the catheter carry no increased risk beyond that inherent in placement of any ventricular catheter.

Ten hydrocephalic children requiring a ventricular catheter have been studied. Indications for ventriculostomy were evaluation of shunt function in eight patients, and treatment of shunt infection in two patients. The catheters were inserted through burr holes using standard techniques, with a silver wire suture in the skin to serve as a reference. The patients were monitored in the waking state while breathing spontaneously during the 24 hours immediately following catheter placement.

During monitoring selected patients were given the following gas mixtures by face mask: 95% O_2 + 5% CO_2; 20% O_2 + 5% CO_2 + 75% N_2; 100% O_2; and room air. Each of the first three gas mixtures was given for a period of 20 minutes, in every case preceded and followed by at least 20 minutes of room air. Measurements were made with the ventricular catheter closed, and in some cases a separate set of measurements was made with the catheter open to drainage set at 20 cm. above ventricular level.

Discussion

Polarographic measurement (3) of oxygen availability (O_2a) is based on the phenomenon of formation of a high resistance layer between tissue and a noble metal electrode, in this case platinum, which hinders electron flow from the electrode through the tissue to a reference electrode, in this case a silver wire. Electrodes are polarized at -600 millivolts and at this voltage O_2 in the region of the electrode act as an electron acceptor. Current flowing through the electrode (O_2a) is then proportional to(O_2) in the region of the electrode as the following reactions occur:

$$O_2 + 2H_2O + 2e^- \rightarrow H_2O_2 + 2OH^-$$

$$H_2O_2 + 2e^- \rightarrow 2OH^-$$

The use of platinum electrodes provides a continuous measurement of O_2 availability. All four electrodes can be monitored simultaneously and independently. A single electrode was chosen for presentation in the examples illustrated. Oxygen current tracings from each of the four electrodes generally moved together, though differences in response time and magnitude of change were seen. We have utilized the necessity of ventricular catheter placement in certain patients to allow placement of intraparenchymal platinum electrodes. The subacute timing of the measurements means that a layer of devitalized tissue lies in contact with the electrodes, providing a diffusion barrier to the passage of oxygen from viable tissue to the electrode. Also, in some cases electrodes may have been surrounded by CSF. Nevertheless, stable and reproducible measurements have been possible probably due to the large size of the electrodes. The layer of injured or non-viable tissue adjacent to the electrodes may explain the lack of response to 5% CO_2 inhalation observed. However, other workers (5) using microelectrodes have reported no difference in brain tissue pO_2 when cats were ventilated with 95% O_2 + 5% CO_2 versus that seen with 100% O_2.

The reciprocal relationship between ICP and O_2a is most apparent in patients with restricted intracranial compliance. These observations suggest that tissue oxygenation may fall promptly and dramatically during periods of elevated ICP. The marked response to increase in inspired O_2 concentration may have important implications in the treatment of brain injured patients.

Results

The following observations were made:

1. Inhalation of 100%O_2 produced an increase in O_2a in every patient regardless of the level of ICP. However, rapidly rising ICP, as seen during "A" waves, could reduce or reverse the expected rise in O_2a (Figure 1, upper).
2. 5% CO_2 inhalation alone produced no increase in O_2a (Figure 2, lower). No difference was seen between the effects 5% CO_2 + 95%O_2, and 100% O_2 (both producing an increase in O_2a), if ICP remained constant (Figure 2, upper). In patients with restricted intracranial compliance 5% CO_2 + 95% O_2 produced "A" waves of LUNDBERG (4) with a fall in O_2a (Figure 1, lower), presumably due to the vasodilator effect of CO_2.
3. The appearance of spontaneous "A" waves (patients breathing room air or 100% O_2) was always accompanied by a fall in O_2a.
4. Patients with restriction of intracranial compliance as demonstrated by appearance of spontaneous "A" waves showed a rise in O_2a with opening of their ventricular drains and a fall in O_2a with drain closure. Patients with "normal" ICP tracings showed no changes in O_2a with drain opening or closure.

5. No change in O_2a was seen prior to appearance of "A" waves, whether spontaneous or induced by 5% CO_2 inhalation.

Summary

Brain O_2a measurements are possible in patients requiring ventricular catheterization at no increased risk to the patient.

5% CO_2 inhalation at normal and at elevated ICP did not produce any rise in brain O_2a. Conversely, the resultant rise in ICP tended to result in a fall in O_2a when compliance was compromised.

100% O_2 inhalation resulted in increased brain O_2a at all levels of ICP except during plateau waves.

References

1. Halsay JH, Clark LC (1970) Some regional circulatory abnormalities following experimental cerebral infarction. Neurol 20:238-246

2. Halsey JH, Galbraith JG, Strong ER, Capra N (1972) A method for monitoring oxygen availability in brain. The Alabama J of Med Sciences 9:444-448

3. Kotchoff JM, Lingare JJ (1952) Polarography. Interscience Publishers, New York London

4. Lundberg N (1960) Continuous recording and control of ventricular fluid pressure in neurosurgical practice. Acta Psych Neurol Scand, Suppl 149, 36:1-193

5. Whalen WJ, Ganfield R, Nair P (1970) Effects of breathing O_2 or $O_2 + CO_2$ and of the injection of neurohumors on the pO_2 of cat cerebral cortex. Stroke 1:194-200

Supported in part by NINCDS Grant # NS08802-10.

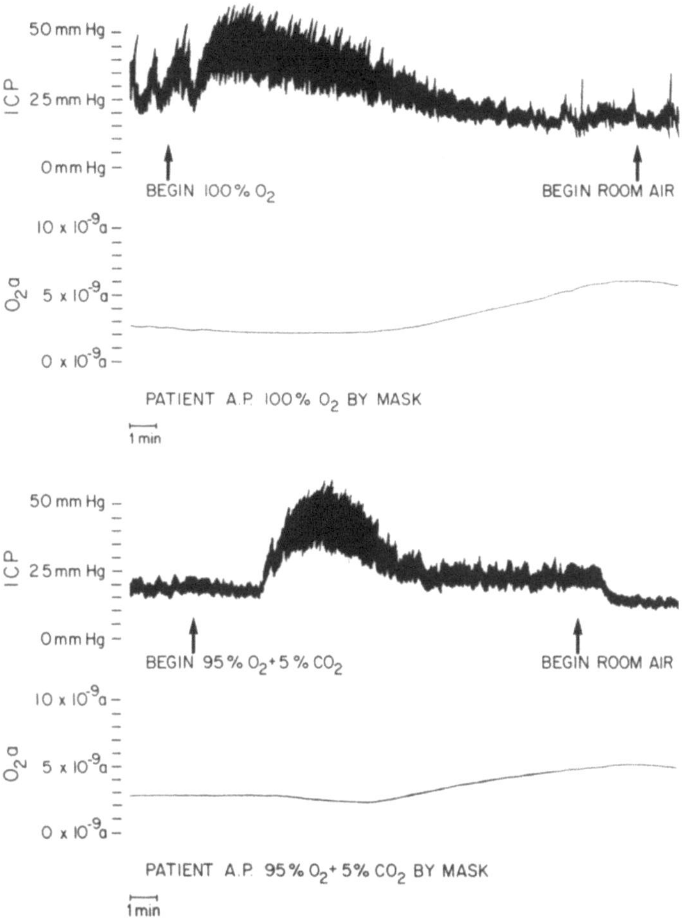

Fig. 1. These records from a hydrocephalic child showed spontaneous "A" and "B" waves during ICP monitoring. The upper tracing shows the appearance of a spontaneous "A" wave at the time the patient was switched from room air to 100% O_2. This resulted in a slight fall in O_2a during the "A" wave, followed by a rise in O_2a as ICP fell. The lower tracing shows an "A" wave produced by inhalation of 95% + 5% CO_2. O_2a fell briefly, then rose as ICP fell. Note that O_2a rises due to 95% O_2, despite an ICP at a higher level due to 5% CO_2.

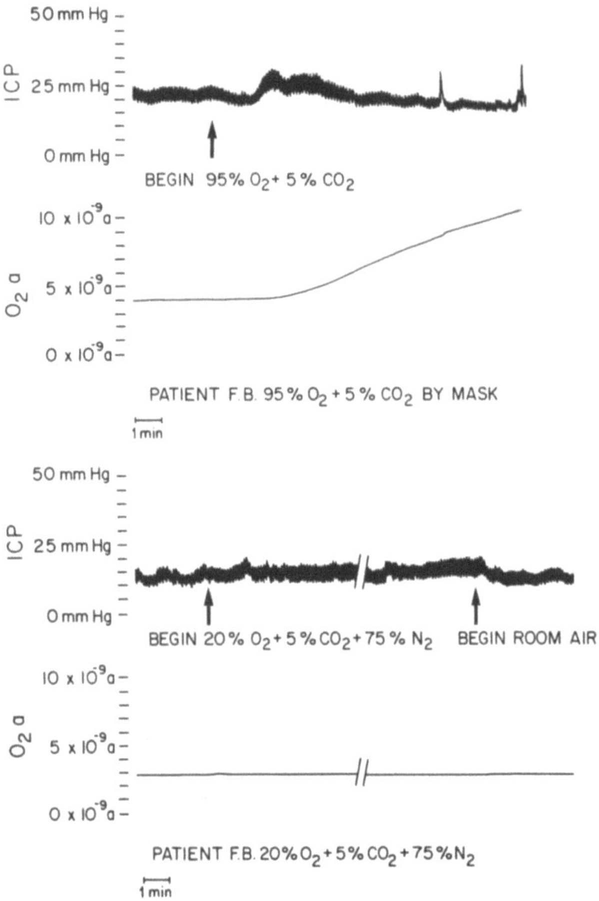

Fig. 2. These records were made in another hydrocephalic child having a functioning ventriculoperitoneal shunt. The upper tracing shows a transient small increase in ICP after the child was switched from room air to 95% O_2 + 5% CO_2. O_2a rose dramatically due to 95% O_2. The lower tracing shows no significant change in ICP or O_2a after the child was switched from room air to 20% O_2 + 5% CO_2 + 75% N_2, and then back to room air.

INTRACRANIAL DYNAMICS ASSOCIATED WITH EXPERIMENTALLY INDUCED PRESSURE WAVES

H. KUCHIWAKI, M. FURUSE, T. NAKAYA, K. TOYAMA, A. IKEYAMA, M. HASUO, M. TERAOKA, AND N. KAGEYAMA

Introduction

The present study was an attempt to induce pressure waves associated with intracranial expanding processes and to examine correlation between changes in intracranial pressure and other related phenomena

Material and methods

Twenty-four adult mongrel dogs were anesthetized with thiamylal-sodium (10-12 mg/kg in total doses), intubated and maintained under spontaneous respiration. Intracranial mass lesions were made by manual intraparenchymal injection of 1) 2 ml of bioresin (6 dogs); homologous blood 2) in unilateral cerebral hemisphere (5 dogs) and 3) in bifrontal lobes (13 dogs). Parameters, including epidural pressure (EDP), respiratory movement by means of impedance pneumograph (RESP), endotidal CO_2 concentration, systemic arterail pressure (SAP), pressure in transverse sinus (Pts) and central venous pressure (CVP). Changes in these parameters were polygraphically recorded throughout the experiments. At the end of experiments, 10-15 ml/kg of carbon black suspension was administered for the microcirculatory study in various stages of pressure oscillation.

Results

Pressure waves appeared in 17 out of 24 dogs, being dominant in bifrontal mass lesions. Pressure oscillations started from the period 2 to 3 hours after lesions (pressure range: 12-40 mmHg). As EDP increased, the oscillation of EDP was gradually transformed into more definitely large pressure waves in the period between 4 and 7 hours. With a further rise in EDP, in the range from 52 to 110 mmHg, they shifted to sustained high pressure without any evidence of rhythmic pressure oscillation.

Occurrence of each pressure oscillation was preceded by a small fall in SAP (10-20 mmHg) and a simultaneous weakening of respiratory movement. No increase of CO_2 in both endtidal air and arterial blood was detected before and after each pressure oscillation. Corresponding to rapid decrease in EDP, SAP as well as respiratory movement instantly returned to previous level (Fig 1).

In the initial stage of increased EDP, a positively synchronized oscillation in Pts was observed in correspondence to the EDP oscillation. In In higher EDP level of typical pressure waves, however, they were accompanied by an adverse decrease in pulse amplitude of sinus pressures. Furthermore, long-lasting plateau waves were accompanied by rapid and continued falls of Pts (Fig 2). During these processes, CVP remained constant. This indicated that disturbances in cerebral venous outflow corresponded to formation of large pressure waves.

Microcirculatory study disclosed fairly preserved tissue perfusion with scattered nonfilling of varying degrees during the stage of pressure waves. This contrasted to diffuse nonfilling in the cerebrum and upper brainstem in the later stage of sustained high pressure.

Discussion

The present study indicated that simultaneous changes in SAP as well as respiratory movement occur consistently corresponding to pressure waves, as noted in clinical study (1). Thereby no distinction in pCO_2 value was detected between the period of plateau waves and the resting level of EDP. This may suggest a possible role of dysfunction of brainstem in the formation of oscillating pressure. It is also interesting that such pressure waves occur under the condition of a fairly preserved perfusion in the cerebrum and upper brainstem, as contrasted to almost total nonfilling in highly sustained pressure without pressure oscillation. These findings also support an initiating role of brainstem, although the exact site and mecahnism remain still undetermined.

Interestingly the mode of sinus pressure oscillation relating to pressure waves in higher EDP differs from that in relatively lower EDP. Decreased Pts level corresponding to large pressure waves likely reveals disturbance or blockage of venous outflow from the cranial cavity. Presumably the duration and pattern of pressure waves are influenced by the states of cerebral venous outflow.

Reference

1. Furuse M, Ikeyama A, Mabe H, Hasuo M, Kuchiwaki H, Nakaya T, Toyama K, Teraoka M, Nagai H, Kageyama N (1979) Relationship between rapid variations in intracranial pressure and changes in respiratory pattern during postoperative monitoring. Neurologia Med Chir (Tokyo) 19:9-16

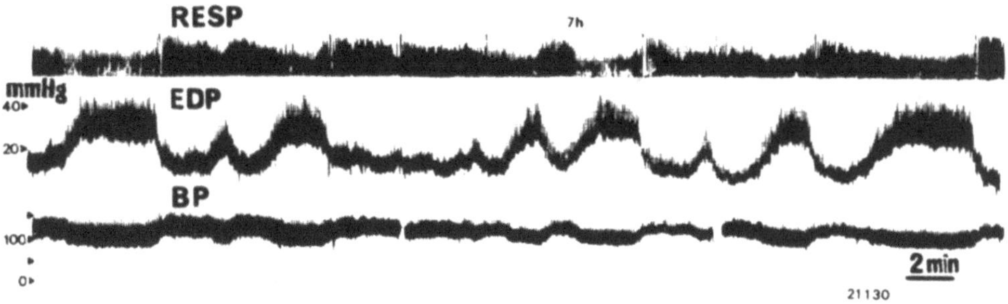

Fig. 1. A polygraphic recording of pressure waves 7 hours after making lesion. Pressure waves appear concomitant with suppression in respiratory movement and blood pressure level.

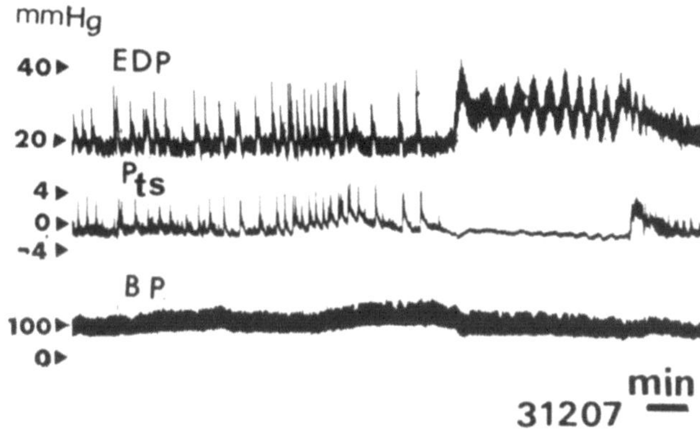

Fig. 2. Changes in epidural pressure and transverse sinus pressure (Pts) associated with occurrence of pressure waves. Note the decrease in sinus pressure during a long-lasting pressure wave.

SYMPATHETIC ROLE OF POSTERIOR HYPOTHALAMUS IN THE DEVELOPMENT OF ACUTE BRAIN SWELLING

Y. NAKAGAWA, M. TSURU, K. OHTUSKA, AND M. MOTOMIYA

Introduction

The purpose of this experiment is to clarify a sympathetic role of the posterior hypothalamusto the cerebral arteries in the development of vasomotor paralysis leading to acute brain swelling (1,2).

Materials and methods (3)

Thirty-two adult mongrel dogs were anesthetized with intravenous thyamyl sodium and $PaCO_2$ and PaO_2 were maintained in the normal range. The intracranial pressure (ICP) was measured by means of a small rubber balloon containing 0.03 cc of water inserted in the posterior parietal subdural space. After insertion of needle, the hypothalamus was destroyed by coagulation for 36 or 72 seconds; the same area was coagulated twice for the same selected time so as to be sure of complete destruction. Before and after insertion of the coagulation needle in the hypothalamus, and also after each coagulation, the systemic arterial (SAP) was elevated by intravenous injection of norepinephrine (NR) ($f \times 10^{-3}$mg/kg) to evaluate whether the ICP increased in accordance.with elevation of SAP. Experiments in 21 dogs were performed under normal ICP, while in five dogs, the ICP was elevated to 300 to 400 mmH_2O (22-30 mmHg), by inflation of a balloon placed over the dura. In the other six dogs under normal ICP, the rCBF in the frontal hemisphere ipsilateral to the destroyed hypothalamus were measured by the hydrogen clearance method before and after coagulation of the hypothalamus.

Results (3)

The extent of the lesion was approximately 7 mm in diameter in all dogs, regardless of the duration of coagulation. The nuclei of posterior hypothalami and dorsomedialis hypothalami (listed under "hypothalamus posterior") were coagulated on one or both sides in all cases. ΔICP/ΔMAP (MAP: Mean Systemic Arterial Pressure) after each procedure increased regardless of normal or elevated ICP (Figure 1) or of uni- or bilateral lesions of the hypothalamus. The correlation between ΔICP/ΔMAP and resting level of ICP was linear and reproducible as far as the resting ICP remained at less than 30 mmHg. Evaluation under higher ICP level than 30 mmHg was not performed. In addition ΔrCBF/ΔMAP after each procedure was not significantly increased following destruction of the hypothalamus.

Discussion

It is very important to clarify whether or not the tonicity of cerebral arteries is regulated by autonomic nervous system of central origin, independent of superior cervical sympathetic system, since studies of this kind eventually contribute to resolution of pathogenesis of vasomotor paralysis and appearance of plateau waves. However, the destruction of posterior portion of the hypothalamus did not cause a change in tonicity of the cerebral arteries. The fact that the ΔICP/ΔMAP and the resting ICP at the time of injection of norepinephrine correlated linearly, also suggests that autoregulation at the time of injection of norepinephrine remained intact. These results indicate that dysfunction of posterior hypothalamus does not play a specific role in the development of vasomotor paralysis leading to acute brain swelling, under conditions of normal or moderately raised ICP with normal $PaCO_2$ levels (3,4).

Summary

Using dogs, the sympathetic role of the posterior hypothalamus in the tonicity of intracerebral arteries was investigated by making destructive stereotaxic lesions in the corresponding areas. The results obtained did not prove a sympathetic role of the posterior hypothalamus to the cerebral arteries.

References

1. Ishii S, Takagi S, Sakurada O, Chigasaki H (1975) Analysis of factors contributing to cerebrovascular autoregulation. In: Lundberg N, Ponten U, Brock M (eds) Intracranial Pressure II. Springer, Berlin Heidelberg New York, p 268

2. Langfitt TW, Weinstein JD, Kassell NF (1965) Cerebral vasomotor paralysis produced by intracranial hypertension. Neurol 15:622-641

3. Nakagawa Y, Motomiya M, Tsuru M, Bando M. Tabata M (1977) Role of the posterior hypothalamus in the development of acute brain swelling. J Neurosurg 46:723-730

4. Nakagawa Y, Tsuru M, Ohtsuka K (1979) Behavior of the intracranial vascular tone following destruction of posterior thalamus. In: Gotoh F, Nagai H, Taxaki Y (eds) Cerebral Blood Flow and Metabolism. Munksgaard, Copenhagen, p 178

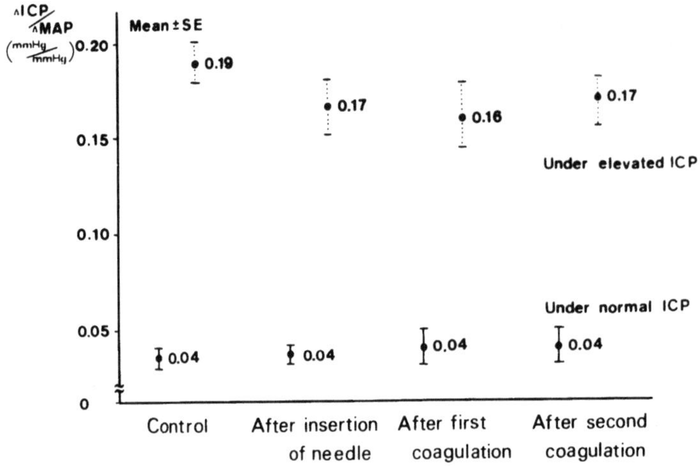

Figure 1

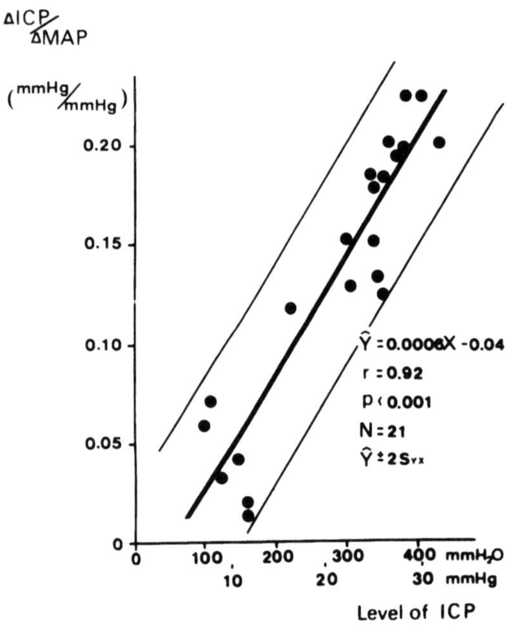

Figure 2

THE CSF PULSE PRESSURE IN RELATION TO INTRACRANIAL ELASTANCE AND FAILURE OF AUTOREGULATION

J.H.M. VAN EIJNDHOVEN, C.J.J.AVEZAAT, AND D.J.WYPER

Introduction

Analogous to the volume-pressure response (VPR), the CSF pulse pressure (CSFPP) is determined by two factors (1): 1. the transient increase in cerebral blood volume per cardiac cycle (ΔV); and 2. the shape of the craniospinal volume-pressure (V/P) curve. The CSFPP can therefore be used as a measure of craniospinal elastance, provided ΔV is constant. Observations in patients have shown a linear relationship between CSFPP and intracranial pressure (ICP) implying a constant ΔV in the individual patient (2). At elevated ICP, however, some authors (2,3,4) have found a break point in this relationship above which the CSFPP increased more rapidly. The meaning of this break point is not yet fully understood. In order to study the concept of CSFPP as a parameter of craniospinal elastance, CSFPP was compared with VPR during cerebral compression in dogs. Special attention was paid to the occurrence of a break point and its physiological significance.

Material and methods

In 6 anesthetized, ventilated and normocapnic dogs, extradural balloons were inflated at a steady rate of 1 ml/15 min until ICP approached arterial pressure. Ventricular fluid pressure (VFP), cisterna magna pressure and systemic arterial pressure (SAP) were continuously recorded. Each 5 minutes VPR was measured by injecting an aliquot of 0.05 ml into the ventricle. The CSFPP before and after each V/P test was related to the pre- and post-injection VFP. The data were analyzed on the basis of a mono-exponential V/P function. From this function the relationships of both CSFPP and VRP with the ICP were derived (1,5).

$$\Delta P = \{P - P_0\} \{\exp (E_1 \ \Delta V) - 1\}$$

where ΔP = CSFPP or VPR, P = ICP, E_1 = elastance coefficient, a constant defining the slope of the V/P curve, ΔV = transient increase in cerebral blood volume per cardiac cycle or injected volume during a V/P test and P_0 = a constant equal to the intercept of this function with the pressure axis. This is a linear function if E_1 and ΔV are constant in which case these parameters can be computed from the slopes of the VPR-ICP and CSFPP-ICP relationships.

Results

Both VPR and CSFPP showed a linear relationship with the VFP with a break point occurring at the same pressure (Fig. 1). Above this break point both variables behaved differently: VPR remained constant, whereas CSFPP continued to increase linearly and even steeper than before. A second break point was observed at the level of the blood pressure, above which VPR started to rise again and CSFPP did no longer increase. This last pressure range was not further studied. The break point could not be attributed to changes in arterial pressure, arterial pulse pressure or heart rate. These variables remained fairly constant (Table I). Nor was the break point related to the occurrence of transtentorial herniation. The linear relationships below the break point implicate a constant E_I, in agreement with a mono-exponential V/P model, and a constant ΔV (Table I). Above the break point, however, the constant VPR implies a linear V/P relationship and the increase in CSFPP consequently indicates a continuous increase of ΔV with rising ICP.

Discussion

The results of this study demonstrate that between individuals the CSFPP is not an accurate measure of the V/P relationships, because of the biological variation in ΔV. However, under controlled conditions in the same individual, ΔV remains constant during rising ICP and the CSFPP can consequently be used to monitor alterations in intracranial elastance. This is only true below a break point ICP, as beyond this point ΔV is no longer constant, which can be explained by considering the origin of ΔV (Fig. 2). The magnitude of ΔV is determined by the difference in pulsatile shape between the arterial inflow and venous outflow curves and is thus proportional to changes in inflow and outflow resistances. The inflow resistance is most dramatically reduced when vasoparesis occurs resulting in a sudden increase in ΔV. The break point may therefore be attributed to failure of autoregulation. ΔV continues to increase because of further compression of the venous outflow tract. It might be argued that also below the break point ΔV cannot be truly constant because of an autoregulatory decrease in inflow resistance. However, the effect on ΔV is apparently so small, that a constant ΔV is a valid approximation for this pressure range. The paradox of a decrease in cerebral blood flow (CBF) and an increase in ΔV when autoregulation becomes impaired can be solved by looking at the cerebral inflow section. A decrease in CBF does not necessarily mean a decrease in the arterial inflow of blood but merely an increase in arterial reflux (4). This also explains why large pulse pressures could still be recorded when the ICP was raised above the level of the blood pressure and CBF had completely ceased. In this case both in- and outflow take place at the arterial side. The finding of the conversion of the V/P curve from an exponential to a linear shape is in agreement with the results of LOFGREN (6), who reported a constant elastance at elevated ICP, using a rapid infusion technique. The time interval, in which the V/P curves were recorded was too short for the autoregulatory response to develop and these experiments were thus conducted under conditions of decreasing CBF. It may therefore be concluded that the V/P curve derives its exponential shape from the integrity of the autoregulatory mechanisms, yielding another argument in favor of relating the break point to failure of autoregulation.

During clinical ICP monitoring the relationship between CSFPP and ICP can be automatically processed and may thus be used as a continuous parameter of alterations in intracranial elastance. An important finding of this study was that a marked increase in CSFPP may indicate loss of autoregulation. In that case the VPR may be expected to be relatively low. Consequently, in non-autoregulating patients, the CSFPP is a more reliable parameter of the clinical state than the VPR.

Table 1. Systemic arterial pressure (SAP), systemic arterial pulse pressure (ΔSAP), heart rate (HR), volume change per cardiac cycle (ΔV), elastance coefficient (E_l) and elastance in relation to the ventricular fluid pressure (VFP) at the break point (M±SD)

	BELOW THE BREAK POINT				BREAK POINT		ABOVE THE BREAK POINT				
Animal No.	SAP mmHg	ΔSAP mmHg	HR beats/min	ΔV	E_l l/ml	VFP mmHg	SAP mmHg	ΔSAP mmHg	HR beats/min	Increase in ΔV ml/mmHg	Elastance mmHg/ml
1	160±8	56±8	114±11	0.047	1.9	66	145±12	54±6	114±12	0.0041	110
2	126±3	40±1	152±11	0.033	4.0	52	122±3	40±5	135±4	0.0013	142
3	119±6	34±2	132±3	0.082	1.5	42	120±5	35±2	135±3	0.0018	74
4	152±4	46±2	145±5	0.029	2.0	58	156±6	44±3	175±14	0.0010	114
5	136±3	54±7	165±2	0.072	1.5	60	131±9	50±2	168±2	0.0023	94
6	168±2	51±4	168±7	0.081	1.3	81	158±5	46±4	156±10	0.0027	64
Mean	143±19	47±9	146±21	0.057	2.0	60	139±17	45±7	147±23	0.0022	100

Summary

The interrelation between CSF pulse pressure and volume pressure response was studied during cerebral compression in dogs. Below a break point ICP, the CSF pulse pressure was shown to be a useful parameter to monitor changes in intracranial elastance. The break point was attributed to vasoparesis and failure of autoregulation. Above this pressure, CSF pulse pressure is a more reliable guide of a patient's clinical condition than the volume pressure response.

References

1. Eijndhoven JHM Van, Avezaat CJJ (this volume) The analogy between CSF pulse pressure and volume pressure response. Intracranial Pressure IV

2. Avezaat CJJ, Van Eijndhoven JHM, De Jong DA, Moolenaar WCJ (1976) A new method of monitoring intracranial volume pressure relationships. In: Beks JWF, Bosch DA, Brock M (eds) Intracranial Pressure III. Springer, Berlin Heidelberg New York, p 308

3. Janny P (1974) La surveillance de la pression intracranienne en neuro-chirurgie. Neuro-chirurgie 20:521-534

4. Nornes H, Aaslid R, Lindegaard KR (1977) Intracranial pressure dynamics in patients with intracranial hypertension. Acta Neurochir 38:177-186

5. Avezaat CJJ, Van Eijndhoven JHM, Wyper DJ (1979 to be published) The cerebrospinal fluid pulse pressure and the intracranial volume-pressure relationships. J Neurol Neurosurg and Psychiat

6. Lofgren J, Von Essen C, Zwetnow NN (1973) The pressure-volume curve of the cerebrospinal fluid space in dogs. Acta Neurol Scand 49:574-575

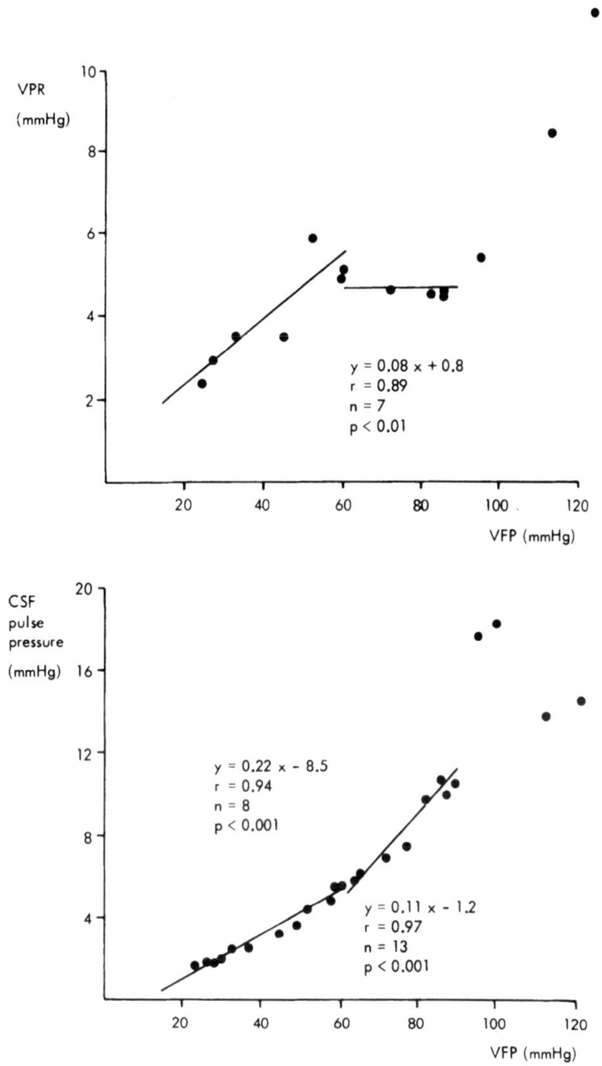

Fig. I. Volume pressue response (VPF) and CSF pulse pressure (CSFPP) plotted against the ventricular fluid pressure (VFP) in a single animal.

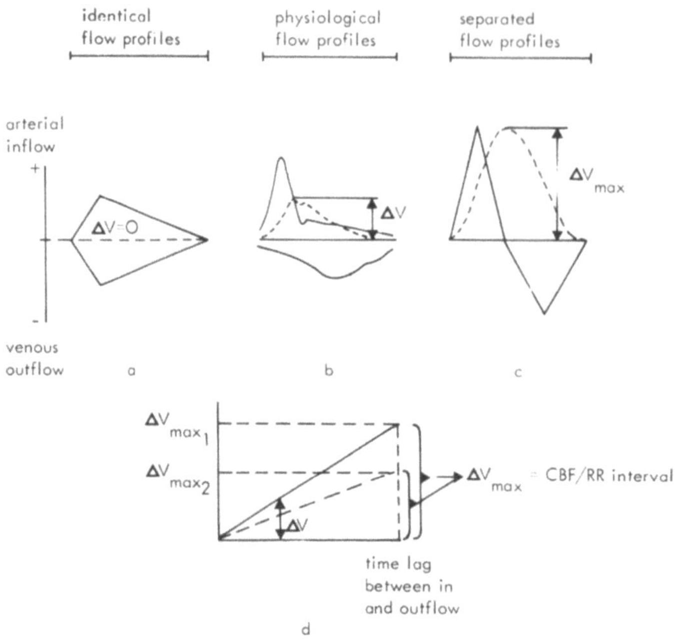

Fig. 2. Diagram illustrating the concept of the transient increase in intracranial blood volume per cardiac cycle (ΔV). The magnitude of ΔV (dashed line) is determined by the interaction between arterial in- and venous outflow. If the flow profiles were identical, ΔV would be nil (Fig 1a). If in- and outflow were completely separated ΔV would be maximal (Fig 1c). In the physiological situation the volume change is intermediate (Fig 1b). Fig 1 d demonstrated the effect of alterations in the cerebral blood flow (CBF) per cardiac cycle on ΔV. An increase in CBF results in a rise in ΔV.

EFFECTS OF HYPERCAPNIA AND SYSTEMIC ARTERIAL HYPO- AND HYPERTENSION ON THE INTERRELATION BETWEEN CSF PULSE PRESSURE AND VOLUME-PRESSURE RESPONSE

C.J.J.AVEZAAT, J.H.M. VAN EIJNDHOVEN, AND D.J.WYPER

Introduction

The interrelation between CSF pulse pressure (CSFPP) and volume-pressure response (VPR) has been previously described (1,2). These studies had been oriented toward clinical applicability: continuous monitoring of intracranial volume-pressure (V/P) relationships by means of CSFPP. A disturbing factor, however, is the variable volume change underlying CSFPP: the transient increase in cerebral blood volume per cardiac cycle (ΔV). The origin of ΔV was attributed to the difference between the pulsatile patterns of the cerebral arterial inflow and venous outflow of blood (1). Hemodynamic factors may thus be expected to affect ΔV and consequently CSFPP. An experimental study was therefore designed to investigate the effects of some major clinical variables, hypercapnia and arterial hypo- and hypertension, on the interrelation between CSFPP and VPR.

Material and methods

In 12 anesthetized, ventilated dogs extradural balloons were inflated at a steady rate of 1 ml/40 min. In 6 animals hypercapnia was intermittently induced by adding 5% CO_2 to the inspired gases. In the remaining animals arterial hypo- and hypertension were intermittently induced, throughout the experiment, by intravenous administration of trimethaphan and angiotension. At regular intervals VPR was measured by injection of 0.05 ml aliquots into the lateral ventricle and compared with the pre-injection CSFPP. The following equation was applied to the relationship between CSFPP and VPR:

$$\text{CSFPP} = \frac{\Delta V}{0.05}\ \text{VPR.}$$

Results

In each experimental condition VRP increased linearly with ventricular fluid pressure, until a break point was reached above which VPR remained constant (1). Only the data below the break point were included in the current study.

Hypercapnia. Both during normocapnia and during hypercapnia CSFPP showed a significant linear correlation with VPR (Fig. 1), which implies that in both conditions ΔV was constant. ΔV was computed from the slopes of the regression lines using the above equation. Hypercapnia produced a significantly larger ΔV: 0.09 ml compared to 0.06 ml during normocapnia (F-test applied to the regression lines: $P<0.01$). The difference in blood pressure and arterial pulse pressure between normo- and hypercapnia was not statistically significant.

Arterial hypo- and hypertension. The results of this series are shown in Figure 2. A decrease in ΔV with rising blood pressure was found: 0.07 ml, 0.05 ml and 0.03 ml. The difference between hypo- and hypertension was significant (F-test: $P<0.001$). The differences in ΔV could not be explained by changes in arterial pulse pressures, as these did not significantly differ (Fig. 2).

Discussion

The results of this study are in agreement with the previously developed concept on the origin of ΔV (1). Hypercapnia is a vasodilator stimulus and arterial hypotension induces vasodilatation as part of the autoregulatory mechanism. This results in a reduction of the arterial inflow resistance, by which the pulsatile pattern of the inflow of blood is changed in such a way that a larger intracranial volume change per cardiac cycle is produced. Arterial hypertension, representing an autoregulatory vasoconstrictor stimulus, produces the opposite effect. $PaCO_2$ and blood pressure are routinely monitored in patients in whom continuous intracranial pressure recording is indicated and information on changes in ΔV will thus be constantly available. On the basis of this information it will be possible to interpret changes in the CSFPP to intracranial pressure ratio in terms of changes in intracranial V/P relationships.

Summary

By comparing CSF pulse pressure with volume-pressure response under various experimental conditions, it was concluded that hypercapnia and arterial hypotension cause an increase, and arterial hypertension causes a decrease in the volume change underlying the CSF pulse pressure. These results contribute to a better understanding of the CSF pulse pressure as a parameter of intracranial elastance.

References

1. Avezaat CJJ, Van Eijndhoven JHM and Wyper DJ (to be published) The cerebrospinal fluid pulse pressure and the intracranial volume-pressure relationships. J Neurol Neurosurg Psychiat

2. Eijndhoven JHM Van, Avezaat CJJ(this volume) The analogy between CSF pulse pressure and volume-pressure response. Intracranial Pressure IV

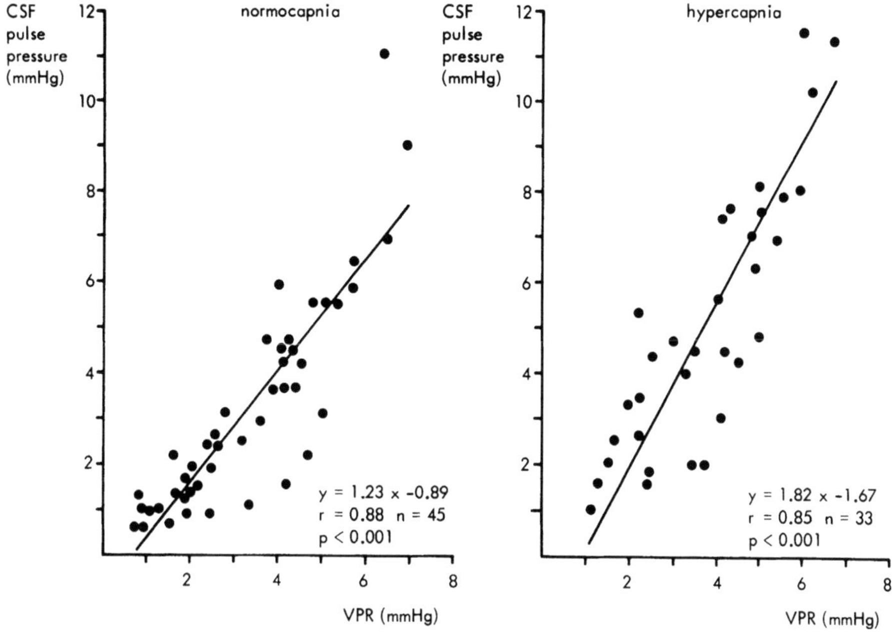

Fig. 1. Composite plots of CSF pulse pressure versus volume-pressure response (VP) during normocapnia (left: $PaCO_2$ = M±SD = 40.8±3.6 mmHg) and during hypercapnia (right; $PaCO_2$ = 57.9±5.5). The ventricular fluid pressure ranges were: 2 to 70 mmHg and 5 to 72 mmHg respectively. The difference between the gradients of the regression lines was statistically significant (F-test: $P < 0.01$).

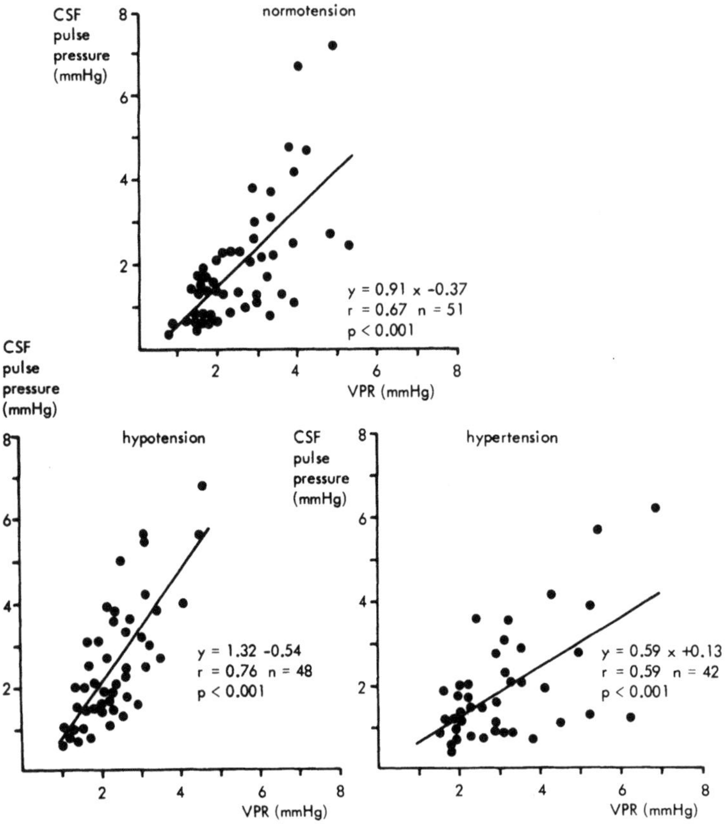

Fig. 2. Composite plots of CSF pulse pressure versus volume-pressure response (VPR) at 3 levels of systemic arterial pressure: 132.2±7.8 mmHg (M±SD: upper), 87.5±7.8 mmHg (lower left) and 173.2±11.0 mmHg (lower right). The corresponding arterial pulse pressures were: 35.1±8.9 mmHg, 30.9±7.0 mmHg and 35.2±13.8 mmHg. The ventricular fluid pressure ranges were 11 to 61 mmHg, 12 to 51 mmHg and 13 to 64 mmHg. The differences between the slopes of the regression lines attained the following levels of significance (F-test): $P < 0.1$ between normo- and hypotension and normo- and hypertension, $P < 0.01$ between hypo- and hypertension.

THE EFFECT OF BLOOD PRESSURE AND $PaCO_2$ UPON BULK COMPLIANCE (PVI)

H.TAKAGI, G.WALSTRA, A.MARMAROU, AND K.SHULMAN

Introduction

Bulk intracranial compliance reflects in part the relative distributions of CBV, CSF, and brain parenchyma. The pressure volume index (PVI) can be used to estimate the entire pressure volume (P-V) curve and to represent compliance as a single number regardless of intracranial pressure (ICP). The purpose of this present investigation is to examine the effect of changes in cerebrovascular dynamics upon PVI in the cat.

Material and methods

Nine adult cats weighing 2.5 to 5.0 kg were anesthetized with pentobarbital (30 mg/kg I.P), paralyzed with gallamine (20 mg/kg, I.V.), tracheostomized and mechanically ventilated on N_2O/O_2 gas mixture with a Harvard respirator. Mean arterial blood pressure (MABP), central venous pressure (CVP) and end tidal CO_2 tension (PCO_2) were monitored continuously. Arterial blood gases were examined frequently during each perturbation. The cisterna magna was cannulated with an 18 gauge needle and used for measuring cisterna magna pressure (CMP) and for bolus injection of fluid to measure PVI. Teflon coated platinum electrodes were inserted in both cerebral hemispheres to measure rCBF using the hydrogen polarographic techniques.

To examine the response of PVI to alterations of cerebral hemodynamics, changes in MABP and $PaCO_2$ were induced. First, MABP was elevated with intravenous levophed (40mg/500 cc), while concurrent exsanguination was used to lower MABP. $PaCO_2$ was controlled during this phase (30 to 32 torr). Incremental elevation of MABP (25-50 mmHg from previous steady state level) was maintained for 10 to 15 minutes. PVI determinations were repeated at each MABP plateau. Next, $PaCO_2$ was decreased by hyperventilation or increased by administration of 5%, 10% or 15% CO_2 or hypoventilation in 5-10 torr increments, while maintaining MABP (115-120 mmHg). PVI determinations were repeated at each plateau.

Following these manipulations, MABP was then elevated above 180mmHg to achieve breakthrough of autoregulation. rCBF measurements were used to confirm loss of autoregulation. PVI was repeated at various levels of MABP and $PaCO_2$.

Results

Autoregulating Animals (n = 7) The PVI was not affected by changes of MABP from 85 to 145 mmHg (Figure 1-A). The PVI was slightly, but significantly affected by changes of $PaCO_2$ ranging from 22-52 torr(Fig.2A).

Non-autoregulating animals (n = 4) The PVI was significantly altered by changes of MABP from 60 to 175mmHg(Fig 1-B). However, PVI did not change when CO_2 was altered over a range of 22-45 torr in these non-autoregulating animals. The linear regression for this group was PVI = 0.001 $PaCO_2$ + 0.72 (r = 0.069, n = 35, P >.01, not significant) (Figure 2-B)

Discussion

Our results show that PVI is affected quite differently by changes of MABP and $PaCO_2$ in autoregulating compared to non-autoregulating animals. During autoregulation, PVI is independent of MABP. Small but statistically significant changes of PVI occur with alterations of $PaCO_2$. When autoregulation is lost, the PVI reflects MABP changes, but is independent of $PaCO_2$. LOFGREN (2), using rapid infusion technique, reported that the P-Vcurve is shifted toward the left by BP changes (25 to 230 mmHg), but not by $PaCO_2$ (24 to 150 torr). When autoregulation was lost his results were similar to ours. Two differences may account for our different results: one, the difference in methods used to estimate the P-V curve, and the other is the extremes of $PaCO_2$ and MABP may have produced loss of autoregulation in these animals. Using the VPR, LEECH and MILLER (1) observed that at normalized BP, the VPR (reciprocal of compliance) did not change with blood pressure alterations from 45 to 178 mmHg. One inference, then, is that as the compensatory processes fails with ICP elevation, the pressure-volume relationship becomes dependent upon changes of blood pressure with loss of $PaCO_2$ responsivity.

During autoregulation, we suggest that CBV remains constant, while MABP is not transmitted to the venous capacitance vessels. Thus, PVI remains independent of MABP changes. However, $PaCO_2$ will increase the volume of the cerebral veins but without impeding the egress of blood from this capacitance system. PVI, which we believe in part assesses the ease of egress from the venous compartment, and also its ability to act as a capacitance system, would thus increase in this setting. When autoregulation is lost, MABP will be transmitted directly to the venous system with a concomitant elevation of transmural pressure. Egress of venous blood volume is impeded, thereby diminishing PVI. The effect of $PaCO_2$ on PVI may be abolished in the non-autoregulating animals because the vascular bed may have already overstretched and there is no further change of blood volume with $PaCO_2$ alterations.

Conclusion

The bulk intracranial compliance will remain independent of blood pressure, but be influenced significantly albeit small, by $PaCO_2$ when autoregulation of CBF is intact. When breakthrough occurs, intracranial compliance and CBF change in reciprocal fashion and become pressure-dependent with loss of $PaCO_2$ reactivity.

References

1. Leech P, Miller JD (1974) Intracranial volume pressure relationships during experimental brain compression in primates. 2. Effect of induced changes in systemic arterial pressure and cerebral blood flow. J Neurol Neurosurg & Psychiat 37:1099-1104

2. Lofgren J (1973) Effect of variations in arterial pressure and carbon dioxide tension on the cerebrospinal fluid pressure volume relationships. Acta Neurol Scand 49:57-69

(A)

(B)

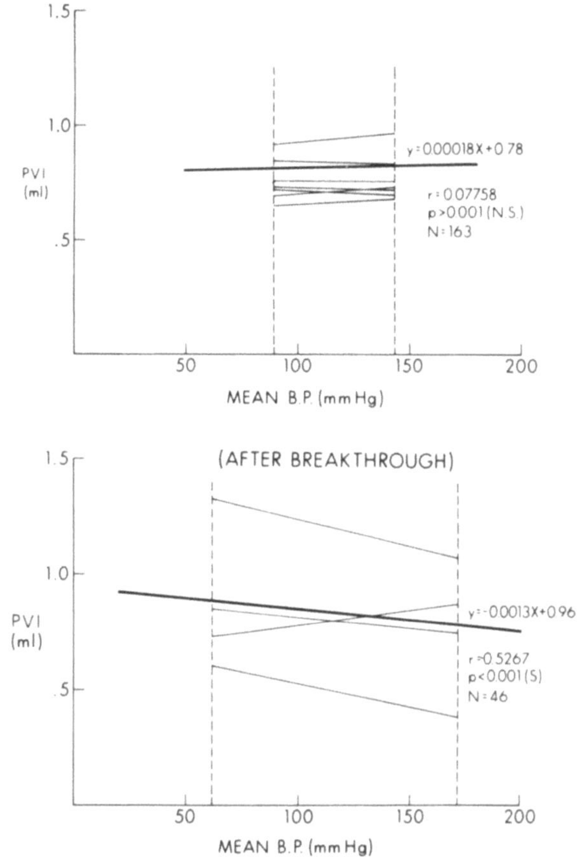

Fig. I. Linear regression of PVI vs MABP in auto and non-autoregulating animals. Data for all animals were randomized and computed as a single regression equation (A) autoregulating (B) non-autoregulating.

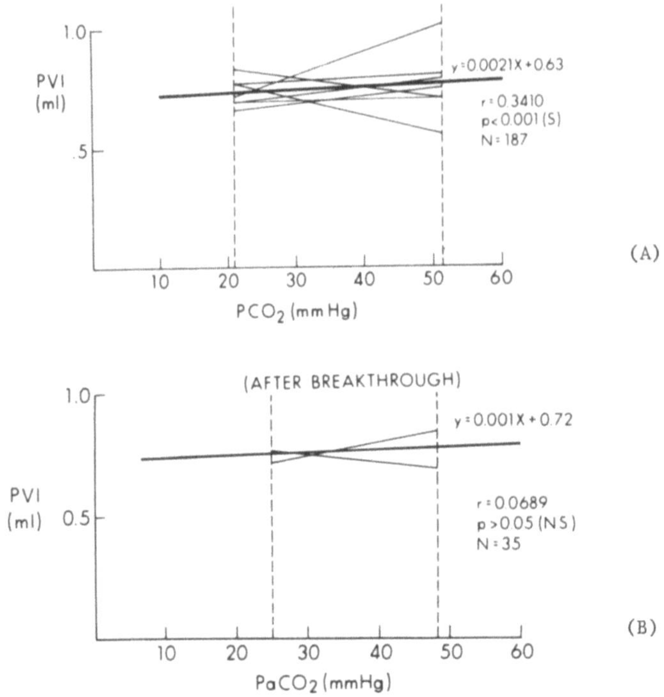

Fig. 2. Linear regression of PCO_2 and PVI. Tests of PVI during large transient changes of BP were excluded. (A) autoregulating (B) non-autoregulating.

SPECTRAL ANALYSIS OF INTRACRANIAL PRESSURE

H.D. PORTNOY AND M. CHOPP

Introduction

Utilizing spectral analysis an unknown system can be characterized by how it responds to a known input signal (1). The intracranial contents can be modeled as an unknown system in which the arterial pulse acts as the known input signal and the ICP pulse acts as the response or output of the system. This technique is utilized in this study to differentiate between an increase in ICP due to epidural balloon inflation (EBI) and intraventricular infusion (IVI).

Material and methods

Ten adult cats were anesthetized with pentobarbital (20 mgm/kg) and all incisions infiltrated with 1% lidocaine. Following tracheotomy and cannulation of the aorta and inferior vena cava, the animals were placed in a stereotaxic frame and mechanically ventilated after paralysis with an infusion of 0.2% succinylcholine. Both ventricles were cannulated and an epidural balloon placed in the right parieto-occipital region.

ICP was increased by alternate injections into the balloon and ventricle. The balloon was inflated by 0.2 ml increments until pupillary dilatation occurred. For each steady state ICP generated by the balloon inflation, the same level of ICP was produced by infusion of Ringer's lactate (RL) solution into the right ventricle after the balloon was deflated. Left ventricular and blood pressure (BP) waveforms were monitored (Tektronix 414) and recorded on an FM analog tape (Sangamo Sabre IV) and a dual strip chart recorder (Brush). After a steady state ICP level was attained, ICP and BP were recorded for 4 minutes following which 0.2 ml of RL was injected intraventricularly and compliance calculated by the method of MARMAROU (3). Spectral analysis was performed on the ICP and BP waveforms utilizing a spectrum analyzer (Hewlett Packard 3582A) and coherence (COH) and transfer functions (XFR) calculated. (Spectral analysis - a decomposition of a complex waveform into its frequency components. Coherence (COH) - the fraction of the system output power directly related to the input power at each component frequency. Transfer function XFR - the ratio of the output amplitude to input amplitude at each component frequency.) Spectral analysis was performed up to 20 Hz. Upon sacrifice the position of the ventricular cannulae were confirmed by injection of Evan's blue dye into the ventricles.

Results

The mean resting ICP was between 4 and 10 mmHg. The maximum mean steady state ICP at pupillary dilatation varied between 39 and 103mmHg with pupillary dilatation usually occurring with a 1.0 ml balloon volume.

Spectral analysis revealed that each waveform was composed of a fundamental and several harmonic frequencies (Fig. 1). A very high degree of coherence was obtained between BP and ICP waveforms at all frequencies and all levels of ICP (COH=0.8-1.0). The high level of coherence is suggested in Figure 1 by the nearly identical frequency components of both waveforms. Because variations in BP alone can induce variations in ICP it is necessary to normalize for any change in arterial input. This is accomplished by utilizing the XFR. The XFR is, therefore the critical parameter in describing the waveform changes within the cranial cavity.

In all animals the XFR determined at resting pressure could be distinguished from the XFR of the subsequent 0.2 ml EBI or IVI sequence even when the steady state ICP was the same.

Reliable XFR data was available for comparing EBI and IVI at the same ICP in 7 cats at 0.2 ml EBI, 5 cats at 0.4 ml, 8 cats at 0.6 ml, and 8 cats at 0.8 ml. At 0.2 ml IVI resulted in a greater XFR than EBI in all animals (Fig. 2). The XFR for EBI, however, was greater in 3 of 5 animals at 0.4 ml, 5 of 8 animals at 0.6 ml, and in 7 of 8 animals at 0.8 ml. In all the animals as the ICP increased so did the amplitude of the XFR (Fig. 2). In addition, with increasing ICP the XFR spectrum increased.

Compliance measurements at each steady state ICP level revealed no difference in compliance between EBI and IVI. All cats exhibited a decrease in compliance up to an ICP of approximately 15 mmHg and above this level the compliance remained relatively constant at 0.012±0.004 ml/mmHg.

Discussion

A system can be characterized by how it responds to an input function. In our model the unknown system is the intracranial contents and the arterial pulse is the known input. Variations in ICP waveform, the output, allows characterization of the system. If there is a change in the output for a given input this indicates a change in the system. The high COH of the various component frequencies of the intracranial and arterial pulses indicates that the intracranial pulse is, in fact, caused by the arterial pulse. With an increase in ICP there is a greater transfer of the component frequencies (Fig.2). At any given steady state level of ICP, there were differences related to whether the ICP elevation was a result of the EBI or IVI. This was readily discernable from the XFR but could likewise be seen by comparing the recorded waveforms as illustrated in Figures 1 and 2. The variations between these recordings indicate that the frequency components of the arterial pulse are being amplified differently, and, therefore, these recordings truly define different intracranial systems.

In contrast to these differences noted on spectral analysis, we were unable to distinguish any change in compliance between EBI and IVI at any given level of ICP, and there was no change in compliance above an ICP of 15 mmHg. Since the compliance at each level of ICP does not change when subjected to either EBI or IVI this implies that the mechanical properties of these systems are the same. This suggests that the difference in XFR are the result of vascular changes with alteration in cerebral blood flow. This is supported by the work of HEKMATPANAH (2) who found that EBI resulted in a decrease in cerebral perfusion.

Our experience in the laboratory led us to observe the waveforms in patients undergoing ICP monitoring. In patients who do not have an expanding mass or cerebral edema, the waveform shows an initial sharp rise and subsequent downward slope similar to the arterial pulse. (Fig. 3). As an expanding mass or edema develops, the waveform becomes more rounded. This can frequently be noted several hours before there are significant changes in the ICP. Though these changes can be seen visually, spectral analysis by on-line computer should enhance our ability to recognize these changes earlier and possibly enlighten us as to their origin.

Summary

Spectral analysis of the intracranial cavity was carried out in cats utilizing the arterial pulse as the known input signal and ICP pulse as the output. The effects of a progressive increase in ICP and the differences between EBI and IVI at the same steady state levels of ICP were evaluated. Changes in XFR were discernable with increasing ICP and between EBI and IVI even when the latter conditions failed to demonstrate differences in compliance. The evaluation of ICP by this technique on patients may have clinical value.

References

1. Bendat JS, Piersol AG (1971) Random Data: Analysis and Measurement Procedures. Wiley Interscience, New York Chichester Brisbane Toronto

2. Hekmatpanah J (1970) Cerebral circulation and perfusion in experimental increased intracranial pressure. J Neurosurg 32:21-29

3. Marmarou A, Shulman K, LaMorgese J (1975) Compartmental analysis of compliance and outflow resistance of the cerebrospinal fluid system. J Neurosurg 43:523-534

Work supported in part by a Research Grant from Crittenton Hospital, Rochester, Michigan; NIH-Biomedical Research Support Grant from Oakland University, Rochester, Mich.

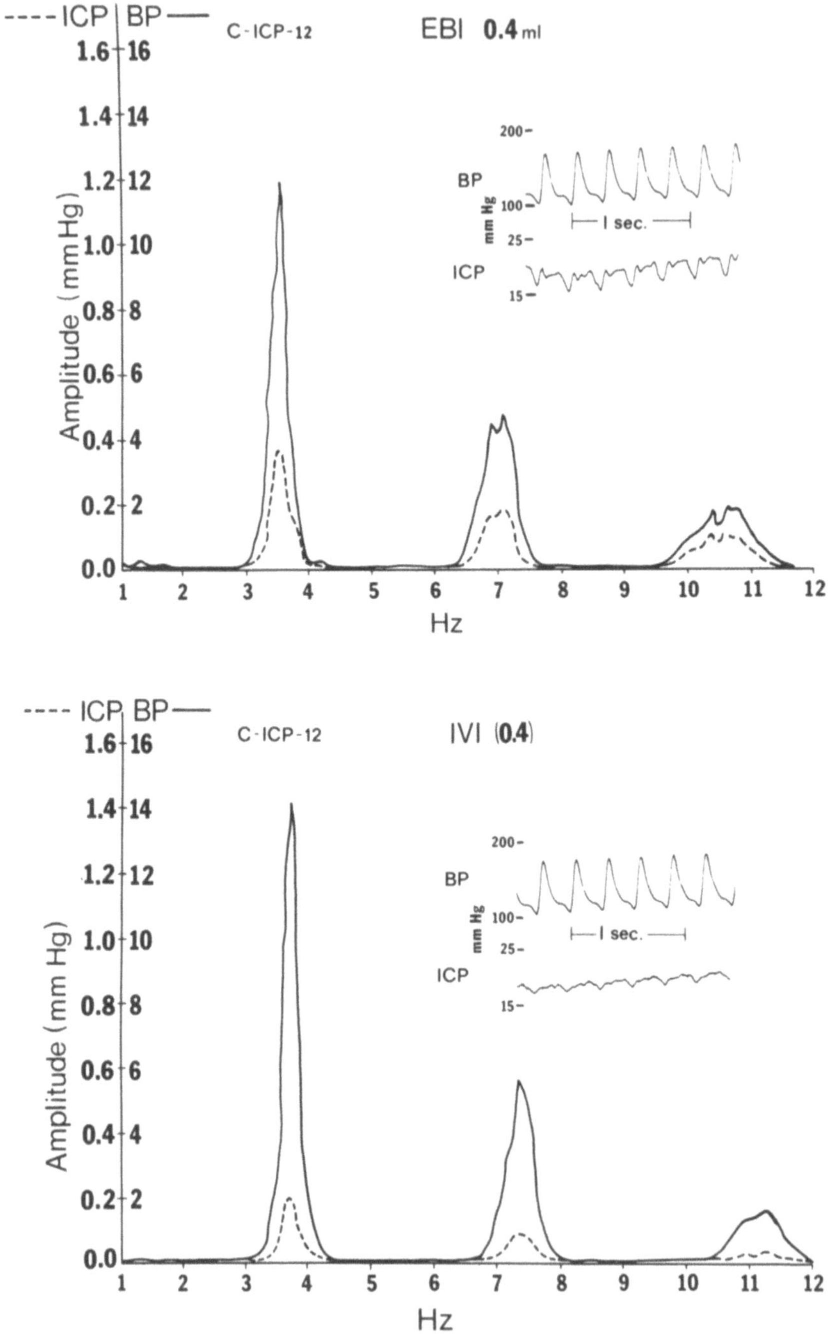

Fig. 1. Spectral analysis and strip chart recordings in typical animal for 0.4 ml EBI and corresponding IVI at same ICP. The frequency spectrum for BP and ICP are nearly identical. The EBI shows a greater proportion of the BP pulse amplitude reflected in the ICP pulse. In the strip chart recordings this is evidenced by the appearance of more structure in the ICP pulse in the EBI record.

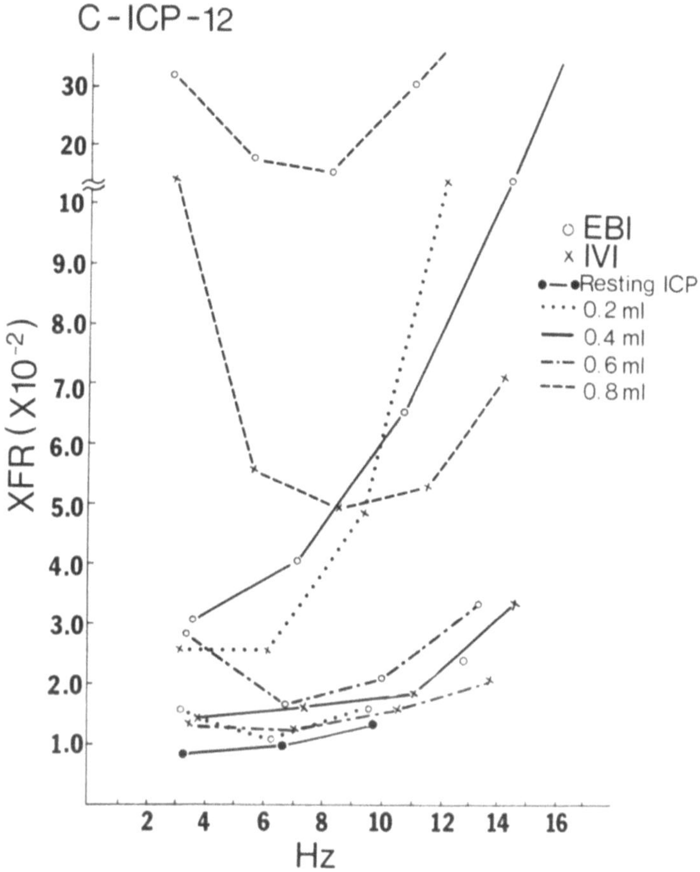

Fig. 2. XFR spectrum for EBI at 0.2, 0.4, 0.6, and 0.8 ml and the corresponding IVI at same ICP. XFR increases with increasing ICP (increasing balloon volume). XFR for IVI greater than for EBI at 0.2 ml, but greater for EBI at 0.4, 0.6, and 0.8 ml.

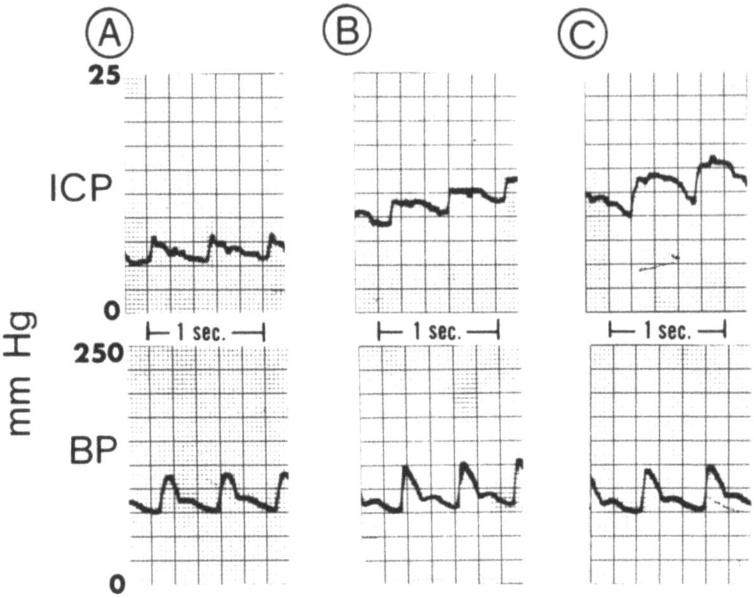

Fig. 3. Progressive changes in ICP waveform in a comatose, 52 year old female with right thalamic hemorrhage from a ruptured internal carotid artery aneurysm at the bifurcation.
3A) ICP normal. ICP waveform shows initial sharp rise and subsequent downward slope similar to blood pressure.
3B) Following initial rise waveform is more flat. This was noted 3 hours before ICP became normal.
3C) Wave becomes increasingly rounded as ICP rises.

THE ANALOGY BETWEEN CSF PULSE PRESSURE AND VOLUME-PRESSURE RESPONSE

J.H.M. VAN EIJNDHOVEN AND C.J.J.AVEZAAT

Introduction

The volume-pressure (V/P) test is widely used to measure intracranial elastance. However, the test has some disadvantages: it increases the infection hazard, may provoke high intracranial pressure (ICP) waves, provides only momentary information and cannot be used in epidural pressure recordings. Another major problem is the varaibility of the volume-pressure response (VPR) due to errors related to the injected volume, spontaneous ICP variations and rapid spatial compensatory mechanisms.

The CSF pulse pressure (CSFPP), on the other hand, is a continuous physiological response containing the same information as the VRP. In contrast with the VPR it is based on an unknown volume change: the transient increase in cerebral blood volume per cardiac cycle (ΔV) (Fig. 1). Factors influencing ΔV will be discussed.

Analytical method and material

The V/P curve can be described by a mono-exponential function (1). A simple mono-exponential curve, however, did not fit the data of all our patients. A model extended with a constant term was more suitable:

$$P = P_{eq} \exp \left[E_1 (V - V_{eq}) \right] + P_0$$

where P = ICP, P_{eq} = a constant equal to the physiological steady state ICP, E_1 = elastance coefficient, a constant defining the slope of the V/P curve, $(V - V_{eq})$ represents the change in total volume of the craniospinal compartments compared to the equilibrium volume and P_0 = a constant, shifting the V/P curve along the pressure axis, without affecting its shape (Fig 1) (2). The relationship of both VPR and CSFPP with the ICP can be derived from this function:

$$\Delta P = \left[P - P_0 \right] \left[\exp (E_1 \Delta V) - 1 \right]$$

where ΔP = VPR or CSFPP and ΔV = the injected volume during a V/P test or the transient blood volume change per cardiac cycle (Fig. 1). If ΔV and E_1 are constant, this is a linear relationship, intersecting the pressure axis at P_0. (N.B. without the constant term, P_0, the relationship should always pass through the origin).

In over a hundred patients, in whom ICP was monitored for various reasons, the CSFPP-ICP relationship was computed at hourly intervals. A number of VPR's was measured at the beginning of each pressure recording.

Results and discussion

The analogy between CSFPP and VPR is demonstrated in a single patient (Fig.2). Both VPR and CSFPP are linearly related to the ventricular fluid pressure (VFP), which implies that E_I and ΔV are constant in the pressure range of the relevant time interval. This was a consistent finding in all the patients. E_I was computed from the slope of the VPR-VFP relationship and varied considerably between patients (range: 0.1 - 0.6 l/ml). ΔV was subsequently calculated from the CSFPP-VFP relationship (range: 0.5 - 5 ml). The VPR data clearly show the earlier mentioned variability demonstrating that elastance and compliance indices calculated from a single VPR are less reliable. The CSFPP data, on the other hand, show less variability and are continuously available. E_I, however, cannot directly be computed from the CSFPP data as these are also dependent on the constant, but unknown ΔV. So, VPR's are still needed to evaluate the initial E_I at the beginning of an ICP recording. Hereafter the patient's ΔV can be calculated from the first CSFPP versus VFP plot. In subsequent time intervals variations in the slope of this relationship are caused by a change either in E_I or in ΔV. Since ΔV is the resultant of the interaction between cerebral arterial inflow and venous outflow (Fig. 1), hemodynamic factors may be responsible for changes in ΔV. Alterations in in- and outflow impedances (autoregulatory mechanisms, venous compression), cerebral blood flow (CBF) and heart rate may thus play an important role in this respect. For an accurate evaluation of E_I by means of the CSFPP-VFP relationship more information is needed on how these factors influence ΔV,

Summary

In individual patients, the CSF pulse pressure is a reliable parameter to monitor alterations in intracranial elastance. The volume change underlying the CSF pulse pressure, however, varies considerably between patients and may be affected by hemodynamic changes.

References

1. Marmarou A (1973) A theoretical and experimental evaluation of the cerebrospinal fluid system. PhD Thesesis, Drexel University

2. Avezaat CJJ, Van Eijndhoven JHM, DeJong DA, Moolenaar WCJ (1976) A new method of monitoring intracranial volume-pressure relationships. In: Beks JWF, Bosch DA, Brock M (eds) Intracranial Pressure III. Springer, Berlin Heidelberg New York, p 308

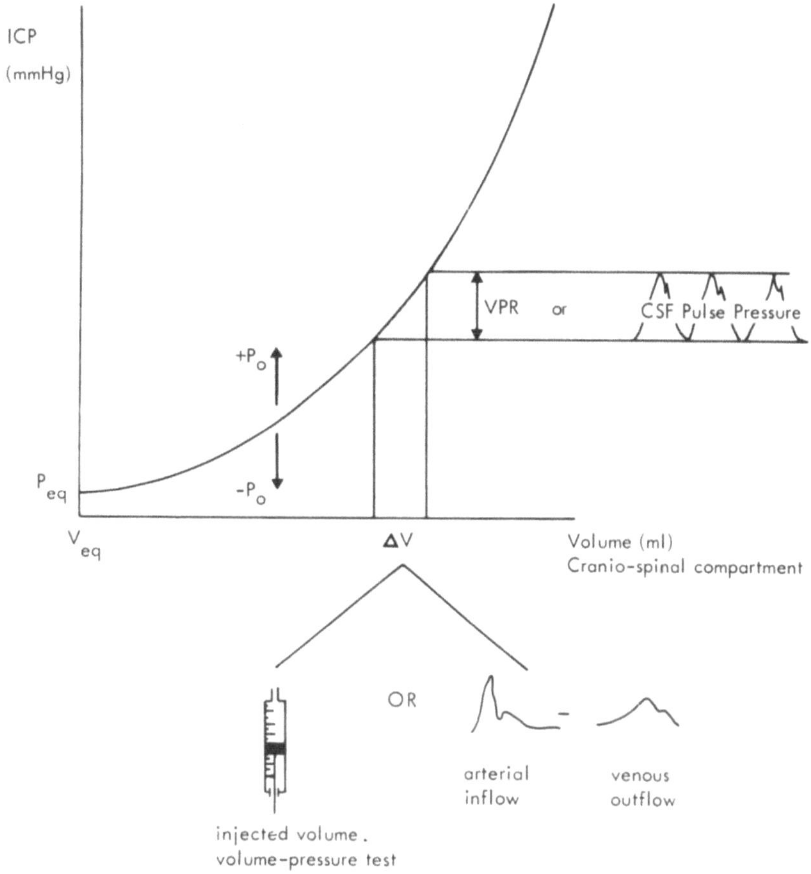

Fig. 1. The CSF pulse pressure and the volume-pressure response are both based on a rapid change in craniospinal volume (ΔV). The magnitude of the responses depends on the shape of the craniospinal volume pressure curve. P_{eq} = equilibrium pressure, physiological steady state ICP; V_{eq} = volume of the craniospinal compartment at which ICP = P_{eq}; P_0 = a constant shifting the volume-pressure curve along the pressure axis.

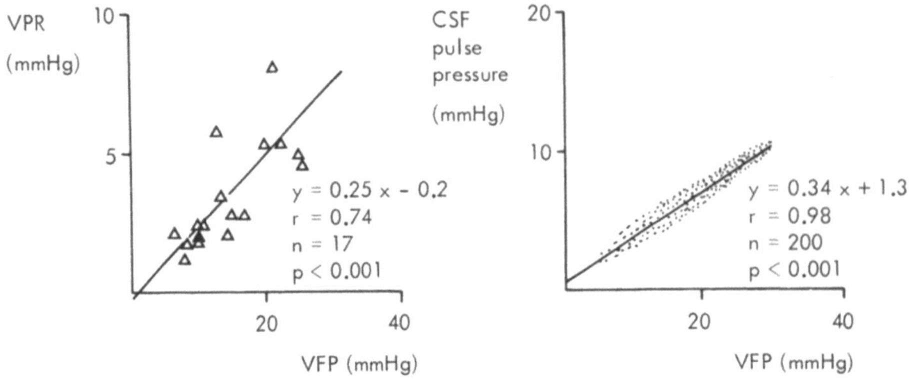

Fig. 2. Plots of the volume-pressure response (VPR) and the CSF pulse pressure (CSFPP) against the ventricular fluid pressure (VFP) in a single patient.

BRAIN STEM - CEREBELLAR AND HEMISPHERIC BLOOD FLOW IN STUPOR AND IMPAIRED STATES OF RESPONSIVENESS WITH AND WITHOUT INTRACRANIAL HYPERTENSION

M. YAMAMOTO, J.S. MEYER, F. SAKAI, AND F. YAMAGUCHI

Introduction

Average or regional cerebral hemispheric blood flow (rCBF) have been reported to be reduced markedly in all comatose patients studied, whether due to apoplexy, trauma, cardiac arrest, or other causes, and in patients with impaired responsiveness (akinetic mutism, "locked-in") syndrome or apallic syndrome (1-3) and are useful in evaluating the prognosis of unresponsive patients (4). It is well known that brain stem injury induces coma and influences prognosis whether primary or secondary to herniation.

The present study was undertaken to measure rCBF of the brain stem region as well as the hemispheres in patients with coma or impaired responsiveness. ^{133}Xe inhalation method enables measurement of brain stem - cerebellar (BSC) regions and both hemispheres simultaneously.

Methods and materials

Regional cerebral blood flow measurements were made in alert normals and compared to stuporous, semicomatose, apallic or "locked-in" patients by ^{133}Xe inhalation (5,6).

Unresponsive states were secondary to ruptured intracranial aneurysm (SAH: semicoma N=3, stupor N=1), massive hemispheric infarction (HI: semicoma N=1, stupor N=2), basilar artery occlusion with "locked-in" syndrome (N=2) and apallic state secondary to temporary cardio-pulmonary arrest (N=4). As controls, rCBF measurements were made in aged-matched normal volunteers (N=15) and alert patients with stroke (N=23). Mean age of all groups were 52-63 years. Semicoma or stuporous states in SAH or HI were associated with papilledema, suspected brain herniation and decerebrate or decorticate states. Patients with locked-in syndrome had no increased intracranial pressure (ICP) and had good collateral circulation of BSC regions by angiography.

Results

Typical "locked-in" rCBF showed mean hemispheric flow (Fg) values of 55 ml/100g brain/min, and BSC flow (Fg) values of 107 ml/100g brain/min. Typical apallic syndrome values were: gray matter flow, 28 ml/100g brain/min in hemispheres, and 98 ml/100g brain/min in BSC regions.

Mean Hemispheric and Brain Stem - Cerebellar Flow in Patients with Unresponsiveness and Alert Patients with Stroke (Figure 1):

Mean hemispheric blood flow (Fg) values were reduced significantly in patients with semicoma, stupor, and apallic syndrome compared to normals and also reduced in alert patients with stroke and "locked-in" syndrome. Brain stem - cerebellar blood flow (Fg) values were reduced significantly in stuporour or semicomatose patients with or without increased ICP compared to normals. However, BSC blood flow values were normal in alert patients and "locked-in" syndrome without increased ICP. In 4 apallic patients, BSC blood flow values were reduced slightly in one patient with increased ICP, some brain stem signs (BSC flow value = 89 ml/100g brain/min), but not in 3 patients with intact brain stem function.

Changes in rCBF Correlated with Changes in Levels of Consciousness in Stroke Patients (Figure 2):

BSC flow values progressively increased in all 5 patients, studied consecutively, whose level of consciousness recovered. However, mean hemispheric flow values remained decreased in 2 of 5 patients despite recovery of consciousness.

Summary

^{133}Xe inhalation rCBF measurements showed reduced hemispheric flow values in patients with unresponsive states confirming reports of others using intracarotid injection methods (1-3). BSC blood flow values were reduced in stuporous or semicomatose patients with increased ICP but not in apallic states unless associated with papilledema and brain stem signs. BSC blood flow values remain normal in patients able to respond without signs of increased ICP or impaired brain stem function and with good collateral circulation. Bruce et al (7) reported that there was poor correlation between hemispheric CBF and neurological states in comatose patients with head injury. Our present data confirm this but demonstrate that changes in BSC flow values correlate well with disturbed levels of consciousness.

References

1. Lassen N (195) Cerebral blood flow and oxygen consumption in man. Physiol Rev 39:183-237

2. Shalit MN, Beller AJ, Feinsod M (1972) Clinical equivalents of cerebral oxygen consumption in coma. Neurol 22:155-160

3 Ingvar D, (1973) Cerebral blood flow and metabolism in complete apallic syndromes, in states of severe dementia, and in akinetic mutism. Acta Neurol Scand 49:233-244

4. Heiss WD, Gerstenbrand F, Prosenz P et al (1972) The prognostic value of cerebral blood flow measurement in patients with apallic syndrome. J Neurol Scien 16:373-382

5. Obrist WD, Thompson HH, Wang HS et al. Regional cerebral blood flow estimated by ^{133}Xenon inhalation. Stroke 6:245-256

6. Meyer JS, Ishihara N, Deshmukh VD et al (1978) Improved method for non-invasive measurement of regional cerebral blood flow by ^{133}Xe inhalation. Description of the method and normal values obtained in healthy volunteeers. Stroke 9:195-205

7. Bruce DA, Langfitt TW, Miller JD, et al (1973) Regional cerebral blood flow, intracranial pressure, and brain metabolism in comatose patients. J Neurosurg 38:131-144

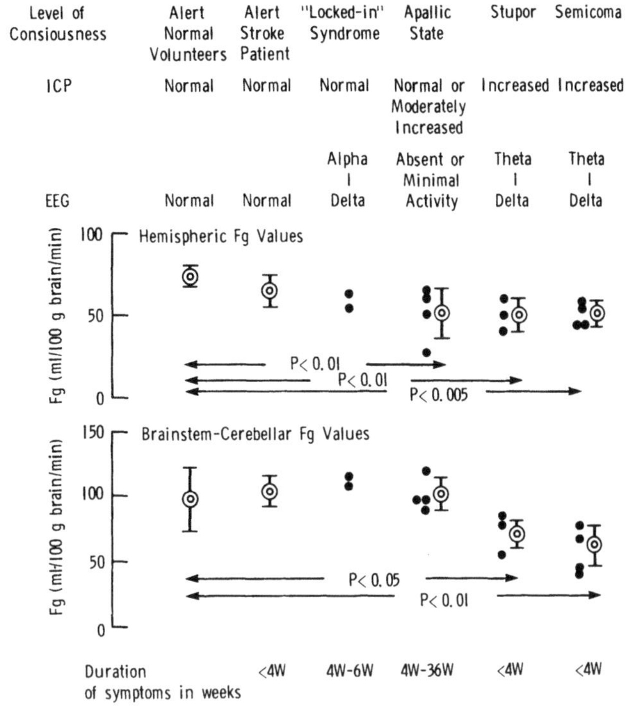

Fig. 1. Shows hemispheric and brain stem - cerebellar blood flow (Fg) values in impaired states of responsiveness with and without intracranial hypertension.

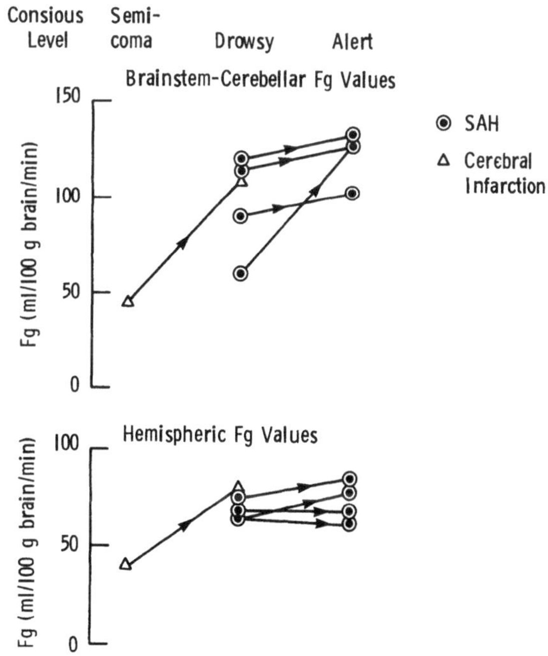

Fig. 2. Shows changes in levels of consciousness in stroke patients.

MEASUREMENT OF REGIONAL CEREBRAL BLOOD VOLUME BY PHOTOELECTRIC METHOD

H. KUYAMA, S. FUJIMOTO, M. TSUCHIMOTO, K. NISHIMOTO, T. AKIOKA, A. MATSUMOTO, AND A. NISHIMOTO

Introduction

The cerebral blood volume (CBF) has been considered as an important parameter in regulation of the cerebral hemodynamics. However, methodological difficulty in measurement of CBV has been well known. This paper is concerned with a photoelectric apparatus which has been developed in our laboratory.

Materials and methods

The sensor of this apparatus is composed of three parts: microlamp, photodiode attached to the gelatin filter which enables us to transmit 520 mμ wave length of light and polyethylene balloon or polyethylene tube for intracranial pressure (ICP) measurement. They are pasted with silicone rubber.

Under ketamine anesthesia, 62 dogs were paralyzed by succinylcholine chloride with controlled respiration. The sensor was applied on the surface of the right parietal lobe. Microlamp illuminated through the brain surface. Subsequently scattered light in the brain was measured by the photodiode. In addition, arterial blood pressure (BP) was recorded from the femoral artery. Cerebral blood flow (CBF) and respiratory rate were measured by the heat clearance technique and thermistor respirometer respectively. To study optical absorption (OA) in the brain tissue, various conditions were prepared, such as retrograde injection of saline or indocyanine green (ICG) into the right brachial artery, compression of the jugular vein, CO_2 inhalation, hyperventilation, occlusion of the descending aorta or ascending aorta and intravenous injection of papaverine or Arfonad.

As an applied experiment, CBV was measured continuously by this apparatus during stepwise increase of ICP. CO_2 reactivity was also obtained from alterations of CBV following inhalation of 10% CO_2. ICP was gradually raised by infusion of saline through a tube connected into the cisterna magna from a bottle of fluid which was elevated to various levels.

Results

All the time, OA was closely related with changes of respiration, BP and ICP. OA decreased immediately after saline injection and conversely increased following ICG injection. Compression of the jugular vein increased OA in spite of decrease of CBF. CO_2 inhalation increased CBF, OA and ICP. Hyperventilation decreased CBF, OA and ICP (Figure 1). Occlusion of descending aorta increased all of CBF, OA ICP and BP. On the contrary, occlusion of ascending aorta produced the decrease of CBF, OA, ICP and BP. Papaverine induced the increase of CBF, OA and ICP. Arfonad caused sudden drop of CBF, OA, ICP and

BP. While ICP was below 50 mmHg, neither CBV nor CBF showed any changes. However, as ICP was raised higher, CBV showed continuous increase while CBF showed continuous decrease (Figure 2). On the other hand, CO_2 reactivities were completely lost at levels of ICP more than 110 mmHg.

Discussion

OA changes in the brain tissue following saline or ICG injection indicated their dependence on the optical characteristic in the vessels, namely hemoglobin. Oxidized hemoglobin and reduced hemoglobin have different optical characteristic except 520 mμ, 550 mμ and 570 mμ wave length. Therefore, OA of the blood measured with gelatin filter is uniform among various conditions of blood gases (1). Both OA in the brain tissue and ICP increased in the state of vasodilatation induced either by jugular vein compression, CO_2 inhalation or papaverine injection. In contrast, both of them decreased during vasoconstriction induced either by hyperventilation or severe arterial hypotension. These results suggest that OA indicates changes of CBV. While ICP was elevated from 50 mmHg to 130 mmHg, CBV increased continuously with decrease of CBF. CO_2 reactivity was completely lost when ICP was more than 110 mmHg, at which stage increase of CBV was thought to be due to vasomotor paralysis (2).

Summary

Although this method still has some disadvantages, several important advantages are as follows: 1) Regional CBV is continuously measured without radionuclide or specific indicators. 2) This method does not require skilled tehcnique. 3) The cerebral transit time is measurable by injection of saline or indicators into the artery. 4) In addition, this device can also measure ICP simultaneously. This method will be useful in measurement of regional CBV with or without increased ICP.

References

1. Kuyama H, Fujimoto S, Nishimoto K, Ninomiya K, Matsumoto A, Nishimoto A (1978) Measurement of regional cerebral blood volume by photoelectric method. Neurol med chir 18:Part II, 655-664

2. Langfitt TW, Weinstein JD, Kassell NF (1965) Cerebral vasomotor paralysis produced by intracranial hypertension. Neurol 15:622-641

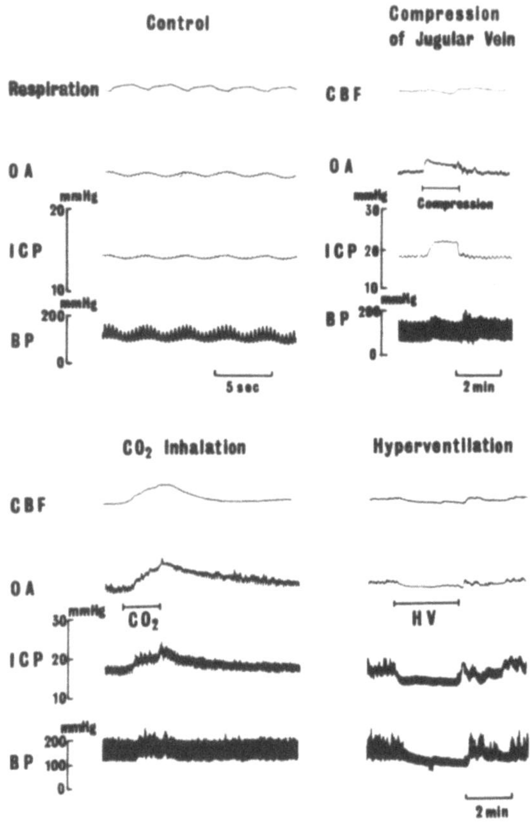

Figure 1

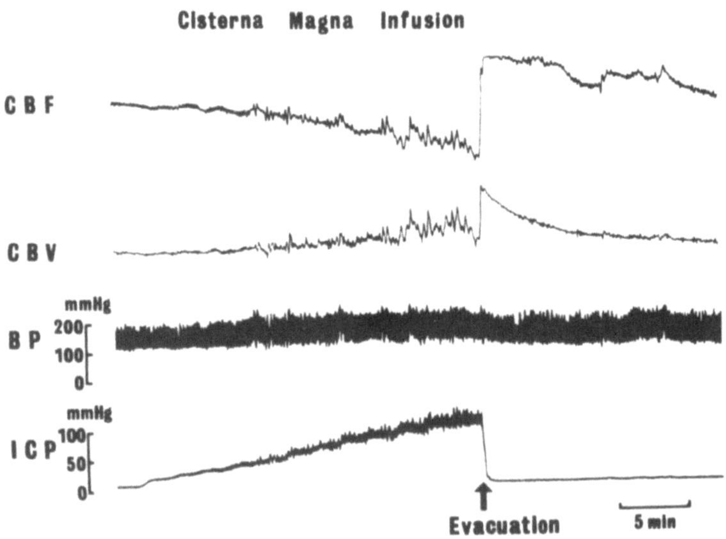

Figure 2

ICP AND EEG IN VARIOUS FORMS OF CEREBRAL SEIZURES

O.E.KNOBLICH, M.GAAB, AND W.WEBER

Introduction

Cerebral seizures lead to an increase in cerebral blood flow (CBF). The increased blood flow is brought about by vascular dilatation created by a reduced pH due to raised CO_2 and increased lactate(1). It can also be observed when clinical convulsions are avoided by controlled respiration and blood pressure crises are suppressed (1). A direct stimulation of the vessels by paroxysmal discharge is also thought to be possible. Both the increase of CBF and also edema (possibly caused by a disturbance of the blood brain barrier (2), lead to a rise in intracranial pressure (ICP). This can have potentially fatal consequences.

It is not clear whether there is an increase in ICP due to every kind of raised electrical activity of the brain. It is also unclear whether progressive brain edema can occur after the status epilepticus subsides in spite of controlled respiration.

Material and Methods

In 30 curarized cats under controlled respiration ($N_2O:O_2/3:2$) the EEG and the parietal epidural pressure (rEP, lEP) were recorded on both sides. Besides central venous (cvP) and femoral arterial pressure (aP), ventricular CSF pressure (VP) was measured after catheterization. We occasionally determined the pressure in the superior sagittal sinus (sssP) and epidurally over the posterior cranial fossa (Pfp). By measurement of the internal carotid blood flow (magnetic flow) cerebral blood flow (CBF) could be estimated. To produce seizures, pentetrazole (400 mg/5-10 sec i.v., 14 animals) was injected or electroconvulsions (EC, continuous current of 5-20 sec duration, 50 volts, current up to 600 mAmp) were applied, in three animals bitemporally and in three unilaterally on the right side. In four animals, the cerebral cortex was frozen with chloric ether on the previous day via a parietal occipital burrhole on the right and the defect closed with a graft.

In 110 patients with tumors or head injuries in whom the EEG and ICP were monitored (assisted or controlled respiration), there were four with clinical seizures and/or paroxysmal electrical discharges. The investigation was carried out preoperatively and/or postoperatively. The epidural pressure in the patient was measured right frontally through a burrhole and the EEG was recorded bilateral fronto-occipitally with needle electrodes.

Results

A few seconds after administration of pentetrazole (Fig. 1a, above), there are "tonic"/"clonic" paroxysmal discharges in the EEG. With the beginning of "clonic" phase, the ICP rises rapidly (Fig. 1b, above).

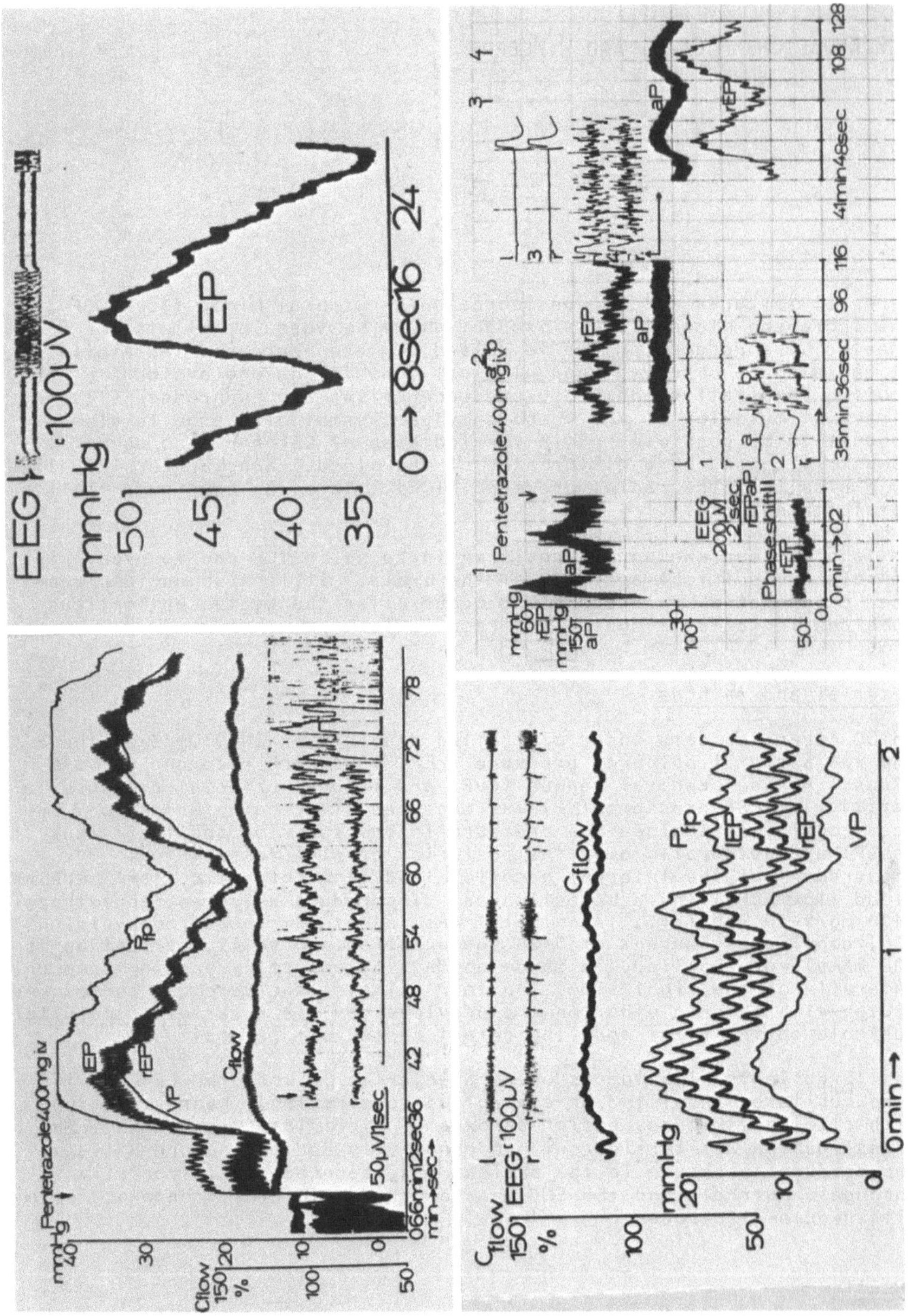
EEG
100μV
mmHg
EP
0 → 8sec16 24
Pentetrazole 400mg iv
Cflow
%
VP
rEP
lEP
Pfp
aP
Phaseshift II
0min →

The ventricular pressure attains a less high peak. The arterial blood pressure rises synchronously with ICP, but the peak blood pressure reached differs from animal to animal (Fig. Ib, below). The typical fluctuations in arterial blood pressure occurring in the same direction as ICP in every paroxysmal EEG discharge often only appear in the later course (Fig. Ib, below). Alterations in carotid blood flow synchronous with the behavior of brain pressure are the rule (Fig. Ia, below). The ICP always falls to the initial value. Only in the unilateral EC (Fig. 2b, above), the ICP is steeper over the simulated hemisphere, and the fall is delayed. The EEG alterations are unilateral. In focal seizures, pressure gradients are lacking 24 hours after freezing (Fig. 2a, above). If one produces further convulsions a short time after a series of seizures, there may be a progressive rise in ICP when a cerebral perfusion pressure of 60 mmHg has fallen below uhder deterioration of the EEG (Fig. 2a, below). A brain edema was verified by autopsy in this animal.

Of the four patients with convulsions, one patient showed a distinct steep rise in ICP of more than 20 mmHg during the electrical paroxysms, and a fall of ICP during the subsequent normalization of the EEG even under conditions of controlled respiration (Fig. 2b, below). Only an elevation of the barbiturate dose lead to normalization of ICP and EEG. In the three further patients, the ICP could be lowered with conventional anticonvulsive therapy.

Discussion

The elevation of ICP is brought about by a cerebral hyperemia induced by a shift in pH. With electrical stimulation, a direct vasodilatation is conceivable because of the rapid effect on ICP. The acute increase in CBF in ictus may be accompanied by rise in blood pressure. We did not always see an alteration in blood pressure synchronous with the rise in ICP. The reason for this is probably a different responsiveness of circulatory centers. Besides the electrical synchronization in tonus-clonus in status epilepticus with subsequent depression, a typical synchronous ICP course is seen which is explained by the increasein CBF (engorgement -3). If the seizures are arrested under conditions of controlled respiration, the brain pressure immediately falls to the initial level. A progressive brain edema only arises when a critical cerebral perfusion pressure is reached.

◁ Fig I a -above. A few seconds after administration of pentetrazole, a desynchronisation, slow hypersynchronous waves, and then "tonic-clonic" paroxysms are shown in the EEG. Rise of rEP and lEP up to 35 mmHg is equal on both sides. The pressure over the posterior cranial fossa is raised, and ventricular pressure shows a lower level. Fluctuations in carotid blood flow in the same direction as ICP. Note the slower chronography of the temporo-occipitally registered EEG. l=left brain, r=right brain EEG.

a -below. Synchronous measurement of ICP, EEG and blood flow in the internal carotid artery.

b -above Synchronous registration of ICP and EEG course,"tonic-clonic" seizure, typical EEG segment, 3 minutes after administration of 400 mg pentetrazole i.v.

b -below. After administration of the convulsive agent, the aP is lower than before. Although the ICP shows typical fluctuations in the same direction as the EEG paroxysms, the aP has an even course; in the later course, fluctuations of aP in the same direction as the EEG. Note phase shift, aP arterial pressure.

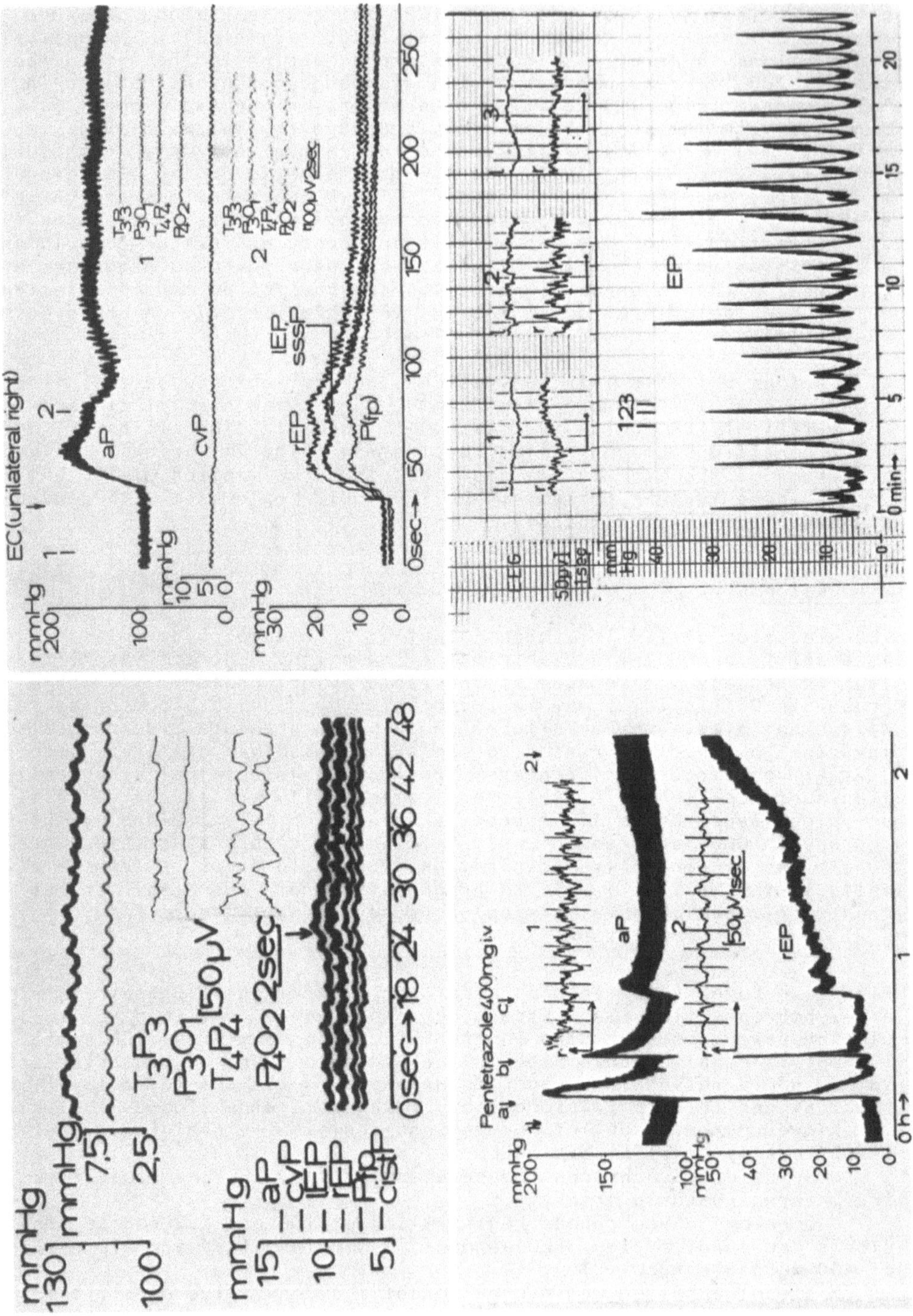

EC (unilateral right)
aP
cvP
rEP
lEP
sssP
P(fp)
Pentetrazole 400 mg i.v.
EP
0 sec→
0 h→
0 min→

Summary

In seizure, the rise in ICP is caused by hyperemia (engorgement). Under controlled respiration conditions, there is no progressive brain edema when a critical cerebral perfusion pressure is not reached.

References

1. Betz E (1976) Blood pressure dependent variations of cerebral blood flow, cerebrospinal fluid pressure and brain volume during and after electrically induced seizures. In: Meyer JS et al.(eds) Cerebral Vascular Disease. Thieme, Stuttgart, p 146

2. Bolwig TG, Hertz MM, Westergaard E (1977) Blood-brain-barrier permeability to protein during epileptic seizures in the rat. Acta Neurol Scand Suppl 64, 56:226-227

3. Jennett B (1978) Clinical brain swellin-oedema or engorgement (Glasgow, Great Britain, Neurological Clinic) Symposium on Brain Edema, Sept 28th, Rotterdam

◁ Fig 2 a -above. Course of ICP and EEG 24 hours after spraying chloric ether on right cortex. Rise of all ICP values with beginning of steep waves in the EEG.

a -below. Course of ICP and arterial blood pressure after repeated i.v. administration of pentetrazole, typical EEG segment. With fresh stimulation after previous administration of pentetrazole, progressive rise in the ICP. At an rEP of 50 mmHg, severe general alterations in the EEG on the right side. A critical cerebral perfusion pressure (mean aP-VP) is reached here.

b -above. Typical course of the brain pressure of an animal with unilateral, longlasting EC (20 sec stimulation), typical EEG segment. The ICP on the right rises markedly over the stimulated side. The epidural pressure over the posterior cranial fossa and the pressure in the superior sagittal sinus do not become so high. There is a rise in blood pressure with marked latency. The EEG on the right shows steep slow waves with faint spike slow wave patterns. sssP pressure in superior sagittal sinus.

b -below. Course of ICP of a patient after left parietal glioblastoma operation, typical EEG segments (fronto-occipital recording) during clinical Jacksonian seizures on the left side. During the attack, brief ICP peaks up to 40 mmHg were measured. There were steep waves and peaks in the EEG on the right side (operation). The pressure fell to the initial level between the attacks. Since the noninvasively measured mean arterial blood pressure did not fall below 110 mmHg during the attacks, the cerebral perfusion was also maintained high during the ICP crisis.

ANALYSIS OF THE WAVE PATTERN OF CSF PULSE WAVE

A.GEGA, S.UTSUMI, Y.IIDA, N.IIDA, AND S.TSUNCDA

Introduction

Even though many studies have been performed to monitor continuous intracranial pressure (ICP) since LUNDBERG (1) reported, the pulsation of CSF has not been precisely studied in the wave pattern. This study aims at analyzing the pressure fluctuation in CSF as the wave pattern.

Materials and method

The pulsation of CSF was recorded as a pulse wave in paper speed of 15 mm or 30 mm per second in comparison with the record in 1 mm per second by STATHAM P37 pressure transducer via a ventricular catheter in 21 patients with ventricular drainage. The CSF pulse wave was named "Ventricular CSF Pulse Wave"(VPW), which was a sawtooth wave composed of small peaks from P 1 to P 5 as shown in Fig. 1.

Among these, P 1, P 2 and P 3 were universally observed and designated the "Component Wave" (CW) of VPW. The notch just before P 3 was named "Dicrotic Notch" (DN) in reference with the concepts of "Carotid Arterial Pulse Wave" (CAR) (2). The length and the height of each CW were measured from the starting point (PO). ICP was measured from the baseline (BL) to P 1 in height. EEG and EKG were monitored. In few cases, spinal CSF pulsation was simultaneously recorded, and named "Spinal CSF Pulse Wave" (SPW).

Results

1. VWP was recorded and observed in 15 or 30 mm per second at the stage of "B-Wave" where ICP was well controlled by drainage, and used as the "Normal ICP Pattern" as shown in Fig. 1. This pattern showed that P 2 was slightly larger in height than P 1, and was affected in the height of CW by respiratory rhythm.

2. Each P 1, P 2 and P 3 were identified in the length by the following formula if it was difficult to recognize the peak of CW:
0-P 1/00=0.347 ± 0.072, 0-P 2/00=0.484 ± 0.045, 0-P 3/00=0.718 ±0.079: 00 showed 0-0 interval of EKG, 0-P 1, 0-P 2 and 0-P 3 show from 0 of EKG to each P of CW in length.

3. The correlation of CW with raised ICP could be demonstrated by compressing the jugular vein. This maneuver caused ICP to raise rapidly as shown in Fig. 2, and changed the wave pattern, making P 1 and P 2 enlarged in height and fused. And then, this caused DN and P 3 to elevate in high position. However, no change of the length of CW was seen during the jugular compression. This pattern was observed in moderate high ICP, but it could not be recognized at the stage of "A Wave" because "A-Wave" was not observed in our series. In the case of Fig. 2, SPW was simultaneously recorded and observed.

Discussion

Recording of the pressure fluctuation of CSF has been performed in slow paper speed (under 1 mm per second) since LUNDBERG (1) reported. However, we have been interested in analyzing the CSF pulsation as the wave pattern, because we thought that the CSF pulsation itself would have significant meaning to the brain function and to express the intracranial pressure responses and the physiological conditions. In general, it has been accepted that the primary generating factor to make the pattern of CSF pulse wave was originated from the arterial pulsation of choroid plexus (3). As was stated by DARDENNE (4), the CSF pulse wave is composed of complex factors such as the intracranial conditions as well as arterial and venous hemodynamics. But the influences and the part of these hemodynamics on VPW has not been thoroughly understood.

The concept of CAR (2) was introduced to understand the pattern by simultaneous recordings between VPW and CAR (5). VPW had a delay of 16 msec to that of CAR, and P 1 of CW corresponded with "Percussion Wave" of CAR, P 2 with "Tidal Wave" and P 3 with "Dicrotic Wave", which was referred with the closing time of the aortic valve. From these observations, P 1 depended on the arterial input, mainly the arterial pressure-volume through the internal carotid artery, and P 2 referred with "Tidal Wave" of CAR was the reflection wave to P 1. Small peaks after P 1 have been the result of "Water Hammer Phenomenon" by the venous pressure (3), but the meanings of small peaks had not been precisely examined and observed.

From the observations by compressing the jugular vein, it could be demonstrated that the venous pressure-volume gave the main influence on DN and P 3 besides enlarging each CW.

The pattern of CSF pulse wave could be classified into three groups: "Normal", "High" and "Low" ICP pattern which was reported previously (5). But as pointed out by CASTEL (6), the relation with different pathological conditions might be considered to relate to the CSF pulse wave. VPW would not only be changed with only raised ICP by increased CSF volume and venous congestion, but by the existence of intracranial pathogenesis.

Summary

The ventricular CSF pulse wave was a sawtooth wave composed of small peaks from P 1 to P 5. Among these, P 1, P 2 and P 3 were universally present and designated "Component Wave" and observed in the wave pattern. The concept of "Carotid Arterial Pulse Wave" was introduced in the understanding of CSF pulse wave.

References

1. Lundberg N (196) Continuous recording and control of ventricular fluid pressure in neurosurgical practice. Acta Psych Scand, Suppl 149, 36:1-193

2. Morton ET (1973) Clinical phonocardiography and experimental pulse recording. Year Book Medical Publishers, Inc.

3. Bering EA,Jr (1955) Choroid plexus and arterial pulsation of cerebrospinal fluid. Demonstration of the choroid plexuses as a cerebrospinal fluid pump. Arch Neurol Psychiat 73:165-172

4. Dardenne G. Dereymaeker A, Lacheron JM (1969) Cerebrospinal fluid pressure and pulsatility. Europ Neurol 2:93-216

5. Gega A, Utsumi S, Terada H, Iida Y, Harada T, Tsunoda S (1977) Continuous observation and analysis of ventricular pulse wave. Brain & Nerve 29:1315-1323

6. Castel JP, Cohadon F (1976) The pattern of cerebral pulse: Automatic analysis. In: Beks JWF, Bosch DA, Brock M (eds) Intracranial Pressure II.Springer, Berlin Heidelberg New York, p 303

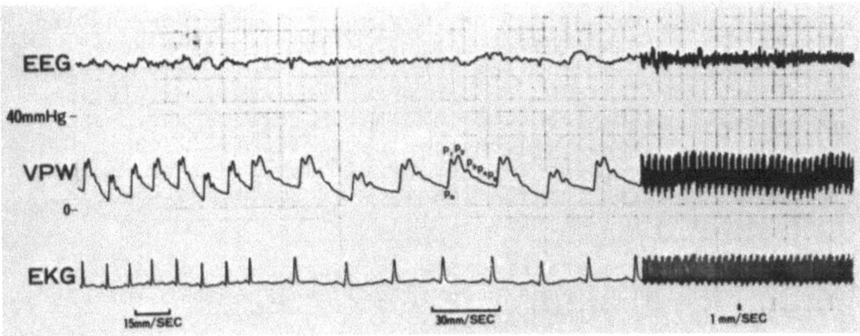

Fig. 1. Recording shows "Ventricular CSF Pulse Wave" (VPW) in 15 mm or 30 mm per second while R-wave in recording of 1 mm per second was observed VPW was a sawtooth wave composed of small peaks frpm P to P5. Among these, P1, P2 and P3 were universally present and designated the "Component Wave" (CW).

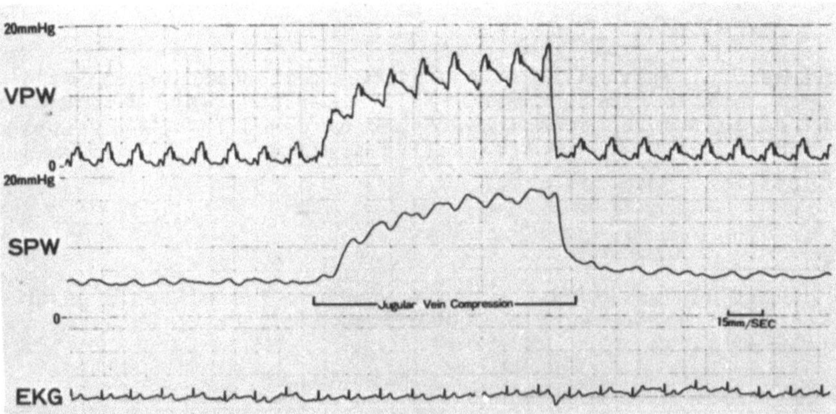

Fig. 2. The close correlation of "Component Wave" with raised ICP could be demonstrated by compressing the jugular vein. Spinal CSF Pulse Wave (SPW) was concomitantly changed with Ventricular CSF Pulse Wave (VPW).

STUDY OF THE CSF PULSATION TRANSFER: APPLICATION TO THE FREQUENCY ANALYSIS

D. GODIN, A. STEVENAERT, AND R. LHOMMEL

Introduction

The ICP is the response to a physical system receiving the various inputs which the general equation may be : $P(t) = H(\alpha_i).E(t)$ where $P(t)$ is the CSF pressure, $E(t)$ the input and $H(\alpha_i)$ the transfer function dependent of parameters α_i related to the physical properties of the cranio-spinal cavity and its contents. The properties have been investigated by the volume/pressure test.

The aim of this study was to define the volume/pressure relationship VPR : $P = \exp B.V + P_l$ (eq. 1) by means of CSF pulse pressure analysis, the CSF pulse pressure representing the pressure response to the net increase in intracranial volume during each cardiac cycle (1,2).

Mathematical Relationships: Before analyzing a wave pattern, the bandwidth of the transmission device has to be verified to obtain absolute characteristics. The transfer function of a hydraulic transmission device was theoretically defined as $H(j\omega) = \cos \phi_l ch\phi_2/ch(\alpha l+a) + j(Bl + b + \phi_l)$
This formula was numerically approximated and experimentally tested with similar results, justifying the use of this equation as a tool in chosing the parts of a system with a convenient bandwidth.

From eq. 1, the elastance/pressure relationship (6) is obtained by derivation: $EPR = dp/_{dv} = B.P$ (eq.3). This equation is normally linear and B remains constant. If in eq. 1 V increases by ΔV, P will increase by ΔP and eq. 1 will become $\Delta P = (P-P_l)(\exp B.\Delta V - 1)$ (eq.4). If ΔV is the volume cahnge per cardiac cycle, P in this equation is P_{dia} which is the low level ICP corresponding to the diastolic arterial pressure and ΔP is the CSF pulse pressure.

If ΔV and B remain constant, this equation is linear. Eq.4 may be changed into a function of the mean pressure Pm:

$$\Delta P = K(P_m - P_l)(\exp B\,\Delta V - 1)/(\exp B\,\Delta V + 2) \quad \text{(eq. 5)}$$

with the introduction of a pattern factor K_p since the mean pressure is a function of the wave pattern. This factor indicates the similarity of arterial pressure to ICP with a maximum of .333. If K_p is independent of the pressure eq. 5 must be linear.

The integration of the power spectrum density (PSD) of a periodic wave represents the energy W(P) (PARCEVAL Theorem). But this energy is also the expected value of the modulus of the squared wave. Thus using eq. 4 we obtain:
expected value of $(P_{dia} - P_l)^2(\exp BV(t) - 1)^2 = W(P)$ (eq. 6).
This equation depends on V(t). We found experimentally that the arterial pressure may be regarded as a Gamma distribution function (5) and consequently V(t) too (4). Introducing V t) we obtain an eq. such as $A_4B^8 + A_3B^6 + A_2B^4 + A_lB^2 + A_0 = 0$ giving B as the slope of EPR. The pressure/volume index (PVI) is calculated according to the method of MARMAROU et al (3).

Material and methods

Fifteen unselected IVP monitorings (probe-transmission catheter-transducer Statham P23Db) and 3 infusion tests were recorded on magnetic tape (Ampex SP700). Five sec. pressure samples were chosen at different levels of mean ICP. For each sample, the mean (P_m), the systolic (P_s), the diastolic (P_{dia}) and the pulsatile (P_{pp}) pressures were computed. By using the FOURIER analysis the PSD was integrated to obtain W(P). A linear regression test was applied to P_{pp}, P_{dia} and to P_{pp}, P_m to find B. V, K_p and P_l. Finally eq. 6 was solved (DEC MINC II).

Results

See Table I.

Discussion

For 3 cases the linear regressions failed (artefacts and baseline shift). For the remaining cases a linear relationship was found between P_{pp}, P_{dia} and P_{pp}, P_m with, in general, high correlation coefficients (mean r = .83 and .88 respectively). The correlation is better for P_{pp}, P_m than for P_{pp}, P_{dia} since P_{dia} is influenced by breathing. The pattern factor K_p is near the maximum (mean difference 3.22%), showing high correlation between arterial and intracranial pressures. The PVI calculations indicate a reduced volume buffering capacity (mean PVI = 10.64 $\pm$ 3 SD) for this group. Average PVI is 42.5% of the normal level (3).

Further studies of larger groups of selected patients will allow us to define the statistical signification of this mathematical method.

Summary

The authors described a method of computerized CSF pressure analysis; this method is able to retrieve the VRP and to give a continuous monitoring of this relationship. Further studies will demonstrate the interest of the clinical application.

References

1. Avezaat CJJ, van Eindhoven JHM, de Jong DA, Moolenaar WCJ (1976) A new method of monitoring intracranial volume/pressure relationship. In: Beks JWF, Bosch DA, Brock M (eds) Intracranial Pressure III. Springer, Berlin Heidelberg New York, p 308

2. Marmarou A, Shulman K, LaMorgese J (1975) Compartmental analysis of compliance and outflow resistance of the cerebral fluid system. J Neurosurg 43:523-534

3. Marmarou A, Shapiro K, Shulman K (1976) Isolation factors leading to sustained elevations of ICP. In: Beks JWF, Bosch DA, Brock M (eds) Intracranial Pressure III. Springer, Berlin Heidelberg New York p 33

4. McDonald DA (1960) Blood Flow Arteries. Williams & Wilkins Co Baltimore

Table I. Results of regressions: B, P_I and PVI calculation

FILE NAME	DAT NBR	LIN.REGRESSION Ppp=APdia+B A	B	R^2	BdV	LIN.REGRESSION Ppp=APmoy+B A	B	R^2	Kp	RANGE Pmoy mmHg from	to	PARAB.REGRESSION W=A0+A1Pm+A2Pm^2 A0	A1	A2	RESULTS SLOPE ELAST ml^-1	P1 mmHg	PVI ml
WAGE	9	.339	2.182	.760	.335	.339	1.739	.830	.346	5.7	14.6	24013	-2667	366	.183	-5.48	10.31
CLAU	14	.129	6.64	.338	.121	.133	6.07	.428	.308	5.5	24.6	72688	-1164	249	.110	-51.62	6.14
COUR	15	.525	-5.619	.922	.422	.408	-4.32	.957	.364	19.3	35.5	260908	-23858	597	.204	10.70	16.36
HORS	14	.417	-.499	.872	.348	.346	-.559	.915	.352	10.8	30.7	-71258	7185	-49	.186	1.19	14.18
SCHO	11	.502	2.21	.929	.406	.398	1.738	.954	.36	4.5	15	30859	-5672	606	.201	-4.41	9.29
HILG	37	.363	-.475	.759	.309	.320	-.811	.827	.336	17.4	31.2	-89985	9564	-94	.175	1.311	14.83
DUMO	16	.103	2.798	.474	.098	.104	2.600	.519	.316	7.0	13.5	-48361	12830	-568	.098	-27.13	11.44
MOTT	18	.318	2.896	.782	.276	.279	2.350	.834	.343	13.2	33.3	-60138	9336	-86	.165	-9.11	12.20
VANP	17	.185	2.530	.586	.170	.172	2.280	.668	.338	4.4	16.1	-7308	4606	-159	.130	-13.65	9.82
PEEV	19	.402	2.400	.313	.338	.424	1.270	.570	.278	7.2	13.6	387608	-8550	4979	.183	-5.96	10.61
THOM	31	.447	5.362	.551	.369	.412	2.431	.689	.314	13.7	65	623750	-32566	668	.175	-11.99	10.03
THOM	37	.488	-.530	.872	.390	.405	-1.140	.911	.345	29	73	76659	-3167	200	.198	1.11	12.86
CASS	29	.922	1.710	.880	.653	.642	1.230	.950	.365	2.3	30	53963	-8349	893	.255	-1.85	7.66
DANT	62	.564	.329	.921	.448	.446	.194	.953	.355	8.1	31.5	22170	101	257	.211	-.58	11.61
JERR	54	.127	3.120	.781	.120	.119	2.960	.807	.340	1.4	44	13590	-299	37	.109	-24.47	4.08
VAND	60	.422	2.079	.663	.325	.368	1.540	.763	.334	3.6	39.5	27068	-3360	367	.187	-4.91	9.20
VAND	8	.654	.746	.477	.503	.524	.216	.720	.341	9.6	14.8	758468	-115607	4701	.204	-1.14	10.76

5. Papoulis A (1965) Probability, Random Variables and Stochastic Processes. McGraw Hill, New York

6. Sklar R, Elashvili I (1977) The pressure volume function of brain elasticity. J Neurosurg 47:670-679

Work supported by the Fonds National de la Recherche Scientifique.

BLOOD PRESSURE FACTORS CAUSING RAISED ICP

A. IKEYAMA, T. NAKAYA, M. TERAOKA, M. HASUO, S. MAEDA, H. KUCHIWAKI, M. FURUSE, AND H. NAGAI

Introduction

It is known that intracranial hypertension accompanies pulse amplitude (PA) increase. Mathematically, if a P-V curve in the intracranial cavity were exponential, the Pa- mean ICP curve would be a straight line. Actually, it is so in many experiments, but the line shows considerable deviations due to pathogenegis. This experiment sought to clarify factors behind increased PA from the concept of the driving pressure (1).

Methods and materials

Experiments were carried out on 27 mongrel dogs. Epidural pressure (EDP), systemic blood pressure (BP) from the femoral artery, transverse sinus pressure (TSP), respiration and ECG were recorded simultaneously. The experiment was performed in 3 groups of animal models, namely, supratentorial epidural balloon expansion (10 ml/min), cisterna magna injection of saline (1.0 ml/min), and neck compression maneuvers. ICP BP dependence was calculated by the following indices: ηHB(=PA of EDP/PA of BP), ηM(=mean EDP/mean BP), the differential waves of EDP (ΔEDP/Δt) and BP (ΔBP/Δt) with time constant 0.01. γHB is defined as the rate of ΔEDP/Δt to ΔBP/Δt. These indices were continuously recorded and the correlation between ICP and BP was observed.

Results

A marked correlation between raised ICP and η increase was observed with cisterna magna injection and supratentorial balloon, but no significant TSP changes were observed (Fig. 1). ηHB and γHB took similar courses in terms of ICP rise. ηM showed a large increment compared with ηHB during injections. In these cases variations of mean EDP approached that of BP. Generally, increase in ηHB with balloon inflation was slightly larger than that with cisterna magna injection(Fig.2). Usually ηHB increase had a close correlation to ICP-TSP difference. When the difference was small, ηHB exhibited little increase in spite of high ICP. When the difference was increased by balloon inflation, ηHB-ICP curve increased from low ICP level and PA greatly increased. If balloon inflation accompanied raised TSP, ηHB-ICP curve deviated in the high ICP direction. ηHB and PA were also affected by the pulse rate and BP level. Bradycardia induced high ηHB and systemic hypotension tended to produce high ηHB.

Discussion

The authors earlier proposed ΔICP/ΔBP as η to represent the pressure transmission rate from BP to ICP. In this study, we added ΔICP/Δt and γHB as a significant index to analyze BP factors of ICP. Since the amplitude of differential waves represents the initial slope of EDP pulse, γHB may express the extent to which ICP is influenced by the stroke volume of the left heart. Normally, ηHB ηM and γHB were negligibly small, but during intracranial hypertension these indices increase. These findings show that ICP/BP dependence increases more or less in terms of raised ICP. Transfer of the pressure from the arterial system to CSF may be influenced by vasomotor tone, CSF circulation, and venous drainage from the brain. It was suggested that the function of the intracranial veno-sinus junction first and foremost played an important role in PA increase in ICP. Heart rate and BP level also contributed to PA increase.

Summary

In order to study factors behind increased pulse amplitude of ICP, ICP BP dependence was observed in animal models. ICP/BP dependence was calculated by the following indices: ηHB, ηM, the differential waves of EDP and BP. In normal condition, ηHB and ΔICP/Δt were negligibly small,but they increased during raised ICP. The transfer of the pressure from the arterial system to CSF was affected largely by ICP-TSP difference. It was suggested that the function of the intracranial veno-sinus junction plays an important role in PA increase in ICP.

Reference

1. Ikeyama A, Maeda S, Nagai H (1976) Analysis of intracranial pressure by the concept of the driving pressure. Brain Nerve 28:157-163

▷

Fig. 2. Regression lines of ηHB-ICP. Slopes with neck compression are extremely moderate compared with the other models. Slopes with balloon inflation are slightly steeper than those with cisterna injection. $p < 0.001$.

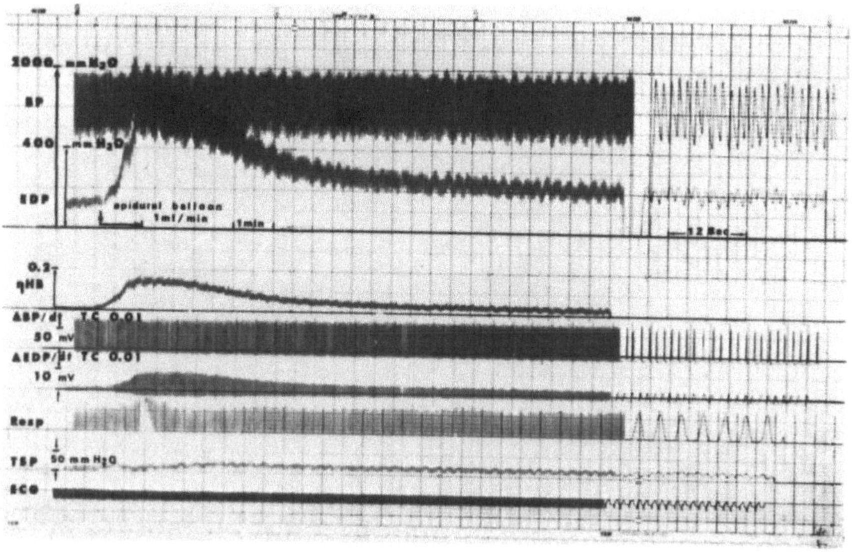

Fig. 1. Continuous recordings of balloon inflation. Balloon inflation produced a rapid increase in EDP, which was accompanied by ηHb and ΔEDP/Δt increase but no significant changes in TSP. The pressure difference of the EDP and TSP was increased.

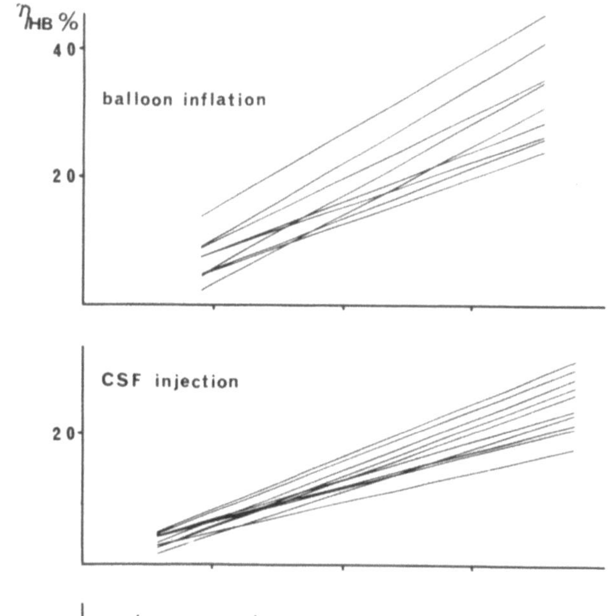

Session IV

INTRACRANIAL HEMORRHAGE

Chairman: M. Brock
Co-chairman: J.A. Jane

SUMMARY

It has become evident from the contributions to Session IV that monitoring of CSFP, CSF drainage and biochemical studies of CSF are of diagnostic, therapeutic and prognostic value in patients with intracranial bleeding, since in this group, outcome appears to be directly related to ICP, to the patency of CSF-outflow pathways and to the amount of blood and lactate in CSF (lactate levels higher than 3.0 mMol/l are usually associated with a bad outcome).

Nevertheless, group-specific differences are noted:

1.) While pathologic pressure waves (A-waves, B-waves, ramp-waves) appear to be rare or not to occur in the presenceof intracerebral hemorrhage, they are frequently observed in patients with subarachnoid bleeding. In this group, vascular spasm, acidosis of CSF, decreased CBF, and impaired CSF resorption, seem to cause overall alterations of cerebral metabolism. Since B-waves are closely associated with periods of REM-sleep and with clearcut changes in respiratory activity, they could, thus, be a sign of "central demodulation".

2.) Intracranial pressure/volume relationship is little altered in patients with intracerebral hematoma, while subarachnoid hemorrhage may profoundly influence this parameter. This underscores the relevance of CSF resorption pathways for intracranial hydrodynamics and constitutes the rationale for shunting procedures in patients in whom CSF resorption remains impaired and ICP does not return to normal one to two weeks after a subarachnoid bleeding.

3.) Shunting procedures will be required more often in patients with subarachnoid bleeding in whom vasospasm is observed. This is in line with the influence of the amount of blood in the CSF both on CSF resorption and on vascular spasm.

4.) Defective CSF resorption following subarachnoid hemorrhage seems to be due to an impairment of vesicular transport across the endothelial covering of the arachnoid villi, apparently related to the macromolecular substances associated with coagulation mechanisms rather than to the presence of corpuscular elements of the blood.

5.) Some patients with subarachnoid hemorrhage do not tolerate well even small rises in ICP, while showing clinical improvement upon CSF-drainage at lower pressure levels. It remains unclear to what extent this effect is due to pressure relief or to clearance of blood from the subarachnoid space. However, reducing ICP prior to eliminating the source of the bleeding (e.g. before clipping an aneurysm), appears to increase the risk of rebleeding.

It would appear that future work in this area should concentrate on the search for substances which, when applied systemically or into the CSF-compartment, promote or facilitate CSF-resorption.

ICP TIME COURSE IN PRIMARY INTRACEREBRAL HEMORRHAGE

I. PAPO, P. JANNY, G. CARUSELLI, G. COLNET, AND A. LUONGO

The criteria for making surgical decisions about primary intracerebral hemorrhages from arterial hypertension are still controversial. The removal of intracerebral hematomas has been advocated to relieve life-threatening intracranial hypertension or to prevent perifocal edema and hemorrhagic infarction from spreading into the surrounding parenchyma, thereby rendering the focal disorders irreversible. Nevertheless, only a few studies on intracranial pressure in such patients are available in literature (1,5). In both reports ICP was measured only once through a lumbar puncture. We have studied ICP time course in a relatively homogeneous series of 79 patients. Our initial results have appeared in previous reports (2,3,6).

Methods

ICP was recorded by LUNDBERG's technique in 75 patients: in 17 of them for periods of 24 to 48 hours over an average of three weeks, in the remainder continuously during the whole critical phase (3 to 12 days). In the last 4 patients with minor neurological disorders ICP was measured repeatedly for periods of 6 to 8 hours through a lumbar needle. Continuous recording was discontinued earlier in the patients who had pressure not exceeding 15 mmHg with stable tracing and normal pulsation. 71 patients had long-standing arterial hypertension. Four were alcoholic and in 4 non-hypertensive patients there was evidence of widespread atherosclerosis. 49 were males and 30 females. The youngest patient was 28 and was suffering from chronic glomerulonephritis and the oldest was 83. Five patients were in the 4th decade, 12 in the 5th, 33 in the 6th, 25 in the 7th, 3 in the 8th and 1 in the 9th. In 43 patients the hematomas were lobar in location: 2 frontal, 2 Rolandic, 23 temporal and 13 parieto-occipital. In the remaining 36 the hematomas were more deeply located, capsular or paracapsular. The ICP recording was begun in the first day of the ictus in 7 patients, between 1 and 3 days in 32 patients, between 3 and 7 days in 27 patients and more than a week after the onset of the stroke in 13 patients. When ICP was first measured 8 patients were alert, 30 confused, 21 drowsy, 11 comatose and 7 deeply comatose. Altogether 26 patients were operated upon: through a craniectomy or small craniotomy the clot was removed under direct vision. In 14 patients (8 with lobar and 6 with more deeply located collection) the operation was performed within 72 hours of the ictus and in the remaining 12 (10 with lobar and 2 with paracapsular hematomas) surgery was delayed 4 to 25 days after the stroke. 27 patients died in the hospital phase, 12 of them for extracerebral complications. The mortality rate was clearly related to the conscious level on admission. (Table 1)

Results

The ICP values on admission correlated with the conscious level are reported in Table 2.

Table 1. Conscious level versus mortality rate

Conscious level	no. of patients	fatal outcome
Alert	8	0
Confused	30	4 (13%)
Drowsy	22	8 (36%)
Comatose	11	8 (73%)
Deeply Comatose	8	7 (87%)

Table 2. Conscious level versus ICP on admission

Conscious level	ICP (mm Hg)		
	<20	20-30	>30
Alert	7	1	-
Confused	10	11	9
Drowsy	8	3	11
Comatose	1	3	7
Deeply Comatose	2	1	5

Table 3. Initial and terminal ICP values in the 14 patients who died with progressive neurological deficits

N.	Age	Sex	Initial ICP (mm Hg)	Terminal ICP (mm Hg)	Day of Death
1	60	F	60	70	7
2	55	M	50	70	4
3	62	F	45-80	90	5
4	55	M	10-80*	20-80	4
5	42	M	40	60	4
6	56	F	45	20	6
7	65	M	25	10	10
8	65	M	20	10	7
9	54	M	35	16	9
10	45	M	35	10	12
11	65	M	15-20	10-80**	9
12	66	F	20	15	3
13	66	F	45	10	5
14	64	M	70	120	2

* Rhythmic plateau waves.
** Agonal vasoparalytic peak (SAP rose from 160 to 240 mm Hg).

ICP time course in the whole series can be summarized as follows:

1) In the 5 deeply comatose patients with signs of vegetative disregulation and huge clots in the basal ganglia, ICP was very high from the onset with tendency to further rise. Therapy, whether medical or surgical, did not influence ICP time course and outcome, which was fatal in all cases.

2) In the majority of patients the pattern of ICP time course was rather typical: in the first phase after the stroke ICP was fairly raised, between 20 and 40 mmHg, save in 4 patients in whom it exceeded 40 mmHg, falling subsequently irrespective of the treatment undertaken. In some patients the slope of the curve of decreasing ICP was steep, in others flatter. There was no strict parallelism between ICP reduction and clinical condition. As a matter of fact, in some patients progressive clinical deterioration did occur despite substantial decrease in ICP, very low pressure was recorded in terminal phase(Table3).

3) In several patients ICP never exceeded 20 mmHg even in the very early phase. Some of these patients showed severe disturbances of consciousness due to huge hematomas with penetration into the ventricles.

4) Early increase in ICP associated with progressive clinical deterioration was observed in 3 patients operated on within 72 hours of the stroke.

5) As far as the postoperative time course is concerned, ICP fell after surgery to normal levels and never rose again only in 4 patients operated on within 72 hours of the ictus. 3 additional patients, operated on early, definitely improved but ICP levels were not significantly modified for several days. After delayed operations in all patients but one, ICP fell for a few hours after surgery only to rise again to its preoperative levels. Only one patient improved quickly after the operation, the remainder behaved as non-operated patients.

6) From the morphological standpoint, rhythmic plateau waves were recorded solely in one patient, who died from a huge capsular hemorrhage extending down to the pons and destroying the ipsilateral half of the brain-stem. Unstable tracing and occasional plateau and ramp waves are fairly common in tracing with baseline exceeding 20 mmHg. Conversely, large amplitude pulsation is very often observed even in patients with normal pressure not exceeding 10 mmHg. In these patients V/P response according to MILLER (4) was always normal.

Discussion

In correlating ICP and clinical time course, we see that the patients with no noticeable disturbances of consciousness have normal or slightly raised pressure. On the other hand, the patients harboring deep located collections and in coma with signs of vegetative disregulation usually exhibit very high pressure uninfluenced by therapy. By contrast, in the vast majority of patients with intermediate disturbances of consciousness no definite parallelism between ICP values and clinical condition was observed. The same symptoms and signs may take place both in patients with raised and with normal ICP. In the normotensive patients, therefore, the symptoms and signs which are usually attributed to intracranial hypertension would depend on other factors, like brain tissue disruption, widespread disturbances in microcirculation, CSF dynamic disorders and so forth. However, as ICP in the very phase of intracerebral bleeding is never recorded it cannot be ruled out that we miss brief stages of acute intracranial hypertension. Conversely, we have observed that several patients are able to tolerate very high levels of intracranial hypertension up 50-60 mmHg or even more surprisingly well, exhibiting only moderate disturbances of consciousness. All these patients have very high SAP and CPP seems to remain within acceptable limits and probably CBF is not too severely impaired. It is worth noting that the patients with massive ischemic brain infarctions are much less tolerant to intracranial hypertension. As regards surgical results, according to our experience, we would say that the most gratifying results were achieved in patients with lobar hematomas operated on within 72 hours of the stroke, even though in some of them ICP takes some days to attain normal levels. On the whole, the patients who underwent delayed surgery showed ICP and clinical time course akin to that of non-operated patients. It might be inferred, thereby, that after the first phase of three or four days at most, perifocal infarction, widespread disturbances in microcirculation and CSF dynamics disturbances are likely to play a more relevant role in producing dysfunction and raised ICP than the clot itself.

References

1. Arana Iniguez R, Wilson E, Bastarrica E, Medici M (1976) Cerebral hematomas. Surg Neurol 6:45-52

2. Janny P, Colnet G, Poppi M (1976) Intracranial pressure in the course of intracerebral hematomas in patients suffering from arterial hypertension. J Neurosurg Sci 20:224-226

3. Janny P, Colnet G, Georget AM, Chazal J (1978) Intracranial pressure with intracerebral hemorrhages. Surg Neurol 10:371-375

4. Millder JD, Garibi J, Pickard JD (1973) Induced changes of cerebrospinal volume during continuous monitoring of ventricular pressure. Arch Neurol 28:265-269

5. Mitsuno T, Kanaya H, Shirakata S, Oshawa K, Ishikawa Y (1966) Surgical treatment of hypertensive intracerebral hemorrhage. J Neurosurg 24:70-76

6. Papo I, Janny P, Caruselli G, Colnet G, Luongo A (to be published) Intracranialpressure time course in primary intracerebral hemorrhage. Neurosurgery

THE EFFECT OF EXPERIMENTALLY PRODUCED INTRACRANIAL HEMATOMA UPON ICP

P. MOHR AND R. LORENZ

Introduction

From the clinical standpoint, it is surprising that there is no clear correlation between the size of an intracerebral hematoma (ICH) and the intracranial pressure (ICP). We have produced experimentally an ICH model to study the effect upon ICP, arterial blood pressure (ABP), heart rate (HR), respiratory rate (RR), and other parameters.

Material and method

A total of 20 cats (weight between 2500g and 3300g) were studied. The preparations were made under general anesthesia (intraperitoneal application of narcorem). ICP was measured epidurally in the parietal region through symmetric burr holes with special MILLAR-tip-catheters. The burr holes were closed with plastics. ABP, HR, RR, and central venous pressure (CVP) were measured in the usual manner. For producing ICH 15 ml venous blood were taken, heparinized and stereotactically injected in the frontal lobe, in the capsula interna, in the hypothalamus, in the mid-brain, and in the basal subarachnoid space. A total of 6 ml blood was injected within 1 hour at a constant rate. After one hour the animals were killed and the brain in situ fixed by intracarotid injection of 5% Formol. The position of the needle, with respect to the ICH was controlled by careful anatomic preparation and section.

Results

The epidural pressure (EDP) rose slowly without any significant difference between the 5 localizations of the ICH, indicating only a moderate lesser rise in cats with lesions in capsula interna and mid-brain. After injection of 1.5 ml and 3.0 ml blood a further slowing of the increase was observed (Fig. 1). Contralateral to the lesion the EDP was somewhat higher. None of the animals died despite the fact that within 1 hour an equivalent of 10% of the total brain volume was injected.

We observed slight alterations of vital organs (Fig.2). In cats with ICH in the basal subarachnoid space, in the frontal lobe, and in the internal capsule ABP increased slightly. In the other localizations (hypothalamus and mid-brain) a slight decrease respectively on alternating course was found. A similar picture results concerning HR and RR. The CVP was stable in all experiments.

Discussion

The most striking fact in our investigations is that a total of 6 ml heparinized blood injected within 1 hour only produced slight alteration. There was no leak where CSF could escape. Compared with results obtained by other authors (1,2,3,4,5) with different methods, we can state that the experimentally produced ICH is similar to those experiments in which physiologic NaCl was used. In all experiments performed with the balloon inflation method a severe increase of EDP and severe vegetative alterations were found. It may be that the CSF resorption rate increased or that the injected blood was resorbed. (6)

Only slight alterations of vegetative parameters could be observed. The slight decrease of ABP, HR, and RR seems to be a local factor, but significant conclusions are not possible. A CUSHING response was not observed.

Summary

ICP, measured as EDP, rises in experimentally produced ICH slower than in experiments with the balloon-inflation method. Despite the fact that at the end of the experiment (1 hour), the injected amount of blood was 10% of the total brain volume, none of the cats died or showed severe alterations of vegetative parameters. This may be due to increased CSF absorption or absorption of the injected blood.

References

1. Asano , Basugi N, Saito I, Sano K (1976) Hemorrhage model in the dog. In: Beks JWF, Bosch DA, Brock M (eds) Intracranial Pressure III. Springer, Berlin Heidelberg New York, p 14

2. Beks JWF, Albarda S, Gieles ACM, Kuypers MH, Franderijn H (1977) Extradural transducer for monitoring intracranial pressure. Acta Neurochirurgica 38:245-250

3. Hamer J, Kuhner A (1976) Pressure response in patients with subarachnoid hemorrhage. In: Beks JWF, Bosch DA, Brock M (eds) Intracranial Pressure III. Springer, Berlin Heidelberg New York, p 157

4. Hase U (1978) Intrakranielle Drucksteigerung. Meßmethoden, Pathophysiologie, Therapie. Neurochir 21:145-157

5. Kassell NF, Peerless SJ, Reilly PL (1976) ICP, aneurysms, and subarachnoid hemorrhage. In: Beks JWF, Bosch DA, Brock M (eds) Intracranial Pressure III. Springer, Berlin Heidelberg New York p 147

6. Lorenz R (1976) The CUSHING response. In: Beks JWF, Bosch DA, Brock M (eds) Intracranial Pressure III. Springer, Berlin Heidelberg New York, p 270

Supported by Sonderforschungsbereich 32 der Deutschen Forschungsgemeinschaft.

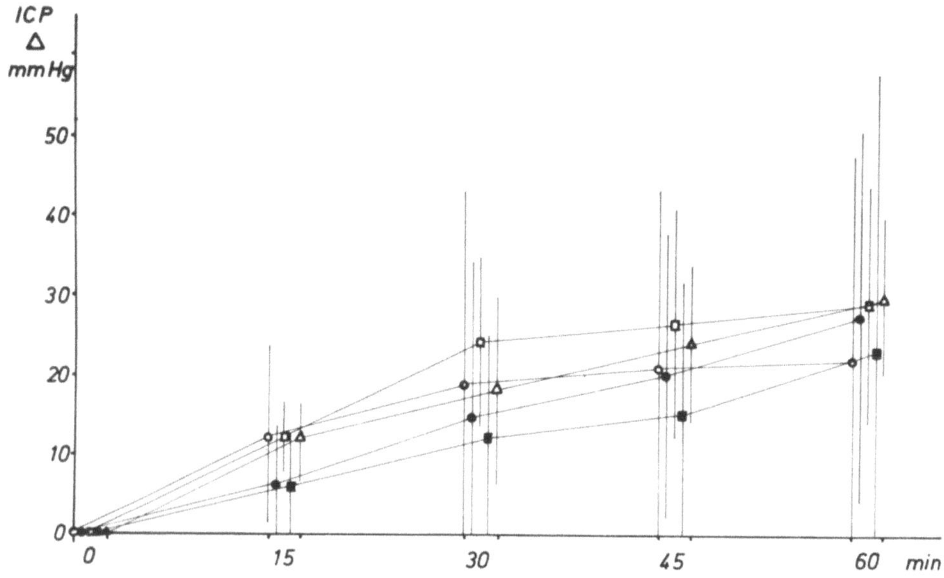

Figure 1. Mean values and variance of ICP with ICH in o frontal lobe, ● capsula interna, □ hypothalamus, ■ mid-brain, and Δ basal subarachnoid space.

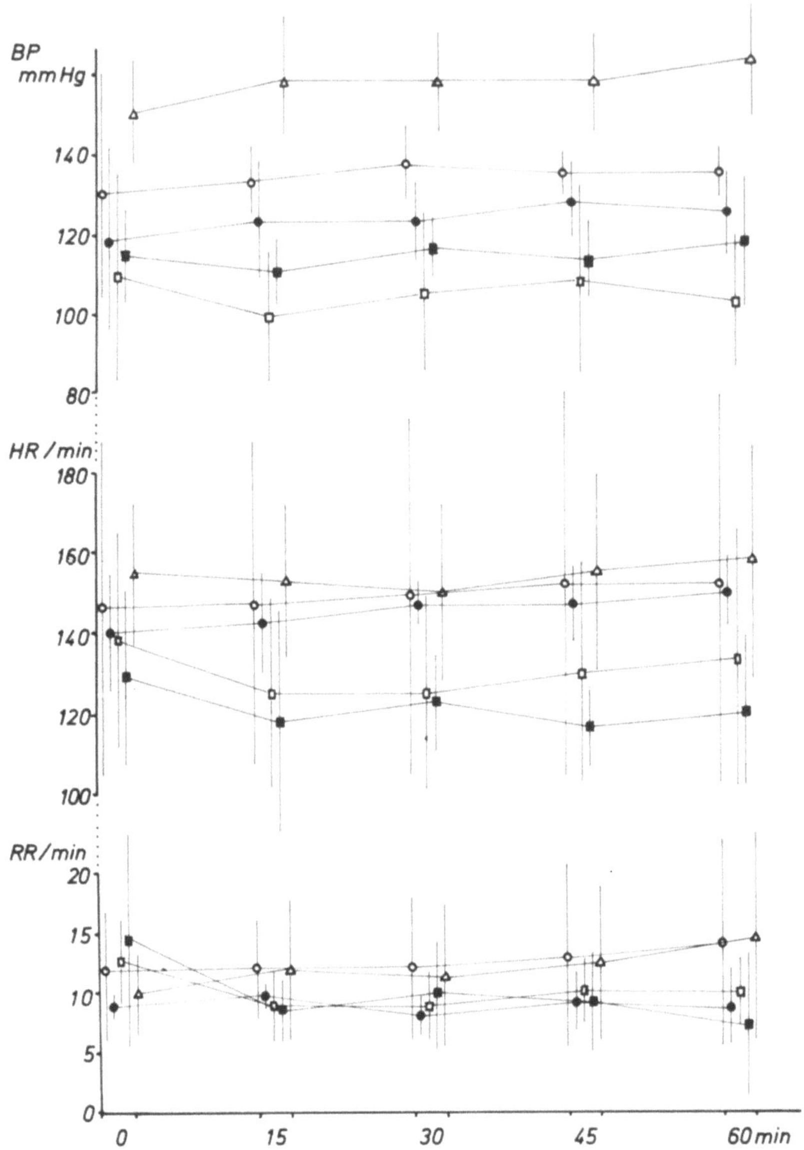

Figure 2. Mean values and variance of blood pressure (BP), heart rate (HR), and respiratory rate (RR) - ICH in o frontal lobe, ● capsula interna, ◻ hypothalamus, ■ mid-brain, and the Δ basal subarachnoid space.

INTRAVENTRICULAR PRESSURE, CSF LACTATE AND VASOSPASM IN RUPTURED INTRACRANIAL ANEURYSM

B. VOLBY AND E.M. ENEVOLDSEN

Introduction

The clinical condition and the age of patients suffering from subarachnoid hemorrhage (SAH) caused by a ruptured intracranial aneurysm are well-known factors of prognostic importance. Complicating events, such as vasospasm, cerebral edema and hydrocephalus, substantially influence the operative risk and carry a high mortality and morbidity. The pathophysiological mechanisms underlying these complications have been the subject of extensive studies during the last few years, and continuous monitoring of the intracranial pressure has especially given valuable information (3,4,6,8). In the present investigation we studied the clincal state of the patients, the intraventricular pressure (IVP), the levels of CSF lactate/pH and angiographic vasospasm in order to assess the value of these parameters for determining the optimal time of operation, and for the prognosis.

Material and methods

The series studied included 50 patients, selected from all patients admitted to the Neurosurgical Department, Aarhus Kommunehospital, since February 1976 with recent rupture of an intracranial saccular aneurysm. The mean age was 48 years (range 17-70). According to the grading system of HUNT and HESS (5), the patients were classified into three groups: I-II alert with no neurological deficit other than cranial nerve palsy. II-III intermittently somnolent or confused, or mild focal deficit. III-V impaired consciousness and/or severe neurological deficit during the whole course. IVP was measured according to the method of LUNDBERG (7), beginning between the 1st and 9th days after SAH, average measuring time being 7 days. Pressure curves were analyzed hourly for mean basal and maximum IVP and abnormal waves, From the intraventricular catheter, samples of CSF were withdrawn daily, if possible. Samples with heavy blood admixture were discarded. The concentration of lactate was determined by enzymatic method after metaphosphoric acid precipitation. pH was measured at the same time in anaerobically obtained CSF. From 2 to 9 samples were taken per patient, and a total of 219 samples were analyzed. Angiography was performed in all patients immediately before or after admission, and in 28 patients angiography was repeated within the first 10 days.

Results

The intraventricular pressure showed a good correlation with the clinical grade (Table 1). The mean pressure of grade I-II patients never exceeded the upper normal limit of 15 mmHg (mean ±SD being 8 ± 3.4). In grade II-III and grade III-IV the mean pressures were within the range of 15-30 mmHg (17 ± 6.8) and 20-40 (25 ± 5.4)mmHg. The maximum pressures showed the same correlations. In most patients with an IVP above 35 mmHg drainage was performed to a level of 25-30 mmHg.

Table 1. Clinical grading, mean IVP and CSF lactate values in 5o patients with ruptured intracranial aneurysm

Clinical grade	No.of Patients	Mean IVP mmHg	Mean Lactate mmol/l	Max.lactate mmol/l
I - II	11	5-15	1.9o ± o.o9	2.16 ± o.13
II - III	19	15-3o	2.52 ± o.13	3.o6 ± o.13
III- V	2o	2o-4o	2.91 ± o.16	3.59 ± o.23

Lactate values are mean ± SEM.

Rebleeding was observed in 7 patients, in 5 of them during drainage. B-waves were a common finding (86%) and their amplitude increased with the severity of symptoms.

All grade IV-V patients had marked B-waves, which disappeared mostly during external stimulation and always during ventilation. In some cases, however, small B-waves reappeared 1-2 days after controlled ventilation was instituted. No plateau waves were seen.

The lactate concentrations of CSF in relation to the clinical grade are shown in Table 1. The mean lactate of grade I-II was within the normal range (1-2 mmol/l) and significantly lower than grade II-III ($p<0.02$), which in turn was lower than grade III-V ($p<0.05$). These differences were even more pronounced for the maximum lactate values. There was a positive correlation between mean lactate and mean ICP (Fig. 1). Generally, lactate values exceeding 3.0 mmol/l predicted a poor outcome but two patients with maximum lactate of 3.3 and 3.6mmol/l recovered.

Cerebral arterial spasm demonstrated by angiography was seen in only two grade I-II patients, but was present in 63% of grade II-III and 75% of gradeIII-V patients. Mean IVP was significantly lower in patients without vasospasm than in patients with slight or severe spasm (Fig. 2). Mean lactate was higher in patients with severe spasm (2.89 ± 0.17) than in patients with slight (2.55 ± 0.16) or no spasm (2.30 ± 0.15).

The early outcome of our patients was: 14 recovered, 13 were more or less disabled and 23 died. Patients who recovered had significantly lower pressure and mean lactate than the other two groups.

Discussion

Our series show that the IVP in patients in satisfactory clinical condition (grade I-II) is within the normal range, whereas patients with some degree of impaired consciousness and neurological deficit (gradeIII-V) had a moderate to severe elevation of IVP with marked rhythmic pressure variations (B-waves). This close relationship between IVP and the clinical condition of the aneurysm patient has been shown by others (3,6,8). Possible mechanisms of significance for the increased IVP are a defective CSF absorption, cerebral edema and altered cerebrovascular reactivity. The role of arterial spasm in this connection is still uncertain. HASE et al (3) could not confirm a close connection between ICP and vasospasm. HAYASHI et al (4) found a suppression of ICP in an early period of the arterial spasm with a secondary increase. Our results show a correlation between vasospasm and IVP as patients without angiographic spasm had significantly lower IVP than those with spasm.

The lactate content of CSF in patients with SAH may be derived from glucolysis in shed blood cells and from hypoxic brain tissue (2). FUJISHIMA et al (1) found that CSF lactate correlated well with the clinical grade and CSF pressure in SAH patients. In the present investigation the level of lactate also showed a good correlation with clinical grade and IVP. In addition, patients with severe vasospasm had significantly elevated lactate levels, which probably reflected the metabolic state of the brain. Our data suggest that patients with lactate levels between 3-4 mmol/l constitute a risk group and that operation in these cases should be postponed.

Summary

Continuous monitoring of the intraventricular pressure and repeated determinations of CSF lactate/pH was performed in 50 patients with recent rupture of an intracranial saccular aneurysm. Patients in good clinical condition had significantly lower mean pressures and lactate levels than patients with impaired consciousness or severe neurological deficit. There was a positive correlation between lactate and IVP. Severe vasospasm was associated with high IVP and elevated lactate levels, and this predicted a poor outcome.

References

1. Fujishima M, Sugi T, Choki J, Yamaguchi T, Omae T (1975) Cerebrospinal fluid and arterial lactate, pyruvate and acid-base balance in patients with intracranial hemorrhages. Stroke 6:707-714

2. Granholm L (1969) The effect of blood in the CSF on the CSF lactate, pyruvate and bicarbonate concentrations. Scand J Clin Lab Invest 23:361-366

3. Hase U, Reulen HJ, Fenske A, Schurmann K (1978) Intracranial pressure and pressure volume relation in patients with subarachnoid hemorrhage. Acta Neurochir 44:69-80

4. Hayashi M, Marukawa S, Fujii H, Kitano T, Kobayashi H, Munemoto S, Yamamoto S (1978) Intracranial pressure in patients with diffuse cerebral arterial spasm following ruptured intracranial aneurysms. Acta Neurochir 44:81-95

5. Hunt WE, Hess RM (1968) Surgical risk as related to time of intervention in the repair of intracranial aneurysms. J Neurosurg 28:14-20

6. Kassell NF, Peerless SJ, Reilly PL. (1976) ICP, Aneurysms and subarachnoid hemorrhage. In: Beks JW, Bosch DA, Brock M (eds) Intracranial Pressure III. Springer, Berlin Heidelberg New York, p 147

7. Lundberg N (1960) Continuous recording and control of ventricular fluid pressure in neurosurgical practice. Acta Psychiat Neurol Scand Suppl 149 36:1-193

8. Nornes H, Magnes B (1972) Intracranial pressure in patients with ruptured saccular aneurysm. J Neurosurg 36:537-547

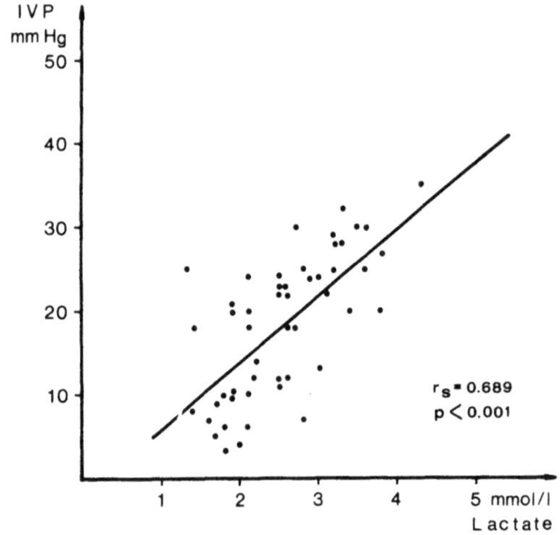

Fig. 1. Relationship between mean intraventricular pressure and mean CSF lactate in 50 patients. Regression line is shown (y=8.02x - 1.99). The correlation is highly significant (spearmann test p<0.001).

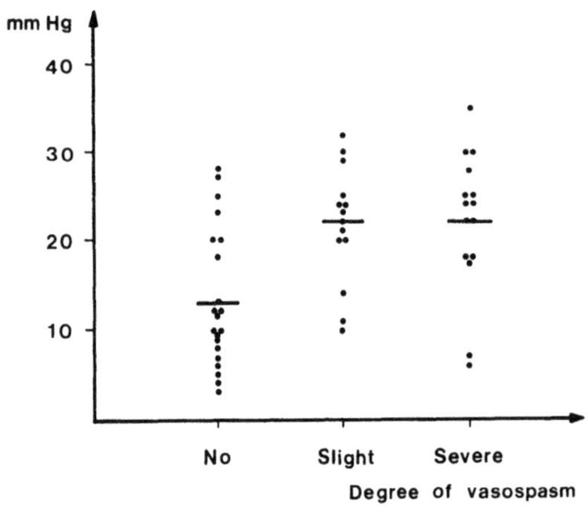

Fig. 2. Relation between vasospasm and mean intraventricular pressure. IVP in patients with slight or severe spasm is significantly higher than in patients without spasm (p<0.02).

INTRACRANIAL PRESSURE CHANGES IN PATIENTS WITH DIFFUSE CEREBRAL VASOSPASM

M.HAYASHI, H.FUJII, T.KITANO, H.KOBAYASHI, S.MUNEMOTO, Y.HANDA, AND S.YAMAMOTO

Introduction

The purpose of this investigation was to study the correlation between intracranial pressure (ICP), clinical status and prognosis in patients with angiographic evidence of diffuse vasospasm after rupture of an intracranial aneurysm.

Material and methods

The series consists of 23 patients with angiographic evidence of diffuse cerebral vasospasm. The patients were admitted within 2 weeks after subarachnoid hemorrhage (SAH). Diffuse vasospasm proved by angiographic study developed during the ICP recording in 11 patients, and it had already been found prior to the recording in the remaining 12 patients. The ventricular catheter was placed in the frontal horn of the right lateral ventricle, and it was connected to a pressure transducer. ICP was registered on a polyrecorder for 1 to 9 days, and when it exceeded a critical level, ventricular drainage was started at a level of about 15 mmHg. Diffuse vasospasm was defined as vasospasm involving the entire anterior cerebral artery or middle cerebral artery or both, in bilateral carotid angiograms, when the caliber of the arteries was reduced by more than 50%. The caliber of the arteries in repeated cerebral angiographic studies on the same patients served as controls.

Results

ICP Course in Diffuse Cerebral Vasospasm

Figure 1 summarizes the correlation between clinical status and mean ICP before and after the development of diffuse vasospasm in the present investigation. An increased ICP in the range of 15-40 mmHg was observed in the acute stage after SAH in 11 out of 23 patients with no signs of angiographic evidence of diffuse vasospasm. While awaiting clinical improvement, the mean ICP began to decrease gradually to a level of about 5-15 mmHg within a few days. Bilateral carotid angiograms at this time showed diffuse vasospasm. Nine of these patients showed signs of recovery in this stage.

A depressed and low ICP was observed in 10 of the patients with angiographic evidence of diffuse vasospasm, in whom the ICP recording was started between 6-11 days after SAH. In this stage, 3 patients showed minor or little neurological deterioration and 7 patients showed impaired consciousness or neurological deterioration.

Thus, the 21 out of 23 patients showed a low and depressed ICP in an early phase of diffuse vasospasm.

On continuing the recording, however, a secondary increase of ICP with or without neurological deterioration throughout the course of diffuse vasospasm. The term "cerebral vasospasm type "II" has been used for this type of ICP tracing. Two patients, in whom the ICP recording was started at the 11th and 13th day after the hemorrhage, had critically high ICP of about 35 mmHg as well as diffuse vasospasm. We believe that these cases may have had a period of low and depressed ICP some time before the vasospasm began. Therefore, we categorized these 2 patients into type I.

ICP Pattern before and after the Development of Diffuse Vasospasm

Figure 2 shows the continuous recording before and after the development of diffuse vasospasm in a type I patient. The beginning of the upper line shows the typical pattern seen in the acute stage of patients who are drowsy or semicomatose after SAH. Rapid variations were superimposed upon an increased ICP base-line. The following ICP began to decrease and the consciousness level improved in this stage. The ICP trace showed a pressure of about 10 mmHg with depressed fluctuations on the 7th day after SAH. Carotid angiograms at this time showed diffuse vasospasm. After 47 hours of low and flat ICP pattern, ICP began to decrease to a level of over 40 mmHg on the 8th day, and the patient became comatose. Continuous ventricular drainage was carried out. The patient survived but had severe neurological deficits.

Other Clinical Findings and Prognosis

Of the 15 patients of diffuse vasospasm type I, 6 patients (40%) were found to show enlargement of the ventricular system and 10 patients (66%) to have widespread low density on CT scan. Continuous ventricular drainage was performed in 12 patients and the administration of mannitol and steroid was made in 3 patients. The quality of survival was good in 6 of them (40%), poor in 5 (33%) and 4 patients (26%) died. On the other hand, 2 out of 8 patients of diffuse vasospasm type II were found to show a circumscribed low density on CT scan. In this group, only the administration of isoproterenol and steroid was made. The quality of survival was good in 6 of them (75%) and poor in 2 (25%).

Discussion

As to the increase of ICP within one week after SAH, we showed that this may mainly be due to an increase in cerebral blood volume as well as edema formation and CSF accumulation (1). On the other hand, in the present investigation, 21 out of 23 patients showed a low and depressed ICP for a period of 6-11 days after aneurysmal rupture. In this stage, angiographic evidence of diffuse vasospasm was observed in all patients. As far as clinical symptoms are concerned, about a half of the patients showed either minor or no neurological signs, or signs of recovery.

Hyperventilation is capable of producing a profound degree of cerebral vasoconstriction, and decreases ICP as well as cerebral blood flow (2). The low level of ICP in the early stage of diffuse vasospasm may reflect the decrease of cerebral blood volume as a consequence of vasoconstriction of the cerebral arteries. It seems likely that when ICP is depressed or remains at a low level, a certain reduction of cerebral blood flow is tolerated in patients with minor or little neurological deterioration, whereas a further reduction of the cerebral blood flow becomes intolerable in patients showing neurological deterioration or impaired consciousness.

In the present study, the patients having the ICP pattern of vasospasm type I showed manifest and serious neurological deterioration at the time of secondary ICP rise, suggesting the presence of ischemic brain swelling or cerebral infarction due to ischemia, or hydrocephalus. In this stage, continuous ventricular drainage or other decompressive procedures may be recommended as well as pharmacological methods. On the other hand, the present investigation shows that the ICP is supressed in the early phase of vasospasm type I and all through the vasospasm type II ICP course. In such a stage of suppressed ICP, drug therapy such as the administration of isoproterenol and steroid may be recommended. These drugs may alleviate the secondary rise of ICP in the type I patients and minimize the neurological deficits in the type II patients.

Summary

An increased ICP which developed in the acute stage after SAH was regularly followed by a depression of ICP between 6-11 days after SAH. Cerebral arteriograms at this time showed diffuse vasospasm. Of the 15 cases, 65% were found to show a secondary rise of ICP with serious neurological deterioration (diffuse vasospasm type I), while in the other 35% there occurred no increase of ICP throughout the course of diffuse vasospasm (diffuse vasospasm type II). The type I patients showed signs of widespread cerebral infarction or hydrocephalus or both in most cases (80%), whereas the type II patients showed signs of circumscribed infarction in only 2 cases (25%).

References

1. Hayashi M, Marukawa S, Fujii H, Kitano T, Kobayashi H, Yamamoto S (1977) Intracranial hypertension in patients with ruptured intracranial aneurysm. J Neurosurg 46:584-590

2. Lundberg N, Kjallquist A, Bien C (1959) Reduction of increased intracranial pressure by hyperventilation. A therapeutic aid in neurological surgery. Acta Psychiat Neurol Scand Suppl 139, 34:1-64

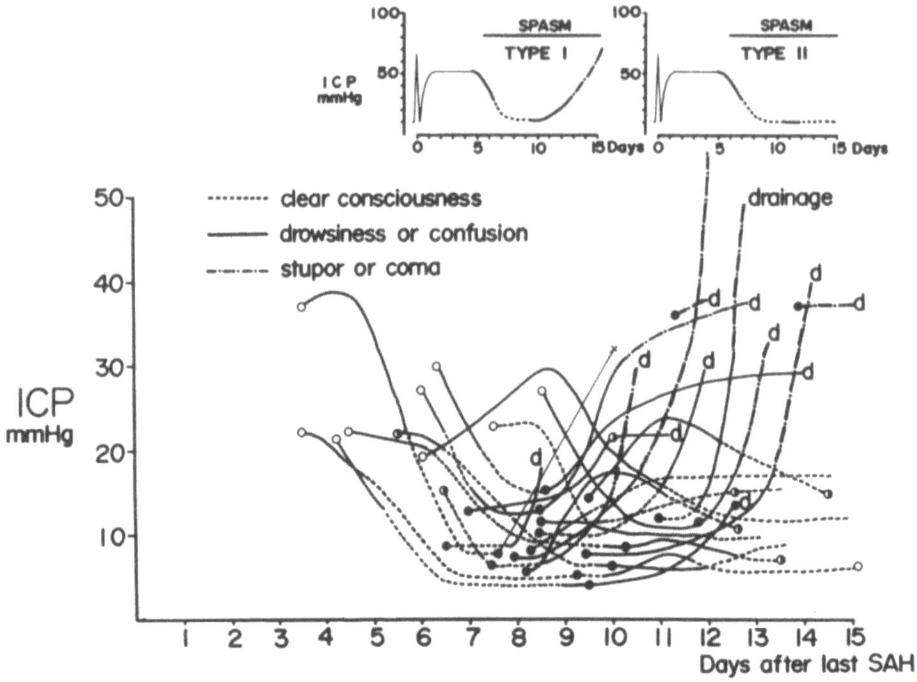

Fig. 1. Correlation between the time course of mean intracranial pressure (ICP) after rupture of an intracranial aneurysm and angiographic evidence of vasospasm in 23 subarachnoid hemorrhage (SAH) patients. Open circle indicates angiographic evidence of no signs of vasospasm. Solid circle indicates angiographic evidence of diffuse vasospasm. Semisolid circle indicates the presence of local spasm in angiogram. Upper 2 graphs show the schema of diffuse vasospasm type I(left) and type II (right).

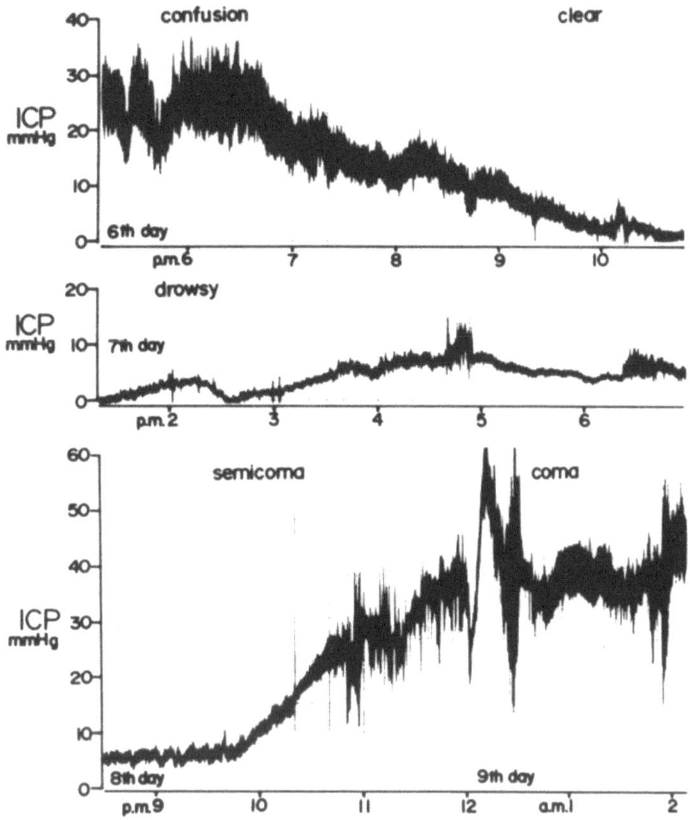

Fig. 2. Intracranial pressure (ICP) recording in a diffuse vasospasm type I patient. High level of ICP with marked fluctuations are seen at the beginning of recording and they are replaced by a low and flat ICP pattern. Carotid angiogram at this time showed diffuse vasospasm. Subsequent course of ICP showed, however, a steep rise to a level over 40 mmHg on the 8th day after aneurysm rupture.

CONTINUOUS MONITORING OF CSF PRESSURE IN ACUTE SUBARACHNOID HEMORRHAGE

A. HARTMANN

Introduction

Since the introduction of selective angiography and microscopic neurosurgery the chances of survival and clinical improvement of patients with subarachnoid hemorrhage (SH) have improved. However, there are still complications during the acute phase which influence the clinical outcome. These complications include development of early or late spasms, resulting in ischemia and eventually brain edema, and blockage of the CSF pathway by blood of leptomeningeal fibrosis.

The operative risks of patients who are classified according to the proposal of HUNT and HESS (5) as being in grade 4 or 5, are high and they are uncertain if the grade is 3. Treatment of the complications should improve the changes of these patients.

In recent years several studies were published evaluating the intracranial pressure (ICP) in patients suffering from acute SAH (1,3,4,6,8 7,10,11,12,13). Some of the authors mentioned report a decline of ICP over the time of monitoring. However, so far there exists no comparative study between CSF pressure data obtained on the first day of the disease and a few days later. We therefore have carried out a study which consists of continuous measurement of cerebrospinal fluid pressure (CSFP) during the acute phase of SAH. The first monitoring was performed on the first or second day after the initial bleeding and repeated between the 6th and 10th day. Our goal was to find an answer to the following questions:

1) Is there a correlation between CSFP and clinical grading and is there a change of grading if CSFP changes over the time?
2) Can monitoring of CSFP during the acute phase of SAH predict the course?
3) Can CSF removal via the lumbar subarachnoid catheter reduce CSFP?

Methods

The study was performed in 25 patients with acute SAH in whom operative therapy was not planned for several reasons. CSFP monitoring was started within 48 hours after onset of symptoms. Diagnosis was performed by lumbar puncture and angiography in all patients and computerized tomography in a few cases. Patients who were suggested as having intracerebral hematomas were excluded from the study. CSFP was recorded over 24 hours via a polyethylene catheter placed with 4 cm of its inner length in the lumbar subarachnoid space after a usual puncture, using a slightly bent needle. The outer end of this catheter was connected to a pressure transducer for recording of CSFP and mean CSFP on a polygraph. QUECKENSTEDT maneuver was normal in all cases. This measurement was repeated between the 6th and 10th day for 24 hours.

The patient was in supine horizontal position with the transducer at the level of the external auditory meatus. On each day of measurement the reaction of CSFP to CSF removal (CSFP drainage factor) was tested in the following way: the 3-way-stopcock of the catheter was opened till 1 ml CSF was drained. This was done 9 times at 3 different pressures. For each mean resting CSFP the mean CSFP-reduction per ml of drained fluid was calculated. This corresponds to the pressure-volume curve as reported by MILLER and LEECH (9), who injected fluid instead of removing it. We did not experience any complication during this study.

Patients were graded on each day of monitoring according to the proposal of HUNT and HESS (5), grade 1 having only minimal headache with slight nuchal rigidity and grade 5 being in coma.

Results

Fig. 1a and 1b indicate the 2 basic patterns which were observed during the period of CSFP recording. In most of the patients a reduction of mean CSFP was recorded from the first to the second measurement(Fig.1a). However, in a few cases mean CSFP did not change significantly(Fig.1b) and showed sometimes even an increased amplitude of the pressure curve. This indicates a reduction of the damping capacity with time.

All patients with clinical grade 1 or 2 presented on the first day with a low mean CSFP range, which, if it was slightly above the upper limit of normal (15 mmHg), came down till the second monitoring (Fig.2). Patients with grade 3 suffered on day 1 from either high or low mean CSFP (Fig.2). Normalization of mean CSFP was not observed in all cases till the 7th to 10th day. A similar pattern was observed in group 4 and 5, where patients presented on both measurements with either high or low pressure.

Figure 2 indicates that all patients with a resting mean CSFP reaching 35 mmHg suffer from low clinical grading (i.e.grade 3-5) but that not all patients with this low clinical grading 3-5 present with high mean CSFP: 2 out of 7 patients who were graded as being in grade 4 or 5 showed normal CSFP. As seen from Fig. 1 there was some variation of CSFP amplitude related to mean CSFP. In general, the amplitude increased with rising resting pressure (Fig. 3). The correlation between the resting mean CSFP and its pressure amplitude followed an exponential regression, which is indicated in Fig. 4. The exponential increase of the CSFP amplitude indicatesa progressive loss of damping capacity with rising resting pressure.

The alteration of the tolerance against additional intracranial volume, which is shown by the "CSFP-pressure amplitude curve" of Fig. 4, can be expressed by the pressure-volume curve or by the CSFP-drainage factor. If the resting mean CSFP was above 35 mmHg, CSFP dropped by up to 7.7 mmHg/ml drained fluid. The maximum reduction was 3.6 mmHg/ml drained fluid if the resting mean CSFP was low. Fig. 5 indicates that slow removal of 12 ml CSF reduced the pressure from 37 mmHg to 17mmHg (CSFP-drainage factor=1.67 mmHg/ml). It should be noted that after the CSF removal CSFP went up again. The variation of CSFP reduction per ml of drained fluid in all patients is shown in Fig. 6. The variation at a certain CSFP point was remarkable and was the reason for the poor regression coefficient in the linear regression correlation. Five to nine days later (the time of the second monitoring) the individual variation of the CSFP-drainage factor was much smaller, thus giving rise to a high regression coefficient in the linear regression(Fig.6.).

However, since resting mean CSFP above 40 mmHg was not observed on the second measurement the CSFP-drainage factor could not be tested to the same extent as during the first monitoring of CSFP.

Discussion

In SAH recording of CSFP with the method here described is a reliable way to control ICP continuously. Several studies including our own in 12 patients have shown that CSFP equals ICP if no herniation is present (4,6).

Regarding the questions mentioned in the introduction the results of this study can be interpreted as follows:

1) Correlation clinical condition and CSFP: Patients suffering from SAH in good clinical condition, i.e., grade 1 and 2, do present with a low CSFP range. The higher the pressure goes up on the first day after the bleeding the lower is the clinical grading. This confirms the observation of HAYASHI et al(4) and HASE et al (3), who described a close correlation between the height of ICP and the level of consciousness or clinical grading respectively. However, looking at Fig.2, it becomes obvious that even in group 4 and 5 a low CSFP can be measured over 24 hours. This indicates that not only ICP influences the clinical grading but other complicating factors also. Both patients of group 5 - one with low and the other with high CSFP - died within the following days without changing their clinical grading.

ICP as one parameter influencing the cerebral blood flow should be closely followed in all patients with acute SAH and bad clinical condition. In our own studies reduction of ICP in acute SAH resulted in increase of blood flow if ICP was elevated (2).

From the results presented here it seems to be unnecessary to monitor ICP in patients who are in grade 1 or 2. In patients with grade 3 through 5, ICP should be followed since reduction of elevated CSFP improves cerebral blood flow and thus the survival chances. In contrast to HASE et al (3) we have observed patients with a mean pressure higher than 30 mmHg who survived. So, even this pressure range should be treated. It should be added that our patient material presents a selected group of those cases who were not submitted for immediate surgery. This is not a randomized study and not a controlled one. We measured CSFP only for 10 days and not beyond that time. Thus, it might be possible that after the 10th day an increase of ICP due to edema or late development of communicating hydrocephalus can occur.

There was no dissociation between course of CSFP over the period of measuring and the clinical grading. That means in cases where CSFP came down from the first to the second monitoring the grading improved and in cases where no change of CSFP range occured the clinical grading remained unchanged. Eight of 10 patients with an increased CSFP on the first monitoring showed elevated values on the second measurement. This indicates that the monitoring of ICP for clinical purposes should be done beyond the 10th day if the clinical condition is poor.

2) Prediction of late complications: Five of our 25 patients developed late communicating hydrocephalus. All of them were classified in the acute phase as being in grade 3-5. Four out of these 5 had on

the initial measurement a CSFP above 20 mmHg (Fig.2). We conclude from this observation that deposition of blood in the subarachnoid space during the acute phase of SAH favors development of late communicating hydrocephalus if the initial CSFP is high. So far it is not proven that early removal of blood or even early shunting can prevent the development of communicating hydrocephalus due to leptomeningeal fibrosis.

3) Reduction of CSFP by CSF drainage: The removal of CSF leads to a reduction of the pressure within the pressure-volume curve. However, due to the variation of the CSF drainage factor the regression coefficient was rather poor. This means that if CSF drainage is chosen for increased ICP it should be done pressure controlled. Acute drainage once or twice a day is not useful since in a short time after drainage CSFP starts to rise again (Fig. 5). A continuous pressure controlled ventricular drainage seems to be the treatment of choice if ICP-elevation in acute SAH is due to obstruction of the CSF pathway. Other causes of elevation of ICP like edema or intracerebral hemorrhage can be excluded by other technical procedures.
Another reason for the continuous monitoring and pressure controlled drainage is the changing of the drainage factor over the time (Fig.6). Between the 7th - 10th day of our study there was a smaller reduction of CSFP per ml of drained fluid (as can be seen from both formulas shown in Fig. 6) compared to the first day.

Conclusion

In conclusion continuous monitoring of CSFP or ICP in acute SAH gives additional insight to the present condition of the patient. Since increased ICP might impair cerebral blood flow it should be treated. One way of handling elevated ICP in some cases is the pressure controlled CSF drainage, for clinical purposes best done from the ventricular system.

References

1. Hamer J, Kuhner A (1976) Mean intracranial pressure, episodic fluctuations, and intracranial volume-pressure response in patients with subarachnoid hemorrhage. In: Beks JWF, Bosch DA, Brock M (eds) Intracranial Pressure III. Springer, Berlin Heidelberg New York, p 157

2. Hartmann, A, Alberti E, Lange D(1977) Effects of CSF-drainage on CBF and CBV in subarachnoid hemorrhage and communicating hydrocephalus. Acta Neurol Scand, Suppl 64, 56:18.10-18.11

3. Hase U, Reulen J.-J, Fenske A, Schurmann K (1978) Intracranial pressure and pressure volume relation in patients with subarachnoid hemorrhage. Acta Neurochirurgica 44:69-80

4. Hayashi M, Marukawa H, Fujii H, Kitano T, Kobayashi H, Yamamoto S (1976) Intracranial hypertension in acute stage of ruptured intracranial aneurysm. In: Beks JWF, Bosch DA, Brock M (eds) Intracranial Pressure III. Springer, Berlin Heidelberg New York, p 162

5. Hunt EW, Hess RM (1968) Surgical risk as related to time of intervention in the repair of intracranial aneurysms. J Neurosurg 28: 14-20

6. Kassel NF, Peerless SJ, Reilly PL (1976) ICT, aneurysms and subarachnoid hemorrhage. In: Beks JWF, Bosch DA, Brock M (eds) Intracranial Pressure III. Springer, Berlin Heidelberg New York, p. 147

7. Klafta A, Hamby WB (1969) Significance of cerebrospinal fluid pressure in determining time for repair of intracranial aneurysms. J Neurosurg 30:217-220

8. Kusske JA, Turner PT, Ofemann GA, Harris BA (1973) Ventriculostomy for the treatment of acute hydrocephalus following subarachnoid hemorrhage. J Neurosurg 38:591-595

9. Miller JD, Leech P (1975) Effects of manitol and steroid therapy on intracranial volume-pressure relationship in patients. J Neurosurg 42:274-281

10. Nornes H, Magnaes B (1972) Intracranial pressure in patients with ruptured saccular aneurysm. J Neurosurg 36:537-547

11. Sundbarg G, Ponten U (1976) ICP and CSF absorption impairment after subarachnoid hemorrhage. In: Beks JWF, Bosch DA, Brock M (eds) Intracranial Pressure III. Springer, Berlin Heidelberg New York,139

12. Troupp H (1975) Intracranial pressure in hydrocephalus after subarachnoid hemorrhage. Zentralbl Neurochir 36:11-17

13. Vapalahti M, Nieminen V, Kari K (1976) Incidence of hydrocephalus and increased VFP in patients with ruptured supratentorial aneurysms. In: Beks JWF, Bosch DA, Brock M (eds) Intracranial Pressure III. Springer, Berlin Heidelberg New York, p. 135

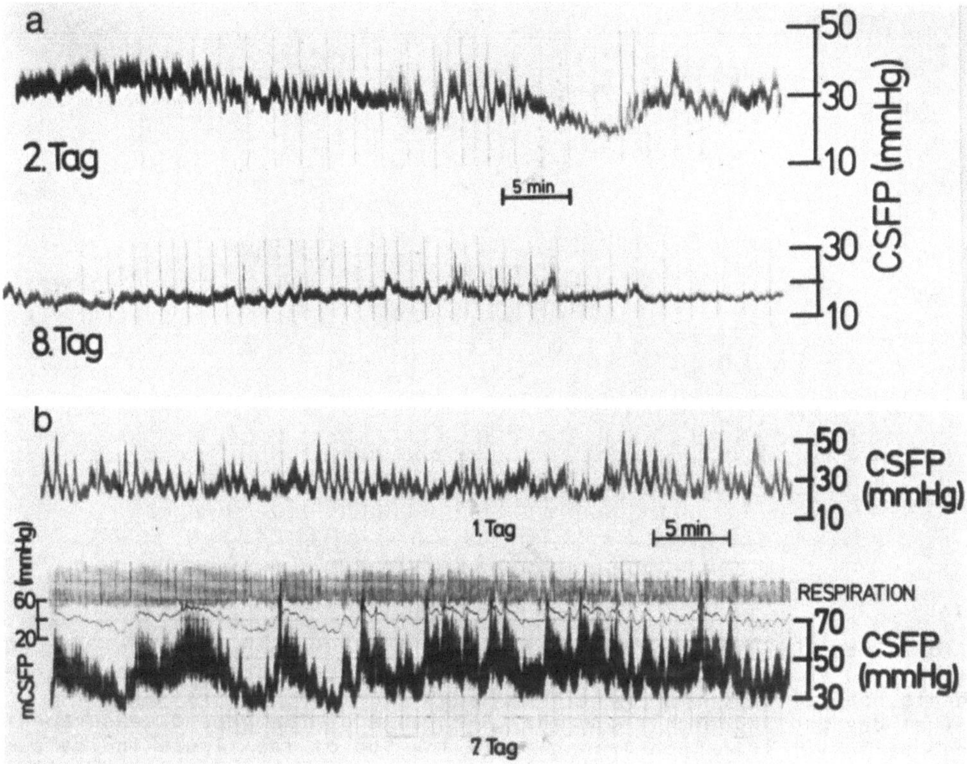

Fig. 1. Continuous monitoring of CSF pressure. The figure reads from right to left. a) shows CSFP on second (2.Tag) and 8th day (8.Tag). There is some reduction of CSFP with narrowing of the pressure amplitude. b) shows CSFP monitoring in another case on the first and 7th day. Mean resting pressure did not change but the pressure amplitude increased as a sign of reduced damping capacity.

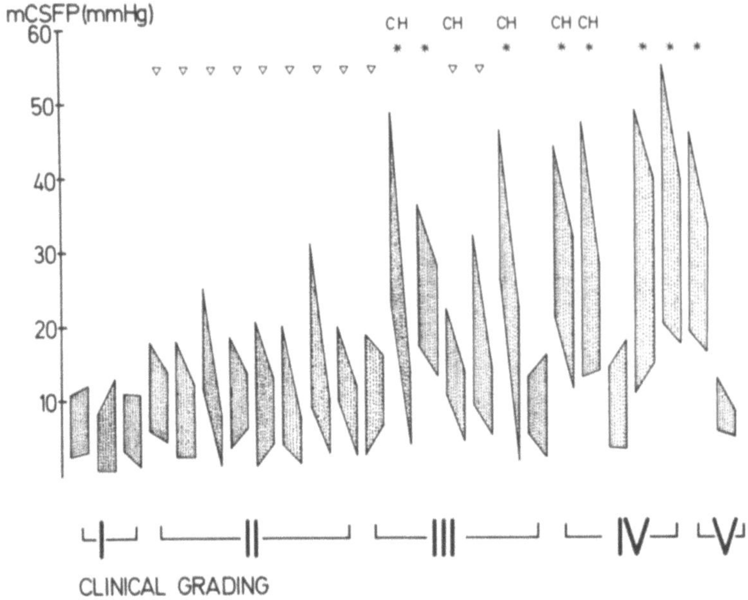

Fig. 2. Mean CSFP range in 25 patients with acute SAH, clinical graded from I to V according to HUNT and HESS (5). Each spotted area represents one patient. The left side shows the mean CSFP range on the first day and the right side the CSFP range of the second measurement on day 7 till 10. Open triangles in the top of the figure indicate those patients where an initially elevated pressure normalized till the second monitoring. Stars indicate those patients where CSFP was still increased on the second measurement. CH marks those cases which developed later on chronic communicating hydrocephalus.

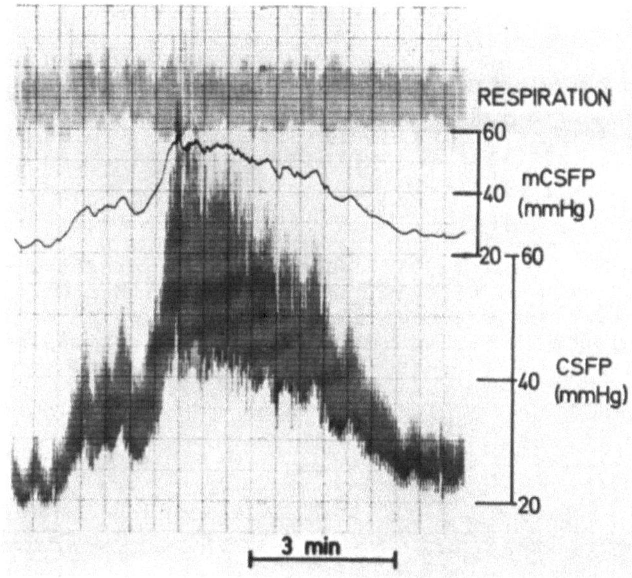

Fig. 3. Rhythmic pressure wave in SAH. Chart reads from right to left. With elevation of CSF pressure an increase of the pressure amplitude was recorded.

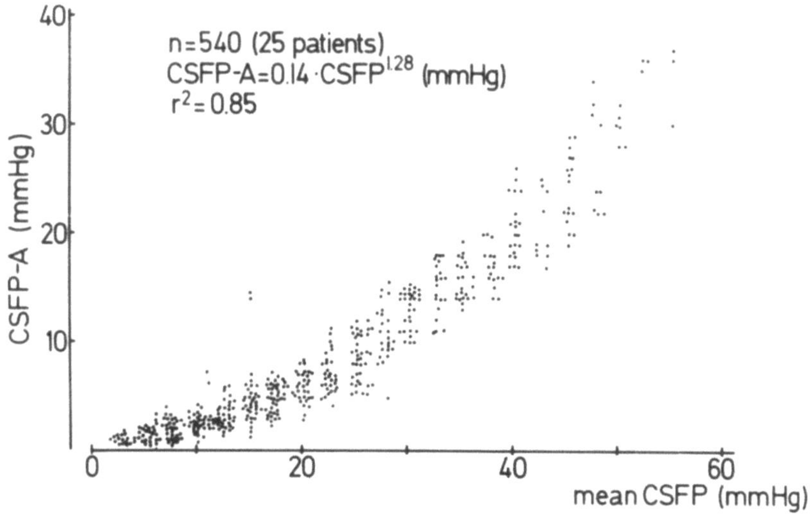

Fig. 4. Correlation between CSF pressure and the pressure amplitude.

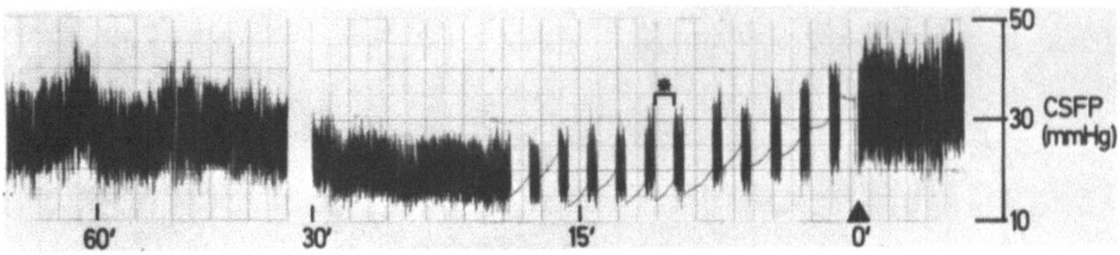

Fig. 5. Effect of CSF drainage on CSF pressure. Chart reads from right to left. I ml CSF was drained 12 times and CSF pressure was recorded between the drainage periods of I ml. The drainage period of one instance is marked with a star. After stopping the drainage new increase of CSF pressure was recorded. Time in minutes.

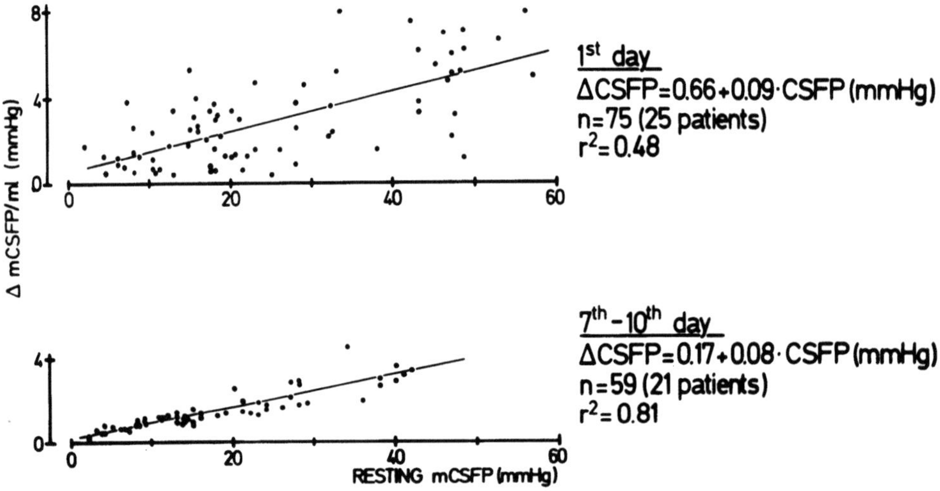

Fig. 6. Effect of CSF drainage on mean CSF pressure. The upper drawing shows the relationship between resting pressure (axis) and CSF pressure reduction per ml of drained fluid (coordinate) on the first monitoring, the lower drawing that of the second monitoring.

POLYGRAPHIC STUDY OF CSF PRESSURE WAVES DURING COMA

F. CALBUCCI, W. DALLOLIO, E. BENERICETTI, A. DORIZZI, AND C. MUNARI

INTRODUCTION

The aim of this study is to ascertain whether cerebro-spinal fluid pressure (CSFP) waves recorded during coma are correlated to modifications in electroencephalogram (EEG) and other variables as reported during sleep (3-7).

Material and method

Thirty-five patients (age 7-67 years) in acute coma, due to head injury (21 cases), subarachnoid hemorrhage (12 cases) and stroke (2cases), have been repeatedly submitted to polygraphic recordings, lasting 1-18 hours, for a total number of 84 recordings over 343 hours.

Seventeen patients were in light coma with appropriate motor responses to pain stimulation; 18 patients were in deep coma with decorticate or decerebrate motor responses. Twenty-four recordings were carried out on patients undergoing assisted respiration.

The recordings carried out on 16 channel ECEM polygraph apparatus (speed 15 mm/s) included EEG, intracranial pressure (ICP)(by ventricular catheter (6) or by MICROFET CV P8 epidural transducer), respiration (Resp) (by thermistor), muscle tone (MT), electrocardiogram (EKG) and eye movements (EM).

ICP was simultaneously monitored on a TECHNICORDER 3047 slow-speed recorder (speed 5 mm/m), synchronized with the polygraph by a time-marker, to obtain a precise visualization of the CSFP waves.

CSFP waves were classified as B-waves and plateau-waves according to LUNDBERG (6) definition, and also as "atypical" plateau waves, which were characterized by progressive and discontinuous increase of ICP with an abrupt fall at the end (Fig. 1 upper).

Results

B-waves: 80 sequences of B-waves (-approx. 50 waves) were recorded during 60 recordings. These waves were always correlated to short periods of EEG modifications. ICP begins to rise 6-9 seconds after appearance of fast desynchronized EEG activity occuring on a background of slow high amplitude activity (Fig. 1). These desynchronizations, sometimes with sleep-patterns, are accompanied by reduction of depth and rate of respiration and heart rate (Fig. 1), and disappearance of MT (Fig. 3). ICP falls 6-9 seconds after the reappearance of slow EEG activity, MT, tachycardia and hyperpnea.

Two sequences of B-waves were related to Cheyne-Stokes respiration with no EEG modifications.

"Atypical" plateau-waves: 46 waves of this type were recorded during 32 recordings, presenting B-waves also. The polygraphic variations which accompany these waves are identical to those described concerning B-waves, but with desynchronizations of longer duration. Falls during rising phase, as well as the end of the wave correspond to an "arousal" polygraphic pattern with reappearance of slow EEG activity and muscle tone, with tachycardia and hyperpnea (Fig. 2). This "arousal" can be spontaneous or provoked by pain stimulation.

Plateau-waves: 9 plateau-waves were observed, during 7 recordings, with no EEG modifications. In 2 of these recordings, EEG changes related to B-waves were noted.

Lack of CSFP waves, in 19 recordings, always corresponded to continuous high amplitude slow EEG activity unresponsive to stimuli. Sixty recordings with B and "atypical" plateau-waves and alternating EEG corresponded to light coma in 17 cases and to deep coma in 10 cases. Mortality rate was 25.9%. Twenty-four recordings with no CSFP waves (except 5 with plateau-waves) and continuous unresponsive slow EEG activity always corresponded to deep coma (8 cases) Mortality rate was 62.5%.

Nine recordings with CSFP waves and alternating EEG were carried out under assisted respiration: CSFP waves during desynchronization appeared attenuated in amplitude, sometimes reduced to a few millimeters, but not disappearing completely.

Discussion

The relationships between rapid ICP variations and changes in EEG and other variables during coma are similar to those described in sleep (3, 7). It is a fact that the periods of desynchronized EEG in coma, correlated to CSFP waves, resemble sleep-like activity (1, 2), due to the presence of sleep and arousal (4) patterns, changes in muscle tone, in depth of respiration and in heart rate. One possible origin of these CSFP waves in coma is the respiratory modifications which almost always accompany the desynchronization phases of EEG. This hypothesis seems to be confirmed by the delay in ICP variations with respect to the changes in other variables, particularly in respiratory depth and rate. This relationship between CSFP waves and respiration has been widely pointed out (5,6,8), but in our recordings respiratory variations are sometimes irrelevant (Fig. 3) and CSFP waves, although attenuated, do not disappear under assisted respiration. However, respiratory variations as well as changes in heart rate (5,8) appear as a partial aspect of the numerous phenomena which accompany the formation of CSFP waves in coma.

Another hypothesis, as suggested by COOPER and HULME (3) concerning sleep is that rapid ICP variations during coma, may depend on cerebral vasodilatation associated with an increased metabolic rate during desynchronized EEG. It cannot be excluded that both these mechanisms may act simultaneously.

Nevertheless, whatever the cause, our data do not permit us to affirm that CSFP waves in coma have a pathological origin, if plateau-waves are excluded. On the contrary they are accompanied by changes in EEG and in other variables which seems to show that capacity to elaborate physiological activities is maintained.

EEG with alternation of slow and fast activity permits a more favorable prognosis in traumatic coma (1). Despite the varying features of cases examined by us, which obviously preclude any definite prognosis, the recordings with CSFP waves and alternating EEG were obtained in lighter coma, with better outcome.

Summary

Thirty-five patients in acute coma were submitted to several polygraphic recordings including ICP, EEK, EKG, EM, MT and respiration, in order to study CSFP waves. B-waves and "atypical" plateau-waves were always correlated to short or longer periods of desynchronized EEG occurring on a background of slow EEG activity. Typical plateau-waves were never related to EEG modifications. The relationships between CSFP waves and EEG are similar to those described during sleep. The authors thus suggest that CSFP waves during coma are not necessarily a pathological feature, if plateau-waves are excluded.

References

1. Bricolo A, Turella G (1973) Electroencephalographic patterns of acute traumatic coma: diagnostic and prognostic value. J Neurosurg Sci 17:278-285

2. Chatrian GE, White LE, Daly D (1963) Electroencephalographic patterns resembling those of sleep in certain comatose states after injuries to the head. Electroenceph Clin Neurophysiol 15:272-280

3. Cooper R, Hulme A (1969) Changes of the EEG, intracranial pressure and other variables during sleep in patients with intracranial lesions. Electroenceph Clin Neurophysiol 27:12-22

4. Evans BM (1976) Patterns of arousal in comatose patients. J Neurol Neurosurg Psychiat 39:392-402

5. Kjallquist A, Lundberg N, Ponten U (1964) Respiratory and cardiovascular changes during rapid spontaneous variations of ventricular fluid pressure in patients with intracranial hypertension. Acta Neurol Scand 40:291-317

6. Lundberg N (1960) Continuous recording and control of ventricular fluid pressure in neurosurgical practice. Acta Psychiat Neurol Scand 36: Suppl 149

7. Munari C, Calbucci F, Versari P, Benericetti E, Columella F (1975) Pressione endocranica e variazioni del livello di vigilanza. Riv Neurol 45:35-44

8. Tindall GT, McGraw CP, Vanderveer RW, Iwata K (1972) Cardiorespiratory changes associated with plateau-waves in patients with head injury. In: Brock M, Dietz H (eds) Intracranial Pressure. Springer, Berlin Heidelberg New York, p 227

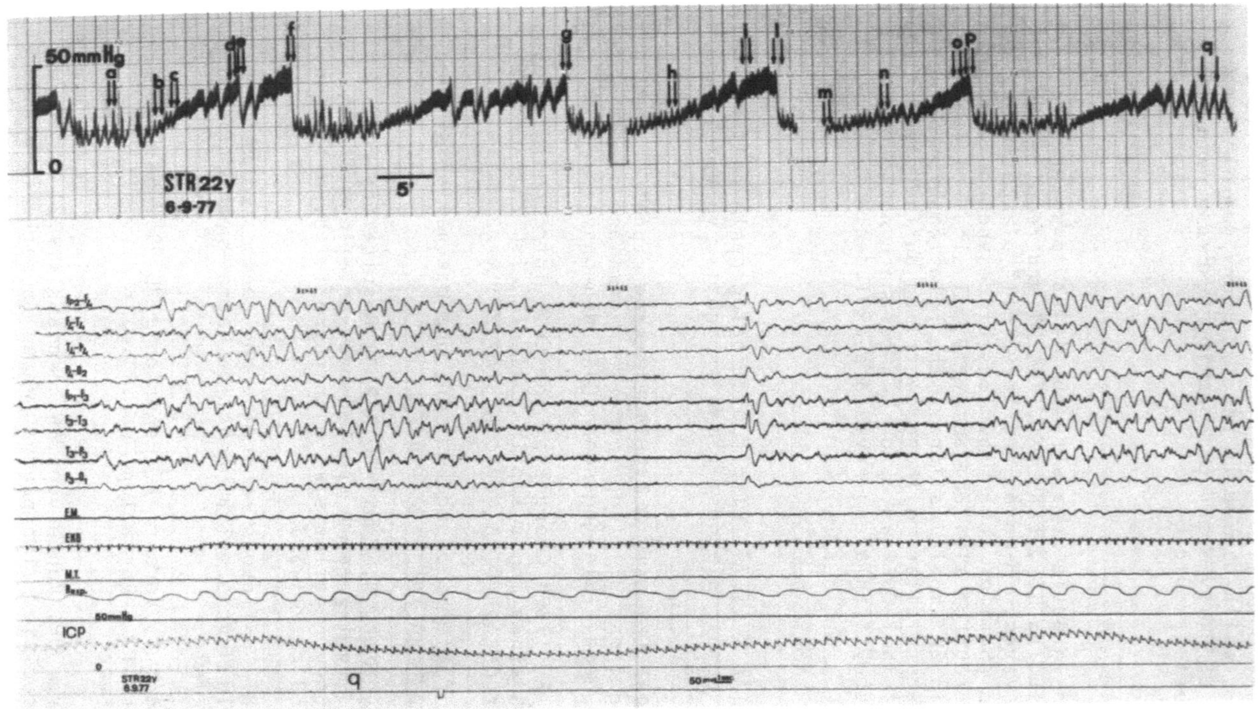

Fig. 1. upper: slow-speed ICP recording: a sequence of "atypical" plateau-waves (b-f, h-l, m-p) and B-waves (q).

lower: Polygraphic recording corresponding to point q. ICP increase occurs on appearance of desynchronized EEG, on a background of flow activity. On reappearance of this activity ICP falls. During desynchronization respiratory and heart rate are reduced.

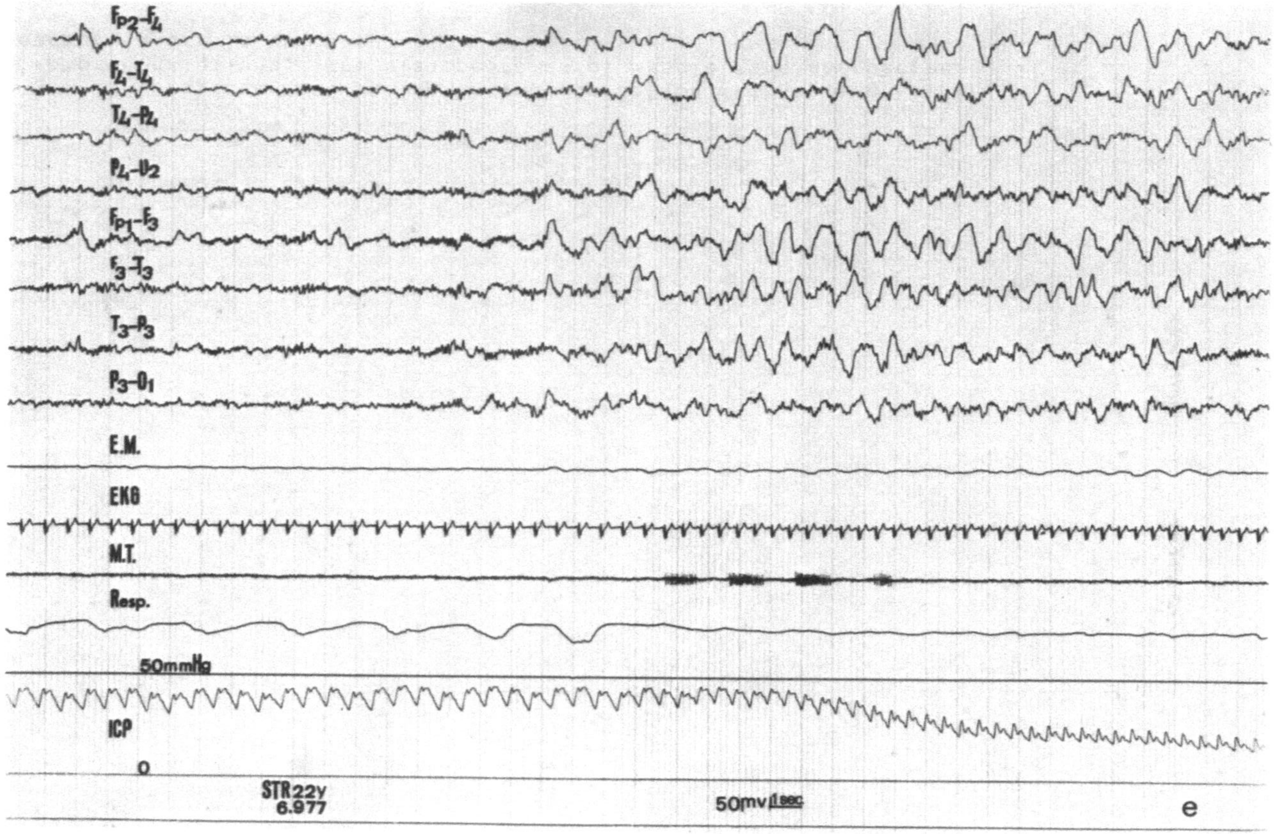

Fig. 2. Polygraphic recording corresponding to point e of Fig.1 upper. Falls during rising phases, as well as the end of the waves (points f, g, l, p) correspond to an "arousal" pattern with reappearance of slow EEG activity, muscle tone, tachycardia and hyperpnear (not recorded due to technical fault), after long duration desynchronization.

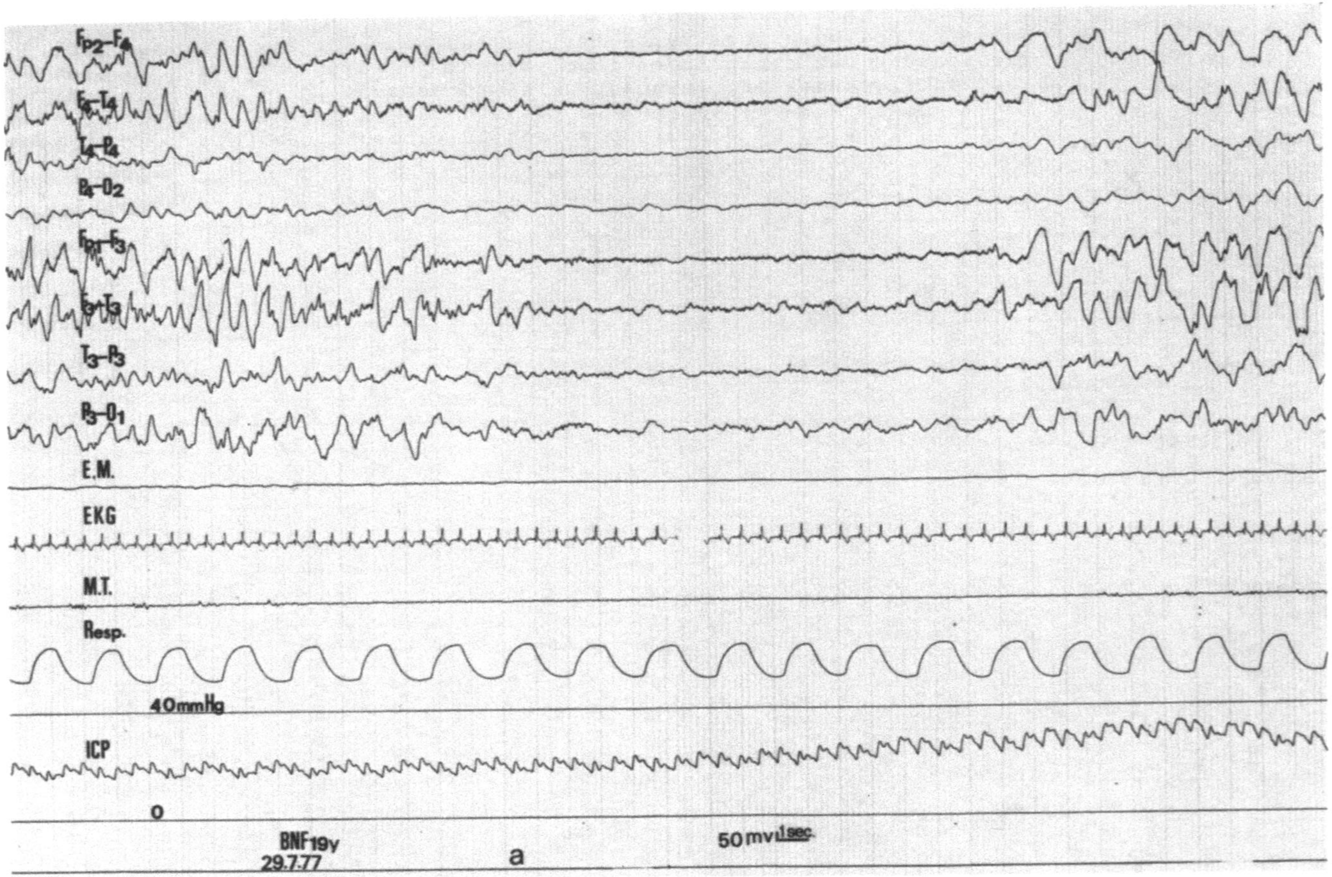

Fig. 3. CSF pressure-wave during desynchronization with no significant respiratory variations; the disappearance of muscle tone and decrease in heart rate are in evidence.

HYDROCEPHALUS FOLLOWING EARLY OPERATION ON RUPTURED CEREBRAL ANEURYSMS: SIGNIFICANCE OF LONG-TERM MONITORING OF INTRACRANIAL PRESSURE

T. SHIGENO, K. ARITAKE, I. SAITO, AND K. SANO

Introduction

The development of normal pressure hydrocephalus (NPH) following an early operation on a ruptured cerebral aneurysm is one of the major complications influencing the prognosis of patients, and its early detection is important in treatment. We have been studying the time course of intracranial pressure (ICP) in patients undergoing early operation, in the hope of gaining greater insight into the prediction of NPH.

Material and methods

A total of 208 patients with ruptured cerebral aneurysms were operated on. One hundred forty-one patients underwent early operation within two weeks after subarachnoid hemorrhage (SAH). The remaining 67 patients underwent late operation two weeks or more after SAH.

In cases of early operation cerebrospinal fluid (CSF) was continuously drained for several days following operation through a catheter set up in the basal cistern. Thereafter, continuous drainage of ventricular fluid was further carried out in a patient with an ICP above 15 mmHg. The development of NPH was assessed from continuous monitorings of ventricular fluid pressure (VFP) and CT scans, which were periodically performed for an average of three weeks after operation.

Results

The incidence of shunt surgery under the diagnosis of NPH was higher in early operation than in later operation; respectively 26% and 16%.

Vasospasm was closely associated with the development of NPH. Thirty-six percent of 73 patients with vasospasm eventually required shunt surgery, as compared to the significantly lower incidence of 16% in 68 patients without vasospasm.

There was also a significant tendency that patients with a large amount of CSF drainage later required shunt surgery. Fifty-nine percent of patients with a daily amount of CSF drainage above 200 ml underwent shunt surgery. In contrast, in patients with a lesser amount of CSF, the percentage was only 22.

VFP was periodically followed in 40 patients from both NPH and non-NPH groups (Fig. 1,2). During the first two weeks following SAH, VFP levels were higher than 15 mmHg in both groups. LUNDBERG'S B-waves(2) appeared frequently in this period. After the third week of SAH, however, there appeared a clear difference in ICP profile between NPH and non-NPH groups. By the end of the third week, VFP fell below 15 mmHg and B-waves ceased to appear in the non-NPH group. In contrast, in all 9 patients from the NPH group, sustained mild elevation of VFP, accompanied by pressure waves, continued beyond the third week after SAH.

The development of hydrocephalus was also followed on CT scans (Fig. 1, 3). During the first week following SAH, seven out of 15 patients showed ventricular enlargement. In most of these seven cases, the ventricles decreased in size during the second week. However, irrespective of the presence or absence of acute hydrocephalus during the first week, there was a tendency of the ventricles to enlarge after the third week in both NPH and non-NPH groups. In this period, the ventricular enlargement was always associated with periventricular lucencies in all patients who developed NPH.

Discussion

The incidence of NPH following SAH is considered approximately 10%. However, acute hydrocephalus is said to occur in a higher incidence during the early period after SAH. In our series, about half of the patients showed hydrocephalus during the first week after SAH. In contrast to the acute hydrocephalus, the period when the chronic hydrocephalus or NPH begins to develop has not been exactly determined. The present study indicates that three weeks are necessary for the development of NPH, for the following two reasons. Firstly, a definite tendency of the ventricles to enlarge in size after the third week of SAH was observed. Secondly, the persistence of increased ICP with pressure waves beyond the third week was seen in patients who later developed NPH.

The fact that many patients who underwent early operation developed NPH posed another problem to be solved. VAPALAHTI et al (5) also documented a similar phenomenon and assumed that it was caused by postoperative vasospasm. The present study also showed the close relationship between NPH and vasospasm. However, it seems more likely that both NPH and vasospasm were brought about by the same cause, i.e., the existence of blood clots in the subarachnoid space. SUNDBARG et al (3) found that as many as 20% of patients undergoing early operation with continuous ventricular fluid drainage for more than three weeks after SAH, required shunt surgery. It may be thus pointed out that both cisternal and ventricular fluid drainage in the acute stage of SAH cause adhesion and closure of the subarachnoid space, because they convert the flow of CSF.

In the initial stages of the development of NPH, other previous studies indicated that the periventricular region suffers the greatest loading (1). Periventricular lucencies observed in the present study are considered to be the result of this mechanism. Furthermore, the ICP was never normal but mildly elevated with pressure waves at this stage.

There is still a controversy as to the indications for shunt surgery, including the significance of pressure waves (4). However, the existence of the periventricular lucency and the above-mentioned pattern of ICP beyond the third week after SAH can be considered as a definite sign of the development of NPH.

Summary

Patients who underwent early operation on ruptured cerebral aneurysms had a higher incidence of NPH. Postoperative CSF drainage appeared to cause the development of NPH. In patients who developed NPH, mildly elevated ICP with pressure waves continued beyond the third week following SAH. The coexistence of this ICP pattern and periventricular lucencies on CT scan can serve as a guide to the indications for shunt surgery.

References

1. Hakim S, Venegas JG, Burton JD (1976) The physics of the cranial cavity, hydrocephalus and normal pressure hydrocephalus: Mechanical interpretation and mathematical model. Surg Neurol 5:187-210

2. Lundberg N (1960) Continuous recording and control of ventricular fluid pressure in neurosurgical practice. Acta Psychiatr Scand 36, Suppl.149:1-193

3. Sundbard G, Ponten U (1976) ICP and CSF absorption impairment after subarachnoid hemorrhage. In: Beks JWF, Bosch DA, Brock M (eds) Intracranial Pressure III. Springer, Berlin Heidelberg New York, p 139

4 Symon L, Hinzpeter T (1976) The enigma of normal pressure hydrocephalus: Tests to select patients for surgery and to predict shunt function. Clin Neurosurg 24:285-315

5. Vapalahti M, Nieminen U, Kari K (1976) Incidence of hydrocephalus and increased ventricular fluid pressure in patients with ruptured supratentorial aneurysms. In: Beks JWF, Bosch DA, Brock M (eds) Intracranial Pressure III. Springer, Berling Heidelberg New York, p 135

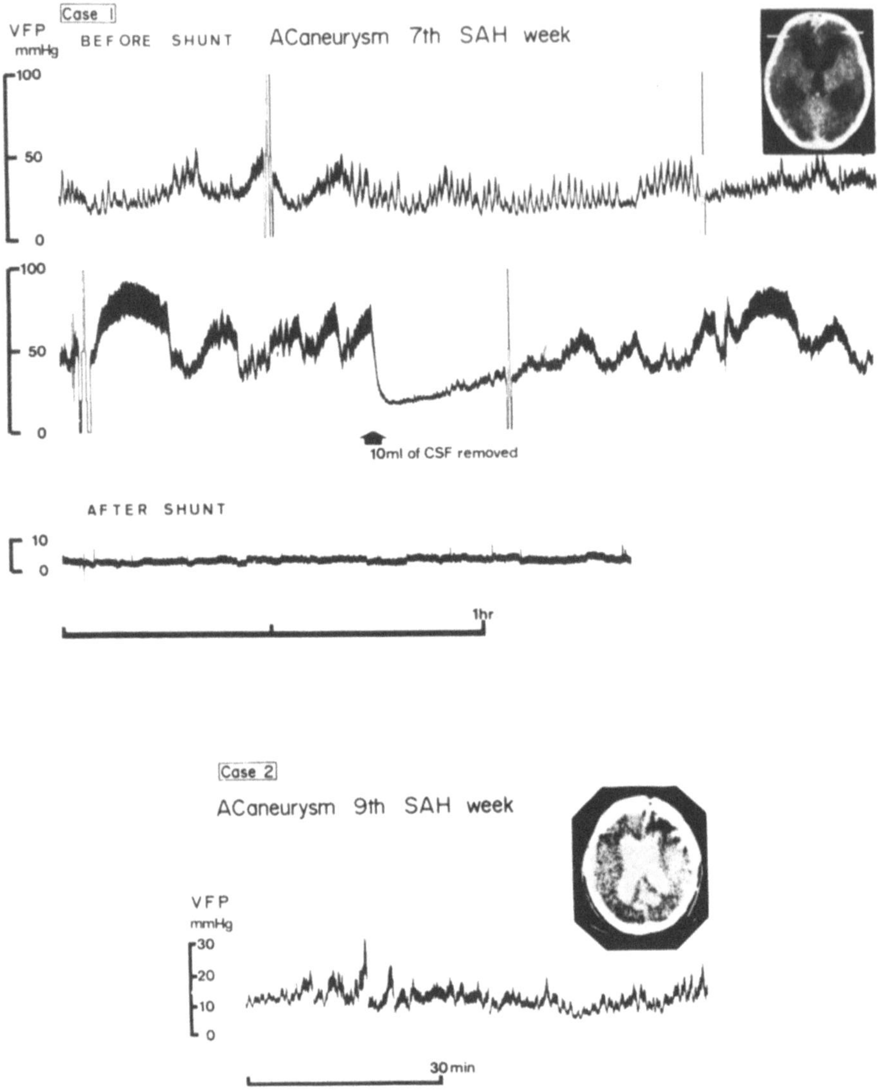

Fig. 1. Recordings of VFP and CT scans in patients with NPH. Several weeks after SAH, mildly elevated VFPs with pressure waves were still observed. Plateau waves were rare; seen only in case 1. Periventricular lucencies were observed (white arrows). The CT scan of case 2 was combined with metrizamide cisternography, showing ventricular reflux.

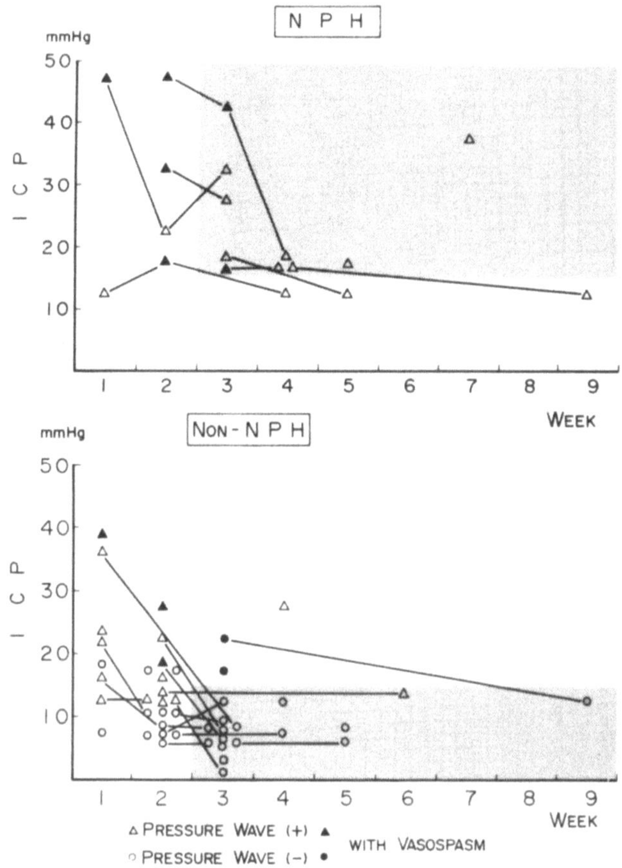

Fig. 2. Mean VFP levels after SAH in NPH and non-NPH groups. Individual pressures are grouped according to pressure intervals of 5 mmHg and weeks after SAH. Shade area differentiates the two groups at the third week, and also the VFP level of 15 mmHg.

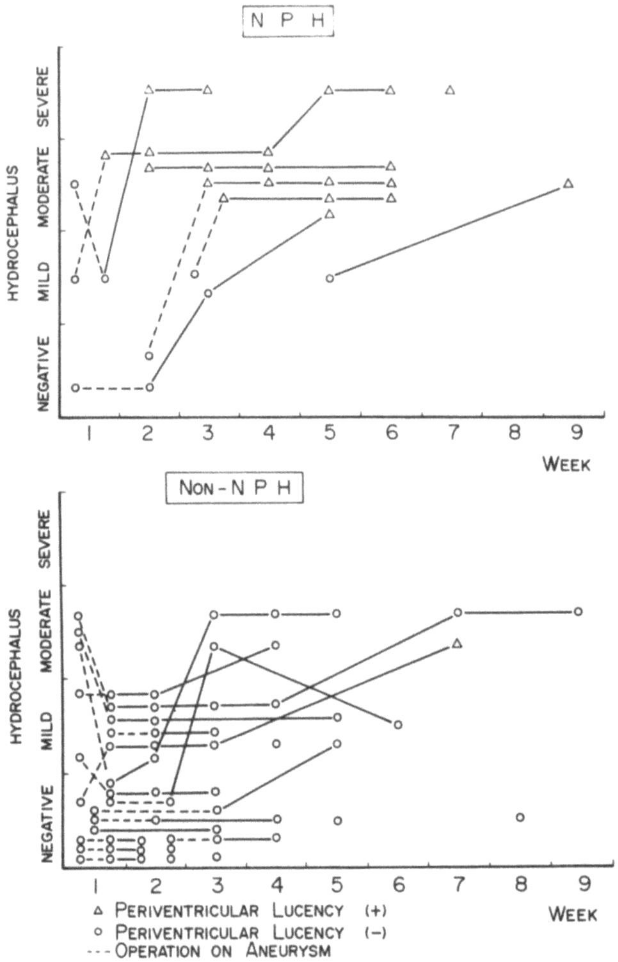

Fig. 3. Follow up of hydrocephalus on CT scans. Individual cases are grouped according to grade of hydrocephalus and weeks after SAH.

ALTERATIONS OF CSF HYDRODYNAMICS FOLLOWING MENINGITIS AND SUBARACHNOID HEMORRHAGE

U. FUHRMEISTER, P. RUETHER, D. DOMMASCH, AND M. GAAB

Introduction

Adult communicating hydrocephalus (characterized by low or normal CSF pressure) develops from an acute stage with increased intracranial pressure. This was demonstrated by various hydrodynamic parameters which were repeatedly determined in 26 patients suffering from purulent meningitis (n = 9), tuberculous meningitis (n = 7), subarachnoid hemorrhage (SAH, n = 10).

Method

A modified constant flow (rates 3, 4 or 5 ml/min) infusion technique using artificial CSF (1,2). Routine lumbar puncture (18 gauge needle), patient in lateral recumbent position, continuous electromanometric pressure monitoring (Statham P 37). Each patient was examined in the acute stage of his disease; 2 to 3 follow up tests were done in intervals of several weeks.

Data Analysis: Composition of the pressure/volume diagram (PV) by computerized elimination of leakage error andendogenous CSF formation. Calculation of mean resting CSF pressure (P_0), pressure at the break point (B) of the PV curve (2), high pressure elastance (E_h), low pressure elastance (E_l) and actual elastance (E_a), defined as slope of the tangent in P_0. Volume of compliance (V_{CO}) denotes that amount of fluid which can be retained in the CSF space without a raise of pressure (Fig. 1) (3). Transformation of typical pressure time absorption curves into volume/time curves. Calculation of outflow resistance (R) from the flow/pressure diagram (1,4).

Results

In the acute stage of SAH and meningitis CSF pressure (P_0) and resistance (R) are markedly elevated. The amplitude of arterial pulse waves is usually high, in SAH 3-fold higher than in meningitis. The onset of pressure decline is frequently delayed, the time of decompression is exceedingly long and the process is often incomplete as the pressure does not return to the original pre-injection level.

Quantitative evaluations were performed separately for three stages: acute = stage I, subacute (from the 20th to the 50th day of illness = stage II, recovery = stage III. Mean values (and range) of data are stated below.

Mean resting pressure (mmHg). Meningitis: stage I 21.9 (18.7 to 35.6) mmHg; stage II 7.2 (-4 to 23.5) mmHg; stage III 13.1 (8.5 to 17.2) mmHg. SAH stage I 28.0 (16.7 to 39.6) mmHg; stage III 8.2 (5.6 to 12.2) mmHg.

Resistance of CSF outflow ($mmHg \cdot ml \cdot ml^{-1}$). Meningitis: stage I 27.1 (16.9 to 37.9), stage III 8.43 (2.0 to 23.3). SAH: stage I 26.7 (19.6 to 31.9), stage III 7.8 (4.6 to 16.5). Flow/pressure relation was not linear in some cases (Fig. 1).

Changes in pressure/volume diagram. Elastance ($mmHg \cdot ml^{-1}$). Break points of the PV curve (2) were localized in a pressure range of 3.95 to 26 mmHg. Mean value of all patients was 14.8 mmHg. CSF pressure at the break point seemed to be an individual property of each patient, since it was not changed in the course of the disease.

E_l (range 0.42 to 0.68 mmHg $\cdot ml^{-1}$) was also seemingly unchanged. E_h in SAH: stage I 7.05 (3.7 to 11.5); stage III 2.37 (1.2 to 3.2). E_h/E_l quotient was approximately 15 in the acute stage, in state of repair it approached the normal or possibly subnormal value of 5.

Volume of compliance (ml). Negative V_{CO} values in acute stage of both diseases. Meningitis: stage I -4.85 ml, stage II 11.8 (3 patients showed increased V_{CO} values of 20, 20.8 and 30.5 ml), stage III 7.11 ml (Fig. 2).

Discussion

Two pathogenetic mechanisms are responsible for the elevation of ICP in the acute stage of meningitis and SAH. 1) CSF pathways are obstructed by blood elements or inflammatory infiltrates. Absorption of CSF is impaired, demonstrated by a 3-fold higher outflow resistance. The increase of resistance causes high CSF pressure. 2) The characteristic shape of the PV curve is altered. The slope of its high pressure segment becomes steeper, caused by edema, infiltration, and vasomotor disturbance. In addition, displacement of raised CSF pressure towards this stiff region of the PV curve abolishes the intracranial reserve space. V_{CO} decreases or becomes negative as evidenced by frequently occurring pressure waves. In the subacute stage all CSF hydrodynamic parameters tend towards normalization. A striking feature in subacute meningitis was subnormal CSF pressure in 2 cases and negative values in 2 other cases. V_{CO} was abnormally high (Fig. 2). Possibly an inflammatory aliquorrhea is the underlying phenomenon.

If only the mean values are interpreted, pressure and resistance are surprisingly normalized in the phase of recovery. Such normalization cannot, however, be demonstrated in each individual case. Five postmeningitis patients showed a borderline pressure. In 3 other cases pressure was slightly elevated to 15.7, 16.8 and 16.3 mmHg. Two of these patients showed an increased outflow resistance. It has to be noted that borderline CSF pressure and increased outflow resistance are the two main pathophysiological features of NPH.

The finding of a non-linear flow/pressure relation (Fig. 1) in some cases must be stressed. Calculation of R over the total pressure range (R_1) may lead to an incorrect assumption of normal resistance. Actually, high speed drainage ends in a high pressure range of 30 mmHg, where it is replaced by a slow operating system (Fig. 1, R_2). High outflow resistance of the second, slow-operating system has to be noted.

Summary

Alterations of CSF hydrodynamics following acute meningitis and subarachnoid hemorrhage were studied by a modified constant flow infusion technique. In the acute stage of the disease CSF pressure was high caused by high outflow resistance. The shape of the pressure volume curve changes by an increase of high pressure elastance. Pressure flow relation was found non-linear in some cases. After recovery post-meningitis patients showed borderline or slight elevated CSF pressure and an impediment to normal CSF drainage.

References

1. Ekstedt J (1978) CSF hydrodynamic studies in man. 2 normal hydrodynamic variables related to CSF pressure and flow. J Neurol Neurosurg Psychiat 41:345-353

2. Lofgren J, Von Essen A, Zwetnow NN (1973) The pressure-volume curve of the cerebrospinal fluid space in dogs. Data neurol Scand 49:557-574

3. Shulman K, Marmarou A (1971) Pressure-volume considerations in infantile hydrocephalus. Develop Med Child Neurol, Suppl 25, 13:90-95

4. Sokolowski SJ (1976) Bolus injection test for measurement of cerebrospinal fluid absorption. J neurol Sci 28:491-504

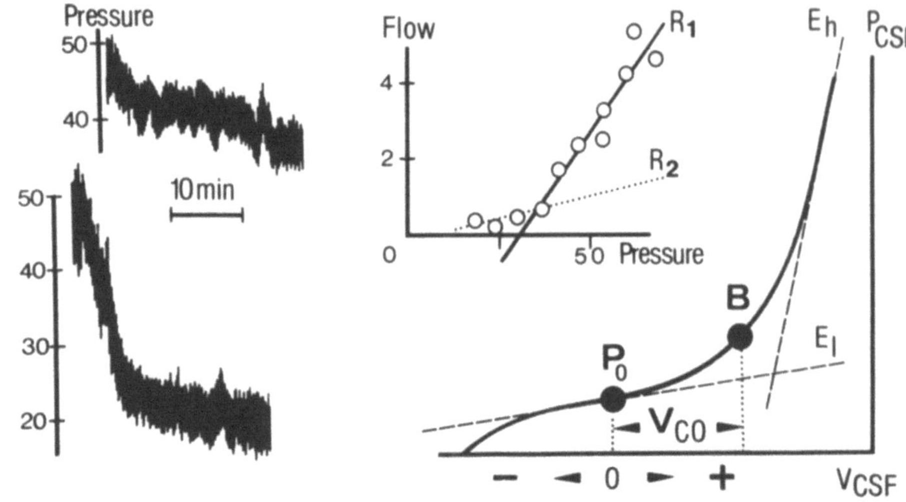

Fig. 1. Pressure/time curves, upper left: high pressure defect in acute meningitis. Lower left: low pressure defect in acute SAH, typical bi-compartmental resorption (4). Flow/pressure diagram: non-linear flow pressure relation, R_l = computerized calculation of regression line on the assumption of linear regression R_l crosses pressure axis (abscissa) at 30 mmHg, R_2 = proposed regression line separately calculated for the lower pressure range. Pressure/volume diagram: compliance volume (V_{CO}) is the amount of CSF necessary to shift resting pressure (P_0) to break point (B).

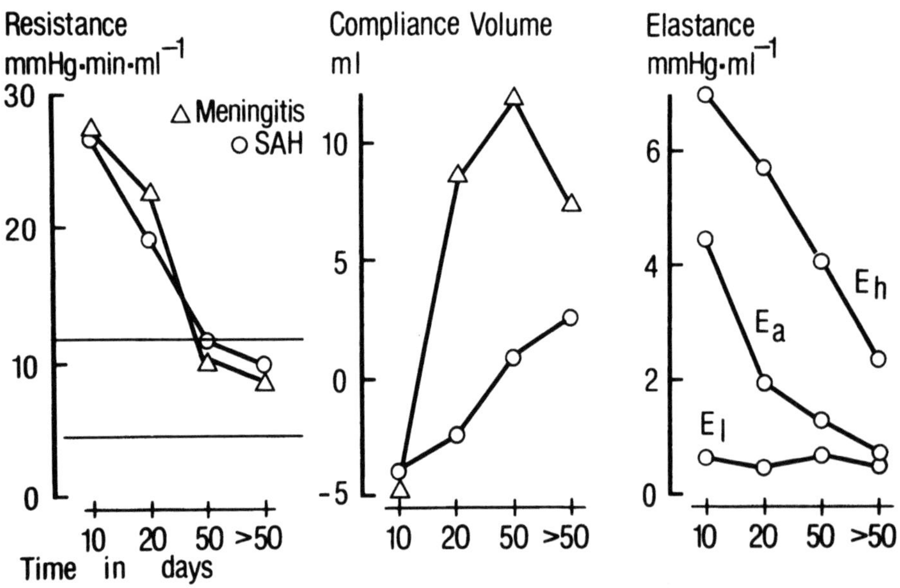

Fig. 2. Resistance, elastance, and compliance volume in the course of meningitis and SAH, mean values. E_h = high pressure elastance, E_a = actual elastance, E_l = low pressure elastance.

IMPAIRED ABSORPTION OF CSF DURING EXPERIMENTAL SUBARACHNOID HEMORRHAGE: EFFECTS OF BLOOD COMPONENTS ON VESICULAR TRANSPORT IN ARACHNOID VILLI

A.B.Butler, C.J.Maffeo, R.N.Johnson, and N.H.Bass

Introduction

Acute subarachnoid hemorrhage is frequently associated with sustained elevation of cerebrospinal fluid (CSF) pressure presumably caused by abnormal effects of accumulating blood on transport mechanisms regulating the efflux of CSF through arachnoid villi. Identification of the blood component(s) responsible for this increased resistance to CSF outflow has been subject to controversy. In the present study, we have assessed the role of various blood components to induce a disturbance in CSF transport using combined physiologic and morphologic observations to assess CSF transport at the arachnoid villus.

Material and methods

CSF outflow resistance and ultrastructure of the arachnoid villus were studied under conditions of experimental subarachnoid hemorrhage in 50 Sprague-Dawley rats (200-300 gms) before and after displacing 88% of the total CSF volume (250 microliters) with various blood components. After a needle was placed in the lumbar subarachnoid space, catheterization of the spinal SAS was accomplished by advancing a catheter through the needle to the high thoracic level. CSF pressures were continuously recorded during constant rate infusions of aritficial CSF (3). In this way, manometric assessment of CSF outflow resistance(2) was performed before and 15 minutes after constant pressure infusions of equivalent amounts of heparinized whole blood, plasma (fibrinogen content: 440 mgs), plasma dialysate (containing substances <6000 molecular weight), serum (fibrinogen content: 0), and artificial CSF, with and without heparin.

For electron microscopic examination of the arachnoid villus, equivalent volumes of horseradish peroxidase (HRP) and artificial CSF were infused into the subarachnoid space after infusion of the various blood components. The infusion rate of the HRP/CSF was adjusted to achieve a steady-state pressure of 800 mmH_2O in all experimental groups. When steady-state pressure was achieved, transcardial aldehyde fixation was performed to preserve the arachnoid villi in their pressure-induced state. Ultrastructural examination of the villus was performed on single and serial thin sections from all groups of animals.

Results

Intracranial pressure (ICP) more than doubled (221±20 mmH_2O) after infusion of whole blood or plasma into the subarachnoid space (Fig. 1) as compared with rats given plasma dialysate, serum, or saline (93.8 ±2.4 mmH_2O). Elevated ICP in the blood- and plasma-infused animals was associated with a three- to tenfold increase in CSF outflow resistance (Fig. 1), with CSF pressures ranging from 200-800 mmH_2O respectively.

In rats infused with saline, serum, or plasma dialysate, electron microscopic examination of the arachnoid villus endothelium demonstrated numerous HRP filled transendothelial channels seen as either single enlarged cytoplasmic vesicles or as transcellular chains of fused vesicles (Fig. 1). In contrast, rats infused with whole blood or plasma exhibited a marked reduction in the number of transendothelial channels (Fig. 1), despite CSF pressure equivalent to those in the other experimental groups. Additionally, an electron-dense fibrin-like material (Fig. 2) was seen within the arachnoid villi of animals infused with whole blood or plasma, identically prepared for electron microscopic examinationa, but without injection of horseradish peroxidase.

Discussion

The mechanism(s) whereby whole blood or one of its components may be responsible for increased CSF outflow resistance and elevated ICP accom, panying acute SAH has been subject to controversy. Although obstruction to CSF Outflow has been most frequently attributed to accumulation of red blood cells within the villus (1), the results of the present study suggest that blood components other than RBCs may impede CSF absorption. Previous descriptions of fibrin deposition within the subarachnoid spaces with SAH (4) and the results of this study demonstrating: 1) a fibrin net within the arachnoid villus, 2) increased outflow resistance, and 3) decreased endothelial vesicular transport in whole blood and plasma-infused animals suggest that macromolecular substances associated with the clotting cascade are contributory to altered CSF absorption in acute SAH.

Summary

The sudden release of large amounts of blood into the subarachnoid space causes an acute alteration of vesicular CSF transport through the arachnoid villi leading to increased CSF pressure. This dramatic effect on CSF outflow resistance can be simulated by macromolecular substances associated with the clotting cascade in the absence of blood cells.

References

1. Ellington E, Margolis G (1969) Block of arachnoid villus by subarachnoid hemorrhage. J Neurosurg 30:651-657

2. Johnson RN, Maffeo CJ, Mann JD, Butler AB, Bass NH (1978) Intracranial pressure regulation: A comparative model of cerebrospinal fluid systems. T.I.T. Life Sciences 8:79-92

3. Mann JD, Bulter AB, Rosenthal JE, Maffeo CJ, Johnson RN, Bass NH (178) Regulation of intracranial pressure in rat, dog and man. Ann Neurol 3:156-165

4. Suzuki S, Ishii M, Ottomo M, Iwabuchi T (1977) Changes in the subarachnoid space after experimental subarachnoid hemorrhage in the dog. Scanning electron microscopic observation. Acta Neurochirur 39:1-14

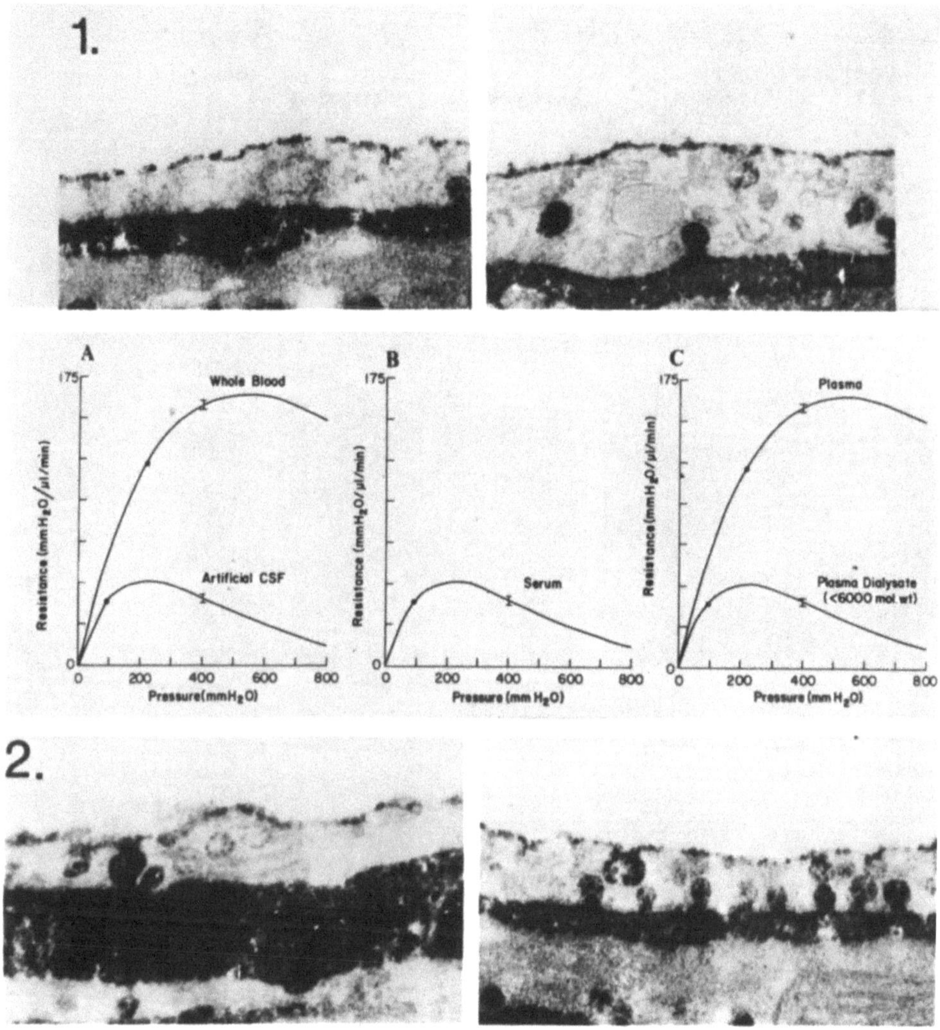

Figure 1
A,B,C: Comparative plots of CSF outflow resistance as a function of pressure in different experimental groups 15 minutes after infusion of different blood components.

1: Vesicular HRP transport through arachnoid villus endothelium after infusion of whole blood or plasma. CSF pressure: 800 mmH_2O. x 50,000

2: HRP transport through transcellular channels in arachnoid villus endothelium after infusion of either artificial CSF, serum, or plasma dialysate. CSF pressure: 800 mmH_2O. x 50,000

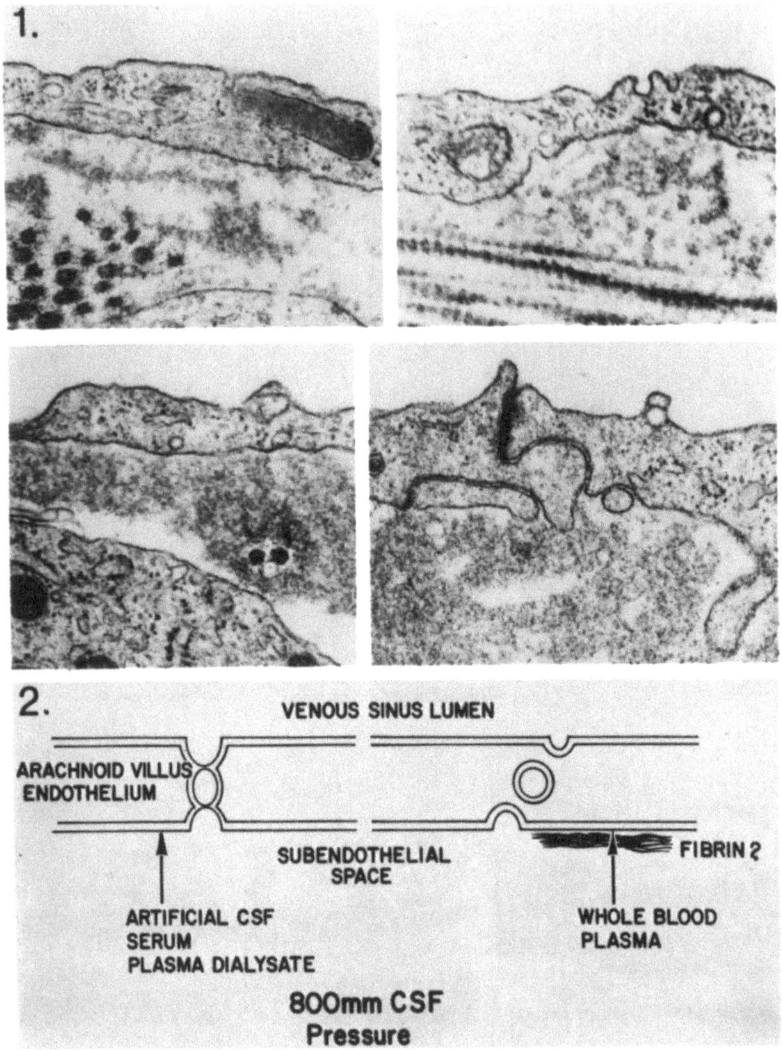

Figure 2
1: Fibrin-like net in subendothelial space of arachnoid villi after infusion of either whole blood or plasma. x36,000.

2: Diagramatic representation of vesicular changes in arachnoid villus endothelium induced by different blood components in experimental subarachnoid hemorrhage.

Session V

BRAIN EDEMA

Chairman: K. SHULMAN
Co-chairman: C.P. McGRAW

SUMMARY

Brain edema, by increasing the volume of tissue within the cranial cavity, induces a rise in ICP. The time course of this intracranial hypertension, pressure gradients and the effect of edema on cerebral metabolism seem to differ according to the model of edema. Attempts to demonstrate therapeutic effects of pharmacologic agents also seem to be model specific. The contributions presented in this session clearly recognize this issue and address it, providing important new information.

If brain edema can be defined as an increase in tissue water, one valid question is whether or not this increased water content, per se, affects blood flow, and is local flow dependent upon changes in tissue biomechanics? Using regional isotope techniques, DICK, NELSON and TURNER show that after a cryogenic injury in the cat no consistent association was seen between changes in glucose consumption, blood flow and edema. These data suggest that increased brain tissue water may not account for all the changes seen in blood flow and glucose consumption. A new model of "pure edema", a simple increase in tissue water content by white matter infusion has been developed to attempt an answer to this puzzle. MARMAROU and his colleagues show no change in CBF_r despite an 8% increase in brain water content. Autoregulation remained intact as well, but a reduction in CO_2 reactivity was a constant finding. With induced hypertension above the autoregulatory range, CBF_r does not rise in areas of increased water content. There is a rise of local tissue pressure and a gradient of 15 mmHg between the local region and ICP. This data suggests that biomechanical changes in brain tissue affect autoregulation and that "false autoregulation" is due to tissue pressure changes. In a separate set of experiments, WALSTRA, TAKAGI, MARMAROU, SHULMAN, and HOROUPIAN further define the biomechanics of the edematous process. These studies indicate that the white matter parenchyma is rather easily distended and that both regional tissue compliance and conductance change in the direction to favor continued spread of fluid and dissipation of pressure gradients. Tissue biochemical parameters were not presented, but need to be controlled in further use of this model.

GARCIA DE SOLA, VAQUERO, CABEZUDO and BRAVO demonstrate an interhemispheric pressure gradient from 8 to 52 hours after a cold injury in goats. CBF increased in both the lesion and control hemispheres associated with the rise of ICP, critical closing of dilated vessels occurring at an ICP of 44 torr. The EDP gradients can be questioned.

The trauma model of CORALES, MILLER and BECKER is dependent upon fluid percussion of the brain with the ICP rise directly related to the force of the percussion. In this model, however, there is no increase in brain water content; the level of ICP correlated best with the degree of traumatic subarachnoid hemorrhage produced. CBV or CBF were not measured. In a study of the comparative mechanics of mammalian brain edema. GARCIA and his colleagues underscore the need for careful neuropathologic analysis of the edematous process. In their models of postischemic brain edema, there was clear topographic separation between foci, showing protein escape and areas of increased water content. This early escape of protein in both hemispheres after untilateral MCA occlusion may deafferent otherwise intact neurons. They showed a perineuronal evacuation in both air emboli and ischemia to cause a neuronal deafferentation with a separation of axonal buttons from the neuronal cell body. Another unique model is that of MESANGEAU, ODILE, LEPAGNOL and AUROSSEAU, which depends upon a blood shift from the thoracic aorta (hypertension). Their animal (dog) developed brain edema and a no-reflow phenomenon. This results from a change of the redox state with an increase of brain lactate.

That brain water, per se, does not affect CBF_r while an equal brain water increase after a freeze lesion does alter CBF and brain metabolism strongly suggest plasma factors as potential edema agents. To address this issue, BAETHMAN et al studied CSF pressure during ventriculo-cisternal perfusion in rats using glutamate or plasma in their perfusate. In animals perfused with plasma, the perfusion pressure rose significantly above that of controls. This suggests to the authors that plasma-borne compounds of a yet unknown nature cause vasodilatation which enhances vasogenic edema mechanisms. The depth of penetration of the "active edema" factors remain unresolved.

The four papers dealing with the therapy of brain edema further underscore the need to choose specific edema models to answer specific clinical questions. Bony and dural decompression by craniectomy have been popular for some time. CZERNICKI, using a model of balloon compression in the cat, proposes that decompression is dangerous when it is done during the decompensation stage (when ICP is rapidly rising). His animals showed white matter hemorrhages and edema. Simiar results are reported by COOPER, HAGLER and CLARK. After a cold lesion in the dog, area of edema measured by Evans blue staining was significantly larger in animals with a craniectomy than in those without. The mechanism of increasing the differential pressure from intravascular space to interstitial fluid space is proposed. A valid question is that of "plateau wave" amelioration without decompression in patients. Treatment of the cold lesion in rabbits with multiple therapeutic modalities is the basis of the report of JAMES et al. Mannitol, Furosemide, alone or with mannitol, pentobarbital and acetazolamide all lowered ICP. All agents reduced water content but in a non-statistically different fashion; all increased hemispheric sodium content; but only pentobarbital reduced potassium significantly. In a model of ischemia, NEMOTO, GILBERTSON and ALEXANDER postulate that an increase in brain free fatty acids during such ischemia could contribute to brain edema. A critical concentration of barbiturate seems to prevent ischemia-induced lipolysis. Whether such lipolysis is a factor in edema requires further documentation.

THE TIME COURSE OF BRAIN TISSUE COMPLIANCE AND RESISTANCE IN A CONTROLLED MODEL OF BRAIN EDEMA

G. WALSTRA, H. TAKAGI, A. MARMAROU, K. SHAPIRO, AND K. SHULMAN

Introduction

In traumatic brain edema, the spread of fluid from the site of injury is in part determined by the biomechanical properties of the brain parenchyma. This study describes the changes of brain tissue compliance (TC) and resistance (TR) that occur in areas of brain tissue as fluids are infused using an edema simulator.

Methods

Fourteen adult cats under pentobarbital (30mg/kg,i.p.) were tracheostomized, paralyzed with gallamine (2mg/kg) and maintained normocapnic under nitrous oxide anesthesia. Femoral arterial and venous catheters were inserted for blood pressure monitoring and drug administration. An 18-gauge scalp vein needle was inserted for cisterna magna pressure (CMP) which was recorded using low compliance strain gauges.

Either plasma (4 animals) or saline (10 animals) tagged with Evan's blue was infused directly into the brain through a 25-gauge needle, connected to an infusion pump via stiff plastic tubing. A low compliance strain gauge was interposed between the needle and the infusion pump by a T-connector in order to measure inflow pressure (IP). Stereotaxic needle placement was either in deep white matter, cortical gray or basal ganglia

A total of 0.5ml was infused over 4 to 5 hours in each experiment. The infusion rate was adjusted so that inflow pressure did not exceed CMP by an established level for each experiment (10mmHg). The infusion rate in the first hour was 0.00075ml/min; the second hour 0.0015ml/min; and thereafter 0.0030ml/min. At selected intervals, estimates of regional tissue compliance and resistance were made in each animal by doubling the inflow rate over a short span.

Brain tissue resistance (TR) was defined as the change in steady state pressure per change in inflow rate (mmHg/ml/min). Tissue compliance was calculated by dividing the change in inflow volume (ΔV) by the observed increase in the inflow pressure (ΔP) and correcting for gauge compliance (GC). For comparison, TC was also computed by first measuring the time required for the inline pressure to reach 63% of its final value (equivalent to one time constant τ), and dividing by the measured TR, correcting for gauge compliance (TC = $[\tau/TR - GC]$). Following completion of infusion, animals were sacrificed, the brains removed and placed in formalin. Sections were taken to confirm needle placement.

Results

At the start of each experiment, prior to infusion of significant volumes values of TR with infusion of saline were the highest ($6.42 \times 10^3 \pm 0.61$ SE mmHg/ml/min, n = 10) for each experiment. This value, obtained in white matter, was similar to those obtained in gray matter of cortex and thalamus. Infusion of plasma showed a similar TR for all white matter areas studied. TR decreased rapidly as the infused volume approached 100 microliters; a more gradual decrease of TR followed as more fluid was infused, falling to ($0.81 \times 10^3 \pm .08$ SE mmHg/ml/min, n = 10) after infusing a volume of 0.5ml (Figure 1).

Initially, TC was low ($5.29 \times 10^{-5} \pm 1.34$ SE ml/mmHg, n = 10), but increased four-fold as the accumulated volume approached 200 microliters. TC was $32.7 \times 10^{-5} \pm 4.83$ SE ml/mmHg, n = 10, at an infused volume of 0.5ml, having increased five-fold from the initial value (Figure 2a).

We compared the two methods of computing brain compliance (slope and time constant). Slope calculations of TC evaluated through the time course of infusion were higher by a ratio of 4 to 1 (Figure 2b).

During the four hours of infusion the inflow pressure (IP) described the following course. At the start of infusion, IP increased to a peak of 30mmHg and within a span of 5 to 20 mintues, gradually decreased to approach the value of the CMP. The infusion rate was then adjusted so as not to exceed a 10mmHg gradient between IP and CMP. Blood pressure, CMP, and bulk brain compliance, as measured by the Pressure Volume Index (PVI) remained constant throughout all experiments regardless of the fluid used in the infusate.

Discussion

This study uses a point source generator to infuse fixed volumes of fluid through brain parenchyma. As such it is an edema simulating model which gives the investigator control over the artificial edema process. Having control not only of the process but also of the "edema fluid", one can control several variables in the study of edema.
This study was undertaken solely to investigate the mechanical properties of the brain as a response to this edema model. A fixed volume of fluid was infused corresponding to the amount accounted for in a cold injury as measured by gravimetric technique (2).

Two methods were used for computing brain tissue compliance. As shown by comparison of Figures 2a and 2b the slope method differs from the time constant method. Values for the slope method were 3 to 4 times greater than those computed by the time constant technique. We considered the slope method less accurate, since it involves a linear approximation of an exponential function and would tend to yield a larger estimate of TC. Comparisons of TR and TC (Figures 1 and 2) during continued infusion show a reciprocal relationship between these two parameters. This would suggest that, as the infusion of fluids occurs, the extracellular space within the brain is distended, allowing for easier migration of fluid. However, as seen in Figure 1, tissue resistance plateaus in spite of increasing volumes of fluid. It is clear from the increase of infused volume over time, that more rapid infusion of fluid can occur with a tissue resistance remaining relatively low during this period of more rapid "edema" accumulation. This would support the concept that relatively small tissue pressure gradients are required to propel fluid (3).

Two infusates were used in this series of experiments. The profiles for both plasma and saline are similar with equal TR being encountered initially and with similar decreases in TR as the infusion volume increases. Since the inflow pressure and CMP did not differ significantly between these two series, it appears that the viscosity (plasma vs saline) of the infusate did not alter the biomechanical properties of the brain parenchyma.

Difficulty was encountered in the stereotaxic positioning of the needle tip in cortical gray matter. However, needle positioning in basal ganglia was accurate. TR and TC in basal ganglia were of the same order of magnitude as white matter.

The similarity of basal ganglia and white matter biomechanical profiles suggests that both types of tissue are equally distensible and should accommodate the spread of edema. However, in both laboratory and clinical settings, it is clear that for certain types of edema (vasogenic) white matter is more vulnerable to the spread of edema (1). Infusion pressure in gray matter remained at the same levels as white matter. Tests indicate that no excessive resistance was offered by the tissue. This would suggest that the restriction of edema fluid to the white matter in vasogenic edema may be due primarily to fibre tract orientation.

Conclusion

These studies show that the brain parenchyma is easily distended and that, in white matter edema, both regional tissue compliance and conductance change in a direction which tends to favor the migration of edema fluid.

References

1. Klatzo I, Wisneiwski H, Steinwall O, Streicher E (1967) Dynamics of cold injury edema. In: Klatzo H, Steitelberg F (eds) Brain Edema. Springer, Berlin Heidelberg New York, p. 554

2. Marmarou A, Poll W, Shulman K, Bhagavan H (1978) A simple gravimetric technique for measurement of cerebral edema. J Neurosurg 48:530-537

3. Shapiro K, Shulman K, Marmarou A, Poll W (1977) Tissue pressure gradients in spinal cord injury. Surg Neurol 7:275-279

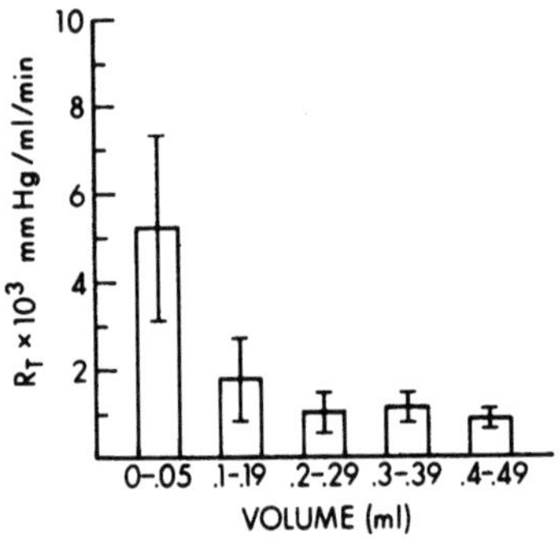

Figure 1. Brain tissue resistance decreased rapidly with infusion of fluid into brain tissue. The reduction of tissue resistance favors the migration of edema and may account for dissipation of tissue pressure gradients

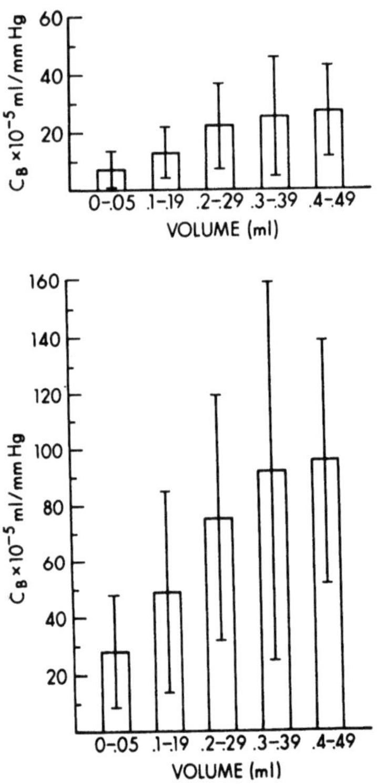

Figure 2a, 2b. Brain tissue compliance increased with edema. This softening of tissue would tend to reduce local increases of tissue pressure. The slope method (ΔV/ΔP) for compliance determinations produced a similar time course (Figure B)

THE ROLE OF BRAIN TISSUE PRESSURE IN AUTOREGULATION OF CBF IN AREAS OF BRAIN EDEMA

A. MARMAROU, H. TAKAGI, G. WALSTRA, AND K. SHULMAN

Introduction

The laboratory model of brain edema produced by cryogenic injury produces a rise in the intracranial pressure and a uniform reduction of cerebral blood flow in the area of the lesion (3). Both these events have been attributed to the compressive effects of the increased tissue volume. The objective of this study was to isolate pressure and volume effects and test the autoregulatory dynamics in the edematous area to help clarify the interaction between local pressures and mechanisms of CBF control.

Method

Platinum electrodes for hydrogen clearance determination of regional CBF were implanted adjacent to the lesion (Probe 1) and at 3 control sites (Probe 2,3,4) in brains of cats maintained normocapnic under nitrous oxide anesthesia. Fluid was infused slowly through a 25-gauge needle positioned 3 mm from a hydrogen electrode in the white matter of the left frontal lobe. By this technique it was possible to infuse a pre-set volume of fluid (0.5 ml) at a controlled rate (100microliters/hr). Intracranial (CMP), tissue pressure (TP) in the area of edema and blood pressure were monitored using conventional pressure transducers referenced to the aural line. Autoregulation of CBF to hypotension (exsanguination) and drug induced hypertension (norepinephirine) was tested. The mean level of CBF was measured in both control and edematous areas under conditions of normal, raised ICP (CMP infusion) and local increase in pressure (balloon inflation).

Results

The amount of edema produced by this method was determined by gravimetric technique and 0.5 ml infusion resulted in an 8% increase of water which was confined to the white matter. Despite the increase of tissue water, CBF in the area of edema (Probe 1) remained constant and the time course of CBF in all areas was remarkably stable. The level of CBF in the area of edema and all control sites was not affected with a generalized increase of ICP by cisternal infusion when ICP was raised from a value of 9.0±3.2 to 46.3±4 mmHg (Fig.1). Autoregulation to hypotension and hypertension appeared to remain intact in the edema area, and at all control sites. Suspecting that this autoregulation was false, we increased the BP above 180 mmHg to achieve "breakthrough. Under this condition the CBF in all areas increased with the exception of the flow in the edematous region (Figure 2). In a few animals where local tissue pressure was measured, this "apparent" autoregulation to a rise in blood pressure was accompanied by a rise in local brain tissue pressure above the level of CMP. When local tissue pressure in the area of edema was increased by balloon inflation (to an average level of 32.1±6.2 mmHg) rCBF of the edematous area decreased to 60%.

Discussion

The widespread derangement of CBF seen in cryogenic injury such as hyperemia and/or reductions of flow in areas of edema have been documented by several investigators (2,4). The fact that flow was maintained constant in a verified area of edema produced by this model suggests that the accumulation of fluid in the brain in the absence of a pressure increase is a benign event. When the increased tissue volume was combined with a generalized increase in ICP, flow in the edematous area remained constant. Perfusion pressure (90 mmHg) was adequate in this situation. However, perfusion pressure was not altered significantly when local tissue pressure was increased (CPP = 115mmHg); yet rCBF was markedly reduced. We concur with others (1,4) that the perfusion pressure concept (CCP = BP - ICP) must be altered in situations where an expanding mass acts directly on the vasculature and under these conditions the capillary to local tissue pressure gradient may be the controlling factor. This may account for the reduction of rCBF that was observed with the relatively mild increase of local TP.

With breakthrough of normal autoregulation, the induced rise in BP was accompanied by a rise in local brain tissue pressure in the area of edema above the level of the CMP. We conclude that the effect of the increase in local tissue pressure seen with hypertension tending to collapse the vessel may explain the false autoregulation phenomenon.

Summary

The dynamics of regional white matter cerebral blood flow and effects of of intracranial pressure were studied in a controlled model of brain edema. Mean CBF levels remained constant in a verified area of brain edema. The apparent autoregulation to MABP changes was shown to be false and attributed to changes in local tissue pressure. Differential effects of generalized and local increase of ICP upon CBF in the edematous area were observed suggesting a modification of the perfusion pressure concept.

References

1. Brock M, Furuse M, Weber R, Hasuo M. Deitz H (1975) Brain tissue pressure gradients. In: LundbergN, Ponten U, Brock M (eds) Intracranial Pressure II. Springer, Berlin Heildelberg New York, p 215

2. Bruce DA, Vapalahti M, Schutz H, Langfitt TW (1972) CBF, $CMRO_2$ and intracranial pressure following a local cold injury to the cortex. In: Brock M, Deitz H (eds) Intracranial Pressure. Springer. Berlin Heidelberg New York p 85

3. Marmarou A, Shulman K, Shapiro K, Poll W (1976) The time course of brain tissue pressure and local CBF in vasogenic edema. In: Pappius HM, Feindel W (eds). Dynamics of Brain Edema. Springer, Berlin Heidelberg New York p 113

4. Reilly PL, Farrar JK, Miller JD (1977) Vascular reactivity in the primate brain after acute cryogenic injury. J Neurol Neurosurg Psychiat 40:1092-1101

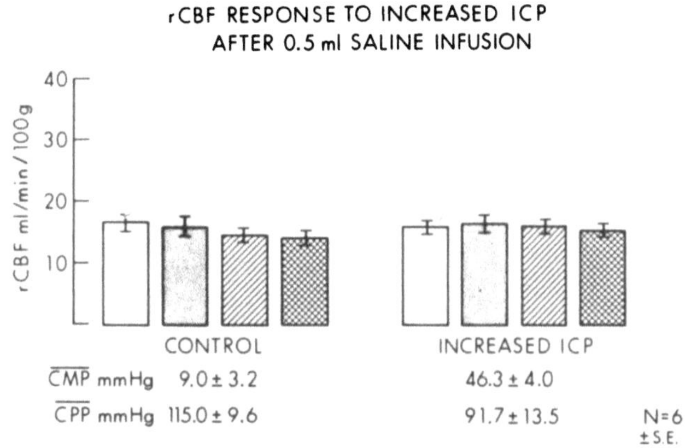

Fig. 1. White matter CBF in area of verified edema (clear bar) and all control sites remained constant with generalized increase of ICP (CMP infusion).

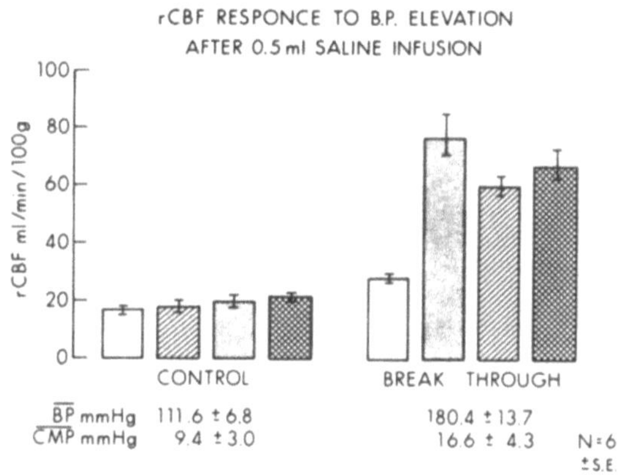

Fig. 2. After breakthrough, CBF increased at all control sites with the exception of edema area (clear bar.

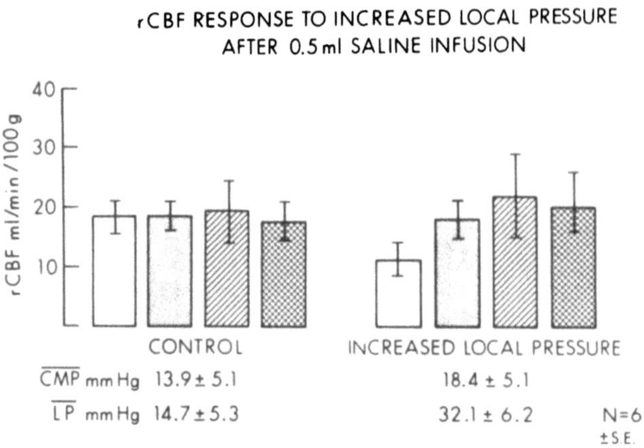

Fig. 3. CBF in area of edema decreased with increased local tissue pressure (LP) despite cerebral perfusion pressure of 110 mgHg.

QUANTIFIED REGIONAL CEREBRAL GLUCOSE CONSUMPTION, rCBF AND EDEMA, AND THE EFFECTS OF PAPAVERINE, IN CATS WITH CORTICAL COLD INJURY

A.R.Dick, S.R.Nelson, and P.L.Turner

Introduction

Two questions were addressed by this study: What is the effect of vasogenic brain edema on rCBF and glucose utilization: will a vasodilating drug, papaverine hydrochloride, alter the effects of the edema or the degree of edema? A "couple" has been shown for brain function and metabolism with rCBF (9), which may be disrupted in brain injury (8). Edema is an additional variable. Changes in energy metabolism in vasogenic edema have been reported (10,5). Diminished CBF in vasogenic edema is reported to be directly related to brain tissue water content (1,2,4). Others however, have been unable to correlate water content of brain tissue and changes in CBF (7). The rate of edema formation may be more important than the amount of edema formed, in terms of clinical deficit and the EEG (3). It appears therefore, that brain water content alone may not explain CBF and metabolic changes. Little is known of the effect of a vasodilating drug on these variables in edematous brain.

Methods

This study employed simultaneous direct tissue counting of iodo(^{14}C) antipyrine and ^{3}H 2-deoxyglucose (^{3}H 2-DG) for CBF and glucose utilization measurements (11,12). Specific gravity measurements were used to assess brain edema (6). Adult cats, 6 control, 3 lesion alone and 3 lesion plus papaverine animals, weighing 2.2 to 4.75 kg, were anesthetized with 1% halothane and a 78% N_2O-22% CO_2 mixture. A right fronto parietal trephine and cold injury lesion through the intact dura were created. Controls were sham operated. Animals recovered from anesthesia, and 1 hour after injury, the lesion plus papaverine animals received papaverine, 1.45 mg/kg by a 1 minute i.v. infusion. Four hours after injury or sham operation, animals were re-anesthetized, mechanically ventilated and paralyzed with i.v. Flaxedil. Arterial blood pressure was monitored ocntinuously and arterial pH, pO_2 and pCO_2 were monitored at regular intervals.

Six hours after lesion or sham operation, and at least 1 hour after halothane was discontinued, 300 microcuries of ^{3}H 2-DG was given by i.v. bolus, and 45 minutes later, 200 microcuries of iodo (^{14}C) antipyrine was given by constant i.v. infusion over 1 minute. Appropriate arterial samples were obtained for ^{3}H and ^{14}C counting as well as for serum glucose. Animals were killed with i.v. KCl, the brain removed and frozen in freon chilled to -80 degrees C.

Four coronal planes approximately equidistant from each other were reached by cryostat sectioning at -20 degrees C. Plane One was most anterior and included the frontal poles. The lesion was contained in Planes Two and Three (fronto-parietal). Plane Four was well posterior to the lesion. Tissue samples weighing 10-20 mg were carved from each plane for simultaneous ^{3}H-2 DG and iodo(^{14}C) antipyrine determinations, and an adjacent sample, 5-10 mg, removed for density gradient column measurement. A total of 86 brain regions were sampled. Areas on the lesion side were numbered 1-43, and on the contralateral side, 51-86. This report concerns 9 brain regions. They are: In Plane One, anterior to the lesion, 2 cortical and 1 white matter area each, on the injured and uninjured side: In Plane Two, near the lesion, 1 cortical and 2 white matter areas on the injured side.

Results

For each of the three variables, an analysis of variance for repeated measures was performed. For rCBF and specific gravity, the three groups--control, lesion alone and lesion plus papaverine--were found to be significantly different ($p < .03$ and $p < .001$ respectively). The mean values for the three groups for glucose utilization were not significantly different. Trends in rCBF are shown in Figure 1. In lesion alone animals, rCBF (open bars) was decreased in all areas. In lesion plus papaverine animals, rCBF(striped bars)was always increased above lesion alone values. In Plane Two, near the lesion, rCBF increased, but did not reach control levels. Figure 2 illustrates trends in brain water content. Values less than control indicate increased brain water content (edema). In lesion alone animals (open bars), edema was seen in all areas. In lesion plus papaverine animals (striped bars), there was less edema in Plane One, with values near control. In Plane Two however, edema became more severe. Regional glucose utilization is shown in Figure 3. Variable changes were seen in lesion alone animals (open bars), with some areas in Plane One above control levels and some below. All areas in Plane Two were below control. In lesion plus papaverine animals (striped bars), areas in Plane One which were high in lesion alone animals, tended to decrease, and those low in the lesion alone animals, tended to increase. In Plane Two, glucose utilization in animals receiving papaverine tended to fall even further or remain unchanged.

Correlations between the three variables were studied. Only in the case of specific gravity and rCBF were consistently positive correlations seen. The most strongly positive correlations were for areas in Plane One where they ranged from .8332 to .3427.

Discussion

In lesion alone animals, rCBF was decreased and edema present in all 9 brain regions. Glucose utilization was variable, and seemed uncoupled from rCBF. While edema and rCBF were positively correlated, the degree of edema (% volume increase of brain tissue) was not a good predictor of the degree of rCBF decrease in lesion alone animals,and was not a good predictor of the degree of rCBF increase associated with papaverine. Papaverine increased blood flow in all areas and diminished edema distant to the lesion. In the vicinity of the lesion, however, edema was increased. The increased rCBF seen with papaverine was associated with glucose utilization values that tended to move toward control levels anterior the lesion, but fell even further in the vicinity of the lesion. Thus, rCBF, edema and glucose utilization distant to the lesion appeared to improve with papaverine. In the vicinity of the lesion, however, these variables became "uncoupled" in that edema became worse and glucose utilization fell, in spite of increased rCBF.

These data are based on a small number of animals and must be considered preliminary. They do suggest however, that in vasogenic edema, factors in addition to brain tissue water alone may be important in altered rCBF. They also suggest that a vasodilator drug may have quite different effects near a lesion as compared to more distant areas.

Summary

The effects of vasogenic edema on rCBF and glucose utilization, and the effects of papaverine on these variables was studied in adult cats. Cryogenic brain injury resulted in edema and decreased rCBF, with variable changes in glucose utilization. Papaverine animals showed improvement in these variables distant from the lesion, but an "uncoupling" near the lesion.

References

1. Frei H, Wallenfang TH et al (1973) Regional cerebral blood flow and regional metabolism in cold induced oedema. Acta Neurochirurg 29: 15-28

2. Grote J, Reulen HJ, Schubert R (1978) Increased tissue water in the brain. Influence of regional cerebral blood flow and oxygen supply. Adv Neurol 20:333-339

3. Marshall LF, Bruce DA, Graham DI, Langfitt TW (1976) Alterations in behaviour, brain electrical activity, cerebral blood flow and intracranial pressure produced by triethyltin sulfate induced cerebral edema. Stroke 7:21-25

4. Meinig G, Reulen H, Magavly C et al (1972) Changes of cerebral hemodynamics and energy metabolism during increased CSF pressure and brain edema. In: Brock M, Dietz H (eds) Intracranial Pressure. Springer, Berlin Heildelberg New York, p 79

5. Nelson S, Mantz M (1971) Energy reserve levels in edematous mouse brain. Exp Neurol 31:53-59

6. Nelson S, Mantz M, Maxwell J (1971) Use of specific gravity in the measurement of cerebral edema. J Applied Physiol 30:368-371

7. Overgaard J, Tweed WA (1976) Cerebral circulation after head injury. Part 2: The effects of traumatic brain edema. J Neurosurg 45:292-300

8. Raichel ME, Gado MH, Grubb RL, Eichling JO (1975) In vivo correlation between regional cerebral blood flow and oxygen utilization in man. Seventh Int Symp on Cerebral Circulation and Metabolism. (Abst.) Aviemore, p 143

9. Reivich M (1974) Blood flow metabolism couple in brain. Res Publ Assoc Res Nerv Ment Dis 53:125-140

10. Reulen HJ (1976) Vasogenic brain oedema. Br J Anaesth 48:741-752

11. Sakurada L.Kennedy C, Jehle J, Brown JD, Carbin GL, Sokoloff L (1978) Measurement of local cerebral blood flow with iodo{^{14}C}antipyrine. Amer J Physiol 234:59-60

12. Sikoloff L. Reivich M, Kennedy C et al (1977) The (^{14}C) deoxyglucose method for the measurement of local cerebral glucose utilization: Theory procedure and normal values in the conscious and anesthetized albino rat. J Neurochem 28:897-916

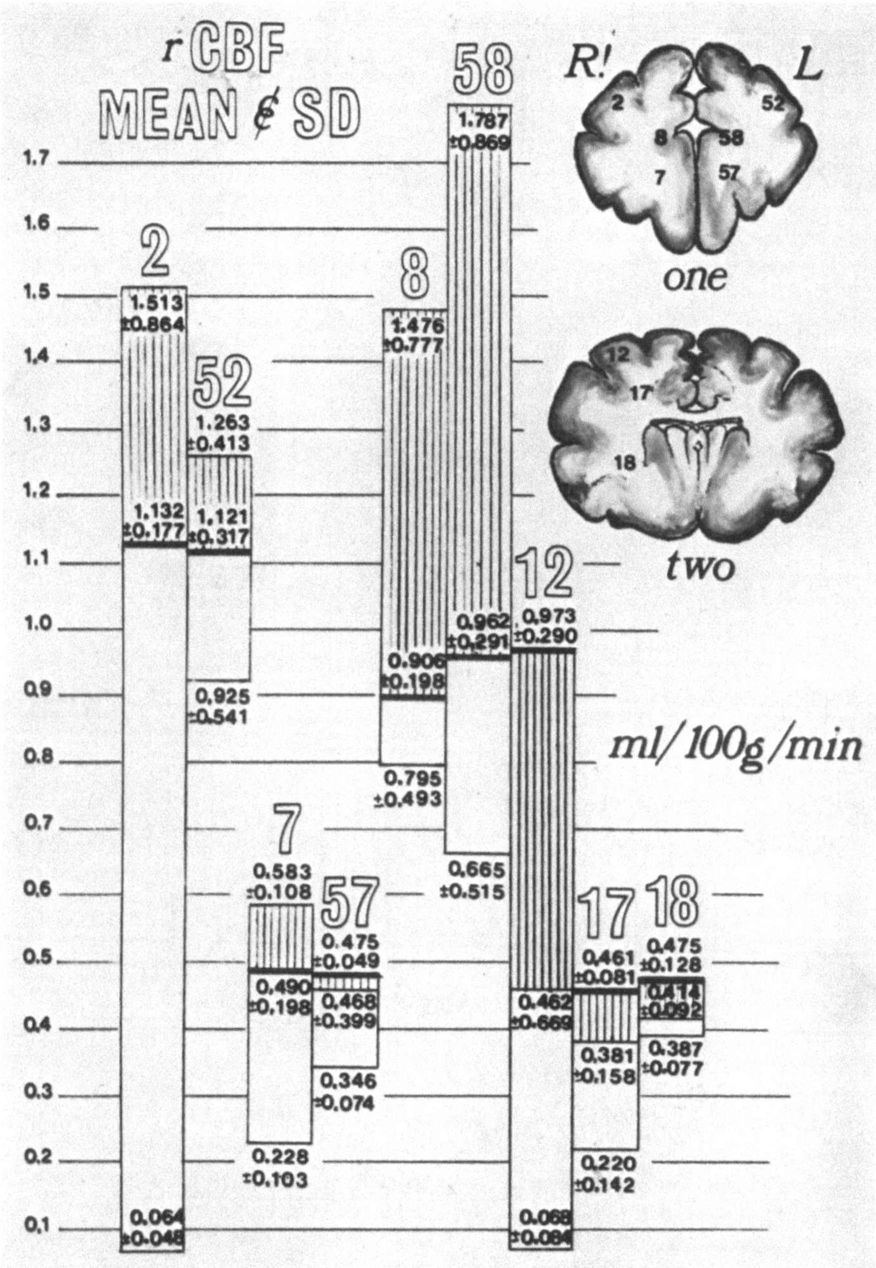

Fig. 1. rCBF by direct tissue counts of iodo (^{14}C) antipyrine. Planes One and Two with 9 brain areas analyzed are shown in upper right. R = right, R! = side of cold lesion, L = left. Control values are indicated by a heavy black horizontal line, lesion alone by open bars, and lesion plus papaverine by striped bars. Means and SD are given. The data represent 6 control, 3 lesion alone and 3 lesion plus papaverine animals.

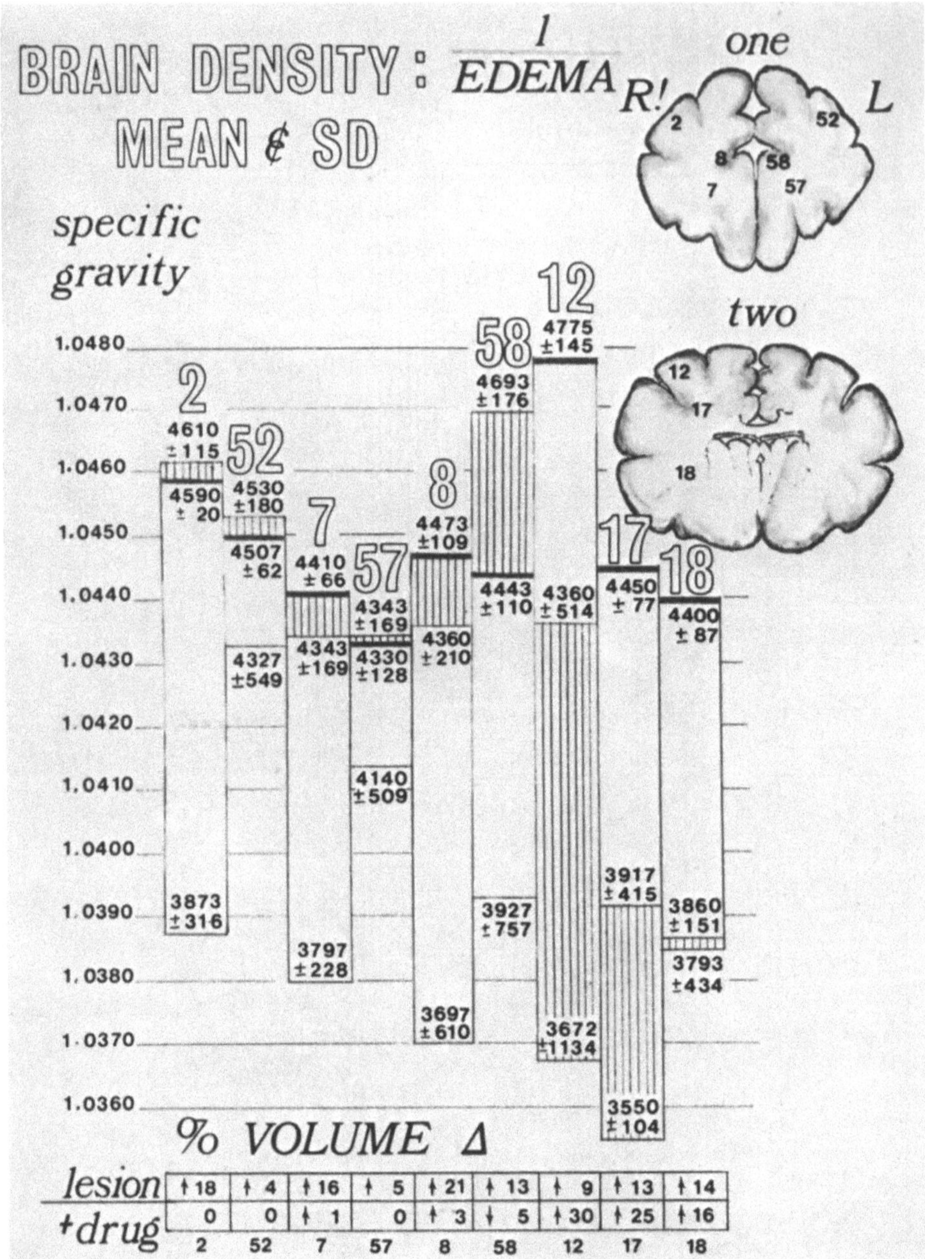

	2	52	7	57	8	58	12	17	18
lesion	↑18	↑4	↑16	↑5	↑21	↑13	↑9	↑13	↑14
+drug	0	0	↑1	0	↑3	↓5	↑30	↑25	↑16

Fig. 2. Brain specific gravity by density gradient column. PlanesOne and Two with 9 brain areas analyzed are shown in upper right. R=right, R!=side of cold lesion, L=left. Control values are indicated by a heavy black horizontal line, lesion alone by open bars, and lesion plus papaverine by striped bars. Means and SD are given. Values below control represent increased brain water content (edema). % volume change of brain tissue = $\frac{\text{control - experimental}}{\text{experimental}} \times 100$. The data represent 6 control, 3 lesion alone and 3 lesion plus papaverine animals.

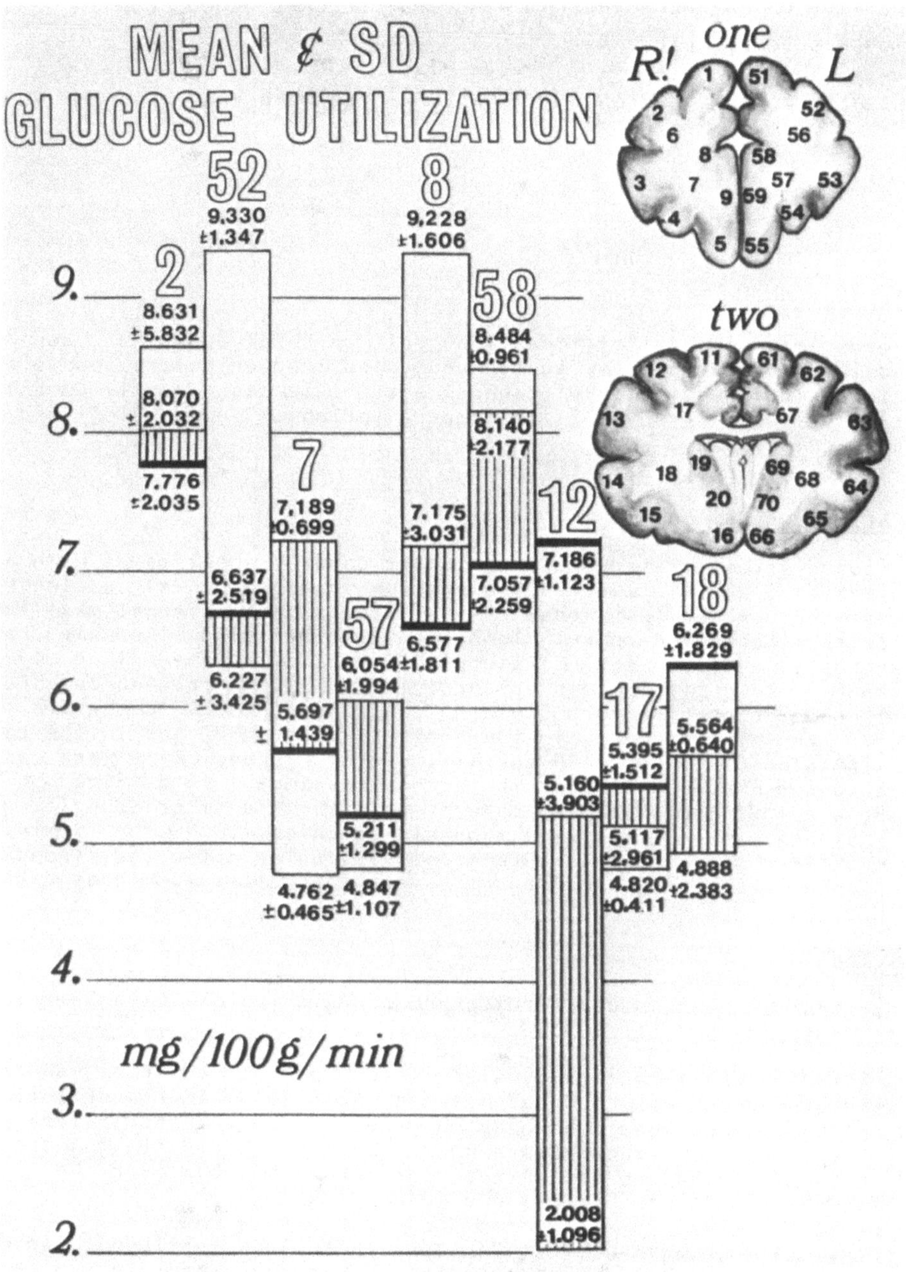

Fig. 3. Regional glucose utilization by direct tissue counts of ^{3}H 2-DG. The 9 brain areas analyzed in Planes One and Two are the same as shown in Figures 1 and 2. R=right, R!=side of cold lesion, L=left. Control values are indicated by a heavy horizontal black line, lesion alone by open bars and lesion plus papaverine by striped bars. Means and SD are given. The data represent 6 control, 3 lesion alone and 3 lesion plus papaverine animals.

EVOLUTION OF INTRACRANIAL PRESSURE AND CEREBRAL BLOOD FLOW IN CRYOGENIC CEREBRAL EDEMA

R. GARCIA DE SOLA, J. VAQUERO, J. CABEZUDO, AND G. BRAVO

Introduction

An experimental model of focal vasogenic cerebral edema has been developed in order to achieve, in the unanesthetized animal, a double goal: 1) to avoid the effect that general anesthesia has directly upon the parameters under study; 2) to compare variables between left and right hemispheres.

Material and method

Six goats were operated on twice, under general anesthesia, with a minimum of 5 days between each operation to implant: a) an electromagnetic flowmeter (Biotronex BL-160) around both internal maxillary arteries (the only cerebral blood input) after tying its extracranial branches so as to measure bilateral CBF, following the method of RIEMANN(7) (Fig. 1); b) an epidural latex balloon on each cerebral hemisphere, connected to a Statham transducer (P23Gb) to measure ICP; c) two femoral catheters, in the aorta to measure BP and in the cava for infusion of fluids. BP and bilateral ICP's and CBF's were registered under basal conditions in the awake animal. In a third operation, a cold injury (CI) was made by applying a 4 mm cryosurgical probe on the dura mater of the left frontal region at -160°C for 10 min. The animals were sacrificed for histological studies after the already mentioned parameters were measured every four hours for three days.

Results

A hemispheric homogenous necrotic-hemorrhagic lesion 20 to 22mm in diameter was provoked.

ICP (Fig.2). A statistically significant ($p<0.05$) interhemispheric pressure gradient was recorded between the 8 to 52 hours post-CI, ICP of the injured hemipshere being greater. By the end of the third day this gradient tended toward normalization. Forty-eight hours after CI, maximum values of ICP are registered (53 mmHg over the injured hemisphere and 34 mmHg over the uninjured one).

CBF (Fig.2) During the first 24 hours there is a continuous increase of the left CBF, being greater in the second day, returning to basal or even lower values by the beginning of the third day (when ICP is highest), returning to baseline levels by the end of the experiments. The right CBF shows a discrete increase that is maintained during the 72 hours.

CVR (cerebrovascular resistance) There is a more pronounced lowering in the injured hemisphere, that is greatest and statistically significant during the second day ($p<0.05$ from 20 to 44 hours post-CI). During the third day there is a progressive return to basal values.

Discussion

As our goal was to compare the variations of CBF between both hemispheres in the normal awake animal, we ligated the extracranial branches of both internal maxillary arteries instead of producing thrombosis of them as proposed by REIMAN et al (7) so as to avoid blindness in the animals. Quantitative measures of CBF gave an extracranial contamination of a 24.8% when compared with these authors' results(3).

The spontaneous evolution of ICP with a maximum value after 48 hours, and the later trend toward normalization, shows a close similarity with the evolution of the weight increase of the injured hemisphere in the experiments carried out by PAPPIUS and McCANN (6). The progressive increase of ICP causes first a progressive decrease of the CVR in preventing a vascular collapse (2), until a situation of maximum vasodilation is reached in the beginning of the second day. Maximum increases of ICP in this situation causes a progressive decrease of CBF that can be avoided by increasing BP (32 Hours). But as ICP continues increasing, this BP increase is not enough to maintain CPP and CBF decreases. The mean value of ICP that starts causing a decrease in CBF is 44mmHg. This value coincides with the one reported by DEWEY et al(2) working on the Critical Closing Pressure.

The fact that the variation of CBF depends directly on the values of ICP is seen also in the results from the uninjured hemisphere. In this hemisphere there is an increase of CBF as a response to increase of ICP. But these variations are less marked than in the injured hemisphere, due to the lower increase of ICP. In no moment CBF decreases below basal values because ICP does not each the Critical Closing Pressure values. This different behaviour of both cerebral hemispheres is essential for a better understanding of the action that the different drugs have upon the evolution of cerebral edema (4, 5).

Summary

Cryogenic edema in the awake animal causes a rise of ICP with a vasodilatation and consequent increase of CBF. If ICP surpasses the Critical Closing Pressure and if BP does not change or its variation does not cause a net increase of CPP, a trend toward vascular collapse with decrease of CBF starts. In this manner ICP is not only a true reflection of the evolution of the amount of existing edema, but also can be an index of the cerebral hemodynamic situation.

References

1. Anderson B, Jewell PA (1956) The distribution of carotid and vertebral blood in the brain and spinal cord of the goat. Quart J Exp Physiol 41:462-474

2. Dewey RC, Pieper HP, Hunt WE (1974) Experimental cerebral hemodynamics. Vasomotor tone, critical closing pressure and vascular bed resistance. J Neurosurg 41:597-606

3. Sola GR, Castillo Olivares JH, Vaquero J, Bravo G (1977) Effects of prolonged use of hyperosmotic agents upon vasogenic cerebral edema. 12th Congress of European Soc for Surgical Research. Apr23-27 Warsaw. Europ Surg Res 9, Suppl I

4. G.Sola R (1977) Thesis. Univesidad Autonoma de Madrid

5. Sola GR, Carrillo R, Cabezudo J, Rodriguez Montes JA, Castillo Olivares JL (1979) Long term action of dexamethasone on intracranial hypertension provoked by vasogenic cerebral edema. 14th Cong of the European Soc for Surgical Research. May 6-9, Barcelona. Europ Surg Res (to be published)

6. Pappius HM, McCann WP (1969) Effects of steroids on cerebral edema in cats. Arch Neurol 20:207-216

7. Reimann C, Lluch S, Glick G (1972) Development and evaluation of an experimental model for the study of the cerebral circulation in the unanesthetized goat. Stroke 3:322-328

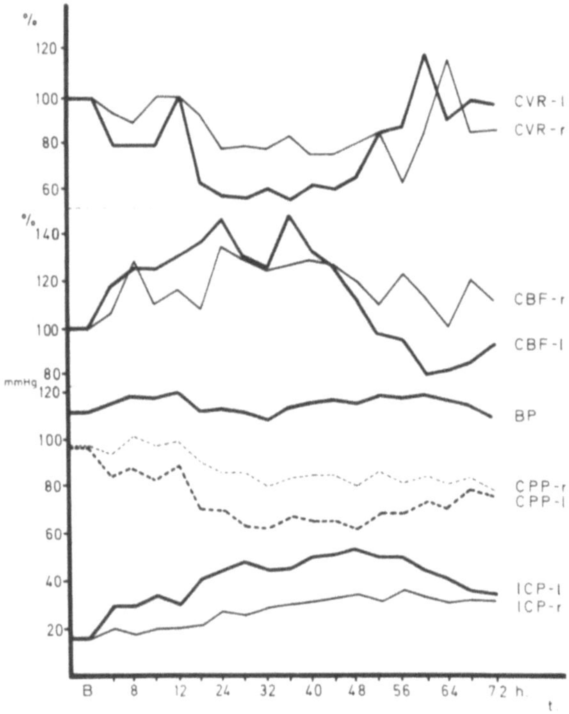

Fig. 1. Evolution of BP, ICP's, CPP's, CBF's and CVR's in the injured hemisphere (left-L) and in the healthy one (right-R). In "B" are the basal values before CI was done.

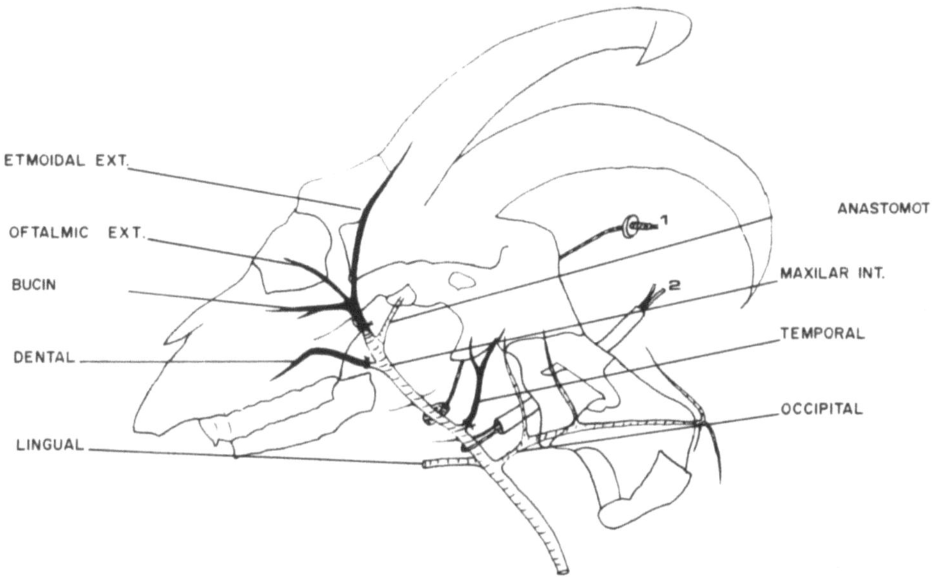

Fig. 2. Schematic representation of the cranial vascular distribution of the goat and of the exact location of the flowmeter (1) and occlussor (2) in the internal maxillary artery after tying the extracranial branches.

THE RESPONSE TO MULTIPLE THERAPEUTIC MODALITIES IN EXPERIMENTAL VASOGENIC EDEMA

H.E.JAMES, R.D.HARBAUGH, L.F.MARSHALL, H.M.SHAPIRO, AND R.LAURIN

Introduction

Multiple therapeutic modalities have been and are presently being employed in the treatment of intracranial pressure secondary to cerebral edema and to brain swelling. While many of these therapies have been shown individually to be efficacious, little attention has been directed toward a systemic evaluation of combined therapies. This study is to analyze the acute response in cryogenic vasogenic edema (1,10) of various parameters following intervention with multiple therapeutic combinations of diuretics.

Material and methods

Albino rabbits weighing 2-3 kg were anesthetized with intravenous sodium thiopental (20 mg/Kg) and underwent a standard cold lesion over the left parieto-occipital region (1) through a trephine hole. The bone was sutured again to the skull, the skin incision closed. At the time of the lesion, 1 mg/kg of 2% Evan's Blue was administered intravenously. Twenty-four hours following the production of the lesion to allow for maximum edema (7) drug therapeutic trials were begun. All animals were reanesthetized, tracheostomized and continuously ventilated with a small animal respirator with a mixture of oxygen and nitrous oxide. They were then paralyzed and femoral arterial and venous lines placed for continuous monitoring of systemic arterial pressure (SAP) and central venous pressure (CVP). $PaCO_2$ was maintained in the range of 37-43 torr. The animals were placed in a stereotaxic device and a #20 gauge plastic catheter was inserted into the cisterna magna for continuous ICP recording and elastance measurements (E_m). Bilateral anterior and posterior screws were placed for EEG recording. The first group of animals was the sham population, and they were monitored until $PaCO_2$ was stabilized, and sacrificed 45 minutes later. A second group (untreated controls) had a freeze lesion performed. Following stabilization of $PaCO_2$ they were also sacrificed 45 minutes later. The remaining groups were treated with various diuretics and combinations of the same, sacrificed five minutes following attainment of a stabilized reduced ICP level. The therapeutic agents, dosages and time of stabilized ICP reduction are summarized in Table 1. A measurement of cerebral compliance was obtained prior to therapy being administered, at the time of the ICP nadir in some animals, by the injection of 0.1 ml of sterile saline through the cisternal cannula (8). The peak pressure recorded following the injection was subtracted from the pre-injection baseline ICP and the value computed. At the end of the experimental period, all animals were sacrificed, the brains rapidly removed, and the hemispheres isolated and weighed. Two samples of brain tissue, each weighing 0.63 ± 0.18 gm including white and gray matter, but excluding areas of lesion necrosis and/or hemorrhage, were taken from the region of the surrounding brain in the left hemisphere. Homologous samples were systematically dissected from the contralateral hemisphere outside any area of visible Evan's Blue extravasation. Water

Table 1. Drug dosage, administration, time to maximum reduction and percent reduction of ICP*

Drug	Dose	Administration	Time to Maximum Reduction+ (minutes)	% Reduction°
Acetazolamide	20 mg/kg	Intravenous 20' infusion	71.4 ± 15.5	$26.82 \pm 38.$
Furosemide	5 mg/kg	Intravenous rapid bolus	38.3 ± 1.23	$156.6 \pm 100.$
Mannitol	1 gm/kg	Intravenous rapid bolus	27.0 ± 9.8	$107.8 \pm 32.$
Acet. & Furos.	same as single doses	First furosemide bolus, then acetazolamide, intravenous	64.7 ± 25.3	88.8 ± 53.8
Furos. & Mann.	same as single doses	Intravenous bolus	36.0 ± 8.2	86.8 ± 52.8

* $PaCO_2$ 37-43 torr.

+ From initiation of administration.

° Percent reduction from baseline value.

Table 2. Water and electrolyte content of both hemispheres

Groups	h	n	Water Content (% dry weight)	p	n	Sodium Content (mEq/kg wet weight)	p	n	Potassium Content (mEq/kg wet weight)	p
Sham	L	16	79.19±1.25	---	10	60.73±4.29	---	10	105.88±3.14	---
	R	16	79.07±1.22	---	10	60.09±4.27	---	10	103.35±4.73	---
Untreated Control (UC)	L	12	81.85±1.24	<.005 from sham	15	67.13±8.88	<.025 from sham	15	78.75±8.72	<.005 from sham
	R	12	80.25±1.13	<.01 from sham	15	60.69±5.47	NS from sham	15	92.0±8.7	<.005 from sham
Acetazolamide & Furosemide	L	16	81.17±0.92	NS from UC	14	72.29±6.4	NS from UC	14	80.34±6.66	NS from UC
	R	16	79.63±1.13	NS from UC	14	62.13±3.96	NS from UC	14	95.50±7.94	NS from UC
Furosemide & Mannitol	L	30	81.46±0.88	NS from UC	14	73.57±5.61	NS from UC	14	78.15±8.32	NS from UC
	R	30	79.78±1.2	NS from UC	14	60.65±6.01	NS from UC	14	90.39±9.06	NS from UC
Acetazolamide & Mannitol	L	28	81.70±0.79	NS from UC	14	73.17±5.87	NS from UC	14	72.65±6.98	<.025 from UC
	R	28	79.84±1.19	NS from UC	14	60.24±5.43	NS from UC	14	85.61±9.34	NS from UC
Acetazolamide	L	26	81.38±1.33	NS from UC	14	77.05±8.87	<.005	14	76.45±9.15	NS from UC
	R	26	79.41±1.31	<.05 from UC	14	60.24±5.67	NS from UC	14	94.04±8.37	NS from UC
Furosemide	L	26	81.37±1.07	NS from UC	14	74.92±9.63	<.025	14	78.47±9.16	NS from UC
	R	26	79.78±0.77	NS from UC	14	63.07±8.87	NS from UC	14	88.02±6.04	NS from UC
Mannitol	L	24	81.47±0.97	NS from UC	14	73.79±7.37	NS from UC	14	78.15±5.84	NS from UC
	R	24	79.73±1.38	NS from UC	14	62.23±8.54	NS from UC	14	93.57±6.47	NS from UC

content was calculated after drying the tissue at 110°C constant weight. Tissue sodium and potassium were determined from the samples.

Results

Most animals who survived from the day of lesion to the experiment demonstrated noticeably intact behavior. There was an overall mortality of 25% the night following the lesion. On the EEG, the lesioned animals revealed pronounced slowing and high-voltage waves over the lesioned hemisphere, and normal fast activity was present over the unlesioned right. There was no gross morphological change between the untreated controls and the therapy groups. Mean SAP in the sham animals, untreated and treated groups, at a $PaCO_2$ of 37-43 torr ranged between 100 and 140 torr. Mean ICP for the sham animals was 2.15 ± 1.53 torr and 8.38 ± 6.26 for the untreated control ($p<0.01$). All therapeutic modalities reduced ICP. The maximum reduction of ICP time ranged from 27.0 ± 9.8 to 71.4 ± 15.5 minutes (Table 1). The E_m measurement was 2.63 ± 1.27 torr (n=8) in the sham group, and 5.65 ± 3.76 torr (n=27) for the untreated controls ($p<0.05$). In all therapeutic modalities not employing acetazolamide, E_m decreased by a mean of 31.72 ± 17.02 percent from pretreatment values save for one trial. In nine of twelve E_m measurements employing acetazolamide alone or in combination with other diuretics, this rose by a mean of 76.07 ± 71.06 percent of pretreatment values, and decreased (one) or remained unchanged (two) in the other three trials. The mean water content, sodium and potassium tissue concentrations are summarized in Table 2.

Discussion

Hypertonic diuretics (2,8,9,12), acetazolamide (4,11), and furosemide (3,5,6) have been employed for the control of clinical and experimental cerebral edema and brain swelling. ICP was reduced when single and multiple diuretic agents were employed, but the reduction was not magnified when two diuretics were administered simultaneously (Table 1). Furthermore, the time to maximum reduction of ICP following the administration of the agent demonstrated no significant difference when two diuretics were employed simultaneously. However, acetazolamide consistently produced an initial rise in ICP, interpreted to be due to an increase in cerebral blood volume secondary to CO_2 release through the carbonic anhydrase mechanism, and furosemide administered immediately following acetazolamide blocked this initial rise in ICP.

Tissue water content of gray and white matter sampled in this series revealed no statistical difference between the diuretics administered alone or in combinations. Though previous authors (5,11) have demonstrated a significant decrease in water content of cold injury induced cerebral edema, it must be noted that in those studies the administration of the agent was subacute or chronic and not in the acute form administered in this present series. It must be noted that a significant reduction of water content of the white matter in cold lesion injured hemispheres at a peak reduction of ICP following hypertonic urea and mannitol has been reported (2). The opposing results in reference to water content of that series with those of the present study may be explained, at least in part, by the fact that the timing of the experimental run following the cold lesion was different. HERMANN et al (7) demonstrated that the peak cerebral edema from cold lesion occurs at 24 hours following the insult. Prior to and following this peak, there is a rapid fall in the degree of edematous tissue. In the present study, the experimental run was always performed in the period which ranged from 22 to 25 hours after the lesion had been applied.

References

1. Bakay L, Haque IU (1964) Morphological and chemical studies in cerebral edema. I. Cold induced edema. J Neuropathol Exp Neurol 23:393-418

2. Beks J, ter Weeme C (1967) The influence of urea and mannitol on increased intraventricular pressure in col-dinduced cerebral edema. Acta Neurochir (Wien) 16:97-107

3. Bergland RM, Page RB, Howland WS (1975) Furosemide: A non-osmotic diuretic for neurosurgical use. Presented at the 43rd Ann Meeting American Association of Neurological Surgeons, Miami Beach, Fla. April 8

4. Buhan S (1972) Effect of furosemide on sodium-22 uptake into cerebrospinal fluid and brain. Exp Brain Res 14:503-510

5. Clasen RA, Pandolfi S, Casey D Jr (1974) Furosemide and pentobarbital in cryogenic cerebral injury and edema. Neurol 24:642-648

6. Cottrel JE, Robustelli A, Post K Turndorf H (1977) Furosemide and mannitol induced changes in intracranial pressure and serum osmolarity and electrolytes. Anesthesiol 47:28-30

7. Herman H, Neuenfeldt D (1972) Development and regression of a disturbance of the blood-brain barrier and of edema in tissue surrounding a circumscribed cold lesion. Exp Neurol 34:115-120

8. James HE, Bruce DA, Welsh F (1978) Cytotoxic edema produced by 5-aminonicotinamide and its response to therapy. Neurosurg 3:196-200

9. James HE, Langfitt TW, Kumar VS, Ghostine SY (1977) Treatment of intracranial hypertension: Analysis of 105 consecutive, continuous recordings of intracranial pressure. Acta Neurochir (Wien) 36:189-200

10. Klatzo I (1972) Pathophysiological aspects of brain edema. In: Reulen H, Schurmann K (eds) Brain Edema. Springer, Berlin Heidelberg New York, p 1

11. Long DM, Maxwell R. Choi K (1976) A new therapy regimen for brain edema. In: Pappius HM, Feindel W (eds) Dynamics of Brain Edema. Springer, Berlin Heildelberg New York, p 293

12. Pappius HM, Dayes LA (1965) Hypertonic urea: Its effect on the distribution of water and electrolytes in normal and edematous brain tissue. Arch Neurol 13:395-402,

DECOMPRESSIVE CRANIECTOMY, ICP AND BRAIN EDEMA

P.R.COOPER, H.HAGLER, AND W.CLARK

Introduction

Decompressive craniotomy has been advocated as a method of treatment for the massive edema often associated with severe head injury (6). Removal of bone over large areas of the calvarium converts a "closed box" with a finite volume into an open one. ICP is controlled and cerebral perfusion pressure is maintained at adequate levels to prevent ischemic injury. Edematous brain may herniate through the craniotomy opening rather than through the tentorial incisura and brain stem compression may be avoided.

Our clinical impression, however, (utilizing serial CT scanning and palpatation of the craniectomy defects) has been that decompression markedly enhances cerebral edema. Because of the variability of human case material it has not been possible to objectively document that an increase in brain edema was a result of decompressive craniotomy. The following experimental study was therefore performed.

Material and methods

Anesthesia was induced in adult mongrel dogs using chloralose. ICP and blood pressure were monitored. A burr hole was made in the left posterior frontal area. A 4 mm in diameter cryo-probe was applied against the dura for periods of three minutes and temperature was maintained at -110° centigrade. Immediately after production of the lesion Evans blue dye was injected intravenously. Intravenous fluids were controlled at 2 cc/kilogram/hour. Systolic arterial pressure was continuously monitored. Five animals were maintained in the post-lesion period as described above. In five additional animals a large craniectomy was performed ipsilateral to the side of the cold lesion. All animals were killed eight hours after production of the cold lesion. Brains were formalin-fixed and sliced in a coronal plane at 1mm intervals. Volumes of edema as defined by Evans blue staining were measured using an image analysis facility built around a PDP 11/05 computer.

Results

Physiological parameters are seen in Table I. ICP was lower in craniectomized animals as expected. pCO_2 was similar in control and craniectomized animals. Blood pressure was somewhat higher in the craniectomized animals but this difference was not statistically significant. The mean volume of edema in five control animals was 0.27 ± 0.19cc's. The mean volume of edema in the five craniectomized animals was 1.96 ± 1.989cc's or over seven times that of the controls. This difference is statistically significant at the .05 level.

Table 1

	Mean B.P (mmHg)	Mean ICP (mmHg)	pCO_2 (mmHg)
Control animals (n=5)	165±31 (S.D.)	10.2±10.8	28.6±2.6
Craniectomized animals (n=5)	188±12	6.3±4.3	27.8±2.3

Discussion

The driving force for the formation of edema is the pressure gradient across the injured brain capillary. This gradient is the difference between intravascular and interstitial fluid pressure. It is probable that decompression of the brain in our experimental animals resulted in a decrease in interstitial fluid pressure and subsequent edema enhancement. The long-term effects on the neuropil of this edema enhancement are unknown.

There is no evidence that outcome is improved by decompression. Following experimental head injury in animals, MOODY et al (5) showed that craniectomy improved mortality (30% in craniectomy vs 100% in controls). Morbidity, however, was unaffected and all craniectomized animals remained comatose.

Similar results have been noted in humans treated with decompression. Recently, HASE et al (4) showed a beneficial effect on the volume-pressure curve following craniectomy in humans. However, this effect was not translated into improved outcome although craniectomy and noncraniectomy groups were not identical. In the series of BRITT and HAMILTON and RANSOHOFF et al(6) (decompressive craniectomy) 70% of the patients had a bad outcome. This was no better than a similar group of patients treated without decompression by FELL et al (3) and BECKER et al (1).

Summary

Craniectomy enhances cold induced edema formation in experimental animals. In humans craniectomy will effect a reduction in ICP and favorably alter the volume-pressure relationship but enhances edema formation. There is no clinical evidence that decompressive craniectomy improved mortality or morbidity in human head injury.

References

1. Becker DP, Miller JD, Ward JD, Greenberg RP, Young HF, SakalasR (1977) The outcome from severe head injury with early diagnosis and intensive management. J Neurosurg 47:491-502

2. Britt RH, Hamilton RD (1978) Large decompressive craniotomy in the treatment of acute subdural hematoma. Neurosurg 2:195-200

3. Fell DA, Fitzgerald S, Moiel RH, Caram P (1975) Acute subdural hematomas: review of 144 cases. J Neurosurg 42:37-42

4. Hase V, Reulen HJ, Meinig G, Schurmann K (1978) The influence of the decompressive operation on the intracranial pressure and the pressure-volume relation in patients with severe head injuries. Acta Neurochir 45:1-13

5. Moody RA, Ruamsuke S, Mullan SF. An evaluation of decompression in experimental head injury. J Neurosurg 29:586-590

6. Ransohoff J, Benjamin MV, Gage, EL Jr, Epstein F (1971) Hemicraniectomy in the management of acute subdural hematoma. J Neurosurg 34:70-67

INTRACRANIAL PRESSURE AND BRAIN WATER CONTENT IN ACUTE GRADED EXPERIMENTAL CEREBRAL TRAUMA

R.L.CORALES, J.D.MILLER, AND D.P.BECKER

Introduction

Elevated intracranial pressure (ICP) is common following severe head injury (5). It is unclear whether this is due to vascular engorgement, intracranial masses, or an increase in brain water content (1,2,7,9). Our objective was to determine whether the early increase in ICP seen in a fluid-percussion model of experimental head injury is associated with increased brain water content.

Material and methods

Forty adult cats (2.5 - 3.5 kg) were anesthetized with 1% methohexitol sodium and 1% lidocaine, tracheotomized, and placed on a Harvard apparatus ventilator on 60% N_2O and 40% O_2. Arterial pressure and blood gases were monitored from a femoral artery cannula. Arterial CO_2 was held in the range 33 - 37 mmHg with normoxia and normothermia. Cerebral trauma was applied using the fluid percussion model (8). A variable pressure pulse callibrated in atmospheres (atm = 760 mmHg)of 20 msec duration is delivered through an 11 mm diameter craniectomy made over the posterior part of the saggital sinus. ICP was measured with an epidural balloon and a needle in the cisterna magna. Animals were randomized into 8 non-injured controls 16 low injury (0.9-2.6 atm.) and 16 high injury (2.9-5.5 atm.). Within each injury group, 8 animals were sacrificed with KCl just after the peak ICP rise (5min) or after the ICP had returned towards baseline values (30min). The brain was rapidly removed and small samples (2-3 mm^3) of white matter (centrum semiovale), gray matter (both caudate and cerebral cortex), and cerebellum were taken. Water content was determined from the specific gravity using the density gradient column method (6) and calculated from the conversion factors of MARMAROU (4).

Results

INTRACRANIAL PRESSURE: Baseline ICP values ranged from 6 to 9 mmHg in all animals. Immediately following trauma, ICP rose to a mean of 26 mmHg in the low injury group and to 76 mmHg in the high injury group. This peak ICP rise occurred within 3 minutes of injury, returned to near baseline values by 30 minutes and was closely related to the force of injury. For animals sacrificed at 5 minutes, mean ICP at the time of sacrifice was 14 mmHg in the low injury group and 55 mmHg in the high injury group. For the groups sacrificed at 30 minutes, the mean ICP at the time of sacrifice was 11 mmHg in low injury and 15 mmHg for high injury (Table 1).

BLOOD PRESSURE: Following trauma, there was an immediate, but transient increase in MABP of 82 mmHg in the low injury group and 104 mmHg in the high injury group. At the time of sacrifice at 5 and 30 mins. MABP in the low injury group was not significantly different from

Table 1

		CONTROL	LEVEL PERCUSSIVE BRAIN INJURY			
			LOW (900-1900 mm Hg)		HIGH (2000-4000 mm Hg)	
			5 min.	30 min.	5 min.	30 min.
	n	8	8	8	8	8
	$PaCO_2$	32	33	34	36	33
ICP (mm Hg)	Baseline	8	7	9	7	6
	Peak	8	26*	26*	75*	78*
	Sacrifice	8	14*	11	54*	15
MAP (mm Hg)	Baseline	118	120	115	118	116
	Peak	120	196*	202*	225*	217*
	Sacrifice	115	123	114	152*	98

* denotes significant over control $p<0.001$.

baseline. For the high injury group, the MABP remained elevated at 5 minutes after trauma and had fallen to sub-baseline values at 30 minutes (Table I).

BRAIN WATER CONTENT: Representative samples of grey matter and white matter were taken from animals which were suffering from raised ICP at the time of sacrifice, from animals which had had raised ICP and from animals with normal ICP. No differences in brain water content in any given area were observed in any of the groups of animals, while there were the expected differences in grey and white matter water content (Table 2).

PATHOLOGICAL FINDINGS: No abnormality was seen in control animals. The low injury group exhibited primarily infratentorial subarachnoid hemorrhage (SAH) with petechial hemorrhage of the pontine mesencephalic junction in 9 of 16 animals. The high injury group mostly had a more extensive SAH and brainstem hemorrhage. Two animals had small cortical contusions at the site of the craneictomy. There was close correlation between the amount of SAH and peak ICP.

Discussion

In an experimental model of early concussive brain injury, we found a significant transient increase in ICP, the extent of which correlated well with the force of injury. We found no increase in cerebral water content during elevated ICP or after ICP had returned to normal.

LANGFITT et al (3) described a secondary ICP increase following experimental concussive brain injury similar to that seen in our study: that is, beginning with the onset of arterial hypertension, but climbing more gradually, with the final extent of ICP increase appearing to be independent of the change in blood pressure. LANGFITT concluded that cerebrovascular dilation and increased blood volume was the cause. In our study, a relatively constant increase in systemic blood pres-

Table 2. Specific gravity of brain samples following concussive injury*

	CONTROL	LEVEL BRAIN INJURY			
		LOW INJURY (900–1900 mm Hg)		HIGH INJURY (2000–4000 mm Hg)	
		5 min.	30 min.	5 min.	30 min.
Cerebral White Matter	1.0442±.0005 66.7%	1.0441±.0004 66.9%	1.0440±.0005 67.1%	1.0440±.0007 66.9%	1.0442±.0004 66.8%
Cerebral Cortex	1.0447±.0007 79.3%	1.0447±.0002 79.3%	1.0446±.0009 79.4%	1.0443±.0009 79.1%	1.0443±.0009 79.3%
Caudate Nucleus	1.0449±.0005 79.1%	1.0446±.0005 79.5%	1.0447±.0006 79.3%	1.0447±.0005 79.3%	1.0449±.0009 79.2%
Pons	1.0428±.0014 67.6%	1.0425±.0008 68.3%	1.0430±.0010 67.7%	1.0433±.0014 67.2%	1.0428±.0014 67.4%
Cerebellum	1.0450±.0006 75.8%	1.0447±.0010 76.7%	1.0448±.0006 76.0%	1.0449±.0006 75.9%	1.0448±.0006 76.0%

* Values are means for the group ± standard deviation
Percentages indicate percent H_2O per gm. tissue

sure was observed above a threshold level of cerebral injury and did not correlate quantitatively to the change in ICP. The level of ICP correlated best with the degree of SAH produced. The exact cause of raised ICP soon after concussive head injury remains in some doubt. However, this study adds further evidence against cerebral edema as a cause.

References

1. Eichelberger L, Kollros JJ, Walker AE (1949) Water nitrogen and electrolyte content of brain following cerebral concussion. Am J Physiol 156:129-136

2. Fass FH, Ommaya AK (1968) Brain tissue electrolytes and water content in experimental concussion in the monkey. J Neurosurg 28:137-144.

3. Langfitt TW, Tannanbaum HM, Kassell NF (1966) The etiology of acute brain swelling following experimental head injury. J Neurosurg 24: 47-56

4. Marmarou P, Poll W, Shulman K, Blagaum H (1978) A simple gravimetric technique for measurement of cerebral edema. J Neurosurg 49: 530-537

5. Miller JD, Becker DP, Ward JD et al (1977) Significance of intracranial hypertension in severe head injury. J Neurosurg 47:503-516

6. Nelson SR, Mantz ML, Maxwell JA (1971) Use of specific gravity in the measurement of cerebral edema. J Appl Physiol 30:268-271

7. Pilcher C (1937) Experimental cerebral trauma. The fluid content of the brain after trauma to the head. Arch Surg Chicago 35: 512-527

8. Sullivan HG, Martinez J, Becker DP, et al (1976) Fluid percussion model of mechanical brain injury in the cat. J Neurosurg 45: 520-534

9. WhiteJC, Brooks JR, Goldthwait JC, Adams RO (1943) Changes in brain volume and blood content after experimental concussion. Ann Surg 118:619-634

BRAIN EDEMA IN ISCHEMIC STROKE AND AIR EMBOLISM

J.H.GARCIA AND K.A.CONGER

Introduction

The purpose of this study was to determine differences and similarities that may exist between brain edema secondary to an arterial occlusion and the ultrastructural abnormalities noted after arterial air embolism. The compartmental enlargement produced by the excess water of edematous brain can be defined by structural methods and quantitated by indirect chemical means.

We studied the effects of three acute injuries on the mammalian brain: (a) carotid ligation, (b) MCA embolic occlusion and (c) arterial air embolism. The former two produce marked enlargement of astrocytic processes, large axis cylinders and pre-synaptic terminals. Air embolism results in an immediate enlargement of the extracellular space; this effect is followed, a few hours later, by the development of ischemic-like changes.

Materials and methods

Mongolian gerbils (Meriones unquiculatus) under either Ketamine or barbiturate anesthesia were used for all experiments; controls were subjected to sham-operations. One group had unilateral carotid artery ligation (30 min to 3 hr) while other gerbils were given less than 0.05 ml of air into the right internal carotid artery. Some animals were given horseradish perioxidase, IV, and all were killed by cardiovascular perfusion with aldehydes (1). MCA occlusion was achieved by injecting an embolus into the internal carotid artery of Rhesus monkeys (Maccaca mulatta), which were killed in the same manner as the gerbils. Inulin was added to the fixative used in the monkey experiments. Tissue samples from all animals were processed for electron microscope (2) and biochemistry(3).

Results

Marked, widespread and progressive enlargement of astrocytic processes was seen in all samples obtained from the ischemic hemispheres, regardless of the method used to occlude the artery. No astrocytic swelling was evident in either contralateral hemisphere or sham-operated animals. A considerable increase in the inulin space occurred in those areas where astrocytic swelling was more pronounced, e.g. putamen. In the white matter. fluid accumulation involved both astrocytes and large myelinated axons, principally (2,3,6).

The immediate (10 min) effects of air embolism consisted of multiple foci (each about 1 mm in diameter) in both hemispheres were the ECS was markedly distended. This resulted in "deafferentation" of many neurons and the wide separation of otherwise intact myelinated fibers (Figs 1,2). After 24 hours the effects of air embolism appeared remarkably similar to those seen during early regional ischemia (Fig.3). Protein extravasation, through transendothelial channels or pores (1) was seen in all animals (Fig.4) but this was particularly obvious in the experimental hemisphere and after long (24 hr) survival periods. The sites of protein escape were different from those where swelling was most evident.

Discussion

A good number of experimental models of brain edema,e.g.,tri-ethyl tin and hexachlorophene intoxication, are known to induce "myelin splitting" in the absence of significant mitochondrial alterations (5). In contrast, regional ischemia induces massive nuclear and cytoplasmic astrocytic swelling while neuronal perikaryon shrinks and large axons swell; no myelin alterations are seen during the initial several hours of ischemia (2,6).

We describe a third variety of brain edema, ultrastructually. The initial (2 hr) effect is reflected in focal areas of water accumulation in the extracellular space of gray and white matter. No intrinsic abnormalities in either neuronal soma or axis cylinders are evident at this time. Protein extravasation, a phenomenon that is greatly increased by air embolism (4), occurs through transendothelial pores but at different sites from those affected by abnormalities in water transport.

The delayed (24 hr) effects of air embolism, which are almost identical to those of regional ischemia, may be secondary to intravascular clotting. Although occluded vessels were not seen in the material we examined, this could be a consequence of the methods used in tissue fixation, i.e., cardiovascular perfusion.

Summary

There are at least three ultrastructural patterns of acute brain edema (a) swelling of astrocytes, axons and presynaptic terminals is characteristic of incomplete ischemia (6); (b) massive enlargement of ECS was seen only in animals embolized with air; and (c)myelin splitting at the intraperiod line has been described in several experimental models of brain edema, based on the administration of substances such as hexachlorophene (5). After the first 3 hours the effects of air embolism mimic those of ischemic stroke.

References

1. Lossinsky AS, Garcia JH, Iwanowski L, Lightfoote W(1979 to be published) New ultrastructural evidence for a tubular transport system in endothelial cells of gerbil brains. Acta Neuropathol

2. Garcia JH, Lossinsky AS, Kauffman FC, Conger KA (1978) Neuronal ischemic injury: Light microscopy, ultrastructure and biochemistry. Acta Neuropathol (Berlin) 43:85-95

3. Conger KA, Garcia JH, Lossinsky AS, Bielefeld JH, Fuld RA, Kaufman FC (unpublished) Cerebral ischemia: Changes in selected amino acids as indicators of tissue injury.

4. Lee J, Olszewski J (1959) Effect of air embolism on permeability of cerebral blood vessels. Neurol 9:619-625

5. Lampert P, O'Brien J, Garrett R (1973) Hexachlorophene encephalopathy. Acta Neuropath 23:326-333

6. Garcia JH, Lossinsky AS, Kauffman FC et al (1979) Fine structure and biochemistry of brain edema in regional cerebral ischemia. In: Price TR, Nelson E (eds) Cerebral Vascular Diseases. Raven Press, New York p 169

Supported by USPHS grant NS 06779.

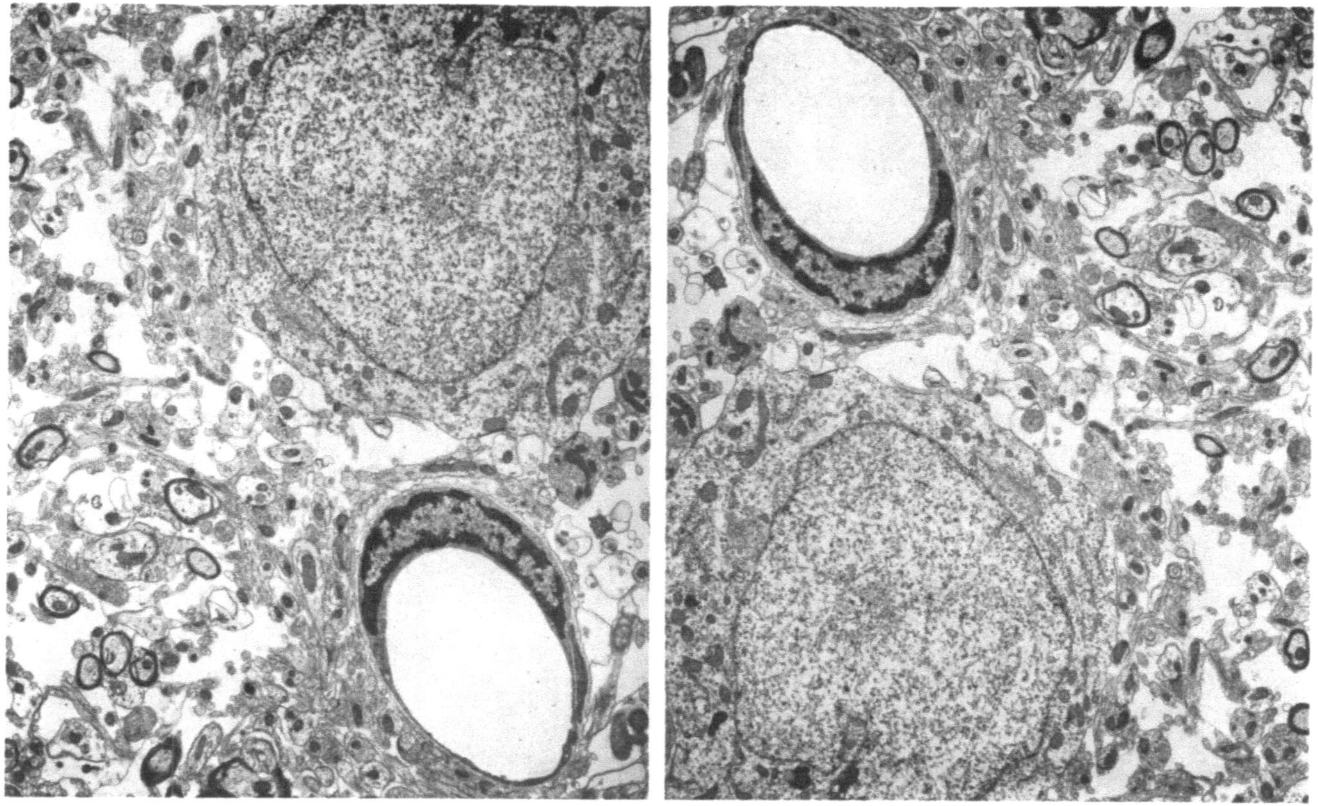

Fig. 1. Gerbil, neocortex. Effects of intraarterial air embolism (10 min). Note marked enlargement of extracellular space, deafferentation of neuronal soma and absence of pericapillary astrocytic processes (original magnification 3,000x).

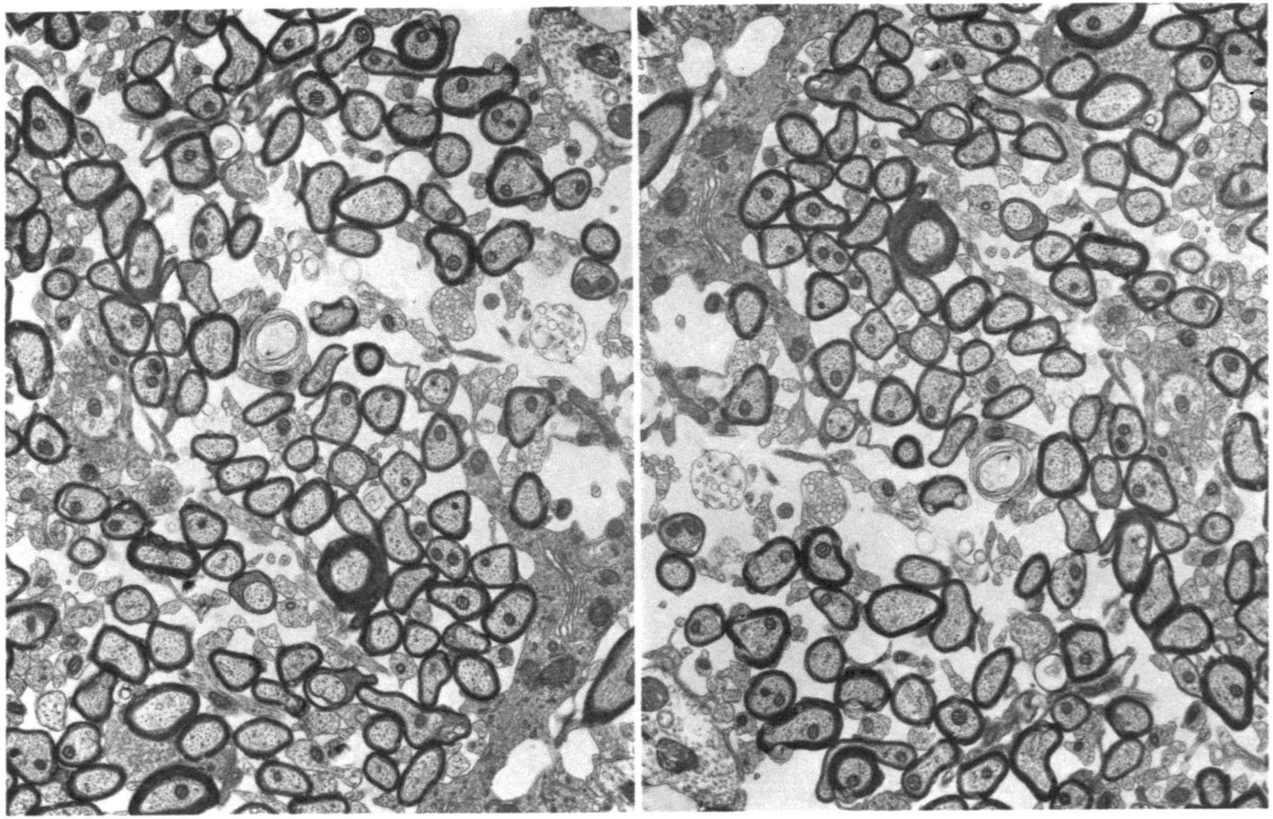

Fig. 2. Same animal as in Fig. 1. Subcortical white matter showing widened extracellular space and intact axons and myelin sheaths. Oligodendrocytic processes contact several myelinated fibers (3,000 x).

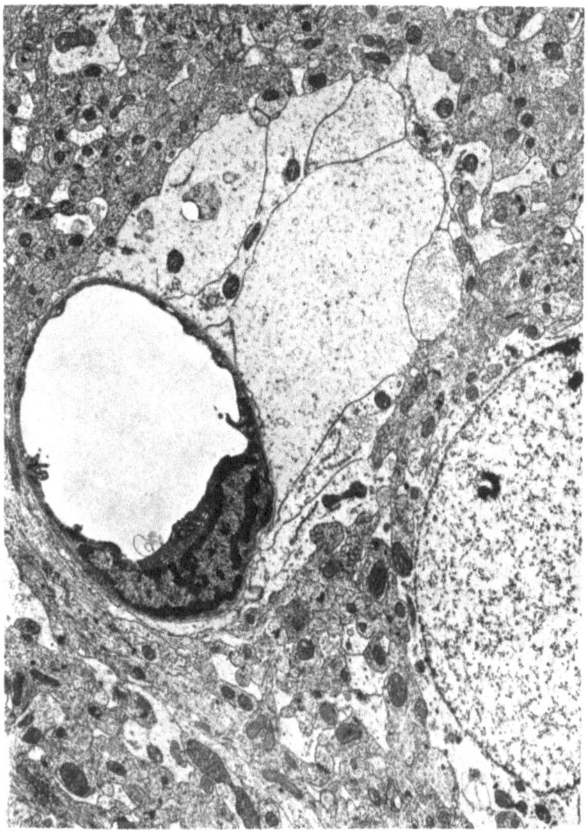

Fig. 3. Gerbil, neocortex. Effects of air embolism (3 hr). The type of swelling has now changed to the intracellular (astrocytic) compartment (3,000x).

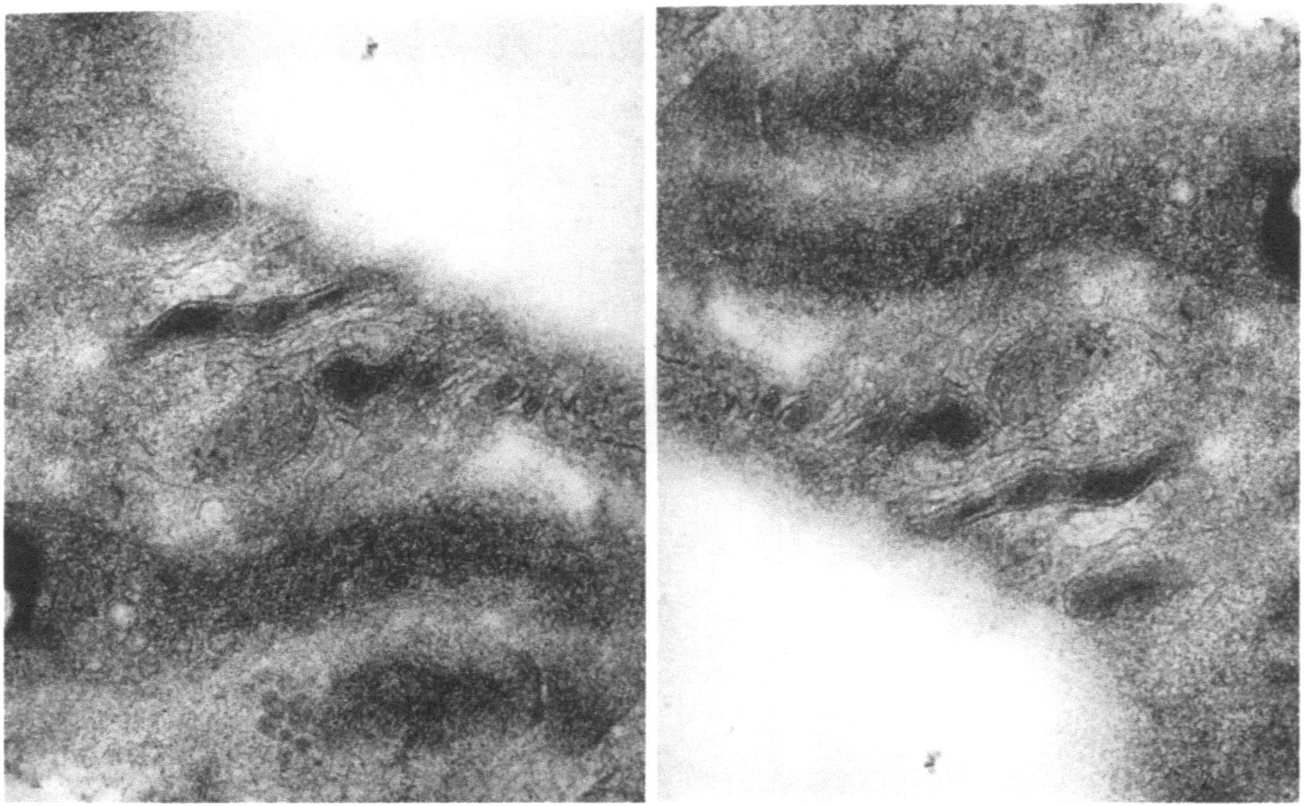

Fig. 4. Gerbil, neocortex, air embolus (arterial) and horseradish peroxidase (intravenous) were injected 3 hr. before death. Close-up view of endothelial pores filled with HRP is demonstrated in this capillary. (40,000x).

CSF-PRESSURE OF RATS DURING VENTRICULO-CISTERNAL PERFUSION WITH POTENTIAL BRAIN EDEMA FACTORS

A. BAETHMANN, W. OTTINGER, W. ROTHENFUSSER, O. KEMPSKI, AND A. UNTERBERG

Introduction

The concept of brain edema enhancing compounds released or activated in the edema process is based on the fact that (a) vasogenic edema fluid penetrating the parenchya constitutes an abnormal environment for cerebral tissue, and (b) that in such a condition swelling of cell elements, i.e., secondary cytotoxic edema is almost always encountered (1,2). Various mechanisms are conceivable but only little is known on how tissue or plasma-factors enhance the brain edema process.

Many compounds present in brain tissue or plasma can be considered to function as edema factors. Table I contains a collection of edema factor candidates, as e.g., lysosomal or other proteolytic enzymes released from damaged tissue, biogenic amines such as serotonin or histamine, or free fatty acids which may accumulate in brain tissue, if demyelinization occurs. For the following reasons we found the kininogen - kinin system and the aminoacid glutamate particuarly promising. Kininogens are constituents of the serum α_2-globulin fraction which along with the plasma-like edema fluid enter the cerebral parenchyma in conditions of gross disruption of the barrier. Formation of kinins may occur, if plasma becomes diluted by CSF (3). Edema fluid penetrating the barrier becomes also diluted by extracellular fluid of the brain which as well could induce kinin formation.

Various secondary effects may result from formation of kinins in brain tissue, e.g., a rise in local tissue blood flow enhancing edema influx, increase in blood-brain barrier permeability, or cytotoxic cell swelling. However, only few specific studies have been undertaken so far which analyze kinin effects in brain tissue. Depletion of the plasma-kininogen content seems to suppress enhanced barrier permeability to the Evans Blue-protein-complex in lymphostatic brain edema, or blockage of the kinin-forming enzyme kallikrein by the proteinase-inhibitor Trasylol(r) to reduce penetration of labelled albumin into brain tissue (4,5). The potential excitatory transmitter compound glutamate may not only mediate cell swelling by rendering nerve- and glia cell membrane more permeable to Na^+-ions but may lead to cerebral tissue necrosis, if extracellular concentrations exceed 8mM (6,7). Such extracellular concentrations are likely to accumulate close to a focus of massive cell destruction. Intracellular glutamate levels can be estimated at 15 mM in normal conditions.

Experiments were carried out to test our hypothesis that glutamate and/or the kininogen-kinin system have a role in the edema process. At first, we studied whether exposure of normal cerebral tissue unprotected by the blood-brain barrier to either potential edema factors induce brain edema. Perfusion of the cerebral ventricle system with both factors served as method to expose brain tissue. This communication reports on the response of the ventricular perfusion pressure to the procedure.

Methods

(a) Kininogen-Kinin System: Ventriculo-cisternal perfusion with diluted and undiluted plasma was performed in male Sprague-Dawley rats anesthetized with chloralhydrate (360 mg/Kg). Animals perfused with mock-CSF served as controls. Prior to plasma perfusion of the ventricular system, the experimental animals were pre-perfused for 10 min with artificial CSF to exclude technical artifacts. In one group, the plasma perfusate was diluted with mock-CSF at a 1:1 ratio. Clotting of the plasma perfusate was prevented by EDTA.

(b) Glutamate: Ventriculo-cisternal perfusion with glutamate was conducted in a similar manner. Two different concentrations (10 or 75 mM) were employed. The glutamate perfusate was buffered (pH 7,4) and isotonic. Ventricle perfusion with plasma was continued for 60 minutes, with glutamate for 120 minutes, respectively. The perfusion pressure in the ventricle system was manometrically monitored throughout perfusion. The cisternal perfusate was sampled after ventricle passage at various intervals to analyze the electrolyte- and the kininogen, or glutamate concentrations in the respective experiments. The kininogen concentration of the plasma perfusion fluid was determined prior to and after ventricle perfusion (8). Glutamate was enzymatically determined. At termination of the experiment and 24 hours later, the animals were sacrificed in order to remove tissue for determination of the water and electrolyte content.

Results

Exposure of brain tissue to either glutamate concentrations, or to plasma led to a significant rise in cerebral water content as shown in Fig. 1. Concurrently, the Na^+-content of brain tissue was significantly increased, while brain-K^+ fell significantly only after perfusion with glutamate, but not with plasma. Both factors seemed to affect K^+ permeability of cell membranes. This was concluded from the increase in K^+- concentrations of the perfusate after ventricle passage compared to mock-CSF where no differences in K^+ between the in- and outflowing perfusion fluid was found. After ventricle passage, the kininogen concentration of the diluted plasma perfusate was significantly reduced for about 26% suggesting formation of kinins during perfusion (9). As shown by pre- and postperfusion concentration profiles of inulin as volumemarker, the reduction in kininogens during ventricle perfusion does not result from mere dilution. The same is true in the case of glutamate, where a dilution independent clearance of approximately 12-15% was observed in both groups. Regression analyses of the cerebral water content and kinin formation revealed the increase in brain water to be the higher, the earlier the maximum occurred in kinin formation after start of plasma perfusion. This would indicate formation of edema to relate with a release of kinins.

Ventricle Perfusion Pressure

(a) Plasma perfusion: Fig. 2 demonstrates the ventricle perfusion pressures (VPP) of controls, and animals perfused with diluted and undiluted plasma. The data of the controls and of the group perfused with diluted plasma have been averaged, while in the group perfused with undiluted plasma the individual curves are shown. Controls hardly exceeded a perfusion pressure of 4 mmHg, while in experimental animals (diluted plasma) the pressure curves revealed a clear tendency to rise. This is particularly prominent in the experiments where undiluted plasma was employed. Upon exchange of mock-CSF against plasma(Fig.2), a dramatic rise in VPP was seen in almost all animals. In 7 out of 11

Table 1. Brain tissue- and plasma-factors potentially associated with formation and persistence of vasogenic and cytotoxic brain edema (from: Baethmann A et al, 1)

1. a) Lysosomes	3. cont'd
- enzymes	- Serotonin
b) Proteolyt. enzymes	- norepinephrine
(e.g. collagenase)	- histamine
	- dopamine
2. Peptides	4. Lipids
- Kininogen-Kinin-system	- lipoperoxydes
	- prostaglandins
3. Biogenic amines	- free fatty acids
- Serotonin	
	5. Free radicals

animals, perfusion had to be terminated in order to prevent brain tissue herniation. Only in this group, brain water content was determined immediately after perfusion, while in all other groups 24 hours later.

(b) <u>Glutamate:</u> In these studies, mean VPP never exceeded 10 mmHg when compared to plasma perfusion. Fig. 3 shows the VPPs of controls and of two groups perfused with 10, or 75 mM glutamate, together with the perfusion rates. As seen, perfusion pressure in controls started at 4,5 mmHg and reached 6,5 mmHg at 120 min. In both glutamate groups, VPP was initially lower ($p<0.02$; <0.001) than in controls. In animals perfused with 75 mM glutamate, VPP appeared to stabilize at this low level throughout the entire perfusion period, while animals perfused with 10 mM glutamate developed an increase in pressure up to the control level during further perfusion. The perfusion rates were generally adjusted, if VPP tended to exceed 10 mmHg. Thus, the perfusion rates were lowered in controls from initially 4 to less than 3 ml/h, and even to less than 2 ml/h in the glu_{10mM} animals, while higher perfusion rates could be maintained in the glu_{75mM} animals (Fig 3).

Discussion

A chemical mediator compound meets the criteria as brain edema factor, if (a) its administration to brain tissue causes edema, (b) it is released in conditions leading to edema, (c) the amount of release is in proportion to the cerebral water uptake, and (d) if interference with factor release influences edema (9). In the case of glutamate and the kinongen-kinin system presented in this report, our experimental data so far obtained demonstrate the candidates to qualify as edema factors, although further evidence is required. The question, how the dramatic increase in perfusion pressure secondary to ventricle perfusion with undiluted plasma is brought about cannot be conclusively answered for the moment. It is , however, conceivable that plasma-born compounds like kinins lead to dilatation of cerebral blood vessels. Kinins were indirectly shown upon activation to increase cerebral blood flow. Moreover, i.v. injection of kallikrein, or bradykinin was observed to increase CSF pressure in man (10). Perfusion of the ventricle system with glutamate did not appear to raise perfusion pressure. To the contrary, perfusion pressure was significantly lower during glutamate perfusion. This effect can be explained with difficulties only, because an increase in ventricle pressure due to metabolically enhanced blood flow after glutamate exposure is to be expected rather than a decrease. Stimulation of cerebral metabolism by glutamate leading to increased blood flow may be indirectly inferred from respective observations in spreading depression, where glutamate is suggested to play an important role (11,12). It may be assumed either that very high extracellular glutamate concentrations constrict cerebral blood vessels, or that upon glutamate entering the ventricle system immediate swelling of periventricular tissue elements prevents diffusion of the aminoacid into deeper layers of the brain parenchyma by blocking of interstitial fluid channels. This would limit acute cerebral glutamate effects during perfusion.

Summary

Ventriculo-cisternal perfusion with glutamate, or plasma was found to induce a moderate, but nevertheless significant increase in brain water content in rats. This observation provides first evidence for glutamate and the plasma kininogen-kinin system to function as brain edema factors making further studies promising. During ventricle perfusion with plasma, a significant, often dramatic rise in ventricular perfusion pressure compared to mock-CSF was observed, which was probably mediated by vasodilatory response of the cerebral vasculature. Ventricle perfusion with glutamate did not increase perfusion pressure. As to the kininogen-kinin system, it is suggested that dilatation of cerebral blood vessels is one mechanism among others which could be entertained by this potential brain edema factor. On the other hand, the ventricular pressure remaining unchanged during glutamate perfusion, does not rule out this compound as one not affecting the cerebral vasculature.

References

1. Baethmann A, Ottinger W, Rothenfusser W, and Geiger R (1978) Biochemical aspects of cerebral edema. In: Mrsulja BB, Rakic LM, Kitazo I (eds) Pathophysiology of Cerebral Energy Metabolism. Plenum Publ Corp, New York

2. Hirano A (1969) The fine structure of brain in edema. In: Bourne GH (ed) The Structure and Function of Nervous Tissue. Academic Press, New York, p 69

3. Sicuteri F, Fanciullacci M, Bavazzano A, Franchi G, DelBianco PL (1970) Kinins and intracranial hemorrhages. Angiol 21:193-210

4. Wendel U and Seidel G (1972) Kinins-Evidence for the involvement in lymphostatic encephalopathy in rats. Pharmacol 7:17-18

5. Blumel G (1969) Beteiligung des Kininsystems bei einem chirurgischen Zustandsbild. In: Haberland GL, Matis P (eds) Neue Aspekta der Trasylol Therapie. Schattauer, Stutgart New York, p 125

6. Harvey JA and McIlwain H (1968) Excitatory acidic amino acids and the cation content and sodium ion flux of isolated tissues from the brain. Biochem J 108:269-276

7. Van Harreveld A, Fifkova E (1971) Light- and electronmicroscopic changes in central nervous tissue after electrophoretic injection of glutamate. Exper Molec Pathol 15:61-81

8. Mann K. Geiger R, Werle E (1976) A sensitive kinin liberating assay for kininogenase in rate urine, isolated glomeruli and tubules of rat kidney. In: Sicuteri F, Back M, Haberland G (eds) Kinins, Pharmacodynamics and Biological Roles. Plenum Publ Corp, N Y p65

9. Ottinger W, Baethmann A, Rothenfusser W, Geiger R and Mann K (1976) Tissue and Plasma Factors in Cerebral Edema. In: Pappius HM, Feindel W (eds) Dynamics of Brain Edema. Springer, Berlin Heidelberg New York, p 161

10. Frey E.K, Draut H, Werle E, Vogel R. Zichgraf G, Trautschold I (1968) Das Kallikrein-Kinin-System und seine Inhibitoren. F Enke, Stuttgart, p 153

11. Rosenthal M, Somjen G (1973) Spreading depression, sustained potential shifts and metabolic activity of cerebral cortex of cats. J Neurophysiol 36:739-749

12. Van Harreveld A (1970) A mechanism for fluid shifts specific for the central nervous system. In: Wycis HT(ed) Current Research in Neurosciences, Topical Probl Psychiatr Neurol. Karger, Basel,p 62

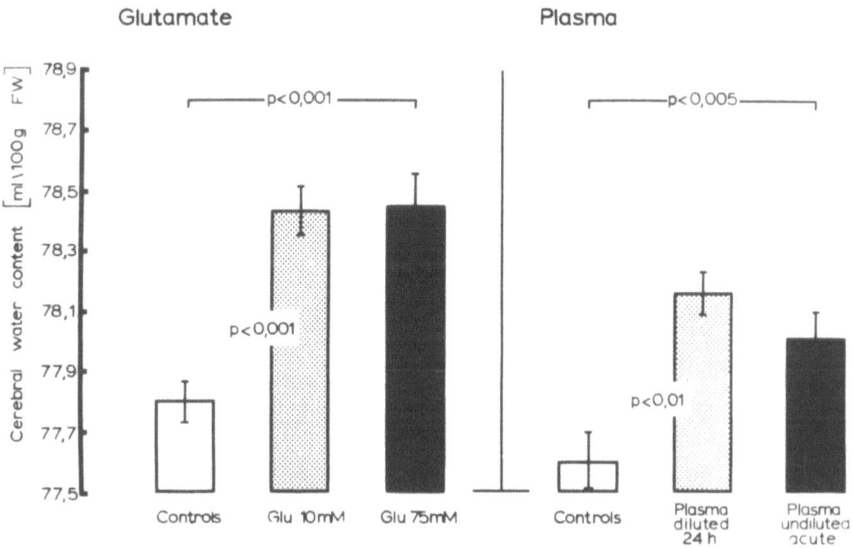

Fig. 1. Cerebral water content ($\bar{x} \pm$ SEM) of rats 24 hours after ventriculo-cisternal perfusion with mock-CSF, glutamate, or plasma. In animals perfused with undiluted plasma, brain water content was determined at termination of the experiment. Two control groups are shown, because the experiments were conducted in two different series.

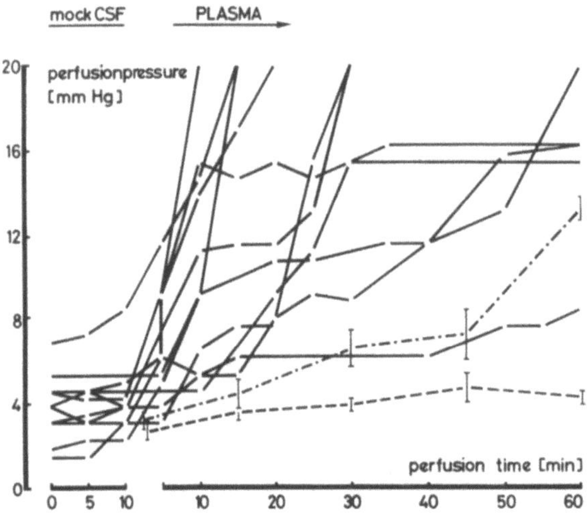

Fig. 2. Perfusion pressure of rats manometrically monitored during ventriculo-cisternal perfusion for 1 hour with mock-CSF (------), diluted (-.-.-.-.) and undiluted plasma (solid lines). The single curves represent the individual pressure responses in animals perfused with undiluted plasma. In all groups, the ventricles were pre-perfused with mock-CSF (from Baethmann A et al, 1).

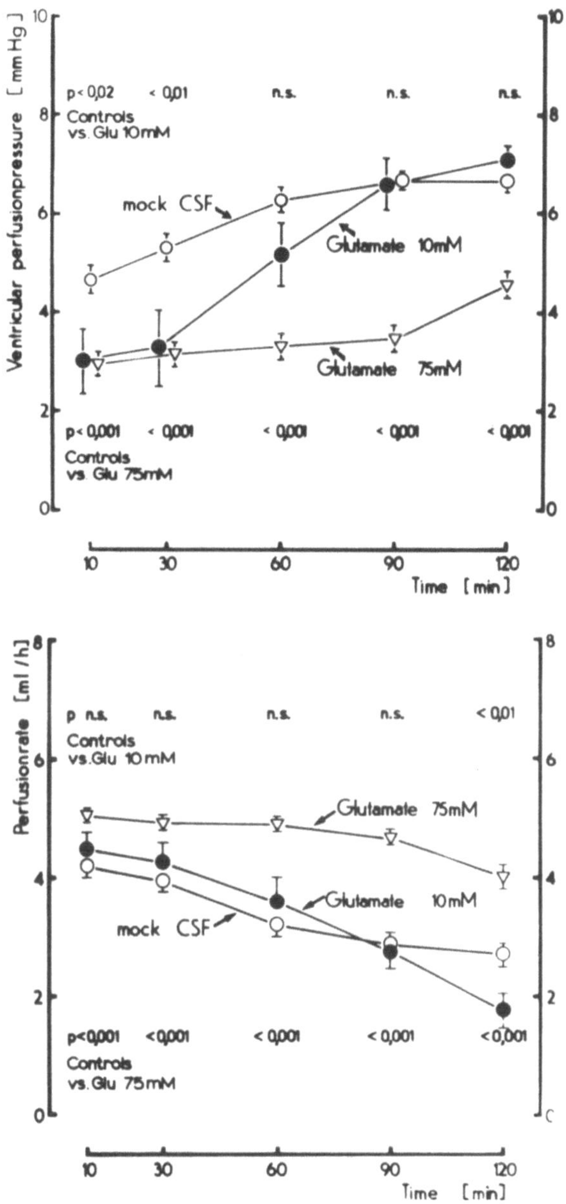

Fig. 3. Manometrically recorded ventricular perfusion pressure ($\bar{x}$ ± SEM) and perfusion rates ($\bar{x}$ ± SEM) of rats perfused for 120 minutes with mock-CSF, or isotonic and buffered glutamate solutions, respectively. All animals were pre-perfused for 10 min with mock-CSF which is omitted from the time axis. The perfusion rates were lowered in controls and animals perfused with 10 mm glutamate to prevent a pressure rise above 10 mmHg. The adjustments necessary in glu_{75mM} animals were minimal.

ICP CHANGES FOLLOWING SUDDEN DECOMPRESSION OF THE CAT BRAIN

Z.CZERNICKI

Introduction

The rapid changes in ICP can be dangerous and neurosurgical procedures usually try to avoid the sudden decompression (SD) effect. Nevertheless, some authors advocate the large decompressive craniectomy in the treatment of the acute subdural hematoma (1). However, the results do not show an improvement in mortality or morbidity and previous experimental data (2,3) confirmed the enhancement of brain edema by the SD. The aim of the present study was to define the conditions under which the SD appear to be harmful to the brain.

Material and methods

The study was carried out on 24 cats weighing 2700 to 3000 gm. The animals were anesthetized with Nembutal 40 mg/kg of body weight, tracheostomized, curarized and artificially ventilated. Mean arterial blood pressure, central venous pressure, and epidural pressure were recorded: blood gases and pH were studied also.

The brain compression was produced by an epidural balloon inflated gradually 0.2 ml every 10 minutes to a total volume of 1.0 ml. An Evans blue solution was used in blood-brain barrier (BBB) studies.

The animals were divided into four experimental groups of 6 animals each: 1-immediate deflation following balloon inflation; 2-deflation after 1 hour of compression; 3-deflation after 2 hours of compression; 4-deflation after 4 hours of compression. All parameters were recorded during the brain compression and 2 hours after decompression. The animals were then sacrificed, brains were fixed in 10% formalin.

Results

The highest ICP values were observed immediately after the balloon was fully inflated, but then, in the nondecompressed animals, the ICP decreased, and about 1 hour after inflation, was only slightly above the control level. The ICP rose after 2 hours of compression. The decompression performed immediately after balloon inflation did not effect an ICP rise while the SD after 2 and 4 hours of compression produced the evident and statistically significant increase of ICP(Fig.1).

The BBB impairment after the SD was observed in the cortex and basal nuclei of both hemispheres in the animals of Group 3 and 4 (Fig.2).

Discussion

The adaptation mechanisms brought down the ICP which had been raised by the inflated ballon and then a steady state was achieved for about

2 hours - the compensation stage. After 2 hours of continued brain compression, the adaptation mechanisms seemed to fail and the decompensation with a rising ICP was observed. The results of SD were found to be dependent on the stage of compression. Immediately after balloon inflation (adaptation), the SD was not harmful to the brain, while at the decompensation stage (after 2 and 4 hours of compression), the SD resulted in the evident and statistically significant ICP elevation. The BBB picture suggests the enhancement of brain edema as a reason for the observed ICP rise. In conclusion the study presented demonstrates the danger of SD performed at the decompensation stage of brain compression.

Summary

Brain compression was produced in 24 cats by a 1 ml epidural balloon. The balloon was inflated and then deflated at different times within four groups of 6 animals. ICP was measured within the epidural space continuously during compression and up to 2 hours after decompression. The blood-brain-barrier was studied using Evans blue. The decompression was found to be harmful with a subsequent high rise of ICP, only when it was performed at elevated ICP - within the decompensation stage after at least a 2-hour compression. In these cats the hemorrhages in the white matter and extensive blue staining of gray matter in cortex and basal ganglia were observed.

References

1. Britt RH, Hamilton RD (1978) Large decompressive craniectomy in the treatment of acute subdural hematoma. Neurosurg 2:195-199

2. Czernicki Z (1977) Disturbances in the blood-brain-barrier and cerebral blood flow after rapid brain decompression in the cat. Acta Neurochir 36:181-187

3. Mead CO, Moody RA, Ruamsuke S, Mullan S (1970) Effect of isovolemic hemodilution on cerebral blood flow following experimental head injury. J Neurosurg 32:40-50

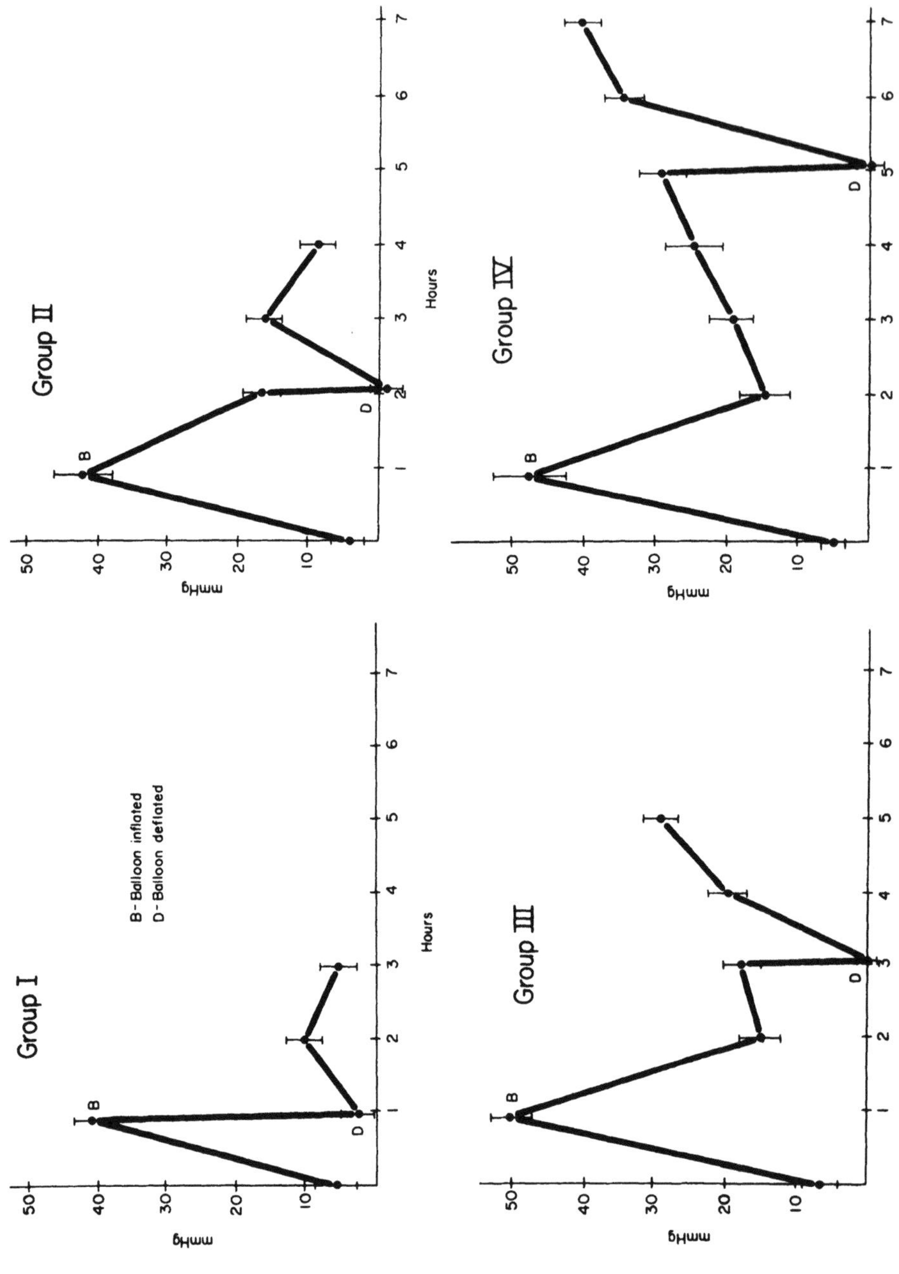

Fig. 1. Epidural pressure and standard deviation. Group 1 - Immediate deflation following balloon inflation. Group 2 - Deflation after 1 hour of compression. Group 3 - Deflation after 2 hours of compression. Group 4 - Deflation after 4 hours of compression.

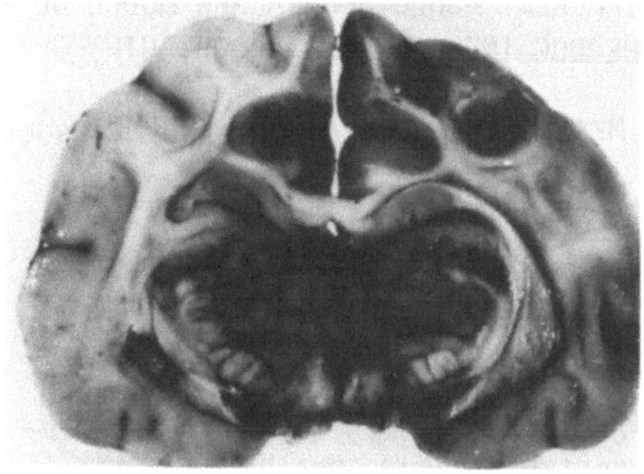

Fig. 2. Frontal cross-section of the brain of cat 5/75. The brain 2 hours after decompression which followed 2 hours epidural compression.

DIFFERENT ASPECTS OF A NEW MODEL OF INTRACRANIAL HYPERTENSION ON THE DOG INDUCED BY A BLOOD SHIFT

D. MESANGEAU, J. LEPAGNOL, AND M. AUROUSSEAU

Introduction

The present study is designed to further study a model of intracranial hypertension due to a blood shift (1,2).

Method

Inflation of a latex balloon situated immediately distal to the left sub-clavian artery caused a blood shift as a result of total aortic obstruction (3). The hypertension obtained in this way lasted for 35 minutes. Measurements were made before, during and after aortic obstruction: in 22 dogs, we measured arterial and venous blood flows, arterial blood pressure, several biochemical parameters in blood and CSF: LDH, α-HBDH, CK-MB, γ-GT, HCO_3^-, glucose, urea, and finally histological studies were performed.

Results

From these first findings, we observed that intracranial hypertension for 35 minutes in the chloralose anesthetized dog with blood shift from thoracic aorta, is able to produce brain edema. The animals present two different post-hypertensive reactions: either a "non-reflow phenomenon" (N.R.P. Group I) or a "luxury perfusion syndrome" (L.P.S. group II) which seemed less injurious to the dog. Our histological findings agree with the differentiation into two pathological groups. The first NRP syndrome, shows an intravascular hyperaggregability inducing thrombosis in pial and intracerebral vessels. The second LPS syndrome, shows disorganized myelin, i.e., a proliferation edema in the white matter.

Haemodynamics: The specificity of our pathological model is proved during the post hypertensive phase by the return at their normal levels of peripheral and cardiac blood flows, whereas the CBF and VBF fall significantly under their control values. In addition, a very weak increase of the cerebral vascular resistance appears after the occlusion.

During the occlusive phase, the intracranial pressure (ICP) increases passively as the mean arterial blood pressure (MABP). But at the balloon deflation, a differentiation between these 2 parameters, appears rapidly, i.e., a significantly high ICP in spite of the sudden fall of arterial pressure. These observations are surely obtained with the formation of brain edema.

Biochemistry: No changes in the level of cardiac and hepatic enzymes have been observed. Thus, the integrity of heart and liver is maintained in spite of the transient blood stasis during the aortic occlusion. The Δ(V-A) LDH increases during the occlusive and post-occlusive phases and is related to a deviation of the glucose metabolism

Table 1

Parameters	Control values	End of inflation	5' after deflation	60' sfter deflation	120' after deflation
Cerebral venous PO_2 mmHg	42.56 ±2.74	51.03 $\pm 3.88_s$	41.40 ±2.84	33.15 $\pm 3.12_s$	31.32 $\pm 5.05_s$
$CMRO_2$ ml/min.	3.03 ±0.17	2.93 ±0.39	2.41 $\pm 0.28_s$	2.63 $\pm 0.09_s$	2.76 ±0.38
CMRg1 mg/min.	5.58 ±0.44	7.28 ±1.51	13.76 $\pm 3.92_s$	3.08 $\pm 1.17_s$	4.82 ±1.36
G/O	1.85 ±0.15	2.55 $\pm 0.42_s$	5.89 $\pm 1.62_s$	2.33 ±0.70	2.17 ±0.65

BIOCHEMICAL PARAMETERS

Blood parameters	Control values	End of inflation 35 min.	2 hours after deflation
Arterial glucose (mM/l)	6.50 ± 0.27	10.81 ± 1.01	5.58 ± 0.77
Arterial urea (mM/l)	6.23 ± 0.78	6.83 ± 0.74	8.30 ± 1.89
LDH (v-a) (U.l./l.)	11.83 ± 2.63	22.80 ± 12.64	23.50 ± 10.30
α-HBDH (U.l./l.)	88 ±10.21	121 ± 12.32	138 ± 13.14
CK-MB (%CK)	2.1 ± 0.62	3.0 ± 0.70	4.2 ± 0.83
Alkalin Phosphatases (U.l./l.)	51.0 ±24.0	55.0 ± 26.4	75.5 ± 26.5
γ-G.T. (U.l./l.)	16.75 ± 2.95	21.5 ± 2.75	19.50 ± 1.32

to anaerobic pathway (Table I). In the same manner, a dimunition of $CMRO_2$ appears conjointly. Though a significant hyperglycemia appears rapidly and is maintained up to 3 hours after occlusion, the CMRgl increases during the blood shift.

All these observations mark a cerebral decompensation. Blood brain barrier rupture is confirmed with Evans blue test and biochemical analysis of the cerebrospinal fluid. The proteins (0,2 → 2,5 g/l.) electrophoresis shows a significant inflammatory state and the leak of HCO_3^- (23,3 → 17,1 mEq/l) shows the rupture as non-reversing and prolonged. (Table I)

Summary

This pathological model seems to approach closely clinical hyper-tensive encephalopathy. The haemodynamic and metabolic studies show an altering of cerebral blood flow autoregulation. As decompensation appears brain edema beginning in the grey matter with the many areas of perivascular edema, diffuses into the white matter.

References

1. Mesangeau D, Maamer M, Aurousseau M (1978) Proc 1st Int Symp on cerebro-vascular diseases. July, Rheims (France)

2. Mesangeau D, Lepagnol J, Albert O, Aurousseau M (to be published) Proc Int Symp on Ergot Alkaloids, March 1979, Paris

3. Simeone FA (1971) Proc 5th Int Symp on CBF regulation, Rome-Siena, p 524

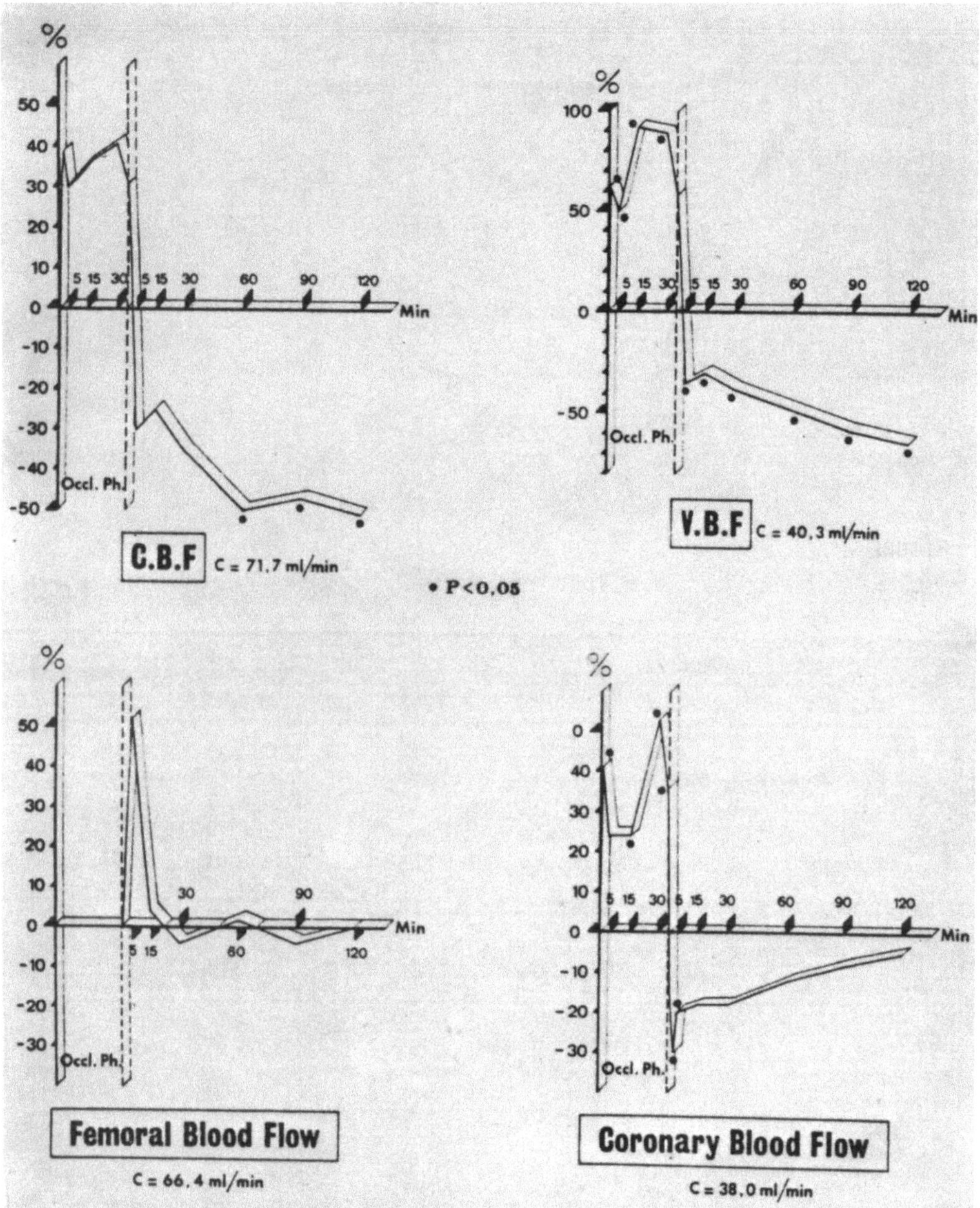
C.B.F
C = 71,7 ml/min
V.B.F
C = 40,3 ml/min
• P<0,05
Femoral Blood Flow
C = 66,4 ml/min
Coronary Blood Flow
C = 38,0 ml/min
• P<0,05
Occl. Ph.
Min
%

FIGURE 1

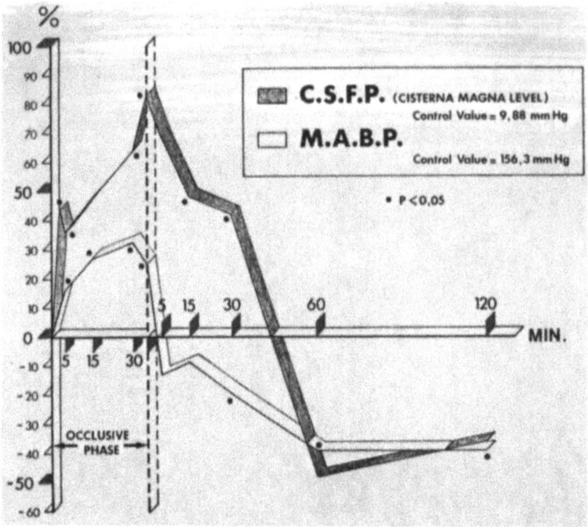

%
C.S.F.P. (CISTERNA MAGNA LEVEL)
Control Value = 9,88 mm Hg
M.A.B.P.
Control Value = 156,3 mm Hg
• P < 0,05
OCCLUSIVE PHASE
MIN.

FIGURE 2

BRAIN FREE FATTY ACIDS AFTER TRANSIENT GLOBAL BRAIN ISCHEMIA WITH POSTINSULT THIOPENTAL THERAPY

E.M. NEMOTO, G.K. SHIU, J.R. GILBERTSON, AND H. ALEXANDER

Introduction

A metabolic basis for barbiturate amelioration of ischemic brain damage is not demonstrable in terms of the rate and magnitude of changes in brain high energy phosphates, glycolytic metabolites and Krebs cycle intermediates during (7,8) or after (9) complete global brain ischemia. Yet, the efficacy of barbiturate therapy in improving neurologic recovery when administered before (4) or after (2) complete global ischemia has been clearly demonstrated.

The severalfold increase in brain free fatty acids (FFA) during cerebral ischemic anoxia (1) including their detrimental effects on mitochondrial oxidation (10), carrier mediated glucose transport (5) and the development of edema (3) are well-documented and may account for some of the pathophysiological and metabolic events occurring postischemia. Our aim was to determine whether the efficacy of barbiturate therapy can be demonstrated in terms of its effects on changes in brain FFA postischemia.

Material and methods

Female albino rats 300 to 400 g body weight were subjected to 16 min complete global brain ischemia during controlled ventilation on 1% halothane in O_2 with continuous monitoring of end-tidal CO_2, rectal temperature and mean arterial pressure (MAP) controlled at 5 to 6%, 36.5 to 37.5°C and 100 to 125 torr, respectively. An arterial blood sample was obtained to verify that blood gases and pH were within normal limits, then ischemia was induced by trimethaphan camsylate hypotension to MAP of 50 torr and a high pressure (1500 torr) neck tourniquet. Halothane was discontinued after 5 min of ischemia. Postischemia, MAP was restored and maintained at about 100 torr by IV norepinephrine infusion. The rat's entire brain was rapidly sampled into liquid N_2 either preischemia, after 16 min of ischemia without recirculation or after 6, 15 or 60 min of recirculation at normal MAP. In thiopental treated animals, IV thiopental (90 mg/kg) was begun at 5 min postischemia. One third the total calculated dose was infused between 5 and 10 min postischemia and two-thirds between 10 and 65 min postischemia.

Brain lipids were extracted in methanol/chloroform, the FFA separated by thin layer chromatography, transmethylated and quantitated by gas-liquid chromatography. Appropriate primary and secondary standards were included to correct for percent recovery, and for quantitation. The t-test for unpaired comparisons were used for all statistical analyses. P values less than or equal to 0.05 were considered significant.

Results

The major FRAs in brain are: Palmitate, sterate, oleate and arachidonate. After 16 min of ischemia without recirculation, palmitate increased by 1.5-fold and sterate by 2-fold (Fig. 1). Both oleate and arachidonate increased by about 2.5-fold (Fig. 2).

Thiopental significantly ($P<0.05$) accelerated the rate of fall of brain sterate, oleate and arachnidonate levels at 15 and 60 min postischemia. Effects on brain palmitate were not significant although mean palmitate levels were lower compared to controls.

The time course and the effects of thiopental on brain FFA appeared to correlate with the changes observed in brain cyclic-AMP (CAMP) in our previous studies (6).

Discussion

Barbiturate therapy after complete global brain ischemia is demonstrable in terms of its effects on brain FFAs and cyclic-AMP. Phospholipases and adenylate cyclases are known to be activated by catecholamines, thus providing further evidence for a role of catecholamines in the pathogenesis of ischemic brain damage.

The finding that the efficacy of barbiturate therapy could be demonstrated by these catecholamine mediated processes suggests that barbiturates ameliorate ischemic brain damage attributable to neurotransmitter dysfunction rather than that due to dysfunction of mitochondrial oxidative processes.

Barbiturate suppression of brain FFA levels postischemia could explain its efficacy in preventing or attenuating the development of brain edema since they are potent edema-inducing agents. Other postischemia pathophysiological processes which may be attributable to FFAs are the inhibition of carrier-mediated glucose transport and delayed postischemic hypermetabolism.

References

1. Bazan NG, DeBazan HEP, Kennedy WG, Joel CD (1971) Regional distribution and rate of production of a free fatty acid in rat brain. J Neurochem 18:1387-1393

2. Bleyaert AL, Nemoto EM, Safar P, Stezoski SW, Mickell J, Moosy J, Rao GR (1978) Theopental amelioration of brain damage after global ischemia in monkeys. Anesthesiol 49:390-398

3. Chan PH, Fishman RA (1978) Brain edema: Induction in cortical slices by polyunsaturated fatty acids. Science 201:358-360

4. Goldstein A Jr, Wells BA, Keats AS (1966) Increased tolerance to cerebral anoxia by pentobarbital. Arch Int Pharmacodyn Ther 161:138-143

5. Hasseblatt A (1971) Interrelations between lipid and carbohydrate metabolism. Naunyn Schmiedebergs Arch Pharmak 269:331-346

6. Kessler P, Nemoto EM (1977) Pathogenesis of postischemic (PI) encephalopathy. Fed Proc 36:588 Abstract #1667

7. Michenfelder JD, Theyre RA (1970) Effects of anesthesia and hypothermia on canine cerebral ATP and lactate during anoxia produced by decapitation. Anesthesiol 33:430-439

8. Nordstrom C-H, Rehncrona S, Siesjo BK (1978) Restitution of cerebral energy state as well as of glycolytic metabolites, citric acid cycle intermediates and associated amino acids after 30 minutes of complete ischemia in rats anesthetized with nitrous oxide or pentobarbital. J Neurochem 30:479-486

9. Nordstrom C-H, Siesjo BK (1978) Influence of phenobarbital on changes in the metabolism of the energy reserve of the cerebral cortex following complete ischemia. Acta Physiol Scand 104:271-280

10. Ozawa K, Seta K, Araki H, Handa H (1967) The effects of ischemia on mitochondiral metabolism. J Biochem 61:512-514

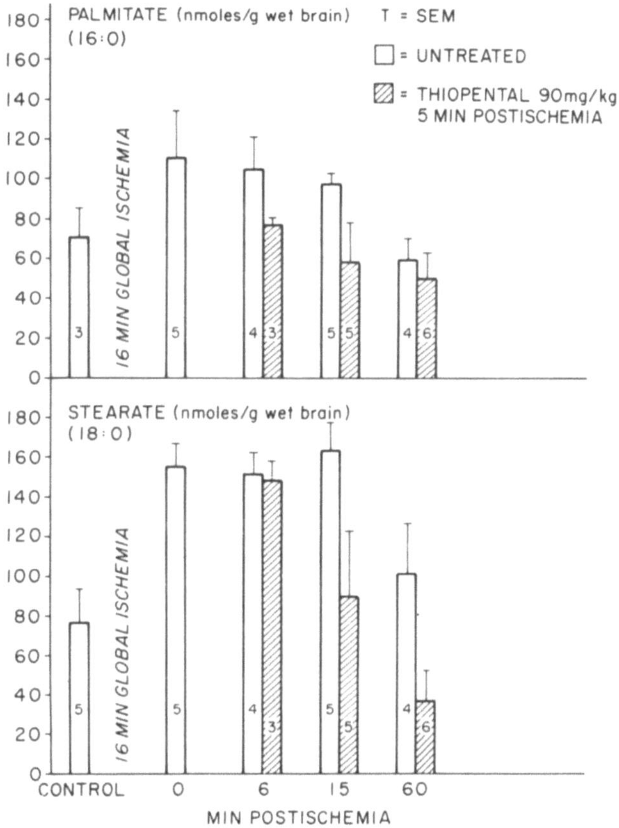

Fig. 1. Rat brain palmitate and stearate before (control) and after 16 min complete global brain ischemia with and without (untreated) thiopental therapy. Global ischemia induced by trimethaphan-induced arterial hypotension (50 torr) and a high pressure (1500 torr) neck tourniquet. Thiopental infusion began at 5 min postischemia. One third the total dose infused in 5 min and two thirds over 55 min. Numbers in columns indicate the number of rats studied.

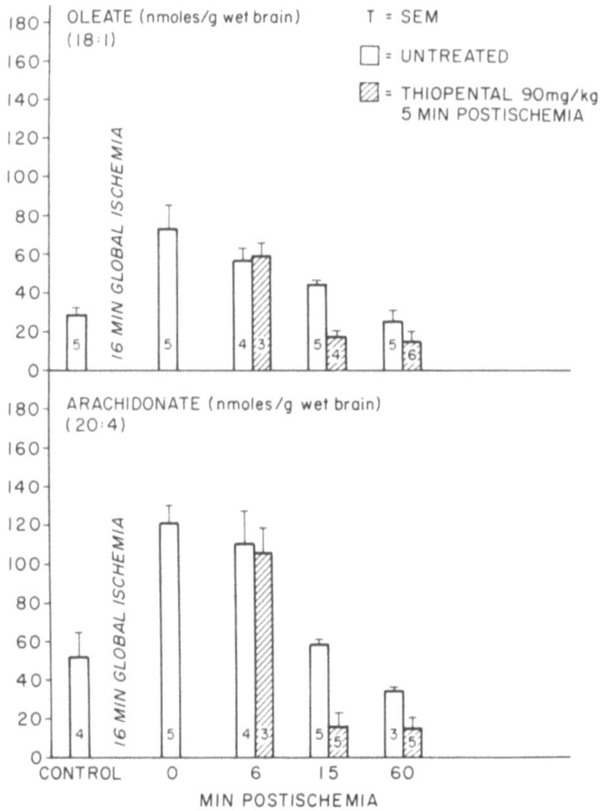

Fig. 2. Rat brain oleate and arachidonate before (control) and after 16 min complete global brain ischemia with and without (untreated) thiopental therapy. See legend of Figure 21 for other details.

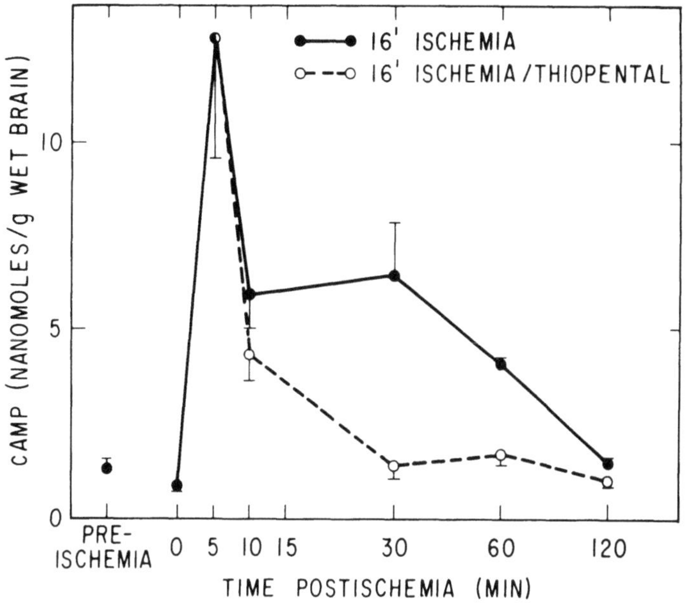

Fig. 3. Rat brain cyclic-AMP (preischemia) and after 16 min global brain ischemia. See legend Figure 1 for other details.

AN AUTORADIOGRAPHIC STUDY OF CAPILLARY PERMEABILITY DURING HYPEROSMOTIC OPENING

J. GAZENDAM, R.G. BLASBERG, C.S. PATLAK, J.D. FENSTERMACHER, AND S.I. RAPOPORT

Introduction

The permeability of the blood-brain barrier (BBB) can be altered by a number of different methods (1). One technique which reversibly opens the BBB without causing gross neurological injuries or measurable brain edema employs an intracarotid infusion of a hyperosmotic solution (2,3,4). This approach has been used to study the penetration of different compounds into brain tissue (4). The present study was performed to evaluate the time course of hyperosmotic induced changes in regional BBB permeability using quantitative autoradiographic techniques.

Material and methods

Sprague-Dawley male rats, weighing 350-400 grm, were anesthetized with sodium pentobarbital (40050 mg/kg, i.p.). The right femoral artery and vein and the right carotid artery were cannulated, as described previously (4). Evans blue which served as a visual indicator of the opening of the BBB, was administered in the femoral vein one min prior to the carotid infusion. A filtered hypertonic solution (1.6 M) of L(+)Arabinose at 37°C was infused for 30 sec at a constant rate of 7.4 ml/min into the cannulated carotid artery in order to open the BBB unilaterally. At various times (0 min to 48 hours) after the hyperosmotic infusion, 100 μCi/mg) was injected intravenously and the arterial plasma activity was serially measured over the course of the experiment (6, 10 or 30 min). At the end of the experiment, the rat was decapitated and the brain was rapidly extracted and frozen(-40°C). Less than one min elapsed from decapitation to complete freezing. Subsequently the frozen brain was sliced into 20 micron thick sections for quantitative autoradiography (5). Local tissue ^{14}C activity was determined densitometrically using calibrated ^{14}C standards and a regional unidirectional capillary transfer constant, K_i, was calculated (6). A computerized densitometer and video display system reconstructed the autoradiograms in whch the K_i values were coded to a color spectrum (courtesy of Dr. Louis Sokoloff, Lab.Cerebral MetabolismNIMH).

Results and Discussion

Gross examination of the cut brain sections demonstrated an intense Evans blue staining of the right hemisphere and light staining of the olfactory, parietal and auditory cortex of the contralateral hemisphere; the latter was due to the vascular distribution of the hyperosmotic infusate through the circle of Willis to the contralateral hemisphere. The blue staining diminished two hours after the BBB opening and had disappeared completely after 48 hours. The clearance of the Evans blue - albumin complex may reflect plasma protein clearance from the brain tissue (7). Several animals studied immediately after the hyperosmotic infusion (0-6 min), showed not only a general increase in the values of K_i throughout the ipsilateral hemisphere but also much greater elevations in K_i in various vertically oriented cortical regions. It is unclear whether these alternating regions reflect differences in the density of capillaries or the distribution of blood flow and the hyperosmotic infusate. The blood to brain transfer constants for AIB in normal grey (GM) and white (WM) matter are 3.7×10^{-5} sec^{-1} and 3.0×10^{-5} sec^{-1}, respectively. Immediately (0-6 min) after hyperosmotic infusion the K_i's increased to 135×10^{-5} sec^{-1} and 60×10^{-5} sec^{-1} for GM and WM, respectively. By 20-30 min after infusion, the K_i's had fallen to 13.8×10^{-5} sec^{-1} (GM) and 6.8×10^{-5} sec^{-1} (WM). After two hours capillary permeability to AIB had virtually returned to normal in both areas.

Summary

A hyperosmotic solution was infused into the carotid artery in order to open the blood-brain barrier (BBB). The magnitude and the time course of the opening was evaluated using ^{14}C labeled aminoisobutyric acid. The blood to brain transfer constant increased 30-40 times the normal values immediately (0-6 min) after hyperosmotic infusion and returned to normal after 1-2 hours.

It is suggested that hyperosmotic opening of the BBB can be used under specific conditions to facilitate drug delivery to the brain.

References

1. Rapoport SI (1976) Blood-brain Barrier in Physiology and Medicine. (1976) Raven Press, New York

2. Rapoport SI, Matthews K, Thompson HK, Pettigrew KD (1977) Osmotic opening of the blood-brain barrier in the rhesus monkey without measurable brain edema. Brain Res 136:23-29

3. Rapoport SI, Hori M, Klatzo I (1972) Testing of a hypothesis for osmotic opening of the blood-brain barrier. Am J Physiol 223: 323-331

4. Chieu CC, Sun CL, Kopin IJ, Fredericks WR, Rapoport SI (1978) Entry of (^{3}H)Norepinephrine, (^{125}I)Albumin and Evans blue from blood into brain following unilateral osmotic opening of the blood-brain barrier. Brain Res. 145:291-301

5. Blasberg RG, Patlak CS, Jehle JW, Fenstermacher JD (1978) An autoradiographic technique to measure the permeability of normal and abnormal brain capillaries. Neurol 28:363

6. Blasberg RG, Patlak CS, Fenstermacher JD (1978) Experimental basis for an autoradiographic technique to measure the permeability of normal and abnormal brain capillaries. Soc Neurosci Abstr 4:243

7. Blasberg RG (1976) Clearance of serum albumin from brain extracellular fluid: a possible role in cerebral edema. In: PappiusHM, Feindel W (eds) Dynamics of Brain Edema. Springer, Berlin Heidelberg New York, p 98

FREEZE LESION OF THE CEREBRUM: LOCAL CAPILLARY PERMEABILITY, BLOOD FLOW AND BULK FLOW OF EDEMA FLUID

R. BLASBERG, J. GAZENDAM, C. PATLAK, AND J. FENSTERMACHER

Introduction

The freeze lesion has been used to model "vasogenic edema" and to study "bulk flow" of edema fluid through the brain (1). However, relatively few studies have employed quantitative measurements (2,3). This report presents preliminary studies of local cerebral capillary permeability, blood flow and the movement of two plasma markers with different molecular weights through the brain after producing a freeze injury in the cerebrum of the rat. Quantitative autoradiographic methods were used which have a resolution capability of 100 microns for the location of tissue radioactivity.

Methods

A freeze lesion in the cerebrum of the rat was induced under halothane-nitrous oxide anesthesia by sequential 5 second applications of liquid nitrogen cooled cotton swabs to the exposed skull (parietal bone above the posterior canthus of the eye) over a 30 second period. Evans blue was administered intravenously. Local blood flow (4) and capillary permeability, expressed as a transfer constant (5,6) were studied in awake animals 30 minutes and 4 hours following induction of the freeze lesion. Bulk flow of edema fluid was studied during a four hour period following the freeze lesion; the activities of two reference compounds, ^{14}C-sucrose and ^{111}In-transferrin, were maintained constant in the plasma (7) and their movements from the freeze lesion through the brain were measured. The activities of the reference compounds in the brain were expressed as apparent tissue spaces realtive to plasma and were determined by quantitative double label autoradiographic methods as developed in our laboratory. Selective absorption of the ^{14}C-beta emission was achieved by placing a sheet of .13 mm thick mylar film between the tissue sections and the X-ray film. Mylar film of this thickness permits a significant fraction of the ^{111}In Auger electrons (e^-) to penetrate and expose the X-ray film. The tissue sections were stored until the ^{111}In decayed away (10 to 12 half-lives) and then reused to expose a second X-ray film in the absence of the ^{14}C-beta absorbing mylar film. The two autoradiograms represent images for each isotope (^{111}In and ^{14}C) separately and were generated from the same tissue section. Local tissue ^{14}C and ^{111}In activity was determined densitometrically using calibrated ^{14}C and ^{111}In standards. A computerized denistometer and video display system transformed the autoradiograms into colored images in which the computed values of the capillary transfer constant, blood flow, and tissue space were coded to a color spectrum (courtesy Dr. Louis Sokoloff, Lab Cerebral Metabolism, NIMH).

Results and Discussion

Increases in capillary permeability, expressed as a blood to brain transfer constant, were limited to the region of the freeze lesion at

0.5 and 4 hours after injury. The increased transcapillary passage of the test molecule (α-aminoisobutryic acid) was less apparent at 4 hours, being approximately one half that measured at 30 minutes, which suggests some "resolution" of the defect and/or a marked reduction in local blood flow. In the 4 hours studies, Evans blue staining was observed in both cortical and white matter (WM) regions remote from the injury site at distances of 2-4 mm and 4-7 mm, respectively. The histological appearance of the blue stained regions demonstrated vacuolation and separation of cellular elements and fiber tracks, implying the presence of "edema".

A marked decrease in capillary blood flow (cc/g/min) was observed within the freeze lesion at 0.5 and 4 hours after injury (.18 and .15 respectively). Blood flow to the hemisphere with the freeze lesion was consistently reduced; cortical flows, remote from but ipsilateral to the lesion, were approximately half (1.2 and 1.0, respectively) that of the contralateral cortex (1.9 and 2.3, respectively) at the two time periods. A marked reduction in blood flow to "edematous" cortex (.22) and WM (.19) adjacent to the freeze lesion and to a lesser extent to "edematous" WM (.24) remote from the lesion was observed in the 4 hour post injury studies: comparable values for "non-edematous" tissue at 0.5 hours were .73, .28 and .32, respectively.

The movement of plasma fluid from the freeze injury through the brain parenchyma was studied using two extracellular fluid reference compounds with significantly different molecular weights and diffusion constants. Limited movement and separation of the marker compounds would suggest diffusion is predominant, whereas, extensive movement through the brain with little separation of the molecules would suggest bulk flow or convective movement predominates. The distribution of the two tracers was greater through WM than through cortex and distribution patterns of the isotopes were essentially equivalent in the two tissue regions. The tissue equilibration spaces were essentially identical reaching 7-13 percent for cortex and 30-45 percent for WM. These observations are consistent with the original concept of "vasogenic edema" and the "bulk flow" of edema fluid (1).

Summary

Quantitative autoradiographic techniques were used to study the progression of changes in local brain capillary permeability, blood flow, and bulk movement of edema fluid in the rat with a freeze injury to the cortex. Increased capillary permeability was limited to the freeze lesion; the capillaries of "edematous" brain tissue remote from the lesion restricted the blood to brain transfer of the test molecule. Blood flow was markedly reduced in the freeze lesion and surrounding edematous tissue; cortical blood flow ipsilateral to but remote from the injury was half that measured for the contralateral cortex. The simultaneous movement of two plasma markers of differing molecular weights and diffusion constants demonstrated equivalent patterns of distribution through cortex and WM as well as equivalent tissue equilibration spaces.

References

1. Klatzo I, Wisniewski H, Steinwall O, Streicher E Dynamics of cold injury edema. In: Klatzo I, Seitelberger F (eds) Brain Edema. Springer, (1967) Berlin Heidelberg New York, p554

2. Reulen HJ, Graham R, Spatz M, Klatz I (1977) Role of pressure gradients and bulk flow in dynamics of vasogenic brain edema. J Neurosurg 46:24-35

3. Gazendam J, Go KE, Van Meer JJ, Zuiderveen F (to be published) Changes in electrical impedance in edematous cat brain.

4. Sakurada O, Kennedy C, Jehle J, Brown JD, Carbin GL, Sokoloff L (1978) Measurement of local cerebral blood flow with (^{14}C)-iodoantipyrine. Am J Physiol 234:H59

5. Blasberg RG, Patlak CS, Jehle JW, Fenstermacher JD (1978) An autoradiographic technique to measure the permeability of normal and abnormal brain capillaries. Neurol 28:363

6. Blasberg RG, Patlak CS, Fenstermacher JD (1978) Experimental basis for an autoradiographic technique to measure the permeability of normal and abnormal brain capillaries. Soc Neurosci Abstr 4:243

7. Patlak CS, Pettigrew Kd (1976) A method to obtain infusion schedules for prescribed blood concentration time courses. J Appl Physiol 40:458-463

INHIBITION OF OXYGEN DIFFUSION AS A MAJOR CAUSE OF PROLONGED CELL ANOXIA AND POSTISCHEMIC ICP ELEVATION

W. ERDMANN, J. BEKS, M. BELOPAVLOVIC, P. J. SALT, S. AGOSTON, AND A. BUCHTHAL

Introduction

Changes in the constitution of the tissue after ischemic anoxia are thought to be the cause of postischemic edema. Edema development leads to an increase of intracranial pressure when the increase in intracranial volume exceeds the buffer capacity of the intracranial compliance. Increase of intracranial pressure is primarily compensated for by increase of arterial pressure, so that the perfusion pressure of the capillaries is maintained constant. Above a determined level this compensation process is exhausted and severe disturbance of tissue perfusion results. This leads to further anoxic damage of the brain tissue and the primary inducing factors of edema are furthermore increased. The osmotic gradient from capillaries to tissue is dependent upon:

1. Protein concentration
2. Mucopolysaccharide polymerization
3. The size of intercellular space and
4. The density of cellular network

The development of brain edema after short-term ischemic insults occurs with a delay after primary recovery of brain tissue. The cause of this delay has never been discussed nor investigated. Recently MORAWETZ et al and CLARK et al (8,1) have shown that short-term ischemic anoxia of tissue results in changes in the oxygen diffusion coefficient. This leads to an embarrassement of the cellular oxygen supply in those areas of intercapillary tissue not directly adjoining the capillaries. Severe and prolonged local intercapillary tissue hypoxia is the consequence(2).

The present study has been designed to investigate the interrelationship of the ischemia-induced primary changes of oxygen diffusion coefficient and the secondary deleterious increases of intracranial pressure which may be fatal. A recently developed micro-electrode system for direct measurement of oxygen diffusion (DO_2) with simultaneous registration of capillary perfusion (via hydrogen clearance) and continuous monitoring of local tissue PO_2(5) has been employed.

Methods

The measuring device is based upon the polarographic principle using micro-electrodes with tip diameters of 5 to 10 µ. Tissue trauma due to electrode insertion is thus negligible. Recently ERDMAN and KRELL succeeded in developing a method for measurement of oxygen diffusion, oxygen conductivity, oxygen concentration and oxygen solubility in the tissue simultaneously with the continuous monitoring of tissue PO_2, intermittent hydrogen clearance (tissue perfusion) and local action potentials (6,7). The system was developed in the form of a double-barrelled electrode with one membrane covered, partial pressure measuring, electrode tip and one bare electrode tip (Fig. 1). These methods are also capable of measuring values two- and three-dimensionally respectively, if multimicroelectrodes are used (4).

The experiments have to be performed in the noise-free atmosphere of a highly shielded chamber (FARADAY cage) as the currents to be measured are extremely small (in the nano- to pico-ampere range). In order to avoid feed back noise from the recording apparatus back into the cage light transmission has to be employed (Fig. 2).

In vivo experiments were performed in the brain of mongolian gerbils. The advantage of using mongolian gerbils is that the carotid arteries represent the only supply of the brain and any collateral blood supply to this tissue can be neglected. Thus it is possible to control the ischemic event. Besides the above-mentioned microphysiologic values intracranial pressure was continuously monitored by introducing a 25 gauge teflon catheter into the ventricles. As control values blood pressure in the arteria femoralis or aorta abdominalis was monitored and connected to a heart rate calculator. In spontaneously breathing animals end-expiratory CO_2 and respiration rate were continuously controlled

Results

Oxygen partial pressure distribution and cellular oxygen supply are closely related to oxygen diffusion (Fig. 3). The initial insult was a short-term ligation of both carotids. The electrodes were inserted through bore holes into the frontal cortex of the brain. Relative changes of tissue perfusion, oxygen partial pressure and oxygen diffusion were registered continuously.

After ligation oxygen partial pressure drops immediately to zero and oxygen diffusion coefficient (DO_2) decreases from 1.72 to 1.4×10^{-5} CM^2/second. After removal of the ligation a primary reactive hyperperfusion of the capillary system is observed with a consequent tissue hyperoxia. The oxygen diffusion coefficient is also increased above normal, thus facilitating oxygen diffusion from capillaries to the cells. However, a secondary postischemic decrease of oxygen diffusion coefficient occurs and DO_2 steadily decreases to values even below the ones during the ischemic period. Simultaneously tissue PO_2 decreases to hypoxic values although tissue perfusion remains normal and even increases compensatorily. Thus, in this phase oxygen diffusion falls dominate and extreme hypoxia in large areas of the intercapillary network is the consequence. Finally tissue perfusion acutely fails with inevitable death. In some animals recovery of diffusion coefficient is observed in the final phase followed by increase of tissue oxygenation until normalization.

Intracranial pressure also decreases during the ischemic phase. However it rises in the postischemic phase reaching values slightly above normal and stays fairly constant until the final phase and then increases rapidly. This occurs after diffusion coefficient and tissue PO_2 have fallen to rather low values. Initially, the final increase in intracranial pressure is associated with a rise in tissue perfusion. However, when a certain value of ICP (≈ 30 mmHg) is reached the tissue perfusion starts to fail. In those animals that survive, intracranial pressure also shows a secondary increase, but values never reach the 25 mmHg mark and return to normal in a parallel fashion to the oxygen diffusion and oxygen partial pressure.

Discussion

The results presented here indicate that changes in tissue pressure diffusion play a role in postischemic brain edema development. Until now it was not possible to determine oxygen diffusion directly in the tissue. Thus, it is understandable that this parameter which decisively controls oxygen supply to the cell has not been previously included in the considerations of the etiology of edema development and intracranial pressure increase.

The described changes in the oxygen diffusion coefficient and the consequent prolonged tissue hypoxia appear to be the main factors in the subsequent development of severe brain edema and the rise in intracranial pressure. The explanation for this sequence of events can only be hypothetical at this stage. However, we would suggest that since oxygen diffusion plays a central role in the vicious circle of cerebral ischemia, it is possible that the enzyme, hyaluronidase, may be important in the etiology of this condition.

References

1. Clark DK, Erdmann W, Halsey JH, Strong E (1978) Oxygen diffusion, conductivity and solubility coefficients in the microarea of the brain. In: Oxygen Transport to Tissue III. Plenum Press, New York and London, p 697

2. Erdmann W (1979) Pathophysiologie der zellulaeren Sauerstoffversorgung in Schock. In: Proc Internatl Shoch Symp. Mainz

3. Erdmann W, Krell W, Metzger H, Nixdorf I (1970) Ein Verfahren zur Hers-ellung standardisierter Gold-Mikroelektroden fur die PO_2 Messung in Gewebe. Pflugers Arch 319:R 69

4. Erdmann W, Kunke S, Krell W (1973) Tissue-PO_2 and cell function - An experimental study with Multimicroelectrodes in the rat brain. In: Oxygen Supply. Urban & Schwarzenberg, Munchen Wien Berlin, p 138

5. Erdman W, Krell W (1976) Measurement of diffusion parameters with noble metal electrodes. In: Oxygen Transport to Tissue II. Plenum Press. New York London, p 225

6. Heidenreich J, Erdmann W, Metzger H. Thews G (1970) Local hydrogen clearance and PO_2 measurement in microareas of the rat brain. Experimentia 26:257-259

7. Kunke S. Erdmann W, Metzger H (1972) A new method for simultaneous PO_2 and action potential measurement in microareas of tissue. J Appl Physiol 32:436-438

8. Morawetz R, Strong E, Clark DK, Erdmann W (1978) Effects of ischemia on the oxygen diffusion coefficients in the brain cortex. In: Oxygen Transport to Tissue III. Plenum Press. New York London, p 629

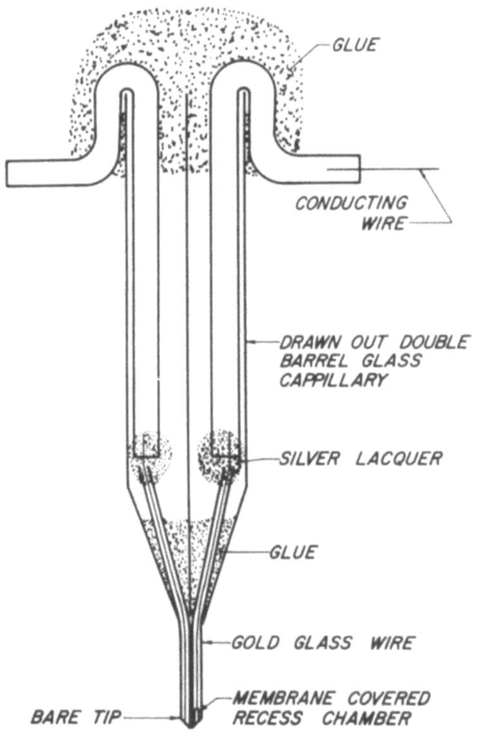

Fig. 1. Schematic of double barrelled microelectrode (Erdmann and Krell, 1976) for simultaneous registration of tissue PO_2, tissue perfusion, unit potentials and the diffusion parameters in tissue:
Two gold wires insolated by glass of 5-10 μ diameter (Erdmann et al., 1970) are connected to conducting wires by means of silver lacquer. One electrode tip is left as a bare noble metal electrode, the other gold wire is ground back into the surrounding glass coat by electrolysis (in concentrated HCl).
A recessed chamber of 5-10 μ depth is formed. The recessed chamber is filled with Rhoplex (Rohm and Haas, Frankfurt/Main, FRG) dissolved in 0.2 molar KCl by diffusion. The two electrode-conducting wire systems are inserted into glass capillaries and fixed with a quick hardening two component glue (Clark et al., 1978). The membrane covered "recessed chamber" electrode is measuring PO_2 with minimal drift, the blanc electrode is used for continuous registration of oxygen concentration and intermittant determination of oxygen diffusion coefficient. The determined values are suitable to calculate oxygen conductivity and oxygen solubility in tissue. In addition, the membrane covered electrode is applied for simultaneous registration of action potentials and intermittant registration of H_2-clearance as a measure for tissue perfusion.

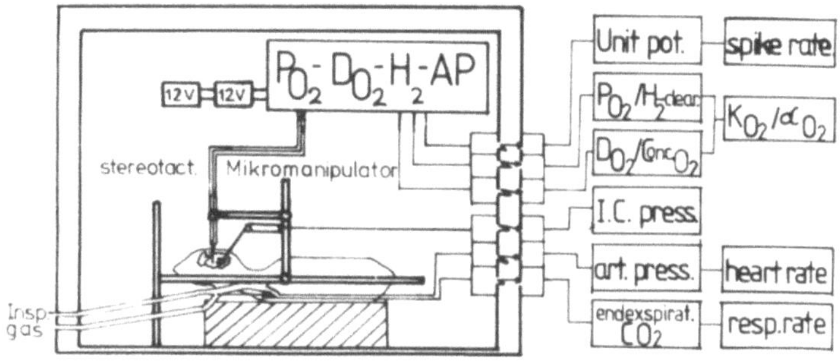

Fig. 2. Diagram of experimental procedure in highly shielded cage: The rat is fixed in a stereotactic holdering inside a highly shielded double walled Faraday cage (Siemens Co., FRG). The microelectrode is driven into the tissue by means of a micromanipulator, and a 25 gauge catheter is placed intraventricularly and connected to a Statham pressure transducer. Microelectrode information is lead to a pre-amplifier system supplied by 12 Volt batteries. As control values function continuous monitoring of arterial pressure in the arteria femoralis and endexpiratory CO_2.
All measured and preamplified signals are led to a chain of light emitting diodes which transmit frequency modulated information through the space between the two walls of the cage to a light receiving phototransistor.Frequency modulation is reversed and information can be recorded.
There exists no galvanic connection between the inside and the outside of the shielded chamber and noise interference - including feed back noise of recorders outside the cage - is totally abolished.

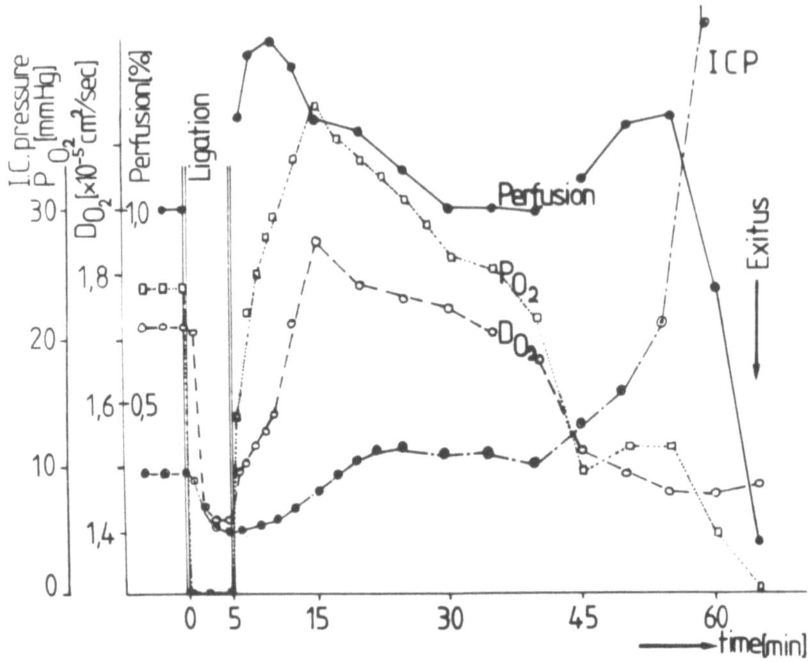

Fig. 3. Simultaneous registration of tissue-PO_2, capillary perfusion and oxygen diffusion coefficient (DO_2) in relation to intraventricular (intracranial) pressure (ICP) in the frontal cortex of the mongolian gerbil.
The registrations are performed before, during and after a two minutes ligation of both arteriae carotides communes, producing total ischemia of the brain.

Session VI

SYSTEMIC FACTORS AND INFECTIOUS PROCESSES

Chairman: J.W.F.Beks
Co-chairman: A.Crockard

SUMMARY

Papers presented in this session fell into three distinct groups:

1) Neurohumoral effects of raised ICP.

The role of the autonomic system in the systemic effects of raised ICP is still not clear. WOOD and MILLIS demonstrated arterial hypoxemia in response to raised ICP and attributed this to an effect on the vasomotor centre. NISHIMURA and HOFF suggested that neurogenic pulmonary edema was coincidental to, rather than resultant from cardiac changes. Unfortunately, none of the models described in this session had exactly the same parameters measured and until simultaneous cardiac, pulmonary and humoral measurements are obtained, the debate will continue. This is also true of the excellent work of RAP et al, who suggest that the Cushing reflex is humoral in origin. Whether this is the mechanism or only one method of initiating the Cushing response requires further work. The role of the endorphins must also be evaluated in this regard.

The elegant studies by JENNETT and NORTH have attempted to isolate the individual effects of PCO_2 and PO_2 on ICP, but we were concerned that some of the changes might in part have been related to changes in respiratory pattern and thus CVP.

2) ICP and intracranial infection.

These very interesting papers show that our knowledge of the pathophysiological consequences of infection require further study and we were particularly impressed with the models. WALLENFANG et al, showed the difference in brain water content before and after the development of the abcess capsule and we are anxious to know what changes in local CBF and blood brain barrier occur so that the possible role of steroid therapy can be investigated. DACEY et al, have shown a 50% reduction in the raised CSF outflow pressure in animals treated with antibiotics and steroids. We were encouraged to have KRISHNAN'S report from India and look forward to further studies in tubercular and tropical conditions.

3) Subdural hematomas.

TABADDOR'S studies confirmed GJERRIS' previously reported findings of the rise in ICP following evacuation of the hematoma. The assumption of GAAB et al, that the hydrostatic effect of patient position would influence subdural membrane transport of fluid and therefore effect the volume of the chronic subdural was interesting but not yet proven.

SYSTEMIC VASOPRESSOR RESPONSES AND THE ARTERIAL HYPOXEMIA ASSOCIATED WITH INCREASED INTRACRANIAL PRESSURE

D.H.Wood, R.M.Millis, and C.O.Trouth

Introduction

The mechanism or mechanisms responsible for the arterial hypoxemia demonstrated in experimental animals (1,5,4) as well as in patients (2,3,6,7) with increased intracranial pressure (ICP) remains somewhat obscure. Intracranial pathological disorders producing chronic elevation of ICP are rarely associated with arterial hypoxemia; whereas those disorders which produce acute elevations of ICP are quite commonly associated with arterial hypoxemia. Additionally, it has been observed that those patients with increased ICP exhibiting decerebrate rigidity appeared to demonstrate this response more consistently and profoundly. This variable correlation between elevated ICP and arterial hypoxemia suggests that the observed arterial hypoxemia may not occur as a direct response or result of the elevated ICP, but is more likely a result of non-specific cardiopulmonary responses associated with ICP elevations. Thus, these investigations were designed to assess the correlation of the development of arterial hypoxemia with the rate of development of increased ICP and the severity of the associated vasopressor responses.

Material and methods

In all experimental groups arterial blood gases were continuously measured in vivo by a mass spectrometer (Medspect, Chemtron). Values were verified in vitro by a blood gas analyzer (Instrumentation Lab Model 113). Arterial blood pressure was measured via a strain gauge pressure transducer (Model 23Db, Statham). For ease in interpretation the mean arterial blood pressure was rounded off to the nearest five torr. In the elevated ICP studies, airway flows were monitored via a heated pneumotachograph connected to a differential pressure transducer (Model PM15e, Statham). Airway gases were sampled via a mass spectrometer (Medspect).

A) Vasopressor responses with elevations of ICP

Mongrel dogs (9-18 kg) were anesthetized with intravenous sodium pentobarbital (25 mg/kg.). A cuffed endotracheal tube was introduced into the larynx, and the animals were mechanically ventilated with a constant volume animal respirator (Harvard instruments, Millis, Mass). Parietal burr holes were drilled in the skull, bilaterally. Through one hole, a catheter (Foley, 12 French) fitted with a 5 ml inflatable balloon was passed into the epidural space. A fiberoptic ICP transducer was inserted through the burr hole into the epidural space contralateral to the Foley catheter for measurement of ICP via an ICP monitor (Ladd).

Each animal served as his own control. Administration of intramuscular atropine sulfate (1 mg/kg) was used to block bradycardia and cardiac arrhythmias. ICP was increased after stabilization of the arterial oxygen tension above 75±2 torr and the carbon dioxide tension below 35±1 torr for 20 minutes, with mechanical ventilation.

(1) Slow elevations of ICP were accomplished by expansion of an epidural balloon, using a syringe infusion pump (Harvard) fitted with a 50 cc syringe containing physiological saline, set to a speed of 1.15 ml per minute.

(2) Rapid elevations of ICP accomplished by the same method described above except that saline was infused at a rate of 2.3 ml per minute. In order to test for reversibility for the observed responses, infused saline was withdrawn at a rate of 15 ml per minute. The students' t-test for independent samples was used to determine the statistical significance of mean differences in the blood gas responses between animals subjected to slow versus fast elevation of ICP.

B) Vasopressor responses without elevations of ICP

(1) Norepinephrine (Levophed, 0.005 mg/kg) was administered rapidly intravenously to mechanically ventilated animals anesthetized with sodium pentobarbital.

(2) The vasomotor center, localized in the medulla oblongata of anesthetized animals (chloralose 40 mg/kg & urethane 200 mg/kg) was directly stimulated (1-4v, 1 msec duration, 40Hz).

Results

Analysis of the changes in mean arterial blood pressure, arterial blood gas concentration and heart rate in ten dogs subjected to slow elevations of ICP revealed that a reduction of the arterial PO_2 occurred in only five animals, and decerebrate posturing was observed in two of these five dogs.

In the 20 dogs whose ICP was raised by the fast method all exhibited reduction in arterial PO_2 and 10 developed decerebrate posturing. Fig. 1 shows an example of the responses recorded when decerebrate posturing was observed (in 10 of 20 dogs) during rapid elevations of ICP.

Decerebrate posturing was associated with a mean decrement in arterial PO_2 of 26±1 (SEM) torr and a mean rise in arterial PCO_2 of 11±(SEM) torr. Although the development of arterial hypoxemia was not found to be dependent upon the development of decerebration, those animals that demonstrated decerebration had a significantly greater fall in arterial PO_2 than those animals which did not ($P<.01$). These studies also revealed that the development of arterial hypoxemia was associated with a greater systemic vasopressor response.

The product of abrupt systemic vasopressor responses by the intravenous administration of norepinephrine in cats and dogs (Fig.2) as well as by direct electrical stimulation of the vasomotor center in cats (Fig. 3) resulted in arterial hypoxemia, hypercapnia, and increased end-expiratory nitrogen tension during controlled ventilation.

Discussion

The arterial hypoxemia accompanying ICP observed in these investigations was more profoundly apparent with rapid elevations of ICP, an effect which is similar to that which has been observed in the production of the Cushing vasopressor response. Slow elevations of ICP in dogs resulted in smaller changes in the mean arterial oxygen tension (7%) and milder systemic vasopressor responses (50%). Whereas, rapidly increased ICP resulted in more pronounced decrements in the mean arterial oxygen tension (14%) and more marked systemic vasopressor responses (68%). Furthermore, no differences in the levels of ICP were detected in animals subjected to slow as compared to those subjected to fast elevations. Therefore, these studies suggest that arterial hypoxemia was better correlated with the level of the mean arterial blood pressure than with that of the ICP. The vasomotor center stimulation and norepinepherine studies further validate this observation.

With rapid elevations in ICP, arterial oxygen desaturation was observed to be greater associated with decerebrate rigidity. The physiological mechanism responsible for this greater decrement is unclear. However, our data indicates that the systemic vasopressor responses could not be invoked to explain this effect since there were no significant differences in the vasopressor responses in the decerebrate versus non-decerebrate preparations. It is conceivable that changes in chest wall rigidity accompanying decerebration may have compromised the effective alveolar ventilation by altering lung compliance even though tidal volume was held constant.

Summary

Slow elevations of ICP produced mild vasopressor responses and no statistically significant reduction in arterial oxygen tension. However, rapid elevations of ICP resulted in marked vasopressor responses coupled with significant decrements in arterial oxygen tension. With fast elevations, the magnitude of the decrement of arterial oxygen tension seemed to be dependent upon concomitant decerebration.

These investigations demonstrate that arterial hypoxemia may be produced by an abrupt, marked elevation of the mean arterial blood pressure with or without an associated ICP elevation; thus, suggesting that arterial hypoxemia may be a nonspecific response to acutely raised ICP.

References

1. Berman IR, Ducker TB, Simmons RL (1969) The effects of increased intracranial pressure upon the oxygenation of blood in dogs. J Neurosurg 30:532-536

2. Froman C (1968) Alterations of respiratory function in patients with severe head injuries. Br J Anaesth 40:354-360

3. Huang CT, Cook AW, Lyon HA (1963) Severe cranio-cerebral trauma and respiratory abnormalities. Arch Neurol 9:545-554

4. Jennett S, Hoff JT (1978) Arterial blood gases during raised intracranial pressure in anesthetized cats under controlled ventilation. J Neurosurg 48:390-401

5. Maxwell JA, Goodwin JW (1973) Neurogenic pulmonary shunting. J Trauma 13:368-373

6. Moss IR, Wald A, Ransohoff J (1974) Respiratory functions and chemical regulation of ventilation in head injury. Am Rev Resp Dis 109:205-215

7. Schumacker PT, Rhodes GR, Newell JC et al (1979) Ventilation-perfusion imbalance after head trauma. Am Rev Resp Dis 119:33-43

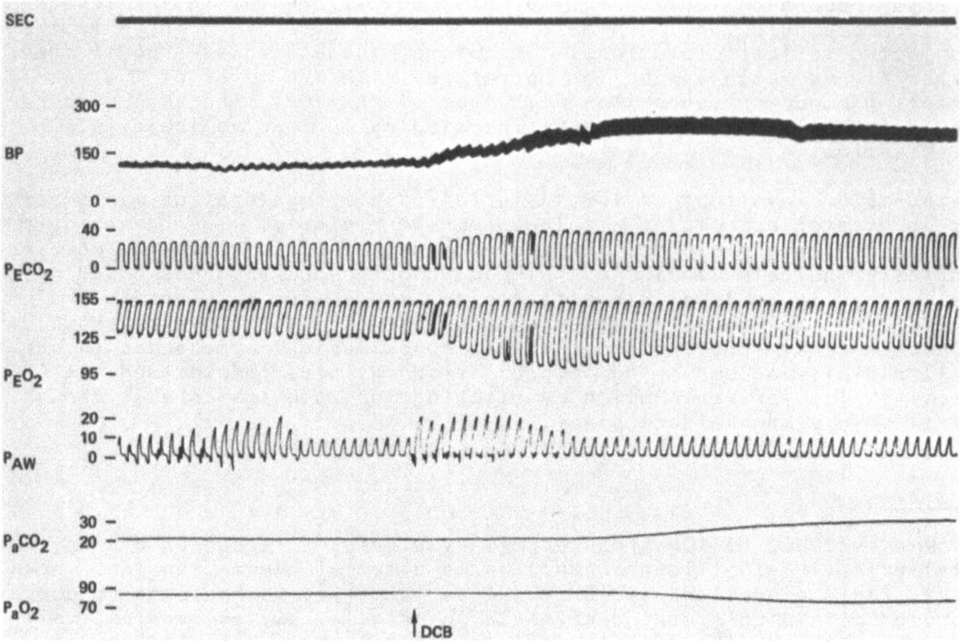

Fig. 1. Responses to rapid elevations of ICP with decerebration Analog recordings of arterial blood pressure (BP) and arterial blood gas (PaO_2, $PaCO_2$) tensions with mechanical ventilation during the vasopressor response associated with rapidly increasing ICP in an anesthetized atropinized animal. DCB indicates observation of decerebrate limb rigidity with opisthotonus.

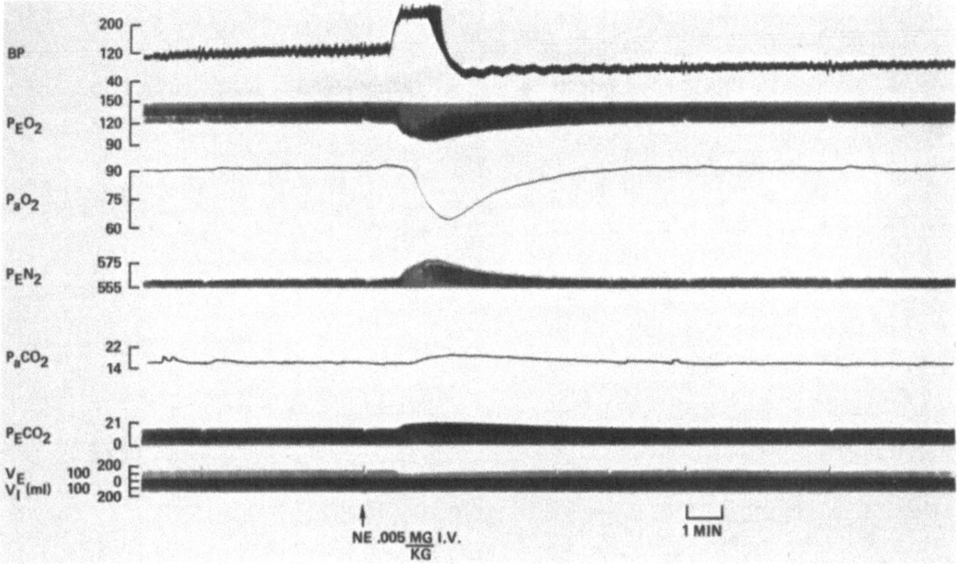

Fig. 2. Responses to norepinephrine-contolled ventilation
Analog recordings of arterial blood pressure (BP) airway flow (RESP) expiratory gas (P_EO_2, P_EN_2, P_ECO_2) and arterial blood gas (PaO_2, $PaCO_2$) tensions from an animal during mechanical ventilation with neuromuscular blockade and subjected to intravenous administration of norepinephrine.

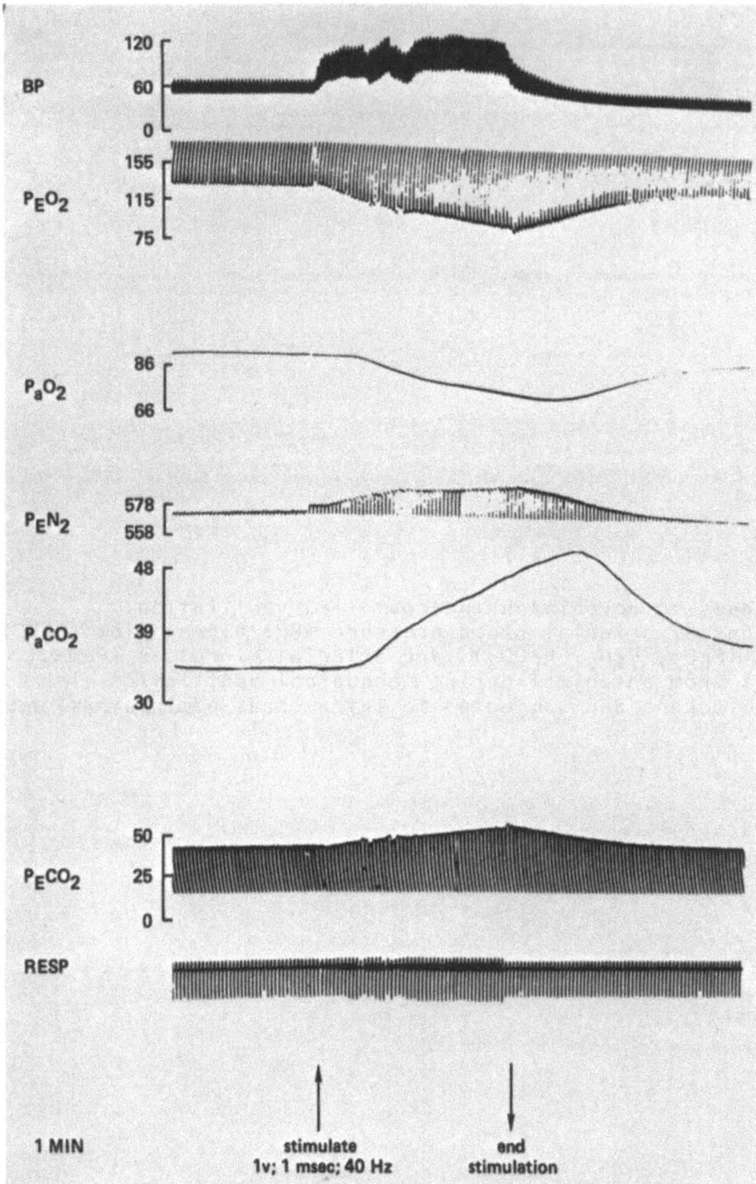

Fig. 3. Responses to vasomotor center stimulation
Analog recordings of arterial blood pressure (BP) airway flow (RESP) expiratory gas (P_EO_2, P_EN_2 and arterial blood gas (PaO_2, $PaCO_2$) tensions from an anesthetized atropinized animal with neuromuscular blockade subjected to mechanical ventilation during electrical vasomotor center stimulation (1-4v, 1 msec duration, 40Hz).

SEQUENTIAL HEMODYNAMIC CHANGES IN EXPERIMENTAL NEUROGENIC PULMONARY EDEMA

M.C. NISHIMURA AND J.T. HOFF

Introduction

Neurogenic pulmonary edema (NPE) may be the final expression of a massive sympathetic discharge, triggered by one of several brain insults, resulting in a progressive rise of systemic arterial (SAP), pulmonary arterial (PAP) and left atrial (LAP) pressures (1,3). The sequential change of pressures which supposedly precedes NPE has not been confirmed, however (5,6). In this study we sought to define those pressure changes.

Material and methods

Twenty-six cats (2.91 kg±0.1SE) were divided into a control group (9) and an experimental group (17), anesthetized (30 mg/kg Na pentobarbital IP), paralyzed and ventilated. Animals in the experimental group were subjected to 150 mmHg intracranial pressure (ICP) for 30 minutes by an intraventricular infusion (rate of rise = 1 mmHg/sec.) of warmed mock CSF. SAP, PAP, LAP, ICP and end tidal CO_2 were monitored continuously (Fig. 1); arterial blood gases and pH, hematocrit, cardiac output (CO) and catecholamines were obtained at fixed intervals. The lungs were removed for gravimetric analysis of lung water 30 minutes after ICP returned to normal (2).

Systemic arterial, pulmonary arterial and left atrial pressures rose as ICP approached diastolic SAP. Within the first 10 minutes of ICP elevation SAP rose 45 ± 4 mmHg, PAP, 9 ± 2 mmHg, and LAP, 10 ± 3 mmHg. Thereafter, PAP and LAP progressively fell but SAP remained elevated. The sequential pressure changes varied with individual animals. PAP rose 57 ± 11 sec and LAP 72 ± 12 sec. after ICP elevation was initiated (Fig.2). Although the PAP responded earlier to increased ICP, LAP rose at a faster rate.

Baseline values of arterial blood gases and pH between groups were comparable. Significant differences occurred during the 20th minute of ICP elevations: $PaCO_2$ rose (28±0.3 to 34±1 mmHg, $p<.001$); pH_a fell (7.40±.01 to 7.32±.02, $p<.001$); and PaO_2 fell (80±2 to 69±4 mmHg, $p<.01$). Cardiac output increased two-fold during intracranial hypertension and returned to baseline at the end of the recovery period (0.145±.026L/min, 0.309±.051L/min and 0.175±.023L/min respectively). Plasma catecholamines increased during elevated ICP and decreased during recovery, but never returned to baseline. Catecholamine levels also increased progressively in control animals throughout the period of anesthesia.

Lung weight (LWt) and total lung water (TLW) were greater in experimental animals than in controls (Table 1). Extravascular lung water(EVLW) was also higher in the experimental group but the difference was not significant by the unpaired t-test.

TABLE I.
GRAVIMETRIC ANALYSES OF LUNG WATER M ± SE

	N	LWt (%Body Wt)	TLW (TLW/Wt)	EVLW (g/g EVDW)	Blood Wt (%LWT)
Control	9	.73±.05	.81±.00	3.55±.13	37.28±4.44
Experimental	17	.99±.08	.84±.01	4.44±.49	41.96±4.93
P		<.025	<.005	<.2	NS

Variable responses to elevated ICP were observed, particularly the rate of rise of SAP. In 56% of cats SAP rose initially, followed by either pulmonary arterial hypertension or left atrial hypertension. In 43% PAP rose before LAP, and in 14% LAP rose initially.

Some investigators have observed decreased cardiac output five minutes after ICP elevation, followed later by an increase (4). We measured CO 20 minutes after ICP elevation began, noting a significant elevation. This increase probably indicates a delayed response to endogenous vasopressors or reduced vasoconstriction after prolonged exposure to elevated ICP. Responses to intracranial hypertension varied from animal to animal, but in most instances (65%) plasma catecholamines rose with increased ICP and fell with decreased ICP, confirming GRAF's observations.

From our study it appears that ICP elevation causes catecholamine release which is then followed by increased SAP; PAP then increases and, finally, LAP rises. Elevation of PAP before LAP suggests that the cascade of pressure changes postulated to follow systemic vasoconstriction may not be the fundamental mechanism of NPE. Rather, the pulmonary arterial tree is probably directly affected by sympathetic discharge induced by elevated ICP.

References

1. Ducker TB, Simmons RL (1968) Increased intracranial pressure and pulmonary edema. J Neurosurg 28:118-123

2. Hoff JT, Nishimura MC (1978) Experimental neurogenic pulmonary edema in cats. J Neurosurg 48:383-389

3. Hoff JT, Mitchell RA (1972) The effect of hypoxia on the Cushing reflex. In: Brock M, Dietz H (eds) Intracranial Pressure. Springer Berlin Heidelberg New York, p 205

4. Malik AB (1977) Pulmonary vascular response to increase in intracranial pressure: role of sympathetic mechanisms. J Appl Physiol 42:335-343

5. Moss G, Staunton C, Stein AA (1972) Cerebral etiology of the "shock lung syndrome". J Trauma 12:885-890

6. Sarnoff SJ, Sarnoff LC (1952) Neurohemodynamics of pulmonary edema. II. The role of sympathetic pathways in the elevation of pulmonary and systemic vascular pressures following the intracisternal injection of fibrin. Circ VI:51-62

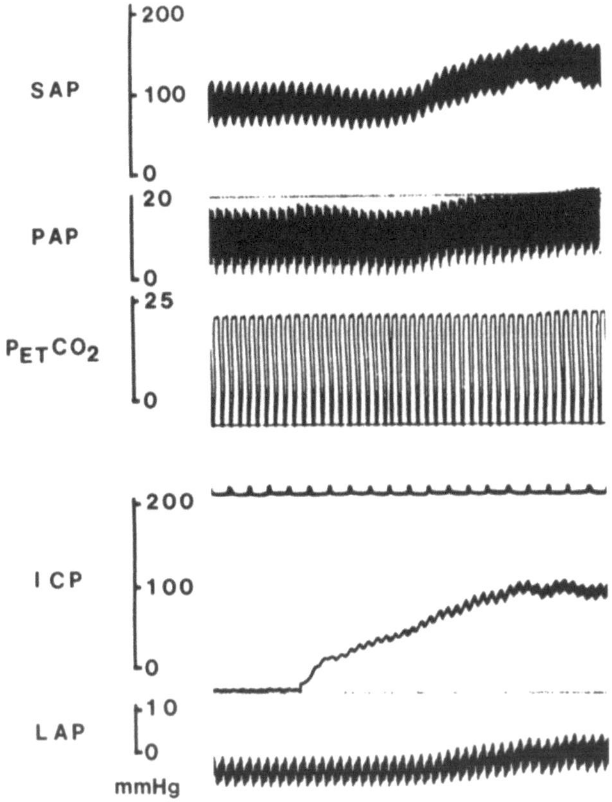

Fig. 1. Recording of an experiment showing the effect of raised ICP on systemic arterial pressure (SAP), pulmonary arterial pressure (PAP), end tidal CO_2 ($P_{ET}CO_2$), intracranial pressure (ICP) and left atrial pressure (LAP).

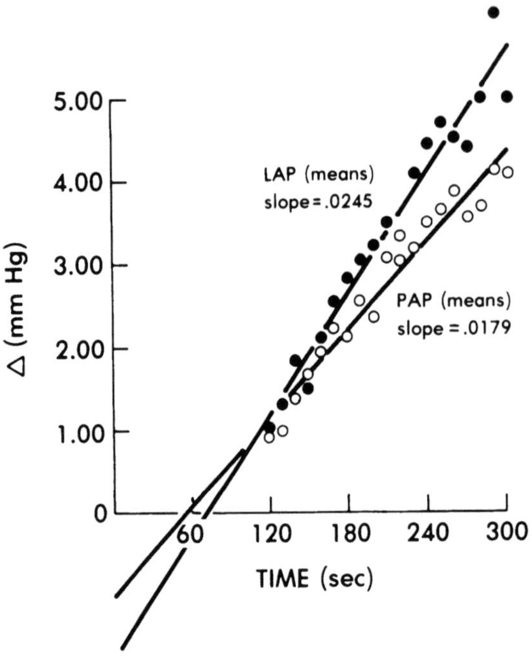

Fig. 2. Effect of elevated ICP on PAP and LAP in experimental NPE. Slopes are determined from mean values obtained from 17 experiments. Closed circles indicate LAP; opened circles, PAP.

SEPARATE AND COMBINED EFFECTS ON INTRACRANIAL PRESSURE OF CHANGES IN PO_2 AND PCO_2

S. JENNETT AND J.B. NORTH

Introduction

The effects of hypoxia and of hypercapnia in raising intracranial pressure (ICP)by virtue of vasodilatation are well known. The effects of each and of arterial blood pressure (BP) on CBF are well documented. It is less clear how oxygen and CO_2 interact in ICP when they change simultaneously in the same or opposite directions; also their separate and combined effects on ICP are likely to be different according to whether or not they cause any alterations in BP.

Rapid responses to brief changes in blood gases have been studied rather than prolonged exposures where secondary changes complicate the picture. Earlier work, in cats, has shown that the vasodilatation which accompanies transient hypoxia can be demonstrated by monitoring changes in ICP (1,2). The present study concerns the effects of similarly brief exposures to hypoxia and to hypercapnia in dogs.

Materials and methods

Ten dogs were anesthetized with sodium pentobarbitone; ICP was measured from a subdural cannula. Tidal volume, airway CO_2, BP, and heart rate were also monitored continuously (Fig. 1). After studies during spontaneous breathing, each animal was paralyzed with succinyl choline and ventilated. Arterial blood gases were measured from time to time using standard electrodes. For hypoxic exposures inspired gas was switched from air to 9% oxygen for 2-3 min; for hypercapnia exposures from air to 5-6% CO_2 in oxygen or air. Each type of test was repeated in each animal during both spontaneous and controlled ventilation (SV & CV).

Results

Hypoxia in SV, led to prompt chemoreflex increase in ventilation, and thus to hypocapnia (Fig.1a); there was a discernible rise in ICP starting 10-15 s after the switch of gases but this was small and often only transient (mean rise 1.65 mmHg); in CV, ICP started to rise after a slightly longer delay attributable to ventilatory dead space, and the rise continued throughout the two or more minutes of hypoxia (mean rise 4.4 mmHg). Although these changes were small they were consistent and significant. For both SV and CV, measurement of arterial blood bases at two minutes of hypoxia showed mean P_aO_2 of 40.1 mmHg (range 34-48); BP rose over 2 min by a mean of 10.75 mmHg (Fig.2). On reoxygenation, a fall in ICP was prompt and consistent, with a latency similar to that for the fall in BP, HR and ventilation (in SV)(Fig.1). Hypercapnia for periods of 1-2 min raised PCO_2 by 5-10 mmHg; ICP increased progressively after a short latency, on average by 1 mmHg per mmHg rise in PCO_2, in both SV and CV.

Discussion

The changes in ICP during hypoxia are likely to be the resultant effect of low PO_2 tending to dilate, and low PCO_2 and high BP tending to constrict. The rise in BP in our experiments was similar in both SV and CV; the three factors virtually cancelled out in SV; it can be concluded that the dilatory effect of P_aO_2 40 mmHg was somewhat greater than the constrictor effect of a reduction of P_aCO_2 by 10 mmHg. This was supported by results of hypoxic exposures during CV in three of the animals after treatment with phenoxybenzamine which prevented or attenuated the hypertensive response; there was a greater rise in ICP. Likewise in chemodenervated cats (2) in which the BP rise was prevented, transient hypoxia caused a greater rise in ICP than in the intact animal. In man BP does not normally rise as part of the chemoreflex response to acute hypoxia (3); more information is required concerning the interaction of these three factors in man. With hypercapnia we did not show any difference in ICP effect between CO_2 in oxygen and CO_2 in air; but the conditions were hyperoxic and normoxic, rather than hypoxic. In recent experiments in cats and rabbits during 1-2 min apnea ICP rose much less steeply when oxygen was diffused into the airway (maintaining a near normal or high P_aO_2) than when P_aO_2 was allowed to fall, despite similar rises in P_aCO_2(JENNETT, unpublished).

Summary

During brief hypoxic exposure in dogs, the effect of a reduction of P_aO_2 to 40 mmHg was counterbalanced by the effect of a reduction of P_aCO_2 by 10 mmHg, so that there was virtually no effect on ICP. A 10 mmHg rise in BP probably contributed to the vasoconstrictive effect; ICP is likely to increase more in species, or in conditions, in which BP does not increase with hypoxia. A 5 mmHg rise in P_aCO_2 had an equivalent effect on ICP to that of P_aO_2 40 mmHg; observations during apnea support the additive nature of effects of rising CO_2 and falling oxygen.

References

1. Jennett S (1975) Changes in intracranial pressure during brief exposure hypoxia in anesthetized cats. J Physiol 251:41-42P

2. Jennett S, Pitts LH (1977) Increase in intracranial pressure with transient hypoxia before and after hemodenervation. J Physiol 266:51-52P

3. Richardson DW, Kontos HA, Raper AJ, Patterson JL (1967) Modification by Beta-Adrenergic blockade of the circulatory responses to acute hypoxia in man. J Clin Invest 46:77-85

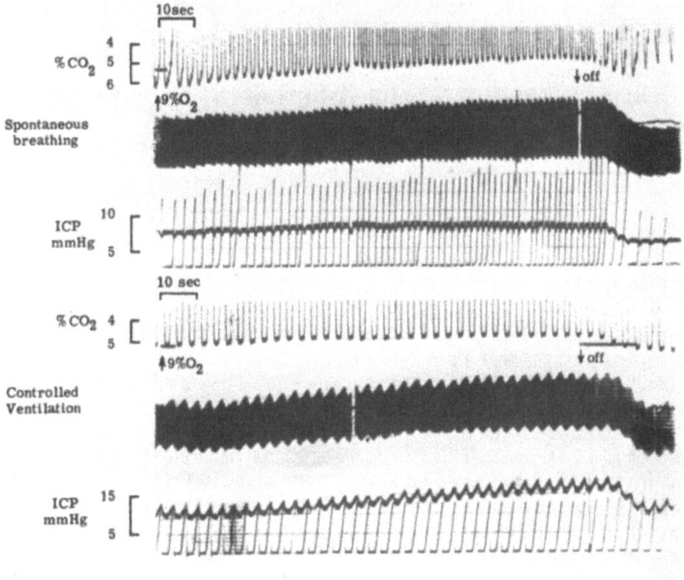

Fig. 1. a) spontaneously breathing animal: 9% oxygen given from arrow to "off" (2 min). CO_2 record (zero offset above edge of trace) shows decrease in end-tidal concentration as respiratory response develops. ICP increases only very slightly. Unlabelled traces show arterial BP, heart rate and tidal volume.

b) the same animal, during a similar hypoxic exposure, under controlled ventilation; ICP rises continuously during hypoxia.

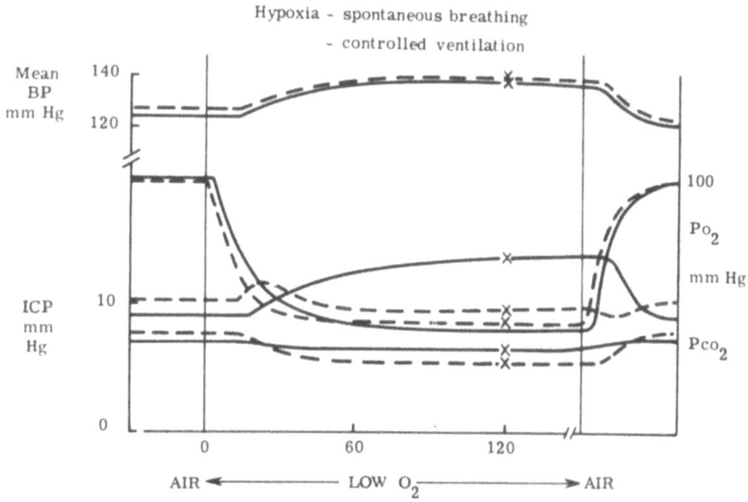

Fig. 2. Composite graph of changes during 2 min hypoxia, from mean results of 2 tests in each of 10 animals. For each variable, broken line shows changes in spontaneous ventilation; solid line shows changes in controlled ventilation. Mean values compared at x (after 2 minutes exposure) show no significant difference in BP, PO_2; PCO_2 and ICP are significantly higher in CV.

THE ROLE OF THE HYPOTHALAMO-HYPOPHYSIAL NEUROSECRETORY ADRENERGIC SYSTEM IN CUSHING REFLEX

Z.M.RAP, L.KROLICKI, AND K.SKOLASINSKA

Introduction

In spite of the great number of publications concerning the vascular response to the rise of intracranial pressure (ICP) its pathogenesis is not quite clear. Most of the investigators point out that elevation of the blood pressure in the Cushing reflex depends on the central and peripheral catecholaminergic system (2,8). On the other hand it is known that the adrenal medulla as well as the hypothalamo-hypophyseal neurosecretory system (HHNS) can modify the blood pressure by synthesizing vasoactive substances and releasing them into the blood. Recent studies demonstrated the high concentration of adrenalin and vasopressin in the blood during the Cushing reflex (6,7). It has been suggested that the above mentioned structures synthesizing these vasoactive substances might play some role in the pathogenesis of Cushing reflex.

In order to verify these observations lesions of median eminence (ME) of hypothalamus, transection of the brainstem, either alone or with bilateral adrenalectomy were performed, and then the Cushing reflex was evoked by cerebral compression.

Material and methods

Experiments were carried out on 20 cats in Nembutal anesthesia(35mg/kg) artificially ventilated for 3-5 hours. The short-term intermittent rise of ICP for 10, 15 sec. was induced by inflation of epidural balloon with 0.5 - 1 ml volume. Intracranial hypertension was produced before and after the following procedure: stereotaxic lesion of ME alone (group I) and with adrenalectomy (group II) pretreatment with Decadron as well as pretrigeminal brainstem transection alone(group III), and with adrenalectomy (group IV). Mean arterial pressure (MABP) in the aorta and cerebrospinal fluid pressure (CSFP) in cisterna magna (group I, II) were recorded continuously. Cerebral blood flow (CBF) was measured by means of ^{133}Xe clearance technique applied before and after the above mentioned procedures. Blood-brain barrier (BBB) was studied using 2% Evans blue solution (2 ml/kg)by i.v. injection. All animals were sacrificed and brains were taken for routine histopathological examination.

Results

The lesion of ME, group I, caused an increase of MABP by 20 mmHg and also of CSFP by 3-5 mmHg, but CBF did not change (37.4±2.8) in comparison with the control values (40.9±4.2). (CBF expressed as ml of blood/100 g brain tissue/min. Results: mean±SD, 5 experiments, ns=non significant changes). The inflation of the balloon evoked the rise of CSFP (100-120 mmHg) and MABP (120-300 mmHg). The CBF measured 30 min later was not changed (37.1±3.9, ns).

Adrenalectomy following the lesion of ME, group II, was accompanied by decrease of MABP (70-100 mmHg) and CBF (36.6±2.7,ns) but CSFP rose slightly (13-20 mmHg). Cerebral compression with CSFP elevation (110-130 mmHg) did not evoke the rise of the MABP (Fig.1). After balloon deflation the CSFP (10-15 mmHg), MABP (60-80 mmHg) and CBF (31.9±4.6, ns) were decreased. Intravenously injected Pitressin(1 IU) and adrenalin (5 ug) elevated both MABP (150-200 mmHg) and CSFP (26-37 mmHg) rapidly.

Morphological examination of brains of groups I and II showed severe damage of BBB in four cases and moderate damage in other six. This was manifested by extravasation of Evans blue-albumin complex into the grey matter of both hemispheres, cerebellum and brainstem (Fig.2). In light microscope irregular necrotic foci in ME of hypothalamus were found. Besides that, secondary vasogenic foci, mainly hemorrhagic, were observed in the both hemispheres being more pronounced on the compression side and in addition in thalamus, posterior hypothalamus and brainstem.

The pretrigeminal transection of the brainstem,group III, was characterized by an increase of the MABP by 20-30 mmHg. It was accompanied by a decrease of CBF (35.2±1.2, ns) in comparison to the control value (38.5±1.8). Cerebral compression caused the rise of MABP (150-320mmHg). After decompression MABP decreased below control level (75-100 mmHg) with a fall of CBF (30.5±0.74, p 0.02).

Bilateral adrenalectomy abolished the elevation of MABP which was observed after brainstem transection, group IV, lowering it visibly (80-100 mmHg) but CBF did not change (38.7±1.6, ns) as compared to control (40.6±2.1). During cerebral compression the elevation of the MABP (80-220 mmHg)was noted. After balloon deflation MABP (60-80 mm Hg) and CBF (26.1±3.8 p 0.05) were decreased.

Macroscopic examination of brains of animals from group III and IV showed blood in subarachnoid space and extravasation of the Evans blue-albumin complex in the mesencephalon at a site of the brainstem transsection. This was accompanied by secondary changes in both hemispheres including thalamus and hypothalamus.

Discussion

Physiological and pathophysiological data indicate that electrical stimulation of the neurosecretory centres or ischemic hypoxia involve almost simultaneously the response of HHNS and adrenal medulla(6,7,9). The destruction of ME, neurosecretory organ, with oxytocin-vasopressinergic tracts caused spontaneously the elevation of MABP and did not eliminate the Cushing reflex. The same symptoms were detected after disconnecting hypothalamo-catecholaminergic cardiovascular pathways in brainstem. This provides evidence that the Cushing reflex could be evoked without brainstem stimulation. The next series of experiments consisted of the elimination of adrenal medulla. It is known that bilateral adrenalectomy did not abolish cardiovascular response to the rise of ICP (8). Therefore, adrenalectomy with brainstem transection and ME lesion was done. These procedures were accompanied by the fall of MABP. Intracranial hypertension induced the Cushing reflex in adrenalectomized animals with brainstem transection but this reflex was abolished after ME lesion and adrenalectomy. These data suggest that both the neurogenic and humoral factors participate in the cardiovascular response. The humoral factors, mainly vasoactive substances, might play more significant role in the regulation of hemodynamics, blood flow or metabolic processes. For example, more recent data showed that vasopressin could dilate cerebral vessels, thereby enhancing the CBF (3). In the present experiments changes of CSFP as well as of CBF in animals in the I and II groups were not considerable both after brainstem transection and adrenalectomy, but in two last groups, III and IV, with repeated cerebral compression CBF was reduced significantly. The morphological observations besides necrotic foci in ME evaluated the secondary vasogenic foci in both hemispheres, thalamus, brainstem and particularly in hypothalamus, which complicated the interpretation of the results from groups I and II. These observations correspond with the secondary vasogenic changes in the hypothalamo-hypophysial system in humans who died after acute intracranial hypertension (5). The congestion of the cerebral vessels with moderate or severe BBB damage in the animals from groups I and II could be connected with their vasoparalysis without reflection in CBF study. Pictures of this type were described after prolonged cerebral compression and sudden decompression (1). Some authors connect these phenomena with brain swelling resulting from damage of posterior hypothalamus (4).

References

1. Czernicki Z, Kozniewska E (1977) Disturbances in the blood-brain barrier and cerebral blood flow after rapid brain decompression in the cat. Acta Neurochir 36:181-187

2. Doba N, Reis DJ (1972) Localization within the lower brainstem of a receptive area mediating the pressor response to increased intracranial pressure (the Cushing response). Brain Res 47:487-491

3. Kozniewska E, Rap ZM, Skolasinska K (to be published) Cerebrovascular effect of vasopressin. International Symposium on CBF and Metabolism. Tokyo, May 1979

4. Nagagava Y, Notomiya M, Tsuru M, Bando M, Tabota M (1977) Role of the posterior hypothalamus in the development of acute brain swelling. J Neurosurg 46:723-730

5. Rap ZM, Zaremba J (1970) Pathomechanism of the secondary morphological lesion in the hypothalamo-hypophysial system in cases of increased intracranial pressure. Pol Med J 10:188-207

6. Rap ZM, Staszewska-Bartczak J (1975) Adrenergic response and morphologic changes in the neurosecretory system and adrenal cortex during intracranial hypertension in cats. In: Kornyey S, TariskaS, Gosztonyi G (eds) Proc VIIth Int Congr Neuropath. Excerpta Med. Amsterdam, p 623

7. Rap ZM, Chwalbinska-Moneta J (1978) Vasopressin concentration in the blood during acute short-term intracranial hypertension in cats. In: Cervos-Navarro J, Betz E, Ebhardt G, Ferszt R, Wollenweber R (eds) Advances in Neurology V 20. Raven Press New York381

8. Roezekrans N, Th P, van Zwietten PA (1977) The role of the adrenergic nervous system in the pressor response due to acute elevation of intracranial pressure (Cushing Response) A pharmacological analysis. Arch Int Pharmacodyn 228:79-91

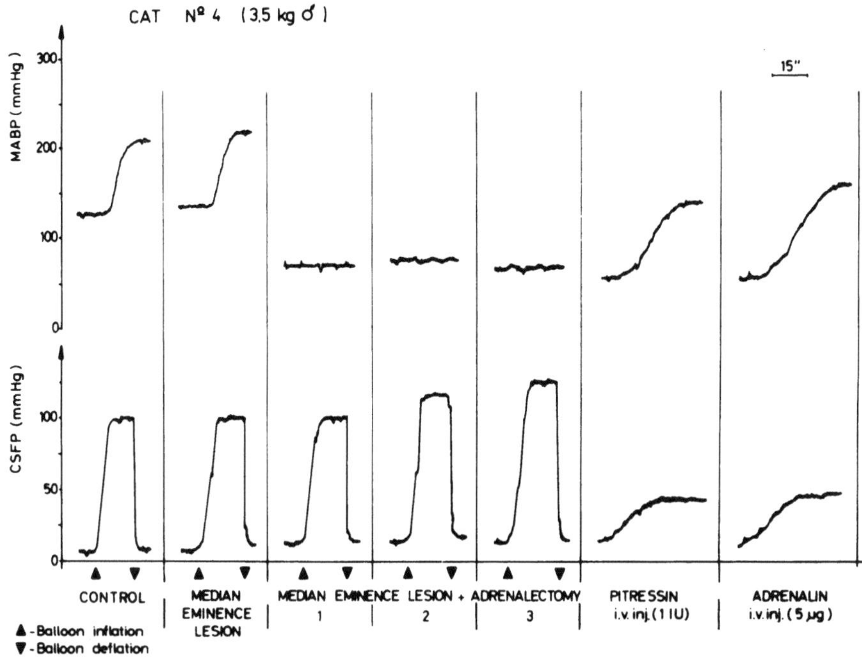

Fig. 1. The response of CSFP and MABP in cats to the rise of ICP in 30 and 15 min intervals (balloon inflation and deflation) after ME lesions alone and with adrenalectomy. Intravenous injection of Pitressin (1 IU) and adrenalin (5ug) in the control test.

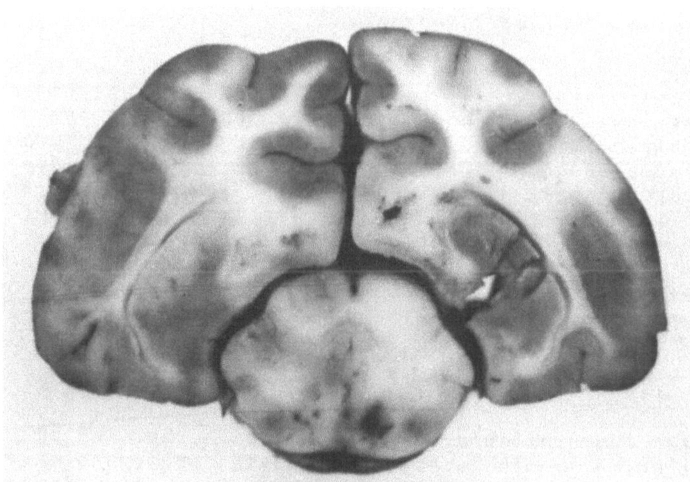

Fig. 2. Coronal section of brain with visible congestion of blood vessels with severe BBB damage in grey matter and secondary vasogenic foci in both hemispheres and brainstem. Cat with ME lesion and adrenalectomy after short-lasting (15 sec) cerebral compression induced 5 times. 10x

INTRACRANIAL PRESSURE, BRAIN EDEMA AND REGIONAL METABOLISM IN EXPERIMENTAL BRAIN ABSCESS IN CATS

TH. WALLENFANG, J. BOHL, M. MAYER, AND K. SCHÜRMANN

Introduction

Despite progress in diagnostic methods (1,3) numerous questions still remained unanswered in the very difficult field of brain abscess. The present investigation employs a reproducible experimental model to study the development of the brain abscess and the alterations of the intracranial pressure correlated with the time course of the edema process. We shall describe the metabolic state of the brain during the development from acute to chronic abscess. Morphological correlates of the dynamics of brain abscess were investigated to gain an insight into the pathophysiology of the inflammatory brain swelling.

Material and methods

Forty-two adults cats 2.5 to 4.5 kg in weight were anesthetized with Ketamine (20 mg/kg). The right hemispheric white matter was inoculated stereotactically with 0.03 ml of a mixture of agar and bouillon containing 1 to 1.5 million Staphylococcus aureus of a high pathogenicity. Besides the comparison with the contralateral hemisphere, there was a control group of 6 cats which had only received agar and bouillon injected into the right hemisphere (2). The extent of edema was visualized by intravenous injections of 2% Evans blue (1 ml/kg). The acute and chronic state of the abscess was observed by means of the computerized tomography.

After 2, 4, 7, 10 and 20 days, a group of 6 animals each was tracheotomized, paralyzed with Flexadil and normoventilated with a conventional Starling pump. Blood gases were analyzed intermittently and kept within normal range (pCO_2 32-36 mmHg). Rectal temperature, arterial blood pressure (MABP) and intraventricular fluid pressure (IVP) were recorded continuously. The brain tissue samples around the abscess and from the contralateral hemisphere were removed to determine water and electrolyte contents and metabolite concentrations (PCr, ATP, ADP, AMP, lactate, pyruvate). Six animals were sacrificed by transcardiac perfusion with 3.9% glutaraldehyde and samples for electron microscopy were taken from the same areas as mentioned above.

Results

After inoculation of Staphylococcus aureau, an abscess developed in all animals. The abscess only extended in the white matter and although there was a rapid increase of abscess diameter until the seventh day, invasion into the ventricular system or into the cortex was extremely rare.

Disturbance of the blood brain barrier by the inflammation, central necrosis, the increase of the acute abscess was detectable by computerized tomography in the first seven days. The maximum of ventricular compression and midline displacement was seen on the seventh day. The first signs of encapsulation were observed between the fifth and seventh day. Neurological symptoms, such as deterioration and hemiparesis in 83% were also most evident around the seventh day.

The increase of abscess and the spreading edema towards the lateral ventricle and the deep white matter was associated with an increase in intraventricular pressure (Fig. 1). On the seventh day the intraventricular pressure was nearly eight times higher than in normal animals and remained significantly increased in the following weeks when encapsulation developed. When intracranial pressure exceeded ten times the normal level, it always resulted in an herniation in the tentorial notch. The increased intraventricular pressure has to be ascribed largely to the increase in the water content around the abscess (4) (Fig.2). Adjacent to the abscess the maximal water accumulation was found from the seventh until the tenth day (82.3 g/100 g w.wt.) and was around 20% higher than in the contralateral hemisphere (68.0 g/100 g w.wt.) and in the control group, which has only received agar and bouillon. The traumatic contribution to the edema was minimal and verifiable on the second day. According to the increase of the acute abscess the spreading edema encroached upon the remote areas later. On the seventh day the water content in the remote area (80.4 g/100 g w.wt) was nearly as high as adjacent to the abscess (82.3/100 g w.wt). With development of encapsulation in the following weeks the water content decreased in the remote area (73.1 g/100 g w.wt.) but only slightly adjacent to the space-occupying mass (80.0 g/100 g w.wt.). There was no significant change in the cortex as regards the water content.

The changes in sodium content in the different areas were similar to those of the water content. There was significant increase until the seventh day; when encapsulation developed the sodium content showed an abrupt decrease in the remote areas after seven days, whereas the decrease in the adjacent areas developed later.

At the time of maximal edema and highest intracranial pressure, there were signs of cerebral hypoxia: increase of lactate and pyruvate and decrease of PCr and ATP. Significant changes of these metabolites were found on the seventh and tenth day. The cellular disturbance is particularly pronounced in the tissue adjacent to the abscess.

On the seventh day, histological and ultrastructural studies revealed in the surrounding white matter an extreme enlargement of extracellular spaces with fibrin deposition, with erythrocytes, macrophages and some leucocytes within the inflammatory edema (Fig. 3). Severe edema was present even in remote white matter areas of the right hemisphere, both with an increase of extracellular fluid and with a remarkable swelling of astrocytic processes. In some areas at the edge of the abscess there was visible an incipient proliferation of small blood vessels with perivascular inflammatory infiltration. On the seventh day many capillaries and venules in the neighborhood of the abscess showed an enlargement of the clefts and furthermore wide gaps between the endothelial cells, sometimes with a splitting and a duplicating of the basal lamina. In the widened perivascular spaces there were often erythrocytes and macrophages, as well as thrombocytes. Sometimes there was a breakdown of the adjacent astrocytic wall, too. These endothelial gaps were still present on the tenth day, but less common. Cellular and vascular proliferation was more pronounced on the tenth day including astrocytic proliferation, but the enlargement of extracellular spaces and the amount of edematous fluid were nearly as high as on the seventh day. On the 20th day the abscess was surrounded by a dense capsule of blood vessels and connective tissue with chronic perivascular inflammation. In the surrounding white matter, a severe loss of myelinated nerve fibres with a pronounced reactive astrocytosis could be observed. Accumulation of extracellular fluid and swelling of astrocytic processes were distinctly reduced on the 20th day compared to acute phase but were still recognizable in the neighborhood of the abscess. Perivascular spaces were enlarged and were sometimes filled with proliferated adventitial cells.

Summary

Brain inflammation caused by inoculated bacteria of high pathogenicity always led to brain abscess and with the spreading inflammatory edema to remarkable neurological deficits. Parallel to the brain swelling, the intraventricular fluid pressure increased. Especially on the seventh day, there is danger of brain stem compression and tissue hypoxia. The most striking morphological changes in the endothelial cells around the abscess correspond with the peak edema on the seventh day. When encapsulation developed, the edema decreased, but the intracranial pressure remained high due to the space occupying mass, persisting as long as bacteria were present.

References

1. Garfield J (1978) Brain abscesses and focal suppurative infections. Handbook of Clin Neurol 33:107-147

2. Thomas L (1942) A single stage method to produce brain abscess in cats. Arch Pathol 33:472-476

3. Wallenfang Th, Reulen HG, Schindling H (1977) Investigation on the prognosis of brain abscess. Advances in Neurosurg 4:296-299

4. Reulen HJ (1976) Vasogenic brain edema. Br J Anaesth 48:741-752

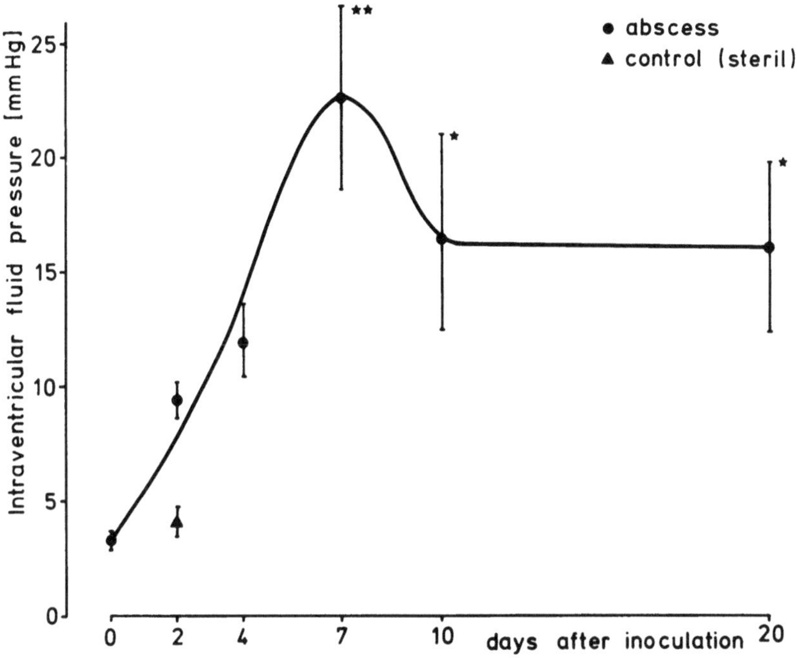

Fig. 1. Intraventricular fluid pressure, measured in the contralateral ventricle on the different days while abscess developed in the right hemispheric white matter. By the encapsulation on the seventh day, the IVP decreased after the seventh day, but was kept high by the space-iccupying mass. $\bar{x} \pm S\bar{x}$ are given.
*, ** = significantly different from control group.
$^{*}p \leq 0.05$, $^{**}p \leq 0.01$ ("Krouskal-Wallis Test").

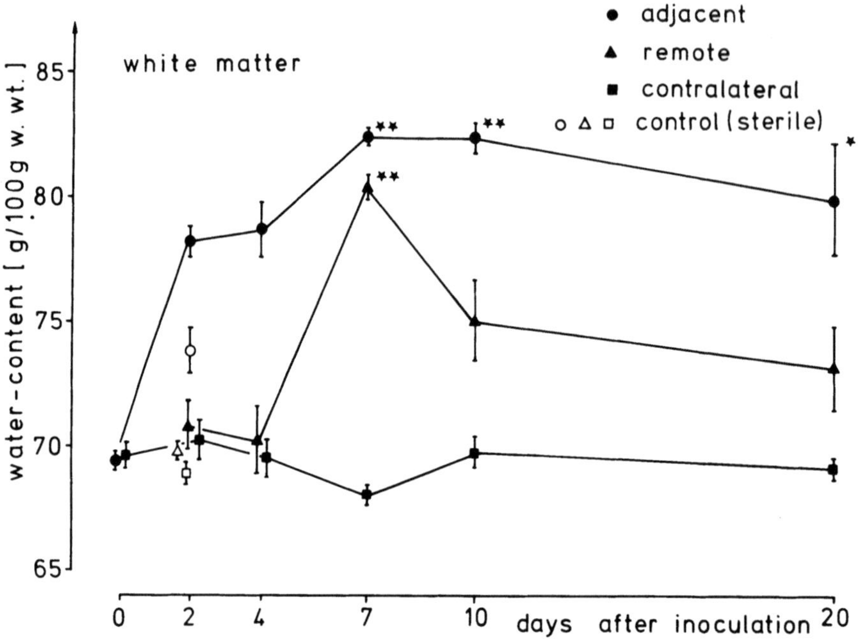

Fig. 2. Changes of water content (g/100g w.wt.) in the different areas of the white matter, while acute abscess developed, followed by the encapsulation from the seventh day onwards. Compared are right and left hemisphere of the abscess group and of the sterile control group (agar-bouillon without Staphylococcus aureus). $\bar{x} \pm S\bar{x}$ are given.
*, ** = significantly different from control group.
*$p \leq 0.05$, **$p \leq 0.01$ ("Krouskal-Wallis Test")

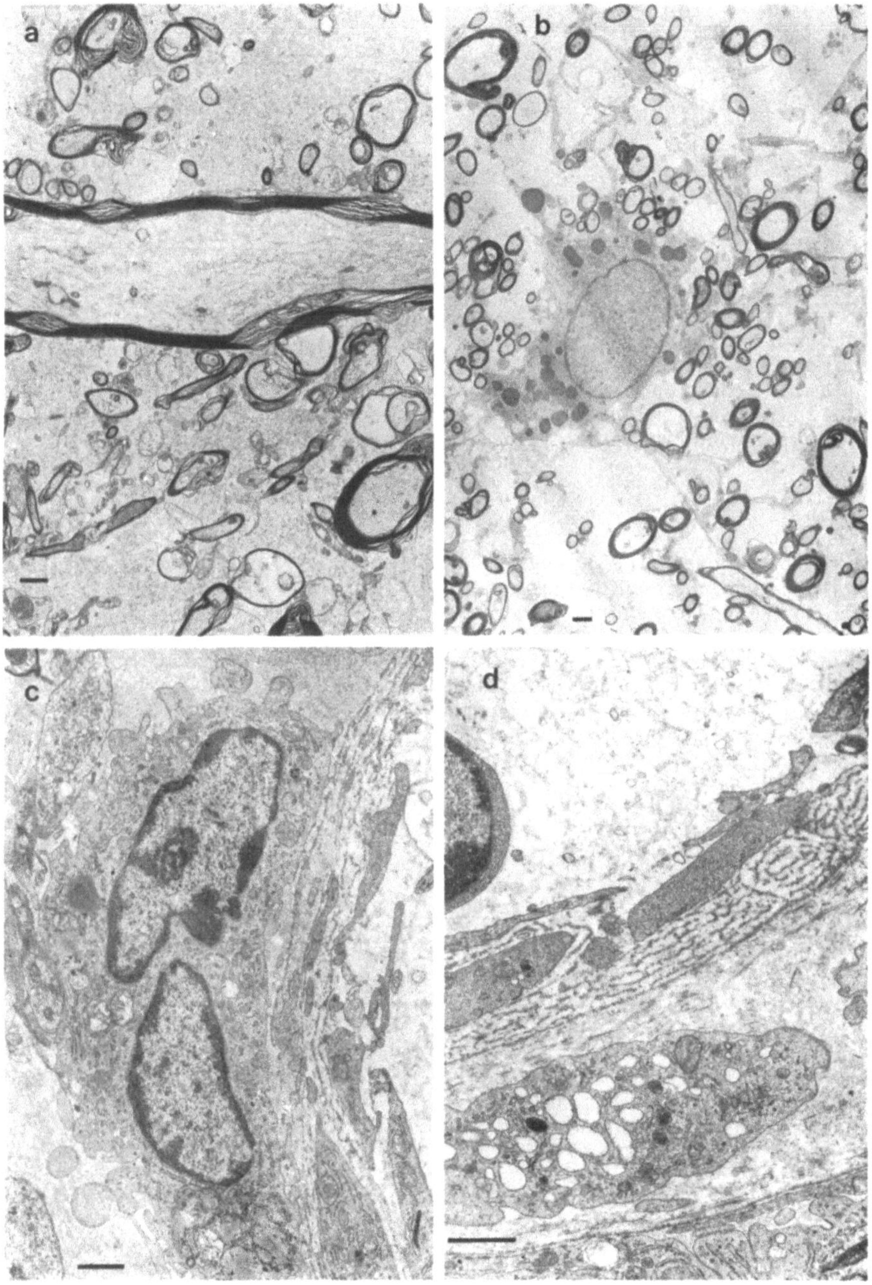

Fig. 3. a + b: Severe edema in the cerebral white matter on the seventh day with extreme enlargement of extracellular spaces in the neighborhood of the abscess (b) and in more distant regions, too (a).
c + d: Some small blood vessels in the vicinity of the abscess (on the seventh day) show side gaps between the endothelial cell processes with an enlargement of perivascular spaces and with an increase of basal lamina material. (The black lines at the bottom of the pictures represent 1 micron).

BACTERIAL MENINGITIS: CHANGES IN CEREBROSPINAL FLUID OUTFLOW RESISTANCE

R.G.DACEY, J.E.WELSH, W.M.SCHELD, H.R.WINN, M.A.SANDE, AND J.A.JANE

Introduction

Although increased intracranial pressure and hydrocephalus frequently accompany bacterial meningitis, the pathophysiology of these complications is not understood. To quantify intracranial volume-pressure regulation in meningitis, we performed manometric infusions in rabbits with experimental bacterial meningitis.

Methods

Single bore pressure screws (4) were implanted into the parietal supracortical subarachnoid space of New Zealand white rabbits. The animals were divided into three groups:

Group I: Uninfected control animals (n = 5)

Group II: Infected but untreated animals (n = 10) In these animals, experimental bacterial meningitis was produced (1) by the intracisternal inoculation of 10^6 Streptococcus pneumoniae, Type III (n = 5) or 10^5 Escherichia coli K_1 (n = 5). Meningitis in all animals was characterized by fever, lethargy, CSF pleocytosis ($0.8 - 2.2 \times 10^3$ PMNs/ml) and CSF bacterial titers of $10^4 - 10^8$ Colony Forming Units (CFU/ml). All animals with untreated experimental meningitis died within 36 hours.

Group III: Infected and penicillin treated animals (n=5). In these animals, experimental S. pneumo meningitis was similarly produced, however, eight hours after cisternal inoculation, intravenous therapy with penicillin G was initiated (1.2×10^6 units/hr for eight hours). At the conclusion of this eight hour course of penicillin therapy, CSF cultures were sterile.

Sixteen hours after cisternal inoculation, manometric infusions were performed on all animals. Artificial CSF was infused via the pressure screw at rates varying from 1.2 to 200 mic.L/min while pressure was simultaneously recorded. At each experimental flow rate, CSF pressure increased with time until an equilibrium pressure was achieved.

The experimental infusion data were analyzed with a non-linear mathematical model of the CSF system described in detail by JOHNSON et al (2). Steady state CSF pressure was plotted against the logarithm of test flow rate. Parameters M and P_R were then determined by least square curve fitting technique according to the relationship between flow and pressure:

$$Q = \frac{1}{M} e^{P/P_R} \qquad \text{(eq. 1).}$$

Table 1

	Number of Animals (n)	Parameter Values M	P_R (mmHg)	Mean Peak Resistance* (mmHg/mic.L/min)
Group I	5	0.02 ± 0.01	29.7 ± 3.1	0.3 ± 0.04
Group II				
S. pneumo	5	1.05 ± 0.79	19.2 ± 7.3	6.8 ± 3.5
E. coli	5	1.92 ± 1.23	13.6 ± 3.2	8.9 ± 4.2
Group III				
Treated *S. pneumo*	5	1.19 ± 1.14	15.1 ± 4.4	5.9 ± 5.7

All values are expressed as mean ± standard deviation.

* $P < 0.05$. P values apply to comparison between control values and Groups II and III values for mean peak resistance.

Resistance was then calculated according to:

$$R = MP\ e^{-P/P_R} \qquad \text{(eq. 2)}.$$

Mean peak resistance values were compared by Student's t test.

Results

In Figure Ia, the experimentally determined equilibrium pressure is plotted against the log of test flow rate for Group I (control) and Group II (S.pneumo. and E.coli) animals. When compared with control animals, animals with S.pneumo and E.coli meningitis achieved the same equilibrium pressure elevations at much lower test flow rates. In Figure Ib, calculated resistance to CSF outflow is plotted against pressure for Group I and Group II animals. Animals with S. pneumo. and E. coli meningitis had a marked increase in CSF outflow resistance over a wide range of CSF pressure.

The parameter values M and P_R as well as the mean peak CSF outflow resistance for all groups are shown in Table I. A significant increase in outflow resistance was noted for S.pneumo. and E.coli animals when compared to control animals. After eight hours of penicillin G treatment animals with S. pneumo meningitis in Group III did not have significantly lowered peak outflow resistance (See Table I).

Discussion

The present study indicates that animals with experimental meningitis have elevated CSF outflow resistance and that after a short period of antibiotic therapy (which erradicated viable bacteria from the CSF) the outflow resistance remains elevated.

There are several mechanisms by which meningitis could elevate outflow resistance. The bacterial organisms could adversely affect arachnoid villus function. SCHELD et al (3) have shown that bacteria are cleared from the CSF to the superior sagittal sinus in experimental bacterial meningitis. However, the abnormal outflow resistance in the present study persisted beyond the erradication of viable bacteria from the CSF. Therefore, it is conceivable that the macromolecular products of inflammation (e.g., albumin, immunoglobins) could alter CSF absorption.

Summary

In animals with experimental bacterial meningitis caused by S.penumo. and E. coli, CSF outflow resistance was found to be markedly increased above control values. Acute treatment with penicillin did not affect this elevation in outflow resistance.

Références

1. Dacey RG, Sande MA (1974) Effect of probenecid on CSF concentrations of penicillin and cephalosporin derivatives. Antimicrobial Agents and Chemotherapy 6:437-441

2. Johnson RN, Maffeo CJ, Mann JD, Butler AB, Bass NH (1978) Intracranial pressure regulation: A comparative model of cerebrospinal fluid systems. T I T J Life Sci 8:79-92

3. Scheld WM, Park TS, Dacey RG, Winn HR, Jane JA, Sande MA (1979) Clearance of bacteria from CSF to blood in experimental meningitis. Inf and Immun 24:102-105

4. Winn HR, Dacey RG, Jame JA (1977)ICP recording.Surg Neurol 8:41-47

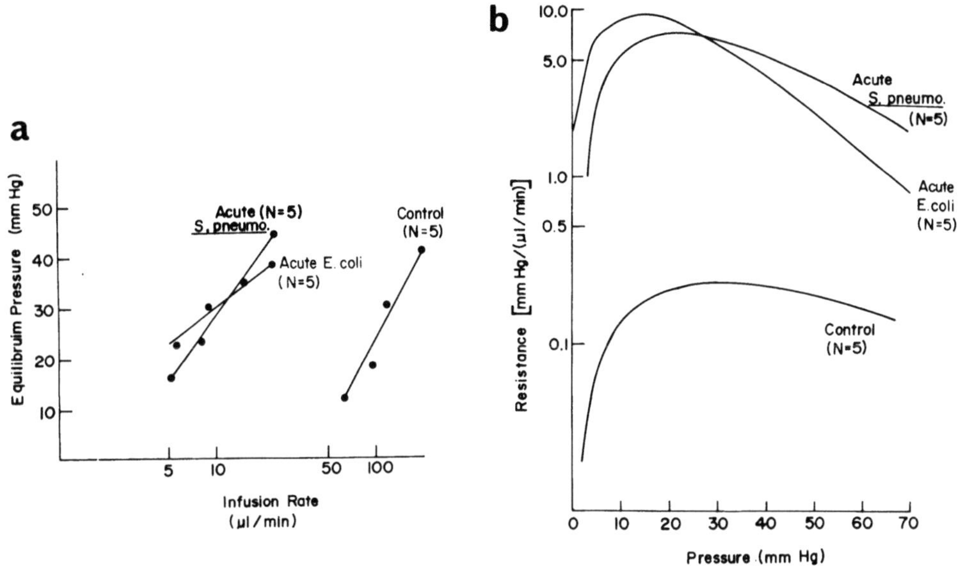

Fig. la. Equilibrium pressure plotted against log of test flow rate for control animals and animals with S. penumo and E. coli meningitis.
lb. Resistance plotted against CSF pressure for control animals and animals with S. pneumo and E. coli meningitis.

EXPERIENCES WITH ICP MONITORING IN INDIA

K.L.M.KRISHNAN

Introduction

In a developing country like India, sophisticated electronic and computerized equipment for ICP monitoring imported from abroad involves difficulties in procurement, maintenance, servicing, etc. Hence, an attempt was made by us, successfully, to develop such instrumentation indigenously (1,2). The method has been applied particularly to the study of ICP profile in tuberculous meningitis and encephalopathy revealing some interesting findings relevant to this disease as also a special feature of brainstem lesions.

Materials and methods

We have found the intraventricular catheter to be the most convenient and reliable, in agreement with the other leaders in this field (3). The Statham P23ID transducer as well as a similar transducer of our own design (2) has been used. The latter has been slightly modified by us to form an implantable epidural transducer (2). We have also designed our own telemetric device (2) based on the principle of induction-power (4) but this is yet to be put to wide clinical application (Fig. 1).

Owing to many limitations, ICP monitoring has not yet become a routine procedure in our set-up. The material presented here comes out of a research project and involves largely patients with tuberculosis of the brain and its coverings to the exclusion of tuberculomas. A total number of seventy-five patients with tuberculosis have been studied; a total of 460 hours of ICP monitoring have been done on these patients.

Results

The ICP profile in these patients has been found, in our experience, to fall into the following patterns:

- I (a) Low state steady.
  - (b) Low state - with fluctuations on manipulations.
  - (c) Low state - with spontaneous fluctuations.
- II (a) Medium state - steady.
  - (b) Medium state - with fluctuations on manipulations.
  - (c) Medium state - with spontaneous fluctuations.
    - i) Response to diuretics, etc.
    - ii) Response to CSF venting alone.
- III (a) High pressure state - response to diuretics etc.
  - (b) High pressure state - response to CSF venting alone.
- IV "S" wave

This classification has helped us to- i) identify the so-called tuberculous encephalopathy - focal and diffuse; ii) establish criteria for the selection of patients for shunt surgery;and iii) assess shunt function as well as the efficacy of other therapeutic maneuvers like osmotherapy, steroids, barbiturate therapy, etc.

We have also come across a peculiar negative deflection - called by us "S" wave - in patients known to have brain stem dysfunction - often associated with simultaneous cardiorespiratory disturbances in the form of sigh and extrasystole (Fig. 2,3). The study of the configuration of the cerebral pulse in these patients is now in progress and will form the subject of another paper.

Discussion

The study of ICP profile in tuberculous meningitis/encephalopathy has proved of great value to us in deciding on and assessing the efficacy of our therapeutic maneuvers. The interesting findings in our study have included - i) the identification of focal and diffuse tuberculous encephalopathy and, ii) the "S" wave which probably indicates brain stem dysfunction.

Summary

Our experience with ICP monitoring in 75 patients with tuberculous meningitis/encephalopathy over a total period of 460 hours as a part of a research project in the Institute of Neurology, Madras, has been presented, along with a brief mention of ICP monitoring equipment including telemetric device of our own design and the "S" wave probably indicating brain stem dysfunction.

References

1. Loga Muthu Krishnan,K (1979) D.S.T. Sponsored Research Project - Continuous Intracranial Pressure Monitoring. Science tech Bulletin 5(1):9

2. Loga Muthu Krishnan,K (1979) Editorial: Proc Inst of Neurol, Madras 8(2):35-42

3. Miller JD (1979) Monitoring of Intracranial Pressure. Guest Article Proc Inst Neurol, Madras 8(2):43-55

4. Rylander HG, Taylor HL, Wissinger JP, and Story JL (1976) Chronic measurement of epidural pressure with an induction-powered oscillator transducer. J Neurosurg 44:465-478

Supported by Grant No.HCS/DST/86/76 of Dept. Science and Technology Government of India, New Delhi-110029, INDIA.

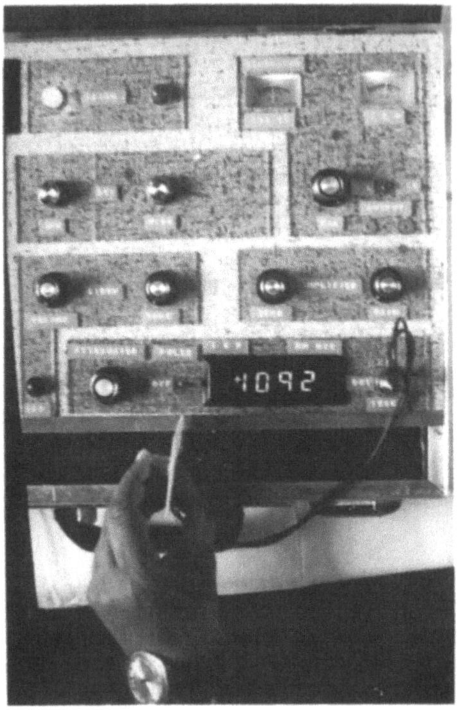

Fig. 1. ICP telemetry - our design; in action - simulation.

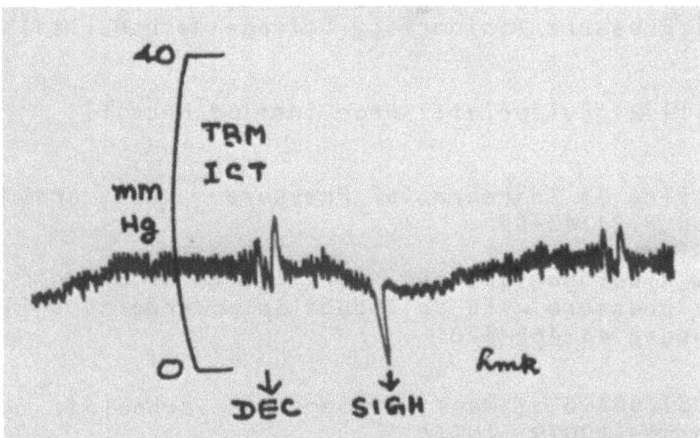

Fig. 2. "S" Wave associated with sigh.

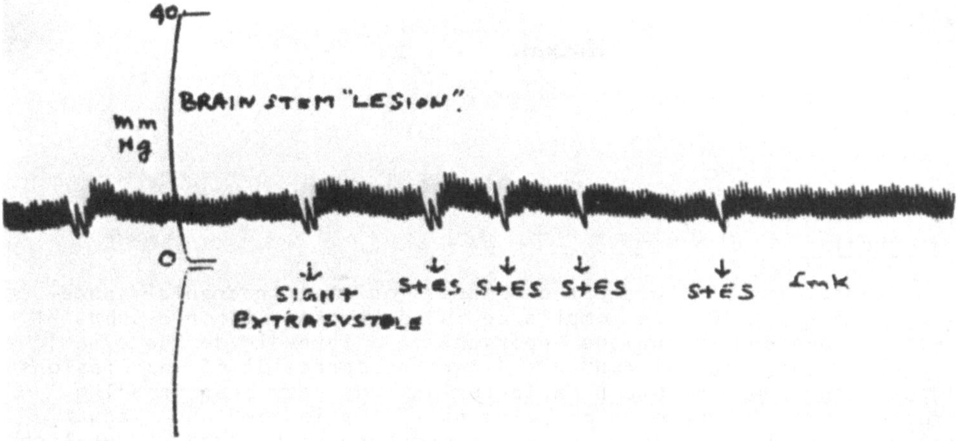

Fig. 3. "S" Wave associated with sigh and/or extrasystole.

ICP AND COMPLIANCE IN CHRONIC SUBDURAL HEMATOMA

K. TABADDOR

Introduction

The dynamic effect of gradual decompression of intracranial space-occupying lesions on ICP and compliance is not known. Chronic subdural hematomas present the unique opportunity to investigate the dynamic changes of intracranial contents after decompression of mass lesions without craniotomy or brain manipulation. We have been treating chronic subdural hematomas by twist drill craniostomy and gradual drainage, enabling us to measure the pressure within the subdural cavity, compare it with subarachnoid pressure, and follow the changes in cerebral compliance after drainage (4).

Method

Twist drill craniostomy was performed under local anesthesia. Dura and subdural capsule were perforated with 18-gauge spinal needles connected to pressure transducers. Subdural pressure was monitored continuously on strip chart recorders. After the steady state opening pressure was determined, drainage into a closed bag system allowed gradual evacuation of the SDH to occur. After the initial subdural pressure was reduced to a safe level (<10 mmHg), lumbar puncture was performed by using an 18-gauge spinal needle connected to a separate transducer referenced to the foramen of Monro. Abdominal and jugular compression was performed to test the transmission of the pressure from spinal dural sac to subdural capsule and vice versa. The pressure volume relation ($\Delta V/\Delta P$) as an index of the compliance was determined in both spaces simultaneously by manipulating the CSF or subdural volume. Once the opening pressure and compliance were determined, the lumbar subarachnoid needle was removed. The subdural needle was replaced by a Scott cannula for a gradual drainage of the subdural hematoma. Complete evacuation commonly required 24 to 36 hours of drainage. Steady state pressure and compliance were again determined in both subarachnoid and subdural spaces, after termination of drainage, and data analyzed to investigate the impact of subdural drainage on intracranial hydrodynamics.

Results

Eight patients, five males and three females ranging from 52 to 80 years of age were included in this study. Three patients presented with bilateral subdural hematomas. The history of trauma was elicited in only half of the cases. The diagnosis was commonly established with CAT scanning. The density of the lesion on CAT scan varied from isodense to hypodense chronic hematoma. Subdural opening pressure ranged from 10 to 18 mmHg (mean ± SE 13 ± 1.2) and gradually declined toward zero as the subdural content was evacuated. Atmospheric pressure was reached after approximately 20% of the total subdural volume was removed. The total volume of fluid drained from the subdural

Table 1

Case #	Subdural Pressure mmHg Pre-evacuation	Post-evacuation	Compliance ΔV/ΔP Pre-evacuation	Post-evacuation
1	11	14	0.83	0.51
2	18	30	0.86	0.36
3	15	22	0.44	0.36
4	13	15	0.53	0.37
5	17	18	0.66	0.44
6	15	22	0.36	0.21
7	10	32	0.65	0.40
8	12	17	0.80	0.71
Mean	13	22	0.64	0.42
SE	1.3	2.1	0.06	0.05

space varied from 120 - 245 ml. Higher opening pressure was observed in patients with subacute SDH's, and clinically presented with a more rapid progression of the neurological deterioration. After subdural pressure was reduced to a safe level (<10 mmHg), spinal subarachnoid pressure and subdural pressure were monitored simultaneously in 5 of the 8 patients. Valsalva maneuvers produced an identical rise of pressure in both spaces. The three patients with bilateral hematoma had no pressure gradient between the two sides; drainage of one side resulted in an equal decrease in the pressure of the opposite side. The ICP measured in the evacuated subdural space ranged from 15 to 32 mmHg (mean ± SE 21 ± 2.1) which is significantly higher than pre-evacuation opening pressure ($p<0.05$). The compliance calculated in the subdural capsule and lumbar subarachnoid space were identical, ranging from 0.36 to 0.86 (mean SE = 0.64 ± 0.06) prior to evacuation and from 0.21 to 0.71 (mean SE = 0.42 ± 0.05) after evacuation (Table 1). This represents a significant decline in the compliance from pre-evacuation values ($p<0.001$). Pressure Volume Index (PVI) as introduced by MARMAROU (2), was computed before and after drainage; although PVI decreased (mean 19.6 - 17.1), these changes were not statistically significant.

Discussion

A free transmission of the pressure was noted from subdural and lumbar subarachnoid fluid spaces in all patients. There have been few reports of simultaneous determination of intracranial and spinal fluid pressure in patients with intracranial pathology. A pressure gradient has been reported in those circumstances where the intercompartmental communication is interrupted by an obstruction to CSF flow. In the absence of such obstruction, the gradient across the brain is negligible (5). These pressure determinations were made in the tissues adjacent to or remote from a space-occupying lesion and not within it.

Chronic subdural hematomas provide a unique opportunity to investigate the pressure communication between the lesion and subarachnoid space. The present data indicates that in the absence of tentorial or foramen magnum herniation, the supratentorial and spinal fluid pressures are identical and alteration in one compartment is reflected in the other. Additionally there was no gradient between the subdural spaces in the three patients with bilateral subdural hematomas. The lack of pressure differences between the two subdural spaces or between subdural and spinal fluid pressure indicates that the inner membrane of the subdural capsules offers no resistance and transmits the intracapsular pressure directly to the brain and CSF compartment. Continuous monitoring in the present study reveals that the opening pressure declines to atmospheric pressure initially and remains at this level as drainage continues. The rate of drainage is expected to follow CSF formation until the subarachnoid volume occupied by the SDH is replaced by reciprocal expansion of the CSF compartment. Upon cessation of the drainage, ICP begins to rise and reaches a new steady state, usually within a few hours. The ICP, however, does not rise in patients with subdural hygroma or whenever the subdural capsule communicates freely with subarachnoid fluid. Under these circumstances a continuous drainage of CSF prevents an increase in ICP.

Four of the 8 patients studied showed an opening subdural pressure of less than 13 mmHg. A similar finding was reported by PLUM and POSNER in 216 patients with chronic subdural hematoma(3). They recorded the lumbar CSF pressure and found it to be less than 150 mm of water in half of the population.

GJERRIS reported the mean VFP twenty-four hours after evacuation of subdural hematomas to be similar to the pressure prior to surgery (1). Our data demonstrate a higher ICP value measured in the evacuated subdural space. This difference may result from the technique of ICP determination. Since intracranial compliances are lower after subdural evacuation, a small leak of ventricular fluid can result in a significant decline in ICP. This leak could not occur with subdural pressure determinations after termination of drainage. Post-evacuation increases in ICP may be explained by increased CBV, CSF outflow resistance or vasogenic edema. A significant decline in compliance without a significant change in PVI indicates that intracranial dynamics are functioning at higher points of the same volume pressure curve.

References

1. Gjerris F (1976) Intraventricular pressure in patients with chronic subdural hematomas before and after evacuation of the hematoma. In: Beks JWF, Bosch DA, Brock M (eds) Intracranial Pressure III. Springer, Berlin Heidelberg New York, p 85

2. Marmarou A, Shulman K, Rosende RM (1978) A nonlinear analysis of the cerebrospinal fluid system and intracranial pressure dynamics. J Neurosurg 48:332-344

3. Plum F, Posner SB (1966) Diagnosis of stupor and coma. Blackwell Scientific Publ, Oxford

4. Tabaddor K, Shulman K (1977) Definitive treatment of chronic subdural hematoma by twist drill craniostomy and closed system drainage. J Neurosurg 46:220-226

5. Weinstein SD, Langfitt TW, Bruno L et al (1968) Experimental study of patients of brain distortion and ischemia produced by an intracranial mass. J Neurosurg 28:513-521

PATHOGNESIS OF CHRONIC SUBDURAL HEMATOMA. ICP, BIOCHEMICAL AND MORPHOLOGICAL FINDINGS

M.GAAB, U.BAUMGARTNER, K.W.PFUGHAUPT, AND R.WODARZ

Introduction

The chronic subdural hematoma is characterized by a clearly encapsulated accumulation of fluid between the dura and arachnoidea (6). Despite its large space-occupation, clinical symptoms only slowly become apparent, and these unique features have prompted several investigations into its pathogenesis. Though a small, often traumatic fibrinous coagulum between the dura and arachnoidea has been established as the initiating factor (6), the pathophysiology of the subsequent massive increase in size remains controversial. Aliquorrhoea with intracranial hypotension (7), inflammatory exudation (4), rebleeding from membranes (9), disturbance of capillary permeability or osmotic and oncotic processes (2,5) are all under consideration.

Material and methods

All 15 patients studied in this investigation had a typical chronic subdural hematoma and to reduce heterogeneity only those with a trauma in anamnesis (at least 4 weeks before operation) and unilateral hematoma, were selected. The mean age was 60 years (range 47-75 years).

Recordings of intracranial pressure (ICP). In all patients, the lumbar CSF pressure was recorded 3 h before, as well as during the operation following catheterization. Throughout the operation (in 2 patients burr holes in local anesthesia; others in normoventilated neurolept analgesia), the epi- and subdural pressures over the hematoma were measured for 30 minutes by miniature force transducers (1), inserted into the burr hole before opening the hematoma. These transducers also allowed registration of the subdural pressure for 3 days after the hematoma operation. In addition, in 4 patients, the epi- and subdural pressures were recorded over the opposite hemisphere as well.

Biochemical and physical investigations. Hematoma fluid, CSF and blood, taken simultaneously during the operation, were analyzed by 19-channel autoanalyzer for electrolytes, glucose, creatinine, urea, triglycerides, cholesterol, bilirubin, total proteins (biuret), albumin and various enzymes. The osmotic (Knauer osmometer) and oncotic (Wescor colloid osmometer) pressures were measured. To study the permeability of the inner hematoma membrane, a 1 cm^2 of membrane was used to separate 2 columns of fluid, the first containing CSF and the other, hematoma fluid, both from the same patient. The resulting levels were then recorded (Fig.1b).

Morphological findings. In the preoperative CT scans, the hematoma thickness and the midline shift were measured. The inner membrane was investigated by light and electron microscopy.

Results

ICP Recordings (Fig. 1a). Despite the size of the hematomas (see below), only moderate ICP pressure values were found. Preoperative and operative pressures in local anesthesia did not differ from values in neurolept analgesia. In the patients where the pressures were measured over both hemispheres, no significant gradients were seen in the horizontal position. However, after operation, the subdural pressure remained lowered by about 10-12 mmHg, compared to preoperative values.

Biochemical and physical investigations (Table). Whereas the osmotic pressures of hematoma, CSF and plasma were equal, the colloid osmotic pressure in the hematoma was considerably higher than that of the CSF. This resulted from differences in protein concentrations. The Na^+ and K^+ concentrations in the hematoma corresponded to the plasma values, but the Ca^{++}, glucose, triglyceride and alkaline phosphatase concentrations were found to be lower. GOT and GPT were not present in hematoma. Increased LDH, bilirubin and Fe resulted from hemolysis. The inner membrane examined in our model osmometer (Fig 1b) showed signs of semipermeability: the difference in height which developed between hematoma (↑) and CSF (↓)fluids, corresponded to 1/2 of the colloid osmotic pressure difference.

Morphological findings. Despite relatively low ICP, all patients had large hematomas (thickness 20 ± 5.5mm, min. 9, max.26mm) and considerable midline shifts (10 ± 4, min.5, max 16.5mm). The ultrastructural examination of the inner hematoma membrane showed a typical collagenous neomembrane with capillaries, macrophages and some remnants of fibrin fibres. No epithelial layer existed.

Discussion

Despite large space-occupation, the relatively low ICP values observed were in good agreement with previous values (3), and indicate only a slow growth of the hematoma, and would appear to exclude repetitive bleeding as a cause of hematoma growth. Whereas no osmotic gradients existed between blood, hematoma and CSF, a constant colloidal osmotic gradient from hematoma to CSF, of about 20 mmHg, was observed, believed to be due to the high protein content of the hematoma, and could result in water absorption by the hematoma from the CSF. This is supported by our in-vitro studies on the hematoma membrane permeability (Fig. 1b), where the fluid flow from CSF to hematoma causes a hydrostatic pressure difference of more than 10 cmH_2O. It is significant that this value corresponds to the mean difference between the pre- and postoperative subdural pressure in the hematoma region, and may be regarded as the hematoma pressure. The structural characteristics of the inner hematoma membrane, i.e., a collagenous network without an epithelial layer, also suggest a semipermeable behaviour. The lower protein, Ca^{++}, glucose and triglyceride concentrations found in the hematoma would further support an in vivo, oncotic water absorption from the CSF, resulting from dilution by absorbed water. The absence of GOT and GPT in the hematoma fluid appears to rule out an increased capillary permeability, i.e., the barrier between the capillaries and hematoma is at least semipermeable, although no colloidal osmotic gradient exists. In conclusion, the correlation of simultaneous investigations on the morphological, physical and biochemical characteristics of these hematomas in our study, favors the hypothesis of "oncotic growth" for chronic subdural hematoma. This would also explain the relatively slow increase in ICP which results from the

Table. Physical and biochemical values measured in simultaneously taken blood, hematoma fluid and CSF. Marked colloid osmotic pressure gradient from hematoma to CSF, caused by differences in protein concentration. Some substrates and most enzymes have lower concentrations in hematoma than in blood(dilution?), with the exception of LDH which is elevated by hemolysis. Values showing differences are underlined.

	osm.pr. (mmol/kg)	colloid osm. pr. (mmHg)	tot.prot. (g/dl)	albumine (g/dl)	glucose (mmol/l)	triglycer. (mmol/l)	bilirubine (umol/l)
blood	296 ± 7,5	20,9 ± 3	6,1 ± 0,5	3,9 ± 0,3	6,63 ± 3,55	1,08 ± 0,2	11,66 ± 5,8
hematoma	294 ± 7,4	21,3 ± 5	5,7 ± 1,1	4,3 ± 0,9	3,73 ± 1,32	0,50 ± 0,2	238,0 ± 55
CSF	297 ± 8,0	0,5 ± 0,5	0,09 ± 0,08	0,07 ± 0,06	4,08 ± 1,11	---------	---------
	Na^+ (mmol/l)	K^+ (mmol/l)	Ca^+ (mmol/l)	GOT (E/l)	GPT (E/l)	alk.Phos. (E/l)	LDH (E/l)
blood	141 ± 3,5	4,2 ± 0,7	2,4 ± 0,23	9,0 ± 3,5	13,0 ± 7,8	185 ± 73	293 ± 172
hematoma	140 ± 2,7	4,3 ± 0,5	1,9 ± 0,45	0,0 ± 0	2,3 ± 4,0	69 ± 20	1642 ± 1147
CSF	145 ± 4,5	3,0 ± 0,3	1,2 ± 0,14	8,0 ± 2,7	2,5 ± 0,7	2,8 ± 0,84	32 ± 17

establishment of a colloidal osmotic gradient between the CSF and hematoma, which is in part counteracted when the patient is in an upright position, due to the fall in CSF pressure.

Summary

In 15 patients with chronic subdural hematomas, the CSF, epi- subdural pressures were recorded pre-, during and postoperatively. Hematoma fluid, CSF and blood were physically and chemically analyzed. The hematoma membranes were studied by electron-microscopy and for permeability, and found to be semipermeable. Despite their considerable space-occupation, only a moderate elevation of ICP (20 mmHg) was seen, which is comparable to a colloidal osmotic pressure gradient between CSF and hematoma, resulting from different protein concentrations. This suggests that chronic subdural hematomas result from "oncotic growth" of small subdural coagula by fluid absorption from CSF.

References

1. Gaab M, Knoblich OE, Dietrich K, Gruss P (1978) Miniaturized methods for monitoring intracranial pressure in craniocerebral trauma before and after operation. In: Fowein RA, Wilcke O, Karimi-Nejad A, Brock M, Klinger M (eds) Advances in Neurosurgery 5. Springer, Berlin Heidelberg New York, p 5

2. Gardner WJ (1932) Traumatic subdural hematoma. Arch Neurol Psychiat 27:847-858

3. Gjerris F (1976) Intraventricular pressure in patients with chronic subdural hematomas before and after evacuation of the hematoma. In: Beks FEW, Bosch DA, Brock M (eds) Intracranial Pressure III. Springer, Berlin Heildelberg New York, p 85

4. Glover D, Labadie EL (1976) Physiopathogenesis of subdural hematomas. Part 2: Inhibition of growth of experimental hematomas with dexamethasone. Neurosurg 45:393-397

5. Goodell Ch.L, Mealey JJ (1963) Pathogenesis of chronic subdural hematoma. Experimental Studies. Arch Neurol (Chirc.)8:429-437

6. Loew F, Kivelitz R (1976) Chronic subdural haematomas. In: Vinken PJ, Bruyn GW (eds) Handbook of Clinical Neurology V 24: Injuries of the Brain and Skull, Part II. North Holland Publ Co, Amsterdam Oxford, p 297

7. Schaltenbrand G (1938) Neuere Anschauungen zur Pathophysiologie der Liquorzirkulation. Zbl Neurochir 3:290-300

8. Weir B (1971) The osmolarity of subdural hematoma fluid. Neurosurg 34:528-533

9. Weber G, Rosemund H, Duckert F (1964) Der Inhalt chronischer Subduralhamatome von Erwachsenen und subduraler Hygrome und Ergüsse von Kindern. Scw Arch Neurol Psychiat 94:348-373

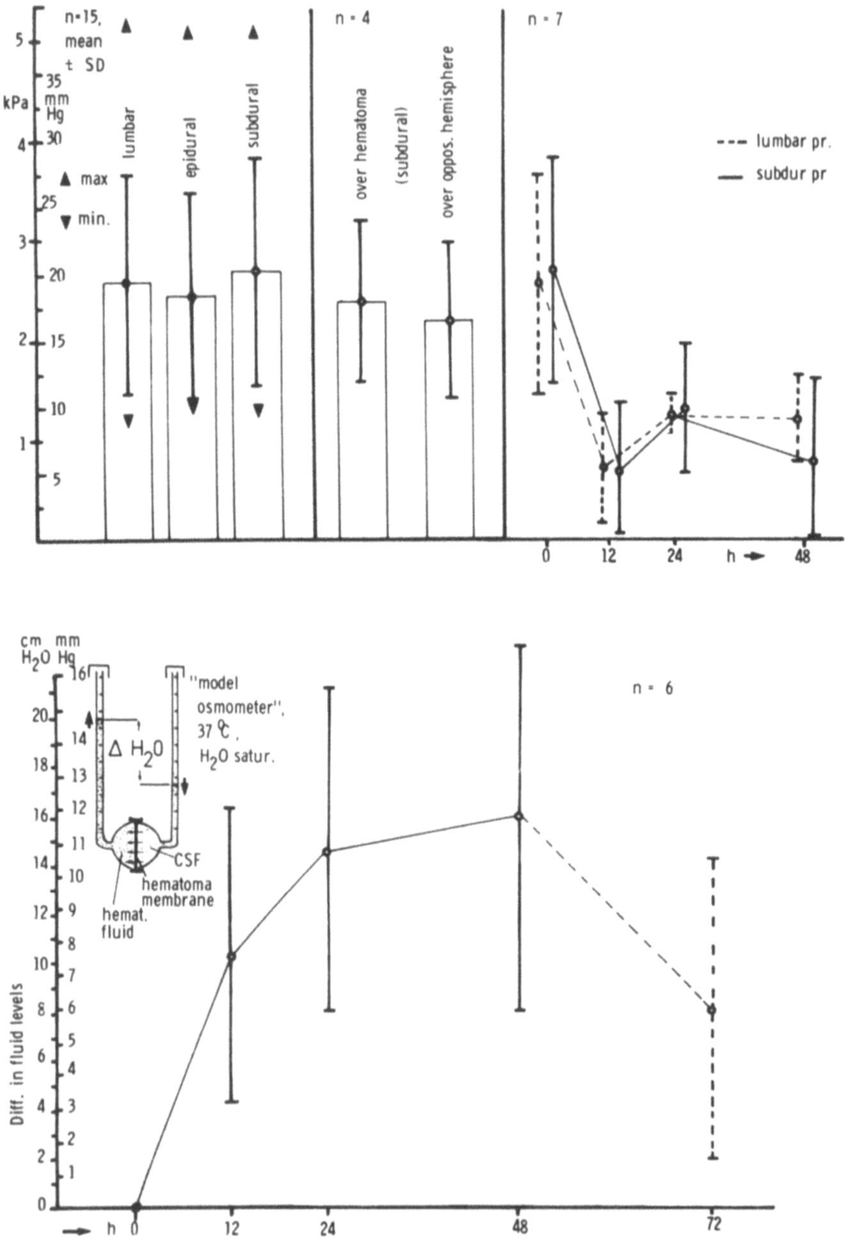

Fig. 1 a and b. ICP (a) and permeability of inner hematoma membrane (b) in chronic subdural hematoma. Despite large space occupation, the ICP is only moderately elevated, no significant gradients exist between hematoma and opposite hemisphere. The hematoma removal results in an ICP decrease of about 10-15 mmHg.
The hematoma membrane tested in a model osmometer(b) shows signs of semipermeability: water crosses membrane from CSF to hematoma fluid due to the difference in protein concentrations (see table).

Session VII

DATA RECORDING AND ANALYSIS

Chairman: J.O.ROWAN
Co-chairman: R.L.GRIFFITH

SUMMARY

By way of introduction the Chairman pointed out that because symposium programs were becoming more and more condensed, there was a temptation for authors when presenting papers to pass quickly over the methodology involved in their study. In order that the variations in reported results can be put into perspective, it is essential that the various ways of recording and analyzing intracranial pressure are critically compared. Furthermore as workers progress towards the situation where more complex measurements will be carried out and microprocessor techniques used, it is also essential that care is taken to ensure that accurate "raw" steady state and dynamic data are collected. Clearly the patient/transducer interface must be studied closely.

The first two papers of this session involved studies comparing, in the main, extradural and intraventricular pressure measurements. They evoked discussion concerning the sources of the pressure differences recorded. Dr.McGRAW emphasized that with solid state transducers sensitivity drift could be as much of a problem as zero reference drift. Dr. MARTIN felt that the geometry of the transducer head was important and should be in the form of a flat coplaner disc. Dr.STALHAMMER was concerned about the variations which can result from differences in dura thickness and their relation to the thickness of the transducer diaphragm and echoed the Chairman's remarks on the topic of well-defined methodology. Dr. BRUCE was disturbed about the lack of good correlation results between extradural and intraventricular pressure measurements at high levels of intracranial pressure, particularly with regard to the calculation of cerebral perfusion pressure levels in critical clinical situations. None of the participants expressed confidence in the acceptance of absolute extradural pressure measurements over a wide range, although it would appear from Dr.DIERSKI's work that the accurate monitoring of pressure trends is a possibility.

Dr. MARMAROU, in congratulating Dr. MATSUMOTO on his group's work, asked for details of the calibration of force vector equipment and the measured time courses of the differences recorded during rapid balloon inflation. Dr. MATSUMOTO indicated that calibration was carried out directly using weights but he had no definite time course data.

Dr.SILVERBERG was questioned on the distance his telemetered signal could be transmitted and on the method used for compensating for variations in barometric pressure. Since with Dr. SILVERBERG's transducer the pick-up loop also acted as the energizer the distance involved had to be very short. With the prototype, barometric pressure was simply measured and correction carried out manually. Dr JAMES commented that with the Ladd system used by Dr. RAJU there was a measurable time lag between intraventricular measurements and those recorded using this transducer. However, more important was the fact that tilt of the transducer plane can result in errors of 5 to 10mmHg.

In answering queries from the Chairman, Mr. PRICE provided details of the safeguards designed into his closed loop system. For example, the syringes containing mannitol were only loaded manually with fixed amounts and the amounts checked by the nursing staff. The varying therapy initiating thresholds were: cerebral perfusion pressure: - 50 mmHg. Fifteen minute mean pressure for the injection of mannitol: - 25 mmHg. Change in ICP pulse pressure: - 15%.

Dr. AVEZAAT pointed out that the level of intracranial pulse pressure depended on more than the brain elastance. Dr. McGRAW felt that the total storage time of 34 hours for Dr. STALHAMMER's microprocessor system was rather limited and one week would be a more practical limit.

In closing the session it was pointed out by the Chairman that a realistic balance had to be struck between the hazard which might result from any particular measuring technique and the hazard which might result from a therapy decision based on inaccurate results.

EXTRADURAL, VENTRICULAR AND SUBDURAL PRESSURE RECORDING COMPARATIVE CLINICAL STUDY

J.ZIERSKI

Introduction

It is generally accepted that the epidural pressure recording (EDP) is connected with the smallest risk of infection and with minimal disadvantages during long-term measurement if compared with intraventricular or subdural method. The principles of correct placement of the epidural transducer have been established (3,11,12); however, the relationships between the EDP and ventricular pressures (IVP) have been studied only in a small number of patients (4,5,6,14,15). On several occasions discrepancies have been found (6,14); some authors reported only very small differences (15). It has been suggested that EDP tends to be higher than IVP at higher values of ICP (4,6), but in general good correlation between both the pressures was reported. Although these problems have been dealt with already 7 years ago, it is still disputed whether existing differences between EDP and IVP are genuine or whether they are caused by methodological factors. The validity of EDP measurement particuarly for study of intercompartmental pressures was questioned (9). The limits of different techniques of measurement have not been sufficiently emphasized and this was certainly one of the reasons of disappointment in several centers where EDP measurement was scheduled to be used in clinical practice. Large variety of techniques used for ICP measurement was documented in a recent review by SAUNDERS (10).

The aim of the present report is the analysis of relations between EDP and IVP and between other sites of ICP measurement occurring during clinical monitoring.

Material and methods

Comparative measurements were performed in 26 patients out of the total of 125 patients in whom ICP was monitored. All EDP/IVP measurements were done in patients with hydrocephalus caused by tumors of the posterior fossa, tumors of the midline, aqueduct stenosis or SAH. Bilateral IVP was recorded in one patient with craniopharyngioma of the IIIrd ventricle. Eleven of these patients had ventricular drainage at some time during the recording. The remaining 9 patients had supratentorial pathology and the pressure was recorded on both sides in the subdural or epidural space.

IVP was recorded by LUNDBERG's method (8) from the right lateral ventricle. The transducer (Statham SP 37) was fixed firmly on the forehead in the midline, 6 cm above the glabella. Calibration was checked at least once in 24 hours or more often if differential pressure to the EDP exceeded 5 mmHg.

EDP was recorded through commercially available Phillips Epidural Transducer (Philips Co., Med.Div., Endthoven, Netherlands) placed in 11 mm burrhole 3 - 4 cm off the midline and mounted in a screw. Particular care was taken to drill the hole perpendicular to the dura and to assure absolute hemostasis. The screw was placed flush with the dura, the transducer indented the dura by 1 mm. The depth of insertion of the screw was checked by a special rod.

SDP recordings were performed in the same manner with the exception that cruciate incision of the dura mater was performed under magnification prior to the insertion of the transducer. Zero point drift of the transducer could not be estimated in situ, however, this proved not to be necessary, and calibration was checked only before and after recording. Over the period of 3 years 2 pairs of transducers have been used for epidural or subdural pressure recordings in 80 patients and only on one occasion a drift of +3 mmHg was noted after 14 days of implantation. During the period of detailed recording the patient's head was elevated by 15 - 20°. Head movements, coughing, changes of body position, etc., were carefully monitored by an observer and entered into a protocol.

Results

Tolerance limits of 5 mmHg were set for the differential pressure after checking that turning patient's head from face-up to lateral position did not influence the differential pressure by more than this value. Significant correlation between the pressures was found independently from the site of measurements in all the recordings(Fig.1). However, almost linear correlation (r 0.9) was not a constant finding and the ratios varied from one patient to another or even in the same patient when analyzed at different intervals. Further analysis of cases in which both the pressure curves showed no significant correlation or negative correlation revealed that this occurred during the time of drainage of ventricular or lumbar fluid. Very high correlation was found between bilateral SDP measurements in the range between 15 - 40 mmHg in a patient with fulminating, strictly unilateral hemispheric edema. The difference between both the sides did not exceed 5 mmHg. High correlation was found between bilateral EDP with pressure difference varying between approx. ± 5 mmHg but changing in favor of one or other side, even when the lesion was strictly unilateral. Good correlation was found between EDP and SDP with constant difference of app. 5 mmHg in favor of the epidural pressure. Correlation coefficients between EDP and IVP were generally also very high over the whole range of pressures but the differential pressure varied between 0 - 2 mmHg and almost 20 mmHg (Fig.2). The differences between EDP and IVP in absolute values are shown in the histogram(Fig.3) In 5 patients the EDP showed values lower than IVP by more than 10mmHg, in 6-higher by more than 10 mmHg and in 5 cases pressure differences did not exceed 5 mmHg for the majority of time. In one patient with combined EDP and lumbar pressure measurement EDP was higher by almost 20 mmHg. Drainage of the ventricular fluid produced a change of differential pressure in 3 out of 11 cases.

Discussion

In spite of the fact that stable non-drifting transducers are commercially available (1,7) reliable measurement of EDP is still connected with difficulties (13). We could confirm that the correlation between EDP and IVP is generally very good (2,3,5) but the range of discrepancies is too disturbing for the routine clinical use. EDP may read higher or lower than IVP. We could not confirm the tendency of EDP reading higher at high values of IVP.

Experimental studies in our laboratory on a model and in animals showed that changing the angle of insertion of transducer by more than 8° produces differences in pressure reading by more than 20% of the control value. The amplitude of pressure and good reproducibility of pulse and respiratory variations as well as that caused by jugular compression were of no help in estimating the correct position of the transducer on the dura. Although at insertion the transducer is placed coplanar and down on the dura the situation may change during the monitoring as evidenced by change of the differential EDP/IVP. The local dural factor, particularly the thickness of the dura plays here an important role. With the present technique of application the reproducibility of a standard difference EDP/IVP could not be assured and the difference varied from case to case. EDP recording seems, therefore, unsuitable for study of intercompartmental pressure differences and pressure gradients. Differences exceeding 5 mmHg and up to 15 - 20 mmHg occurring when measuring EDP/IVP in patients with hydrocephalus are thought to be connected with the technique of application and are not genuine. EDP is a reliable method for monitoring the trend of changes in ICP.

Summary

Comparative EDP/IVP measurements were performed in patients with hydrocephalus and comparative EDP/SDP, EDP/EDP and SDP/SDP measurements in patients with supratentorial pathology. In half the number of cases differential pressures exceeding 5 or 10 mmHg were found, even if correlation between pressures measured at different sites was very good. Local dura condition seems to be the most important factor contributing to the errors of EDP measurement.

References

1. Beks JWF, Albarda S, Gieles ACM, Kuypers MH, Flanderijn H (1977) Extradural transducer for monitoring intracranial pressure. Acta Neurochir 38:245-250

2. Coroneos NJ, Turner JM, Gibson RM, McDowall DG, Pickerodt VWA, Keaney NP (1972) Comparison of extradural with intraventricular pressure in patients after head injury. In: Brock M, Dietz H (eds) Intracranial Pressure. Springer, Berlin Heidelberg New York, p 51

3. Dorsh NWC, Symon L (1972) The validity of extradural measurement of the intracranial pressure. In: Lundberg N, Ponten U, Brock M (eds) Intracranial Pressure II. Springer, Berlin Heidelberg New York, p 403

4. Gobiet W, Bock WJ, Liesegang J, Grote W (1972) Long-time monitoring of epidural pressure in man. In: Brock M, Dietz H (eds) Intracranial Pressure. Springer, Berlin Heidelberg New York, p 14

5. Ikeyama A, Maeda S, Nagai H, Furuse M, Igarashi I, Inagaki D, Kitano T (1977) Epidural measurement of intracranial pressure by newly developed pressure transducer. Neurol medico-chirur 17:1-7

6. Jorgensen PB, Riishede J (1972) Comparative clinical studies of epidural and ventricular pressure. In: Brock M, Dietz H (eds) Intracranial Pressure. Springer, Berlin Heidelberg New york,p 41

7. Koster WG (1978) Edpidurale Gehirndruckmessung. Biomedizinische Technik 23:37-38

8. Lundberg N (1960) Continuous recording and control of ventricular fluid pressure in neurosurgical practice. Acta Psychiat Neurol Scand 36, Suppl. 149

9. Rowan JO, Johnston IH (1975) Intracranial pressure gradients - do they exist? In: Lundberg N, Ponten U, Brock M (eds) Intracranial Pressure II. Springer, Berlin Heildelberg New York, p 239

10. Saunders RL (1978) Intracranial pressure monitoring survey. Neurosurg 3:130

11. Schettini A, McKay L, Majors R, Mahig J, Nevis AH (1971) Experimental approach for monitoring surface brain pressure. J Neurosurg 34:38-47

12. Schettini A, Walsh E (1975) Simultaneous pressure-depth measurements of the intracranial system made epidurally. In: Lundberg N, Ponten U, Brock M (eds) Intracranial Pressure II. Springer, Berlin Heidelberg New York, p 409

13. Stalhamer D (personal communication 1979)

14. Sundbarg G, Nornes H (1972) Simultaneous recording of the epidural and ventricular fluid pressure. In: Brock M, Dietz H (eds) Intracranial Pressure. Springer, Berlin Heidelberg New York, p46

15. Turner JM, Gibson RM, McDowall DG, Nahhas F (1975) Further experience with extradural pressure monitoring. In: Lundberg N, Ponten U, Brock M (eds) Intracranial Pressure II. Springer, Berlin Heidelberg New York, p 397

Supported by Deutsche Forschungsgemeinschaft, SFB 32.

METHODS	NO. OF 2-HRS-INTERVALS	NO SIGNIFIC.	SIGNIFICANT NEGATIVE	SIGNIFIC. POSITIVE R<0.9	R>0.9
IVP/EDP	151	6	5	82	58
IVP/IVP	4	1	-	3	-
SDP/IVP	8	-	-	8	-
SDP/SDP	34	-	-	9	25
EDP/SDP	14	1	-	8	5
EDP/EDP	32	1	2	19	10
EDP/LUMB.	3	-	-	3	-

Fig. 1. Relationship between different methods of ICP measurement estimated at 2-hourly intervals. Mean pressure values sampled every 24 sec.

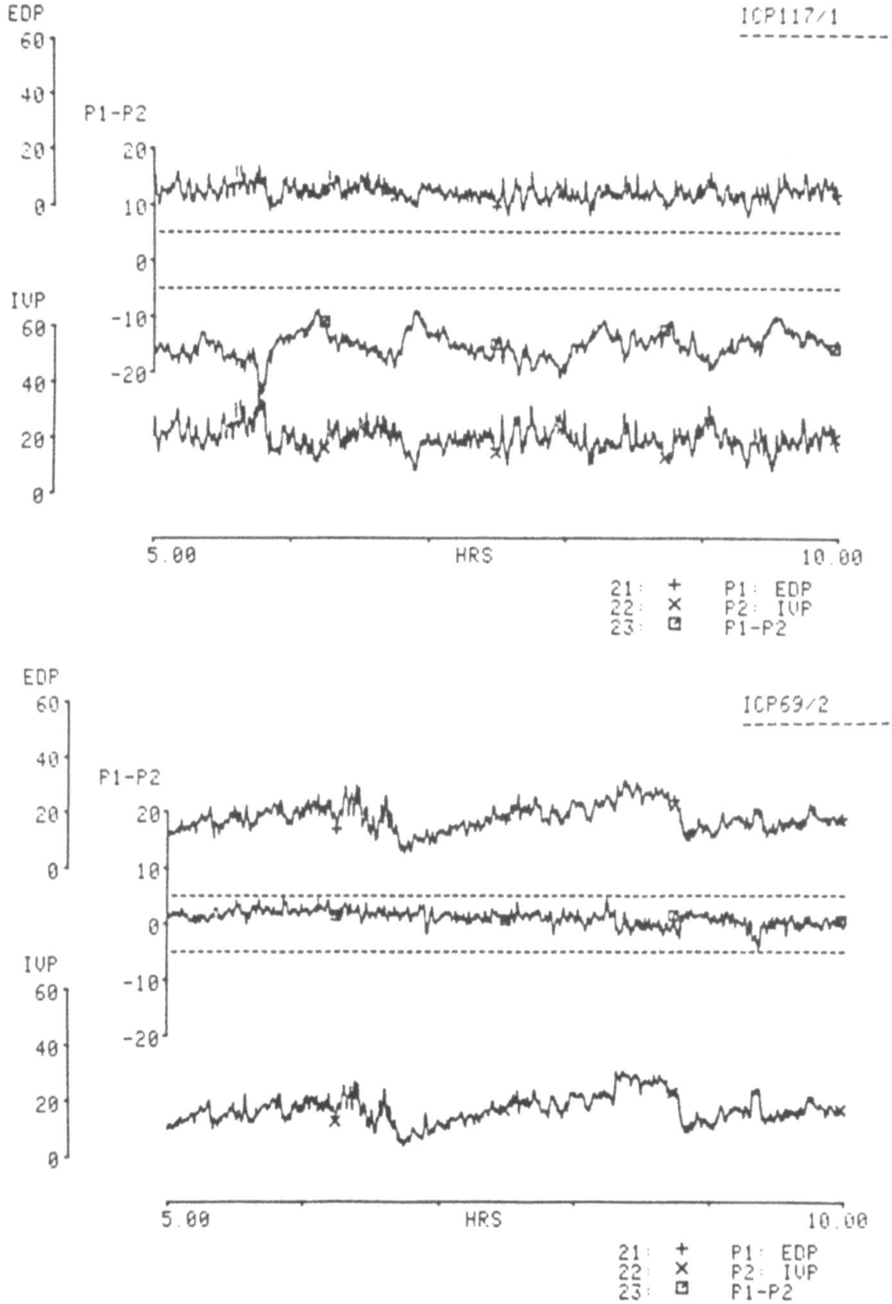

Fig. 2. Upper trace: Differential trace EDP/IVP. Pressure difference above 10 mmHg.
Lower trace: Differential trace EDP/IVP. Pressures equal.

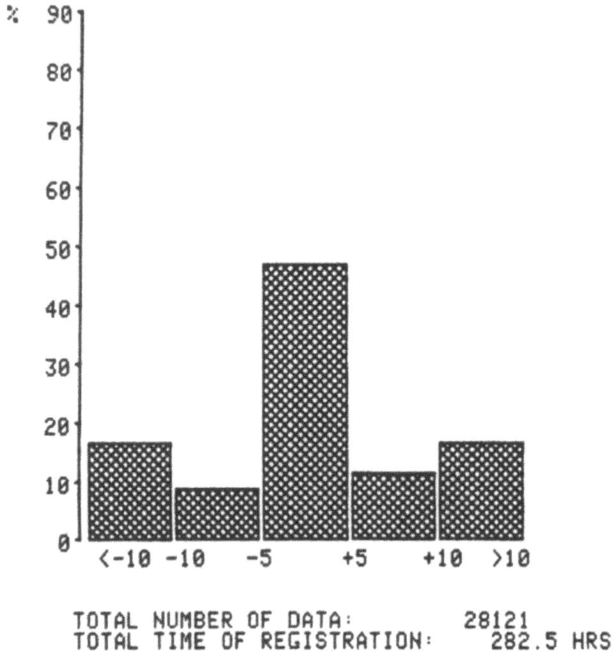

Fig. 3. Histogram of EDP/IVP differential pressure.

SIMULTANEOUS EPIDURAL AND INTRAVENTRICULAR PRESSURE MEASUREMENT DURING THE OCCURRENCE OF SUPRATENTORIAL EXPANDING LESIONS

J. ESPARZA, A. MANRIQUE, R. D. LOBATO, AND E. LAMAS

Introduction

The reliability of epidural pressure measurements has been questioned because the existence of gradients between epidural pressure (EDP) and ventricular fluid pressure (VFP) (1,3,7). Differences between these two pressures have been explained on methodological grounds, and the "coplanar principle" has been argued (2,4,6), as well as the existence of intracompartmental pressure gradients (2). It has been our objective to check the occurrence of EDP and VFP gradients in humans studying at the same time the patency of the CSF circulation.

Material and methods

Intracranial pressure was preoperatively measured in 30 adult patients affected by supratentorial gliomas and metastasis. EDP was continuously recorded by means of a non-coplanar fiber-optic sensor (Ladd Pressure Monitor M-1000/Ladd Research Ind, Inc., Burlington, Vt) placed on the tumoral hemisphere. VFP was simultaneously recorded according with the method described by LUNDBERG; implantation of the ventricular catheter was contralateral in respect to the placement of the epidural sensor. Pressure recordings lasted more than 24 hours in all patients. Zero-point adjustments were performed, and in the case of epidural sensor checked after removal.

RHISA ventriculography was performed in 20 patients injecting 50-100 µCi through the ventricular catheter. It was possible to analyze the diffusion of the isotope over the brain hemispheres in all these cases.

Results

Patients in this series have been classified into two groups. Group A includes cases showing VFP levels under 20 mmHg (10 cases). Group B is formed by those cases with VFP levels above 20 mmHg (20 cases).

EDP and VFP were similar in all patients included in Group A. RHISA ventriculography showed, in the six paients of this group in which it was performed, a patent convexity subarachnoid pathways. Nevertheless a partial block in CSF circulation was found in two cases. In patients pertaining to Group B, variable and sustained differences between EDP and VFP were recorded (Fig. 1). In the fourteen cases of this group in which RHISA ventriculography was performed, no diffusion of the isotope over the pathological hemisphere was observed. (Fig. 2).

Discussion

The existence of intracompartmental pressure gradients depends on several factors (5). Among them are: a) The measurement device employed,

b) The relationship between the subarachnoid pressure and the brain parenchyma pressure, and c) To what extent pressure within the tissue is transmitted to the rest of the brain. As has been shown here, brain displacements produced by supratentorial expanding lesions may cause blocks in CSF circulation. These blocks are able to induce differences between EDP and VFP. We suggest that these differences may be due to local increases in pressure which occur when CSF flow is compromised. To us, pressure gradients observed in this study are genuine. Nevertheless it is possible that they are methodological in part.

Summary

Continuous simultaneous monitoring of EDP and VFP in patients with supratentorial expanding lesions has been performed. Patency of CSF circulation was studied by means of RHISA ventriculography, EDP and VFP were identical in patients showing normal CSF flow over the cerebral hemispheres. Contrarily, gradients between these two pressures were recorded when brain displacements blocked the convexity subarachnoid pathways.

References

1. Coroneos NJ, Turner JM, Gibson RM, McDowall DG, Pickerodt VWA, Keaney NP (1972) Comparison of extradural with intraventricular pressure in patients after head injury. In: Brock M, Dietz H (eds) Intracranial Pressure. Springer, Berlin Heidelberg New York, p 51

2. Dorsch NWC, Symon L (1975) The validity of extradural measurement of the intracranial pressure. In: Lundberg N, Ponten U, Brock M (eds) Intracranial Pressure II. Springer, Berlin Heidelberg New York, p 403

3. Jorgensen PB, Riishede J (1972) Comparative clinical studies of epidural and ventricular pressure. In: Brock M, Dietz H (eds) Intracranial Pressure. Springer, Berlin Heidelberg New York, p 41

4. McGraw CP, Epidural intracranial pressure monitoring. In: Lundberg N, Ponten U, Brock M (eds) Intracranial Pressure II. Springer, Berlin Heidelberg New York, p 394

5. Rowan JO, Johnston IH (1975) Intracranial pressure gradients -Do they exist? In: Lundberg N, Ponten U, Brock M (eds) Intracranial Pressure II. Springer, Berlin Heidelberg New York, p 239

6. Schettini A, Welsh E (1975) Simultaneous pressure-depth measurements of the intracranial system made epidurally. In: Lundberg N, Ponten U, Brock M (eds) Intracranial Pressure II. Springer, Berlin Heidelberg New York, p409

7. Sundbarg G (1972) Simultaneous recording of the epidural and ventricular fluid pressure. In: Brock M, Deitz H (eds) Intracranial Pressure. Springer, Berlin Heidelberg New York, p 46

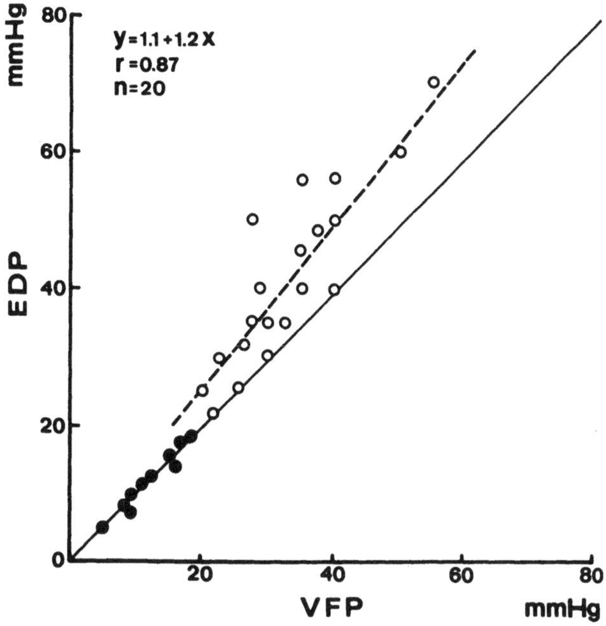

Fig. 1. Correlation between EDP and VFP in patients with normal RHISA ventriculography, (black circles) and in patients with impaired isotopic diffusion over the tumoral hemisphere, (open circles). All cases with normal isotope diffusion fall near the identity line.

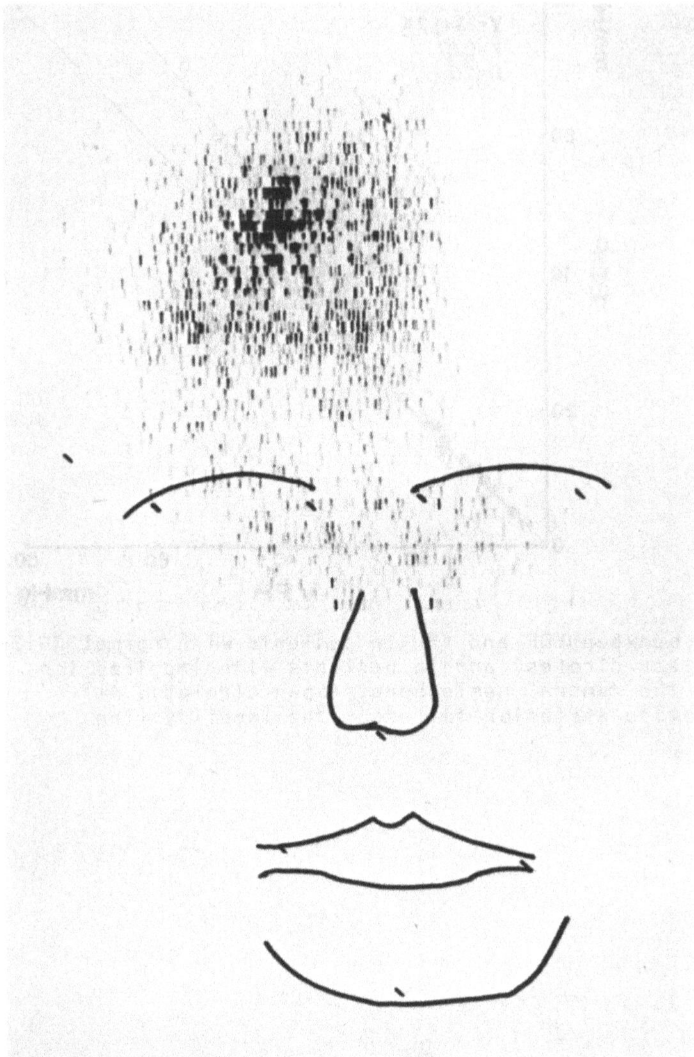

Fig. 2. Isotopic ventriculography in a patient with a left temporal astrocytoma. 24 hours after injection the isotope spread over the right convexity with no radioactivity over the left hemisphere.

MEASUREMENT OF INTRACRANIAL FORCE VECTOR AND ITS SIGNIFICANCE

T. AKIOKA, A. MATSUMOTO, M. TSUCHIMOTO, H. KUYAMA, AND A. NISHIMOTO

Introduction

The existence of pressure gradients within the brain parenchyma has been reported (3,6), but little is known about the mechanism of its development. We have devised the apparatus to measure intracranial force vector (FV). This is a preliminary report to introduce it and to discuss the significance of intracranial FV under the condition of intracranial hypertension.

Materials and Methods

Experiments were carried out on mongrel dogs anesthetized with sodium pentobarbital, paralyzed with succinyl choline chloride, and ventilated on respirator to maintain normal arterial blood gas levels. Epidural pressure (EDP) was monitored by Numoto's fiber optic pressure switches (4) attached to bilateral parietal epidural spaces. Cerebrospinal fluid pressure (CSFP) was also monitored by the catheter inserted in the cisterna magna. Systemic arterial blood pressure was recorded from the femoral artery. FV was measured at left parietal area by our newly devised apparatus. This apparatus consists of a sensor, Wheatstone bridge, D.C. amplifier and recorder. The sensor is made of a needle of 0.5mm in diameter which is inserted into the brain tissue, and four strain gauges which are at right angles to one another around the needle. The force detected by a needle is divided into each directional component by a stress sensor and is continuously recorded on a chart paper (Figure 1). Intracranial pressure (ICP) was increased at various speeds by either inflation of rubber balloon inserted in left frontal epidural space, as a model of space taking lesion, or saline infusion into the cisterna magna, as a model of hydrostatic intracranial hypertension. Intracranial FV was investigated under these two conditions.

Results

I. Epidural balloon compression group: Expansion of an epidural balloon over the left frontal area caused a rise of biparietal EDP and interhemispheric EDP gradients, more often observed in fast inflation speed (0.4ml/5min) than in slow speed (0.2ml/5min). When the balloon volume reached about 3-4ml, about 300mmH_2O of EDP gradients was observed in fast inflation. Increasing the balloon volume at a faster rate caused EDP gradients to decline progressively and finally disappear. The component of FV directing to the temporal (or lateral) side also became maximum at the same point which EDP gradients showed maximum value (Figure 2). At 6ml of the balloon volume, this component of FV began to decrease and became a shearing force along the falx cerebri. Keeping the balloon content at 6ml, FV gradually decreased with time, and then, 20 minutes later when the balloon volume deflated suddenly, FV immediately disappeared.

2. Hydrostatic saline infusion group: In this group interhemispheric EDP graients were not detected, even when CSFP was elevated abruptly by 5ml of saline infusion to the cisterna magna. However, the component of FV directing to the temporal side (i.e. FV from lateral ventricle to cortex) was observed, even though 6 minutes later when CSFP declined almost to the base line (Figure 3).

Discussion

Intracranial hypertension due to space taking lesion causes cerebral circulation disturbance and brain tissue distortion. In recent years there have been several reports describing the development of pressure gradients within the cranial cavity during increased ICP. However, the existence of tissue pressure gradients is still under controversy (5). We have already reported that interhemispheric EDP difference was obviously seen in the epidural balloon compression study, but was not observed in the hydrostatic intracranial hypertension caused by saline infusion into the cisterna magna (2). Why do EDP gradients occur? If the cranial cavity consisted of only CSF, ICP will transmit uniformly according to Pascal's law. But blood and brain tissue are coexistent with CSF and each of these has different viscoelasticity. In addition, it is well known that sensors for measuring EDP are sensitive to not only pure pressure itself, but also the stress/strain. Because of this, we presumed FV would be also present in the condition of increased ICP, particularly due to space taking lesion. To study how FV does act on the development of EDP gradients, we devised this apparatus. The technical aspects and reliability of it were already reported elsewhere (1). This apparatus might be useful to investigate the mechanism of brain tissue distortion and cerebral herniation under increased ICP, in spite of its disadvantages: 1. cerebral tissue damage may accompany insertion of a needle; 2. FV can be only two dimensionally analyzed. Based on our experimental data that FV reached a maximum value in parallel with EDP gradients under the condition of increasing ICP, it was suggested that not only pure pressure itself, but also FV, may play an important role in causing EDP gradients. It is concluded that the appearance of FV may bring about the EDP gradients. Then, brain tissue may shift and/or herniate in the cranial cavity in the direction of greater FV.

Summary

FV was monitored in dogs under intracranial hypertension by our newly devised apparatus. FV was obviously observed in parallel with EDP gradients in the condition of increased ICP due to extradural balloon compression. On the other hand, neither remarkable FV nor EDP gradients were seen in the experiment with hydrostatic saline infusion into the cisterna magna. It is concluded that FV might be a main cause to develop EDP gradients in the cranial cavity under intracranial hypertension produced by mass lesion.

References

1. Akioka T, Nishimoto K, Fujimoto S, Kuyama H, Ninomiya K, Matsumoto A, Nishimoto A, Watanabe H (1976) A new equipment for the monitoring of intracranial force vector. J Japan Med Inst 46:141-143

2. Akioka T, Fujimoto S, Kuyama H, Nishimoto K, Ninomiya K, Matsumoto A, Nishimoto A (1977) A new equipment for the continuous monitoring of intracranial epidural pressure. Neurolog Surg 5:979-984

3. Langfitt TW, Weinstein JD, Kassel NF, Gagliardi LJ (1961) Transmission of increased intracranial pressure within the supratentorial space. J Neurosurg 21:998-1005

4. Numoto M, Slater JP, Donaghy RMP (1969) An automatic method of measuring and recording intracranial pressure. Med Res Eng 8:38-39

5. Rowan JO, Johnston IH (1975) Intracranial pressure gradients--Do they exist? In: Lundberg N, Ponten U, Brock M (eds) Intracranial Pressure II. Springer, Berlin Heidelberg New York, p. 239

6. Shulman K, Marmarou A, Weitz S (1975) Gradients of brain interstitial fluid pressure in experimental brain infusion and compression. In: Lundberg N, Ponten U, Brock M (eds) Intracranial Pressure II. Springer, Berlin Heidelberg New York p. 221

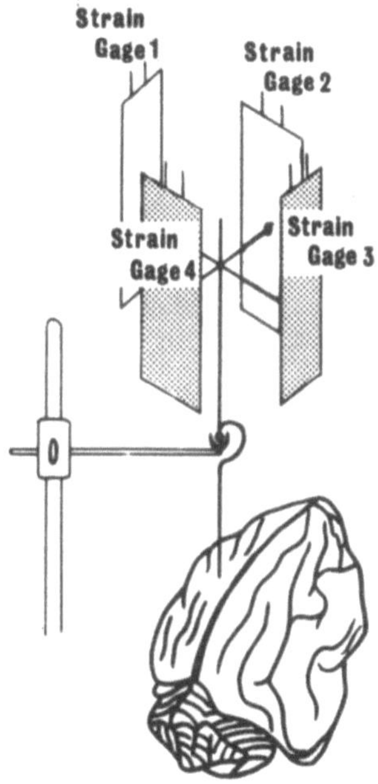

Figure 1.
Schema of the FV sensor. The needle is inserted about 1 cm into the brain parenchyma. Intracranial FV is detected by the needle and transferred to the stress sensors.

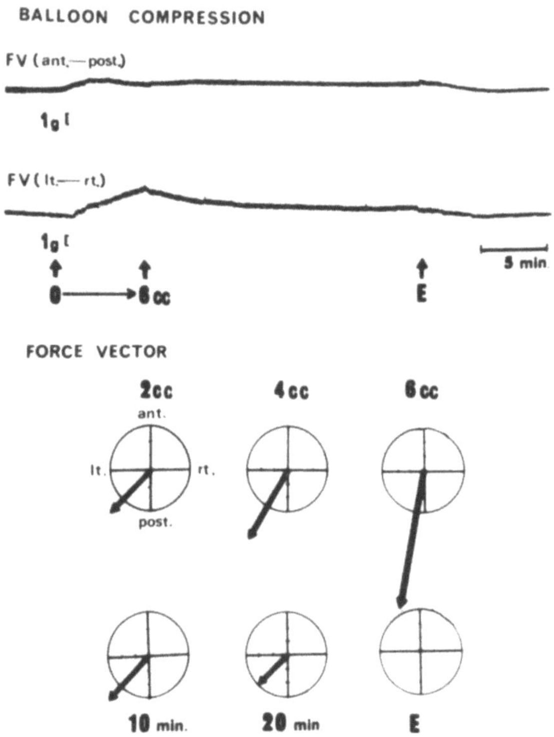

Figure 2.
FV induced by extradural balloon compression. By the balloon compression over left frontal area, FV was induced posterolaterally at left parietal area. Temporal (or lateral) directed component of FV was about 2 grams as maximum at the stage of 4ml balloon volume. By the compression of 6ml of the balloon content, sagittal (or posterior) directed FV became larger than temporal one. This FV, which is a shearing force along the falx cerebri, disappeared promptly after complete evacuation of the balloon content.

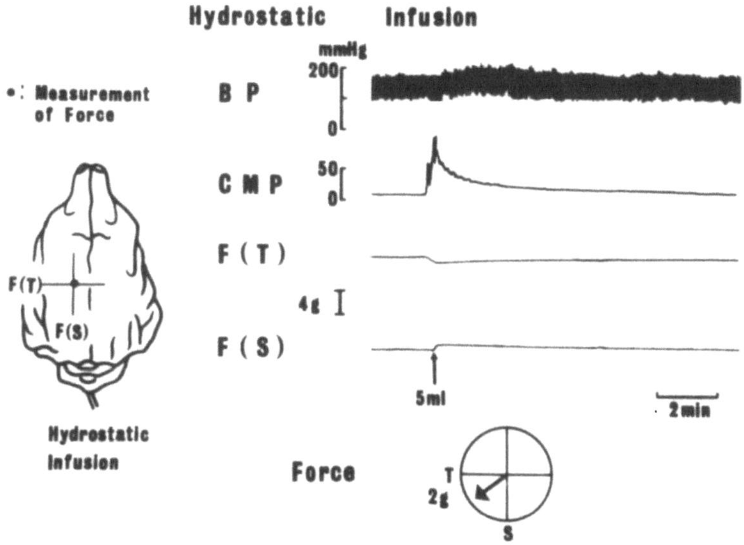

Figure 3.
FV induced by hydrostatic saline infusion into the cisterna magna. 5ml of saline infusion increased abruptly the cisterna magna pressure (CMP). FV directed posterolaterally was observed. It exists for a while after CMP declined almost to the base line.

CLINICAL EVALUATION OF A NEW EPIDURAL PRESSURE TRANSDUCER

F. GJERRIS, S. E. BØRGESEN, AND S. C. SØRENSEN

Introduction

Measurement of intraventricular pressure (IVP) through a ventricular catheter is a well-known method and has the advantage of being a direct method. If the catheter and the transducer are placed correctly, the ICP is measured exactly. The greatest disadvantage is the risk of infection. Therefore a number of epidural pressure transducers have been developed during the last decennium (3,4). PHILIPS Medical System Division has produced a transducer for EDP-monitoring described by BEKS et al (1).

Material, Method and Results

We have tested this epidural pressure transducer in clinical practice. We have compared intraventricular pressure measured through a Seletz catheter using a conventional strain gauge transducer (Statham P23) with the epidural pressure measured with the new epidural transducer, during both spontaneous and induced variations in IVP. The IVP catheter was always placed in a right precoronal burrhole and the EDP-transducer in a left one. The pressures were recorded on a double channel recorder with a paper speed of 160mm/hr. The records were analyzed for spontaneous occurrence of A-waves and B-waves and induced variations in pressures by hyperventilation and Mannitol treatment.

In fifty patients IVP and EDP were measured simultaneously for at least 24 hours. In 42 patients spontaneous variations in IVP caused nearly quantitatively similar variations in EDP. Small differences (3-6mmHg) were seen in periods, but in 8 patients we found great differences. In the 8 cases the discrepancies were caused by the following: Thickness of the skull (4 cases), intentional placement of a piece of Spongostan between dura and transducer (2 cases) and finally break-down of two transducers (prototypes). Following 24 hours monitoring of ICP, IVP and EDP were further measured during stepwise increases in IVP in 20 patients with normal pressure hydrocephalus in connection with a lumbo-ventricular perfusion test (Fiaure 1) (2). The slope of the regression line for corresponding value of IVP and EDP was caluclated for each patient. The mean of the slopes of these lines was 1.14 (range .90-1.5) i.e. $\Delta EDP = 1.14 \Delta IVP$. Thus, EDP increased more than IVP when IVP was elevated by raising the pressure in the ventricle per se. When IVP was raised in this way we also observed a greater increase in the amplitude of pulse pressure waves in EDP than in IVP (Figure 1). More than 24 hours of pressure monitoring disclosed no zero point drift, no temperature drifts and no sensitivity drifts. IVP and EDP were also measured simultaneously during sudden decreases in brain volume during administration of Mannitol or hyperventilation (Figure 2). Few times we found a temporary "undershot" in the EDP-reading, which must be due to failing contact between dura and the transducer following the decrease of brain volume.

Discussion

By measuring IVP and EDP simultaneously in 50 patients for 24 hours or more, we have found that an epidural transducer placed correctly is a reliable method for monitoring spontaneous variations in ICP. Two prototypes of the EDP-transducer broke down, but with the final model, we have had no problems at all. No zero drift has been observed. The discrepancies observed during lumbo-ventricular perfusion and following Mannitol treatment demonstrated that a pressure gradient can exist between the ventricular system and the brain surface, but during the lumbo-ventricular perfusion test, the patient is positioned on the left side (EDP-transducer side). The differences in amplitude of pulse pressure waves can be caused by a damping effect in the IVP monitoring system or one can suggest that this procedure causes a greater decrease in compliance of the tissue mass below the epidural transducer, than in the brain as a whole. In some cases we observed that there was either a decrease or increase in EDP compared to IVP. These discrepancies could mostly be explained by differences in the level of the IVP catheter and the EDP-transducer. In skilled hands these differences are easily detected and give only small limitations in the use of the EDP-transducer. An exact placement of the transducer coplanar to dura is obligatory.

Summary

PHILIPS Medical System Division has produced a transducer for epidural pressure monitoring. The transducer was tested in 50 patients with simultaneously intraventricular and epidural pressure monitoring during spontaneous or induced pressure increases. In 20 patients stepwise increase of IVP by lumbo-ventricular perfusion tests showed good agreement between the pressure measurements. 24 hours of pressure monitoring disclosed no zero point drift and no sensitivity drift. Problems concerning insertion of the transducer were minimal. It was found imperative that the transducer is coplanar and in contact with the dura. This new EDP transducer is stable, reliable, and useful in clinical practice.

References

1. Beks, JWF, Albarda S, Gieles ACM, Kuypers MH, Flanderijn H (1977) Extradural transducer for monitoring intracranial pressure. Acta Neurochir 38:245-250

2. Børgesen SE, Gjerris F, Sørensen SC (1978) The resistance to cerebrospinal fluid abosrption in humans. Acta Neurol Scand 57:88-96

3. DeJong DA, Berfelo MW, DeLange SA, Maas AIR (1979) Epidural pressure monitoring with the so-called Rotterdam transducer. Further in vivo results. Acta Neurochir 45:301-309

4. Dorsch NWC, Symon L (1975) A practical technique for monitoring extradural pressure. J Neurosurg 42:249-257

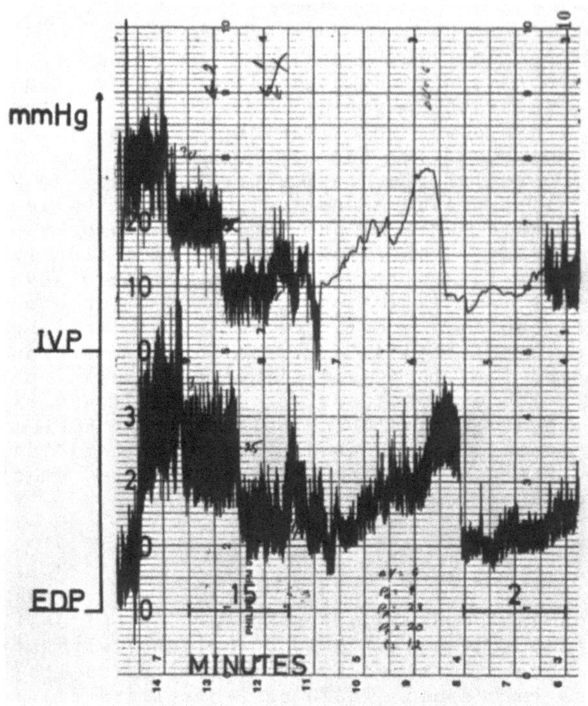

Figure I.
Simultaneous measurement of IVP and EDP during lumbo-ventricular perfusion test. To be read from right to left.

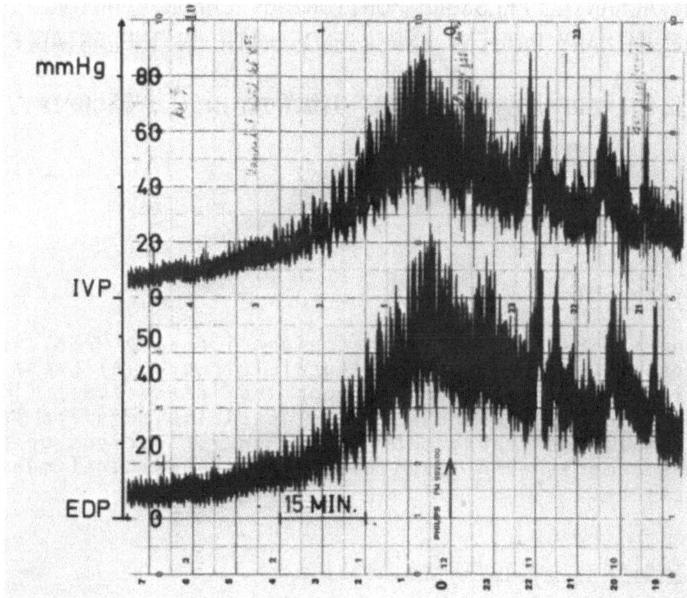

Figure 2.
Simultaneous measurement of IVP and EDP during infusion of Mannitol 0.5 g/kg (vertical arrow). To be read from right to left.

INTRACRANIAL PRESSURE MONITORING: CHRONIC ANIMAL IMPLANTATION AND PRELIMINARY PATIENT EXPERIENCE WITH AN IMPLANTABLE TELEMETERED SYSTEM

G.D. Silverberg, A.K. Ream, S.D. Corbin, E.V. Schmidt, and T.B. Fryer

Introduction

Over the past 4 years, in conjunction with NASA, we have developed a capacitive implantable epidural intracranial pressure (ICP) monitor (Figure 1) telemetered through the intact scalp (1). After acceptable in vitro studies and acute epidural implantation in dogs (CORBIN et al), we implanted transducers in 5 dogs for periods up to 4 months. Multiple measurements were taken comparing the epidural measurements to cisternal pressure.

Materials, Methods and Results

The grouped data showed a mean error of 0.2 torr, while the average error per transducer was 1.9 torr with a standard deviation of 3.8 torr. Several sources of error were uncovered during this study. The most important was the repeated trauma to the units caused by the dog's scratching at the wound (in several cases, they were able to actually unscrew the transducer). In no case was there clinical evidence of infections; all cultures were negative. We found that the error did not increase with time up to the 112 day maximum studied. Fidelity of the epidural signal was excellent, even after 4 months implantation and modest dural thickening. We found that precise implantation of the transducer, so that the guard ring and sensing surface is coplanar with the dura and rigid fixation of the unit to the skull, is mandatory for reliable pressure monitoring (2).

We have since implanted the transducer in 10 patients for an average duration of 4 days (range 1-8 days). The spectrum of neurosurgical problems were as follows: severe head injury with coma (1), cysts or tumors obstructing the CSF pathways (3); aneurysms (2); Reyes syndrome (1); patients with significant cerebral edema associated with tumor, toxic encephalopathy or anoxic/ischaemic encephalopathy (3). In 5 of these patients, we were able to correlate the epidural measurement with a CSF pressure by lumbar puncture. The mean error was 1.8 torr (range: 0.5-3.4 torr). This value compares favorably with the results of bench and animal studies. There were no complications and no infections. In 1 patient with a severe head injury, the transducer initially showed a good pulse tracing but then had to be repositioned a few days later following a decompressive craniotomy and gave erratic readings with a poor pulse tracing. The transducer was removed and found to be separated from the dura by a thin layer of epidural clot.

Discussion

A telemetered epidural ICP monitor has several advantages over fluid coupled systems: 1) minimizes risk of infection because there is no percutaneous pathway; 2) minimizes risk of cerebral infection because the dura is intact; 3) does not become obstructed by swollen brain; 4) increases patient mobility.

These factors outweigh the drawbacks of not being able to withdraw CSF and the somewhat increased surgical time required for exact dural coplanarity and rigid fixation.

The transducer has been particularly helpful in monitoring those patients receiving high-dose barbiturate therapy. Without being able to monitor ICP, the endpoint of therapy is not clear. Using the ICP monitor with intravenous thiopental, we try to keep the ICP below 16 torr. In those patients receiving large doses of thiopental at surgery for difficult aneurysms or cases where elective hypothermia and cardiac arrest is employed (giant aneurysms and hemangioblastomas of the medulla), ICP monitoring is the most sensitive guide to postoperative complications since the patient may not awaken for 24 hours.

References

1. Fryer TB, Corbin SD, Silvergerg GD, Schmidt EV, Ream AK (1978) Telemetry of intracranial pressure. Biotelemetry and Patient Monitoring 5:88-112

2. Ream AK, Silverberg GD, Corbin SD, Schmidt EV, Fryer TB (in press) Epidural measurement of intracranial pressure. Neurosurg

Work supported in part by NASA NGR 05-020-634.
Work carried out at Stanford University School of Medicine.

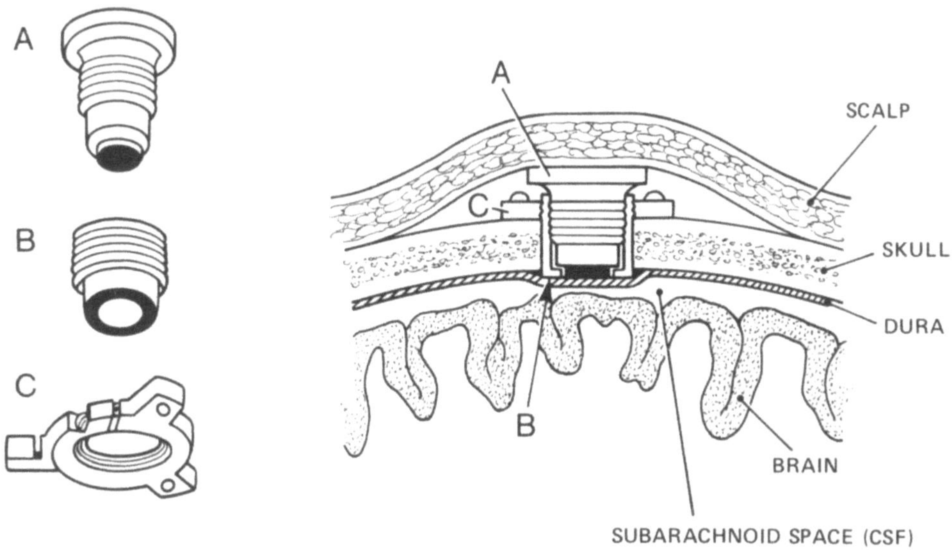

Figure 1.
Transducer configuration. A) Pressure transducer and telemetry package. B) Guard ring. C) Flanged bracket.

INTRACRANIAL PRESSURE STUDIES IN ACUTELY ILL NEONATES USING A NONINVASIVE TECHNIQUE: A THREE YEAR EXPERIENCE

T.N.K.Raju and D.Vidyasagar

Introduction

In the newborn period, the presence of an open anterior fontanel (AF) permits one to assess intracranial pressure (ICP) by palpation. For accurate recording of pressure however, this method is inadequate. We therefore utilized a transducer for placement over the fontanel for measurement of ICP in the newborn.

Materials and Methods

A Ladd fiberoptic transducer, placed on a special holding device, was secured over the AF with Velcro tape. The sensitive surface of the transducer was in contact with the fontanel. A Roche ICP monitor was used to measure ICP. The technique has been published in detail elsewhere (5,6). Over a three year period, we have studied ICP from a group of normal infants and in a variety of sick newborns in the intensive care unit.

Results

Normal newborns: In 46 normal term infants and 6 normal preterm infants the ICP was 9.6 $\pm$ 0.4cm of H_2O (mean $\pm$ SEM). Crying and spontaneous movements of the infant caused wide fluctuations in ICP (Figure 1A). Respiratory distress: In a group of 32 infants with hyaline membrane disease (HMD) the mean $\pm$ SEM ICP was 13.3 $\pm$ 0.6cm of H_2O. Four of these developed neonatal intracranial hemorrhage (ICH) and the ICP rose to 25 $\pm$ 2.6cm of H_2O within 12 to 24 hours after the episode. In 16 infants with HMD without ICH, the pressure returned to 9.4 $\pm$ 0.8cm of H_2O during recovery. Meconium aspiration syndrome and birth asphyxia: (MAS and BA): ICP varied widely in this group. Eleven infants were studied. In 7 who made an uneventful recovery, the ICP was 24.1 $\pm$ 1.8cm of H_2O during the acute phase and 15.6 $\pm$ 3.5cm of H_2O during recovery. In 4 other infants with very severe birth asphyxia, monitoring for a mean period of 8.1 hours was carried out. Mean $\pm$ SEM ICP in these infants was 53.1 $\pm$ 4.5. Three of the four died and the fourth infant has cerebral palsy. In one infant with birth asphyxia, an episode of seizure occurred during monitoring. ICP changes are shown in Figure 1B.

Other disorders: Figure 2 illustrates the ICP values in infants with meningitis, birth asphyxia, ICH and hydrocephalus. In all hydrocephalus infants ICP returned to the normal range (10 cm of H_2O) following shunt surgery, and in one of them, an obstructed shunt was diagnosed when ICP rose to 20cm of H_2O.

Discussion

EPSTEIN et al (2) modified the implantable switch originally described by NUMOTO and associates (3). We used the same sensor for placement over the fontanel. The technique of measuring ICP is simple and noninvasive. Similar values of ICP in normal newborns have been obtained by using a different device by SALMON et al (4). We and others have shown a good correlation of ICP obtained at the fontanel and ICP measured directly at the lumbar and ventricular level (r, 0.95, y = 1.08x + 2.7), (1,5). The explanation for the increased pressure in infants with hydrocephalus and meningitis seems to be obvious. Infants with HMD are susceptible to hypoxic episodes and this could explain raised ICP. Infants with ischemic hypoxic brain damage due to birth asphyxia usually have cerebral edema (7) which might be responsible for elevated pressure seen in this group of infants.

Summary

The noninvasive technique of measuring ICP described here is safe and accurate. ICP monitoring in sick newborn infants is helpful in the clinical management.

References

1. Donn SM, Phillip AGS (1978) Early increase in intracranial pressure in preterm infants. Pediatrics 61:904-907

2. Epstein F, Wald A, Hochwald GM (1966) Intracranial pressure during compressive head wrapping in treatment of neonatal hydrocephalus. Pediatrics 54:786-790

3. Numoto M, Slater JP, Donaghy RMP (1966) An implantable switch for monitoring intracranial pressure. Lancet 1:528

4. Salmon JH, Hajjar W, Bada HS (1977) The Fontogram: A noninvasive intracranial pressure monitor. Pediatrics 60:721-725

5. Vidyasagar D, Raju TNK (1977)A simple noninvasive technique of measuring intracranial pressure in the newborn. Pediatrics 59: 957-961

6. Vidyasagar D, Raju TNK, Chiang J (1978) Clinical significance of monitoring anterior fontanel pressure in sick neonates and infants. Pediatrics 62:996-999

7. Volpe JJ (1975) Neurological disorders. In: Avery GB (ed) Neonatology; Pathophysiology and Management of the Newborn. Lippincott Co., Philadelphia, p. 729-795

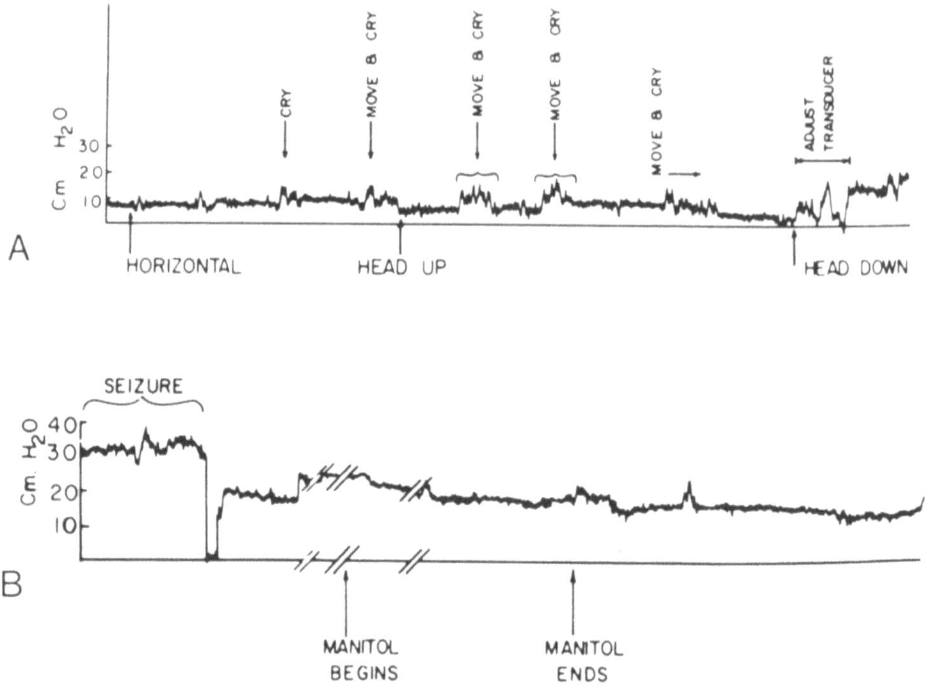

Figure 1.
ICP measured via the fontanel in a normal infant (A), and in an infant with birth asphyxia (B). During the period of recording the infant developed a seizure. Following mannitol therapy over a 2 hour period, ICP started to fall.

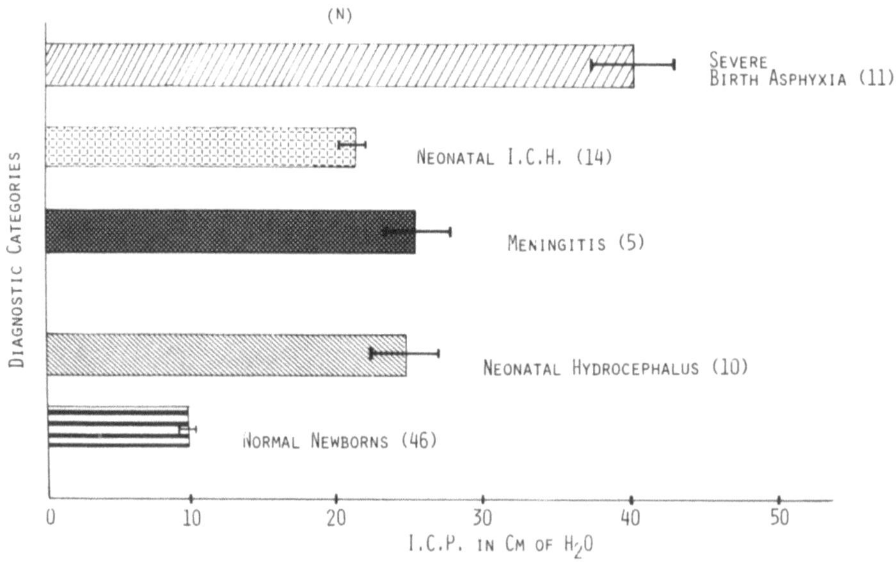

Figure 2.
Mean ± ICP from normal and sick newborns.

THE CONTROL OF ICP USING THREE ASYNCHRONOUS CLOSED LOOPS

D.J.PRICE, R.E.DUGDALE, AND J.MASON

Introduction

The prevention of secondary brain damage after head injury is the ultimate priority in any neurosurgeon's management regime. This protective vigil over a vulnerable traumatised brain includes the detection and adequate correction of midline shift, the immediate recognition and treatment of hypoxia and the continuous maintenance of an adequate cerebral perfusion pressure.

We have shown a reduction in mortality of patients admitted in coma from 51% to 36% and in severe disability from 18% to 3% since applying these principles aggressively and using high doses of steroids and elective ventilation as required.

We hoped we could improve these results further by controlling ICP more effectively. Until then, our treatment of intracranial hypertension had been unstructured and haphazard and our junior colleagues were rightly demanding a more objective approach.

Materials and Methods

Development of data processing methods: At the same time, we were trying to find a sufficiently reliable method of predicting a rise in mean ICP to enable us to treat that prediction and therefore prevent the rise. We purchased a PDP11 minicomputer with 24K of memory and 2 disks with an excellent real time foreground/background operating system. We rather presumed that we could make the prediction by simply applying one of the conventional forms of time-series analysis to the ICP signal. This involved slow sampling speeds and was very economical on computer memory. We soon abandoned this idea as it became apparent that the result would not be sufficiently reliable for application to "prophylactic" therapy. We then used Fast Fourier Transform analysis of the signal expecting to consistently find the cardiac and respiratory components. In the low frequency spectrum, we also found a body temperature regulating signal (2). We observed during continuous saline infusion tests that an increase in the cardiac component preceded a rise in mean confirming the observations of TURNER et al (6) that an increase in standard deviation of the ICP often provides a warning of an impending rise of pressure. As the standard deviation also contains the respiratory wave form with its superimposed influence of nursing and physiotherapy procedures, this secondary signal was too noisy as an input to a therapy model. Along with AVESAAT et al (1) and SZEWCZYKOWSKI et al (5) we increased our sampling rate in order to measure the Pulse Wave Amplitude (PWA) and the Pulse Wave Mean (PWM). We were able to avoid the need to concurrently sample the ECG by setting the sampling window within 1.4 second epochs to the cardiac cycle time as calculated from the heart rate. We were therefore able to produce a systolic and diastolic pressure reading every 1.4 seconds without significant influence from the respiratory wave-form.

In our continuing efforts to calculate a simple factor related to cerebral elastance, we attempted a linear regression on the 600 PWM and PWA pairs every 15 minutes. As most of our severe head injured patients were electively ventilated, the pulse wave components were fairly stable and a linear regression rarely produced a meaningful slope. We found that by dividing the PWA by the PWM each 1.4 seconds and then calculating the overall mean of these quotients at the end of each 15 minute epoch, a useful approximation to an index of elastance was achieved but only if the mean ICP was above 25mmHg. This calculation presumed that the graph passed through the origin and failed to recognize that it has 2 linear components intercepting at a transition point. We found that the transition point remains in a reasonably constant position in an individual patient but we confirmed SZEWCZYKOWKIS'S findings (5) that there was considerable variation between one patient and another. By applying a linear regression to the data pairs during a 60 second period of intermittent jugular compression with maintenance of the PWM above 25mmHg a very good fit is usually obtained. From the slope and intercept and a knowledge of the amplitude prior to jugular compression, the transition point At,Mt can be determined (Figure 1). This calculation is computed automatically whenever we carry out a jugular compression and can update the values of At and Mt. Each 15 minutes, the Pulse Wave Index and its standard deviation is calculated (Figure 2) and recorded on the data base along with the mean and standard deviation if the PWA, PWM and perfusion pressure. The Pulse Wave Index (PWI) is equivalent to the elastivity described by SZEWCZYKOWSKI (5). In the last 100 head injured patients monitored in this way, we have ascertained the ranges of At and Mt.

Manually controlled loop therapy: As soon as we had established the continuous monitoring of perfusion pressure, PWM and PWI, as routine in head injured patients, we tested these with several traditional forms of therapy. Furosemide proved more effective than Mannitol for the control of a rising PWI and we were satisfied that Mannitol remained the agent of choice for reducing the PWM. The only sure way of rapidly preventing falls in perfusion pressure below a presumed danger level of 50mmHg was by releasing the ventricular catheter to allow drainage of just sufficient CSF to return that pressure to above that danger level. This development of 3 asynchronous manually controlled loops each with a precise monitoring parameter linked to specific therapy regime proved useful. As a rise in PWI usually preceded a rise in PWM, Furosemide was administered as a first-line treatment often preventing a rise in PWM and therefore Mannitol was required less frequently. If Mannitol failed to control the mean, the perfusion pressure would fall indicating the need for ventricular drainage and then if control was lost at this stage, we would proceed with urgent decompressive surgery. A reasonably rigid protocol for our junior medical staff and nurses gradually developed and we now had 3 models aimed at prevention and control of intracranial hypertension. Although the instructions were precise, a patient with poorly stabilized ICP could be the cause of several hours of time consuming vigilance by the nursing staff and insomnia by the junior doctors!

Automation of closed loops: Having formulated the treatment regime, automation was a small and logical step forward. By this time, all but 300 of the 2 year $40,000 research grant had been used to purchase and install the hardware and software. Fortunately, this was just sufficient to achieve this next step. We were aware of the work of SHEPPARD et al (4) and their attempts to control arterial blood pressure by closed loop but their model was very different. We used 3 decoupled loops (Figure 3) with non-adapting parameters and elective information time delays appropriate to the response times required and to ensure adequate loop stabilization with minimal resonance. We applied delays of 30 minutes for the PWI/Furosemide loop, 15 minutes for the PWM/ Mannitol loop and 30 seconds for the perfusion pressure/CSF drainage loop.

Our previous experience with single loop control of status epilepticus (3) proved useful and we use similar logic actuated relays to control a syringe pump containing 200 mgs of Furosemide and a standard infusion pump for administration of 20% Mannitol. Both agents are delivered to the intravenous line at a point close to the cannula. The drainage of CSF is controlled by a sterilisable solenoid valve which opens the catheter for intermittent 1 second periods. Therapy data is continuously available on a graphics terminal at the nurses' station with the PWM, PWI and perfusion pressure for simultaneous visualisation of treatment and effect.

Safety precautions: Any excess use of a drug is automatically displayed and the automatic infusion mechanism then becomes disabled. A manual override to allow further drug administration can be applied after the necessary checks of plasma osmolarity and electrolytes have been made.

Software and hardware fail-safe mechanisms are in-built to each part of the 3 loops. We are developin g the use of a conventional home computer as an intelligent terminal with color graphics for linkage through a Modem for retrieval of the ICP and therapy data by the on-call neurosurgeon at his home.

Summary

The isolation of a reliable monitoring index closely related to elastance and formalization of treatment algorithms proved to be a greater challenge than the automation of the closed loops. By using three decoupled loops, control of intracranial hypertension is established with greater ease and precision.

References

1. Avezaat CJJ, Van Eijndhoven JHM, De Jong DA, Moolenaar WCJ (1976) A new method of monitoring intracranial volume/pressure relationship. In: Beks JWF, Bosch DA, Brock M (eds) Intracranial Pressure III. Springer, Berlin Heildelberg New York, p 308

2. Harness JB, Mearns AJ, Mason J, Price DJ (in preparation) The influence of body temperature regulation on the ICP signal.

3. Price DJ, Mason J, Dugdale RE (1979) An attempt at more effective control of status epilepticus by using a computer. J Neurol Neurosurg Psychiat 42:286

4. Sheppard LC, Kouchoukos NT, Kurtts MA, Kirklin JW (1968) Automated treatment of critically ill patients following operation. Ann Surg 168:596-604

5. Szewczykowski J, Sliwka ST, Kunicki A, Dytko P, Korsak-Sliwka J: A fast method for estimating the elastance of the intracranial system. J Neurosurg 47:19-26

6. Turner JM, McDowall Dg, Gibson RM, Khalili HL (1976) Computer analysis of intracranial pressure measurements. In: ICP III. Springer Berlin Heidelberg New York, p 283

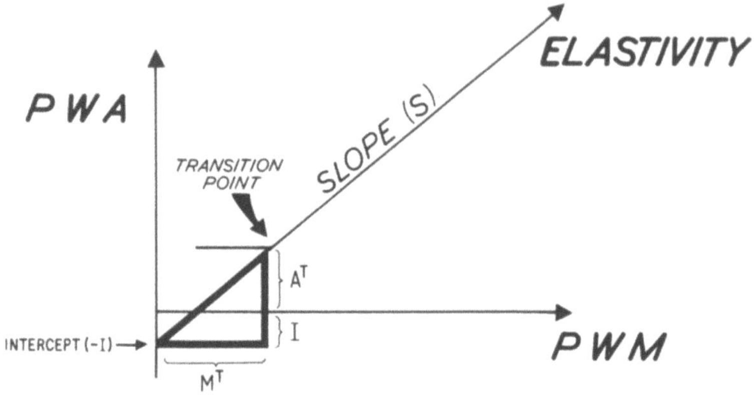

$$M^T = \frac{A^T + I}{S}$$

Fig. 1. Estimation of transition point from linear regression during jugular compression.

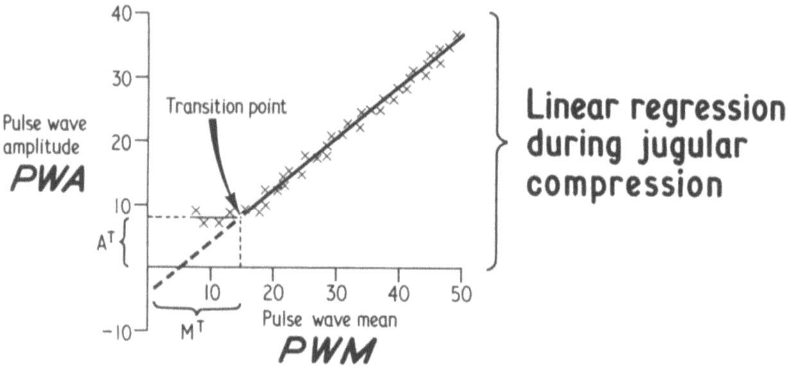

$$\text{ELASTIVITY} = \frac{\sum(\text{PULSE WAVE AMPLITUDE} - A^T)}{\sum(\text{PULSE WAVE MEAN} - M^T)}$$

Fig. 2. Continuous monitoring of elastivity (Pulse Wave Index) from Pulse Wave Amplitude and Pulse Wave Mean.

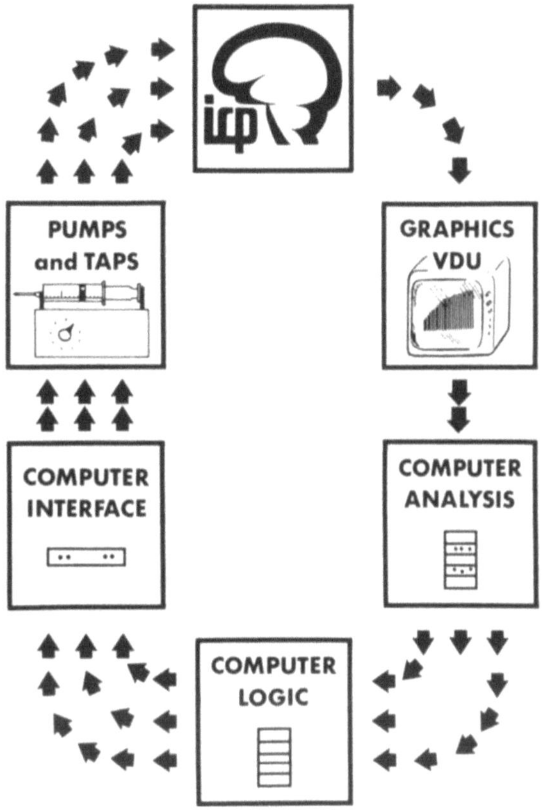

Fig. 3. Automation of 3 decoupled closed loops.

A COMBINATION OF BED SIDE ICP RECORDINGS; HISTOGRAM, TREND-GRAPH, AND DIGITAL PRINT

H. TAKIZAWA, T. CHISHIKI, K. MURAOKA, AND K. SUGIURA

Introduction

Advantages of continuous ICP monitoring are now well recognized. Various methods of recording and displaying ICP data have been proposed, but are mostly experimental.

We have been performing daily ICP data recording in three different ways, namely histogram, trend-graph, and digital print. This report deals with comparative evaluations of these three recording methods.

Material and methods

ICP was detected through a lateral ventricular catheter and a pressure transducer. Fig I is a block diagram of our ICP recording system, containing two microcomputers.

Trend-graph portion records the analog ICP value in a traditional manner. Histogram portion samples ICP value three times per second and accumulates them to calculate the mean ICP and to make a histogram. Accumulation time is presettable in several steps from 5 minutes to 24 hrs. Range of measurement is chosen from four levels: (I) -5~+20 mmHg, (2) -10~+40, (3) -20~+80, (4) -40~+160. Pressure class is 0.5 mmHg in range (I) and (2), I mmHg in (3), and 2 mmHg in (4). The histogram thus classified is shown on an oscilloscope during the accumulation of data, and is recorded on a paper at the end of accumulation time.

Digital print portion samples ICP value every one minute averaged by an integral circuit with a time constant of 5 seconds. The time and the ICP value are printed on a paper and displayed on a monitor TV. The mean ICP value is also shown every ten minutes.

Results

Fig 2 is an example of ICP data recorded with these different ways. (a) is a digital print of ICP value and the time. Mean ICP value of ten minutes is also printed. (b) shows a trend-graph of 6 hrs and (c) is its histogram. This case had abnormally high ICP that had to be controlled by intermittent ventricular drainage. The histogram had double-humped distribution; a high peak of basal pressure level ranges from 0 to 8 mmHg and a lower peak of abnormally increased pressure level ranges from 14 to 40 mmHg. The weight of the abnormally high pressure is about 40% of the whole pressure distribution.

Discussion

Each of these methods for ICP recording has its own merits and drawbacks, and a combination of them will compensate each other for further ICP analysis.

ICP was usually recorded in a trend-graph and analyzed visually to detect the tendency of ICP change in a short-term, and to find a plateau or other abnormal waves. It was, however, difficult to compare objectively the ICP data of a long time course.

BROCK et al (1) stated the biggest advantage of histographic presentation is the high degree of data compression. Comparison of data of long-term for example of 12 or 24 hrs. may become necessary to determine whether intracranial pressure condition is improving or not. A histogram of ICP would be the most convenient for this purpose. It is also easy to know a range of ICP fluctuation, a baseline pressure level or "typical" pressure level, presence and its weight of abnormally high pressure.

Methods of obtaining a histogram of ICP have been different among several authors (2,3,4). Two points should be discussed here: (1) the frequency of data sampling, and (2) the pressure class. Theory of NYQUIST frequency shows that, with our sampling rate of three times per second, it would become possible to analyze correctly the ICP fluctuation of cycles up to 90 per minute. It is obvious that ICP has higher frequency fluctuation mainly under the influence of heart beats. Although higher frequency of data sampling is preferable to make a more correct histogram, it would make the number of data overwhelming. From the clinical standpoint our histogram analyzer was designed to present the distribution of pressure of a long time course totally, and was not aimed to analyze the fluctuations over 90 cycles per minute in a shorter-term. For this purpose the trend-graph would be more suitable.

KULLBERG (2) made a histogram with pressure class of 10 mmHg, and JANNY et al (3) 2 mmHg. Optimal pressure class would depend on the range of measurements to be analyzed, but it should theoretically be as small as possible. Our histogram analyzer has the small pressure classification of 0.5~2 mmHg, and is proved to be very useful for bedside ICP monitoring.

Digital print-out of ICP value is convenient to know the value numerically at a certain time and to perform statistical analysis. Statistical parameters are known to be useful in analyzing the distribution of ICP. JANNY et al (3) studied several parameters and noticed that right and left standard deviation provided a measure of ICP fluctuations. Our preliminary study also showed that the standard deviation was the most suitable in determining the degree of ICP fluctuations, but skewness and kurtosis had only limited value for this purpose.

Summary

We have been performing bedside ICP recording in three different ways: histogram, trend-graph, and digital print-out. Trend-graph is indispensable to known an ICP change in a short-term and to find a plateau or other abnormal waves. Histogram is necessary to compare objectively the data of a long time course such as 12 or 24 hrs. Digital print-out can afford an ICP value numerically and is useful to perform the statistical analysis. A conclusion was drawn that adoption of each one of these methods should not defy the usage of others, and a combination of them would be the method of choice for a detailed analysis of ICP.

References

1. Brock M, Anywietz C, Mock P, Woeganad H, Zilig C, Tamburus WM (1976) Reliability and reproduceability of ICP frequency analysis. In: Beks JWF, Bosch DA, Brock M(eds) Intracranial Pressure III. Springer, Berlin Heidelberg New York, p 288

2. Kullberg G (1972) A method for statistical analysis of intracranial pressure recordings. In: Brock M, Dietz H (eds) Intracranial Pressure. Springer, Berlin Heidelberg New York,p 65

3. Janny P, Jouan JP, Janny L, Gourgand M, Gueit UM (1972) A statistical approach to long-term monitoring of intracranial pressure. In: Brock M, Dietz H (eds) Intracranial Pressure. Springer, Berlin Heidelberg New York, p 59

4. Barnes RW, McGraw CP (1975) A new on-line portable ICP data processor. In: Lundberg N, Ponten U, Brock M (eds) Intracranial Pressure II. Springer, Berlin Heidelberg New York, p 389

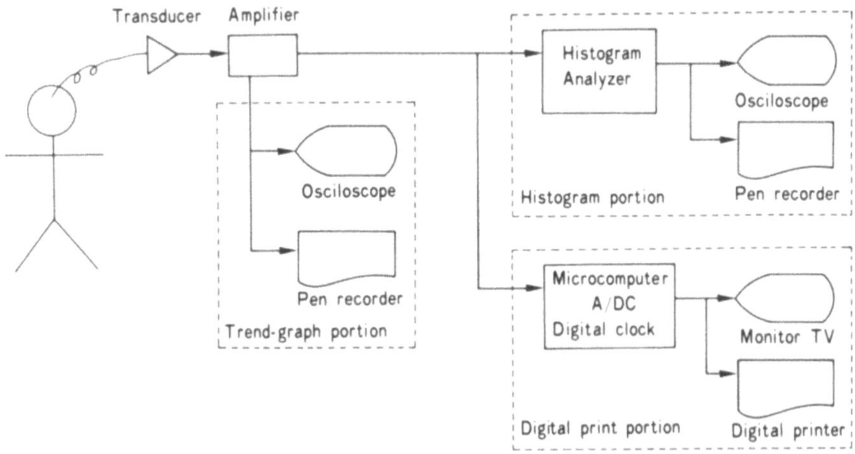

Fig. 1. Block-diagram of the ICP recording system.

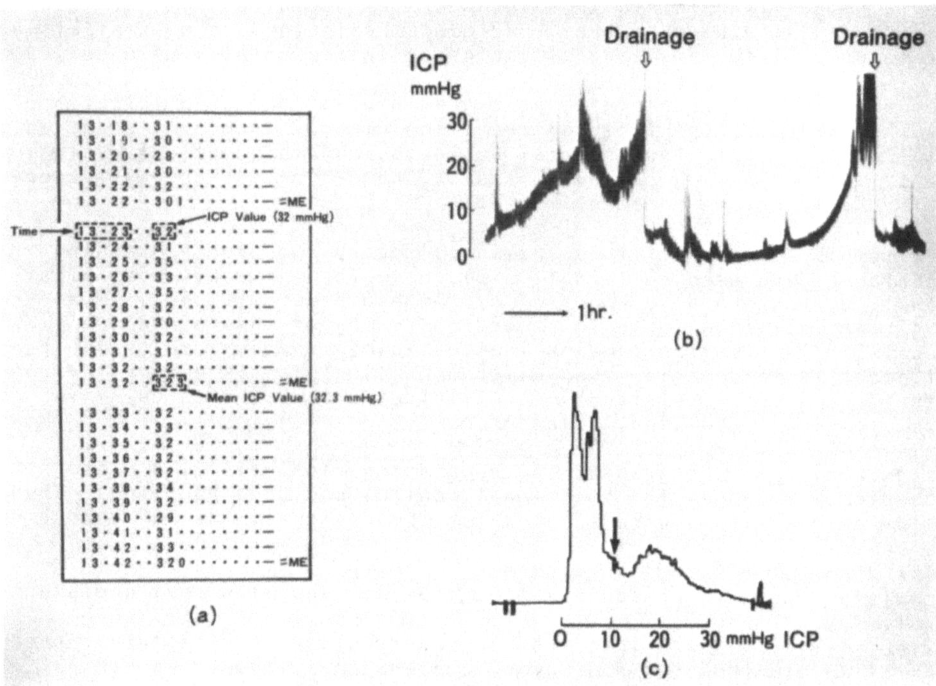

Fig. 2. An example of recorded ICP data. (a) Digital print-out, (b) Trend-graph of 6 hrs and (c) is its histogram. The mean ICP is shown on a histogram with a marker (arrow).

INTRACRANIAL PRESSURE REGISTRATION ADMINISTRATED BY A MICROPROCESSOR

D. STÅLHAMMAR, P. ARKELSJÖ, L. LINDSTRÖM, AND R. ÖRTENGREN

Introduction

There is accumulating evidence that intracranial pressure (ICP) registration is of definite value in routine clinical work for diagnosis, patient monitoring, treatment, and prognosis. However, the success of an ICP registration system depends on whether it fulfills a number of basic requirements and on its handiness in the acute clinical situation.

At bedside the access to the pressure information must be immediate; the pressure should be clearly and continuously displayed and recorded, and the course of the pressure during the past hours, and days even, should be easily retrievable. The clinical usefulness of the information should also be enhanced by automatic calculations of statistical parameters, histograms, and estimates of intracranial elastance(2,4,6).

Adequate documentation of the pressure information for clinical and research purpose must include: reduction of data from single patients, compilation of data from several patients, and mathematical evaluation. The utility of an ICP recording system that is small and easily portable should not be underestimated.

In attempts to meet all these demands, modern computer processing techniques have been applied (1,3,5), but, for the routine clinical situation, no generally accepted system has been developed. Most clinicians still use graphic recordings on paper sheets and great amounts of information remains inaccessible. The purpose of the present paper is to describe the design of a flexible system for ICP registration, primarily intended for clinical use, but with built-in possibilities to be used in research.

Design Features: Because of the demands on flexibility, a microprocessor was chosen for functional control and data handling. The following guidelines were adopted for the design of the ICP recording instrument:

Clear display of current pressure
Immediate access to pressure values from at least the past one and a half day
Portability with low weight, robust construction, and battery operation
Possibility to transfer the memory content to a large computer
Possibility to connect analog recording devices.

The design of the pressure measuring instrument is shown schematically in Fig 1. All communication within the instrument occurs on a common "bus" to which different digital circuits are connected: the microprocessor which controls all events, a memory containing the instructions for the microprocessor, an analog-to-digital converter which on command samples the signal from the pressure transducer and converts it to a binary form, a data memory in which all samples from the transducer are stored, a display unit which presents time and pressure values, an output interface for communication with large computers (for long-term storage of data, statistical evaluation,etc.), and a power control unit which switches off the power supply to the transducer when sampling does not occur.

The microprocessor is controlled by a stable crystal clock. The clock signal is also scaled down in frequency by a divider and used as an interrupt signal to control the timing of sampling. All digital circuits are CMOS-devices characterized by a very low power consumption. Accordingly, liquid crystal displays were chosen because of their negligible power requirements.

The instrument was originally developed for monitoring ICP during transportation of patients. Thus, the following mode of operation was chosen: Once every minute the power to the transducer and its circuits is turned on, the ICP is sampled for 4 s with a sampling frequency of 4 Hz, the mean pressure value is computed and stored. Hereafter, the power is switched off until the next minute period. The present time - in hours and minutes - and the pressure value are displayed.

With buttons on the front panel, scanning through previous data is controlled: fast or slow, backward or forward. The pressure values are then displayed together with the corresponding time of acquisition. Automatic reset to current pressure occurs if manual scanning has not been performed during the past minute. Of course, new sampling occurs independently of the display mode. During the initial phase, i.e., when mounting the pressure transducer on the patient, the microprocessor is programmed to continuously monitor the pressure. The buttons for scanning are then used to set the timer. A photograph of the instrument is shown in Fig 2.

Discussion

It should be emphasized that an instrument with the described configuration is very flexible indeed. By changing the transducer, measurements of other quantities can easily be administered by the same instrument. By changing the program memory, other modes of operation are obtained, e.g., computation of various statistical measures, harmonic analysis, and threshold analysis with alarm signal output. The mode of operation chosen for the instrument described here is, of course, a compromise between power consumption and possibility to retrieve stored data. One pressure datum each minute was considered enough from a clinical point of view; this rather low rate enables the instrument to operate intermittently having units with significant power consumption switched off most of the time. Each stored value represents the mean of 16 samples obtained during appxorimately four seconds. This choice was guided by a power spectrum analysis of ICP signals. As seen in Fig 3, the spectrum shows large peaks yielded by the respiration and the heart beats. A mean pressure value calculated as described will reduce most of these variations.

Clinical tests of the instrument have demonstrated its feasibility in routine work. Monitoring of cases with CSF shunts and "normal pressure hydrocephalus" has proved to be of particular value. The tests have also revealed an immediate need for other functions of the instrument. Such functions, easily obtained by re-programming, are calculation of perfusion pressure with ICP and arterial pressure as input signals, calculation of intracranial compliance from the relative heights of the spectral peaks pertaining to heart activity and respiration, and regression analysis for prediction of the future ICP development.

References

1. Barnes R, McGraw P (1975) A new on-line portable ICP data processor. In: Lundberg N, Ponten U, Brock M (eds) Intracranial Pressure II. Springer, Berlin Heidelberg New York, p 389

2. Brock M, Zywietz C, Mock P. Wiegand H, Zillig C, Tanburus WM(1975) Reliability and reproduceability of ICP frequency analysis. In: Lundberg N, Ponten U, Brock M (eds) Intracranial Pressure II. Springer, Berlin Heidelberg New York p 288

3. Hulme A, Cooper R (1975) Multi-channel data acquisition and analysis in clinical practice. In: Lundberg N, Ponten U, Brock M (eds) Springer, Berlin Heidelberg New York, p 387

4. Janny P, Fontaine J, Maille M, Colnet G, Hullo G, Janny L(1977) Un module d'analyse statistique de la pression intra-cranienne: le systeme A.S.P.I.C. Neurochirurg 3:187-194

5. Szewcykowski J, Korsak-Sliwka J, Kunicki A, Dytko PW, Sliwka S, Dziduszko J (1975) Computer-Assisted determination of optimum ICP levels. In: Lundberg N, Ponten U, Brock M (eds) Intracranial Pressure II. Springer, Berlin Heidelberg New York, p 295

6. Turner J, Gibson R, McDowall D, Nahhas F (1975) Further experience with extradural pressure monitoring. In: Lundberg N, Ponten U, Brock M (eds) Intracranial Pressure II. Springer, Berlin Heidelberg New York p 397

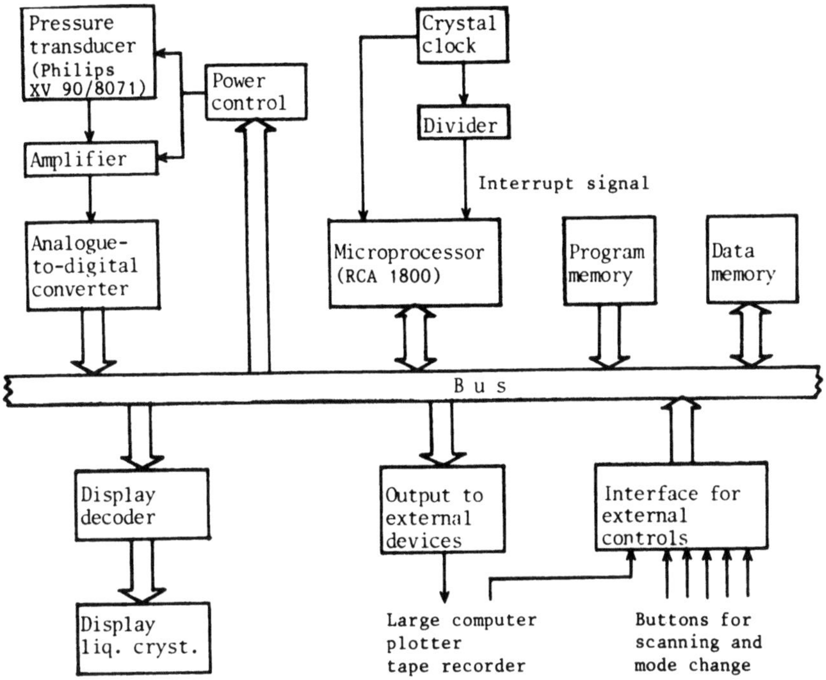

Fig. 1. Architecture of the microprocessor controlled ICP registration instrument.

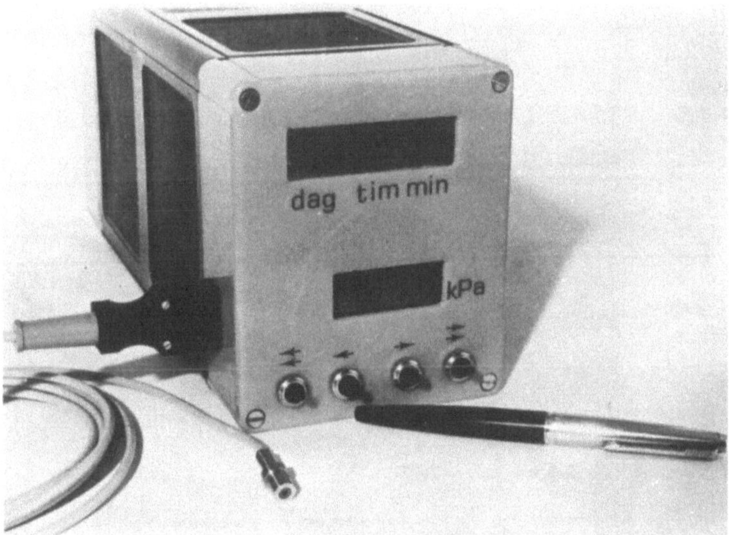

Fig.2. External view of the ICP-registration instrument with an EDP-transducer (Philips XV 90/7081). The total weight is 2.1 kg.

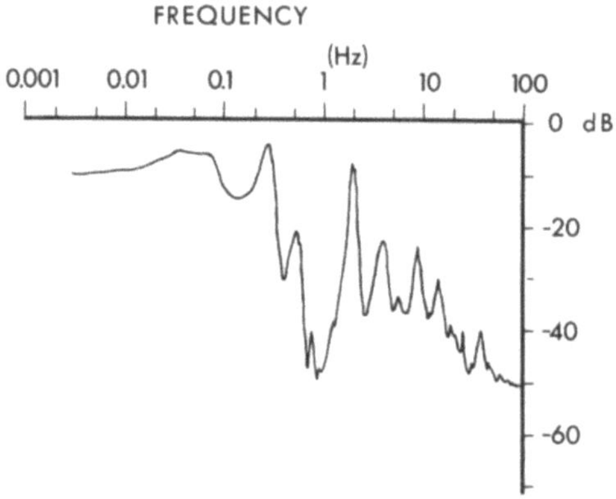

Fig. 3. Power spectrum of an ICP signal with marked peaks caused by respiration and heart activity.

A MICROCOMPUTER SYSTEM FOR ICP ANALYSIS

S.H.GRAHAM, L.E.HACKENBERRY, G.REA, AND M.E.MINER

Introduction

Analysis of ICP has been primarily limited to the evaluation of mean pressure; however the pulsatile component of ICP may also contain useful information. Changes in the ICP waveform have been noted with intracranial hypertension, changes in arterial blood pressure and central venous pressure (CVP), hypoxia and hypercapnia (1,2,3). Analyzing the ICP waveform by chart recorder is impractical for routine measurements; therefore we have developed a microcomputer system to acquire, store, and analyze ICP waveform data.

Material and methods

The system consists of a Z-80 microcomputer with 64K bytes of semiconductor memory, two eight inch floppy disk drives, a CRT terminal, a printer, analog to digital (A/D) and digital to analog (D/A) convertors, and an oscilloscope used to display waveforms. Using timers or the R wave of the EKG to generate interrupts which pass control from one program to another, the microprocessor performs several tasks simultaneously. Maxima and minima of the ICP waveform can be detected and used to continuously monitor ICP pulse height. Data may be sampled every 5 msec, and signal averages with respect to the EKG spike. Waveforms are displayed every 16 msec by outputting data to the oscilloscope via the D/A converter. A BASIC program runs simultaneously that controls all these tasks and displays data to the CRT terminal and stores it on floppy disks.

We used an animal experiment to demonstrate the system. Four dogs were anesthesized with pentobarbital, intubated, and respirated to maintain normal blood PO_2 and PCO_2. A catheter tip pressure transducer was inserted subdurally, and an epidural balloon was tunnelled over the contralateral hemisphere. Arterial pressure, heart rate, CVP, mean intracranial pressure, and the amplitude of the ICP pulsations were recorded by the microcomputer every 30 seconds and samples of waveforms were signal averaged.

Results

Fig 1 illustrates the effect of hemorrhagic hypotension upon the ICP waveform in one animal. At a mean arterial blood pressure (MAP) of 60 mmHg, the amplitude of the ICP pulsations (A) is almost three times the amplitude of the ICP pulse at a MAP of 110 mmHg (B). Fig 2 shows the effect of the inflation of the epidural balloon on pulsatile and mean ICP in one animal. Measurements were made 5 minutes after each mass increment. For the initial increments of mass, pulsatile ICP increases were much more striking than the increases in mean ICP.

Discussion

More detailed and convenient analysis of the ICP waveform is possible with the microcomputer than with traditional means. Even the simplest measure of ICP waveform, the pulse amplitude, may have certain advantages over mean pressure analysis. Two factors may produce increases in pulse height: vasodilation, as in the case of hypotension, and increases in intracranial elastance, as with increasing intracranial mass. Due to the nonlinear nature of the pressure-volume relationship, initial increases in intracranial mass result in small changes in intracranial pressure. Therefore, monitoring of ICP alone does not provide a sensitive means of detecting increasing intracranial mass. Pulsatile ICP is sensitive to increases in intracranial elastance and cerebral vasodilation, two parameters which accompany decompensation and steep increases in ICP.

A microcomputer system has been developed to continuously measure mean ICP and the amplitude of ICP pulsations, and sample and signal average the ICP waveform. Increases in the amplitude of ICP pulsations were seen with hemorrhagic hypotension and with increasing supratentorial mass. Monitoring ICP waveform changes may be a useful adjunct to monitoring mean ICP.

References

1. Dunbar HS, Guntrie T, Karpell B (1966) A study of the cerebrospinal fluid pulse wave. Arch Neurol 14:624-630

2. Hamer J, Alberti E, Hoyer S, Wiedemann K (1977) Influence of systemic and cerebral vascular factors on the cerebrospinal pulse waves. J Neurosurg 46:36-45

3. Hamit HF, Beall AC, Debakey ME (1965) Hemodynamic influences upon brain and cerebrospinal fluid pulsations and pressures. J Trauma 5:174-184

Work supported by NIH Grant SR01 NS 13251.

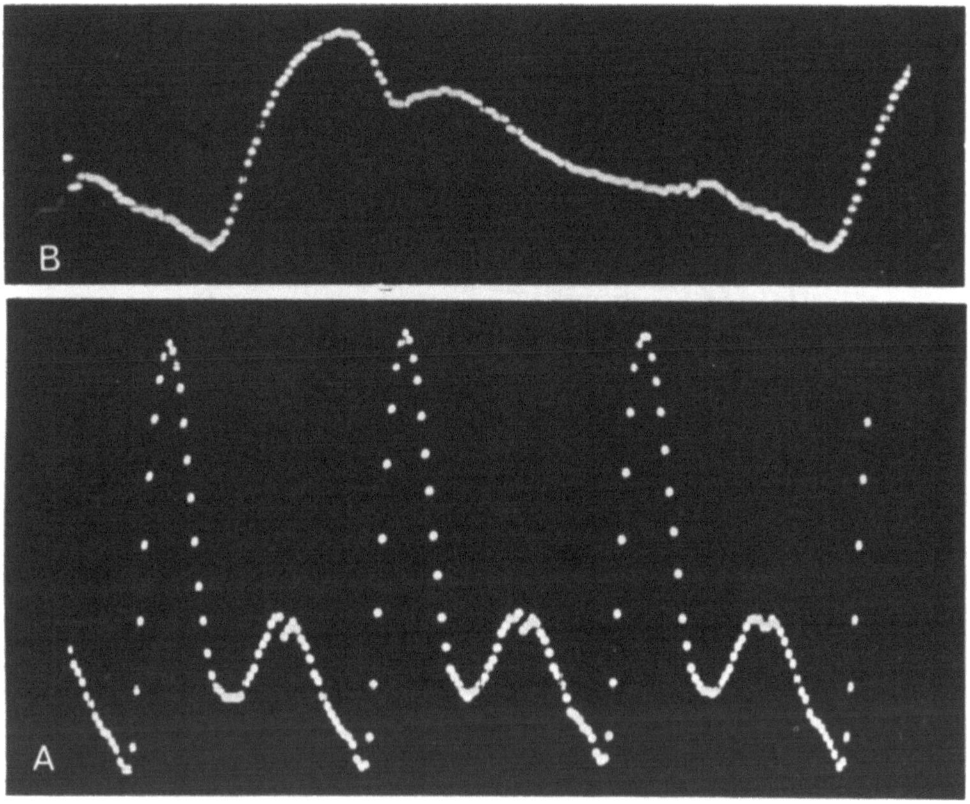

Fig 1. ICP waveforms signal averaged 10 times with respect to R wave of ICP. Sampling interval = 50 msec; 1 second = total frame duration. Vertical resolution = .0234 mmHg, 6 mmHg full scale.

(A). ICP waveform with MAP = 110 mmHg, ICP = 8 mmHg, Amplitude= 1.10 mmHg.

(B). ICP waveform during hemorrhagic hypotension. MAP = 60 mmHg, CIP = 10 mmHg. Amplitude = 3.12 mmHg.

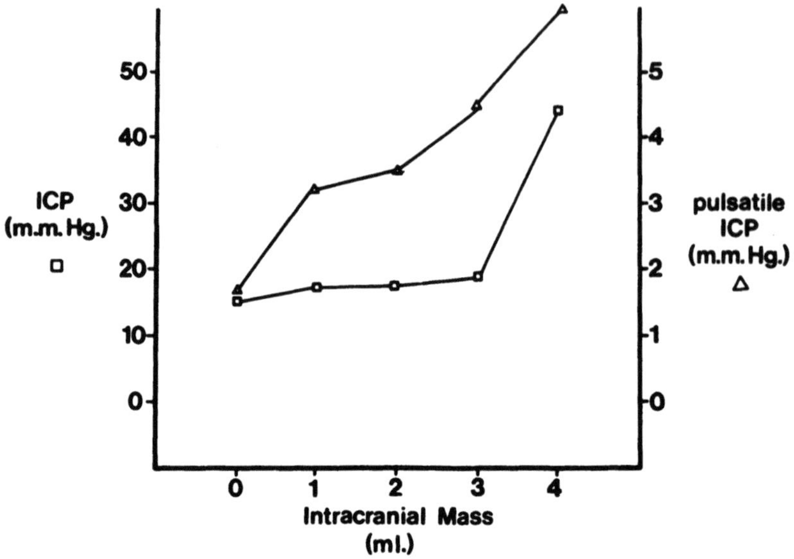

Fig. 2. Pulsatile ICP and mean ICP at intracranial masses 0-4 cc. Measurements were taken 5 minutes after each l cc inflation of the balloon.

EPIDURAL MEASUREMENT OF INTRACRANIAL PRESSURE

W.G.KOSTER AND M.H.KUYPERS

Introduction

Thanks to JANNY (5) and LUNDBERG (7) intraventricular pressure (IVP) can be measured continuously, but routine clinical use of IVP is hampered by the risk of infection, difficulties in puncturing the ventricles of high-pressure patients, catheter blockages, and leakage of fluid. These problems can be avoided by epidural methods, with the dura mater remaining closed and the transducer applied against it; but it is necessary to pay particular attention to the stability of the transducer (and amplifier) and to agreement between ventricular and epidural measurements.

Stability of the Transducer: In the epidural methods, the transducer is zeroed before implantation, and no further adjustments should be made during implantation to avoid infection. Each signal from the transducer is a combination of a pressure signal and a component caused by electrical instability of the transducer. Implantation periods of from a few days to several weeks are required. As normal pressure is about 5 - 10 mmHg, transducer instability should be of the order of 1 mmHg per implantation period if serious errors are to be avoided; with conventional transducers such stability is unobtainable. Using modern semi-conductor technology, the sensitive elements of a Wheatstone bridge can be incorporated in a silicone membrane (2), thus avoiding many of the disadvantages of conventional transducers. Working closely with the neurosurgical department of the ACADEMISCH ZIEKENHUIS in Groningen (head: Prof Dr. J.W.F.BEKS), a transducer with exceptionally high zero stability has been developed. Over an extended period of experiment and development, the packaging of the sensitive part has been improved to give a typical in-vivo zero stability of 0.25 mmHg per week for the complete system (1,4), thus more than satisfying clinical requirements.

Epidural Method: Even with a very stable transducer, the pressure of the volume contained by a biological membrane can only be measured accurately when forces present within the membrane itself are prevented from reaching the sensitive part of the transducer. This so-called co-planarity principle was first described by KLEIBER (6), and is used also in neurosurgery (8).

In Fig 1 the method is presented schematically. A self-tapping screw adaptor is screwed into an 11-mm burr-hole, until the co-planar ring touches the dura. It is given another full turn (1-mm) further intrusion to ensure proper contact with the dura, and the transducer is automatically made co-planar with the ring of the adaptor so as to ensure accurate measurement. This implantation method has the further advantage that the whole set-up is rigidly fixed in the skull so that it cannot be pulled out by the patient. This small appliance causes no discomfort to the patient.

Table I. CLINICAL EXPERIENCE

Name of Clinic	Number of Patients			Duration of monitoring (days)	Literature
	Total	Both epidural and ventricular measurements	Epidural measurements only		
GRONINGEN Prof. Beks Dr. Belopavlovic	>600	80	520	1-7	Beks, ICP III, 251-254 (1976) Beks, Medicamundi 23:156-159(1978) Belopavlovic, Paris (1978)
COPENHAGEN Dr.Gjerris	76	45	31	3	Gjerris, this issue
GIESSEN Prof. Lorenz Dr. Zierski	19	15	4	Max.7 days	Zierski,Medizinelektronik5:2-7 (1977) Zierski, this issue
MAINZ Dr. Hase	19	14	5	2-11	Hase, Neurochir 21:84-90 (1978)
MUNCHEN Dr. Abbushi	19	-	19	Average 6	Abbushi, Medicamundi 23:160-165 (1978)
GOTHENBURG Dr.Stalhammar	17	15	2	2-13	Stalhammar, this issue
CLERMONT - FERRAND Prof. Janny	11	11	-	½-5	Janny, this issue

Clinical Tests: Model studies have shown that with this epidural arrangement intracranial pressure can be measured reliably: it has been used with success on more than 1000 patients distributed over many neurosurgical institutes. Over one hundred comparisons have been made between the epidural and intraventricular systems (Table I), most of them showing a high degree of coincidence. Extensive clinical results are presented elsewhere in this issue (3,9). In cases of communicating hydrocephalus, ventricular and epidural pressures have always been found to be identical (3). In other cases, the two pressures are usually within a few mmHg, but although occasional differences of 10-15 mmHg have been found - whether these are errors in measurement, or are based on real pressure differences (gradients), is not yet established. Only two serious infections have been noticed, and no serious necroses.

Summary

An epidural method is described for measuring intracranial pressure, using a specially developed transducer, with extremely good zero stability (less than 1 mmHg per week), that is rigidly fixed in a hole through the skull. This method has been used with success on more than 1000 patients distributed over more than ten neurosurgical institutes in Europe. Over one hundred comparisons have been made between this system and intraventricular measurement. Most of them show a high degree of similarity.

References

1. Beks JWF (1978) The measurement of intracranial pressure - some considerations. Medicamundi 23:156-159

2. Gieles ACM (1978) Application of IC Technology. In: Regtien PPL (ed) Measuring Techniques: Modern Electronics Measuring Systems. Delft University Press, p 25

3. Gjerris F, Børgesen SW, Sørensen SC. Clinical evaluation of a new epidural pressure transducer. This issue.

4. Hase U (1978) Intrakranielle Druckmessung. Neurochirurgia 21: 84-90

5. Janny P (1950) La Pression Intracranielle Chez l'Homme. Thesis. Aubriere, Clermont Reproduction 1972.

6. Kleiber M (1945) A tympanometer. Rev Scient Instr 16:79-81

7. Lundberg N (1960) Continuous recoring and control of ventricular fluid pressure in neurosurgical practice. Acta Psychiat Neurol Scand Suppl 149, 36:1-193

8. Schettini A, Mahig J (1972) Intracranial pressure measurements and rheological behaviour of the intracranial system. J Neurosurg 37:170-176

9. Zierski J. Extradural: Ventricular and Subdural pressure recording: comparative experimental and clinical study. This issue

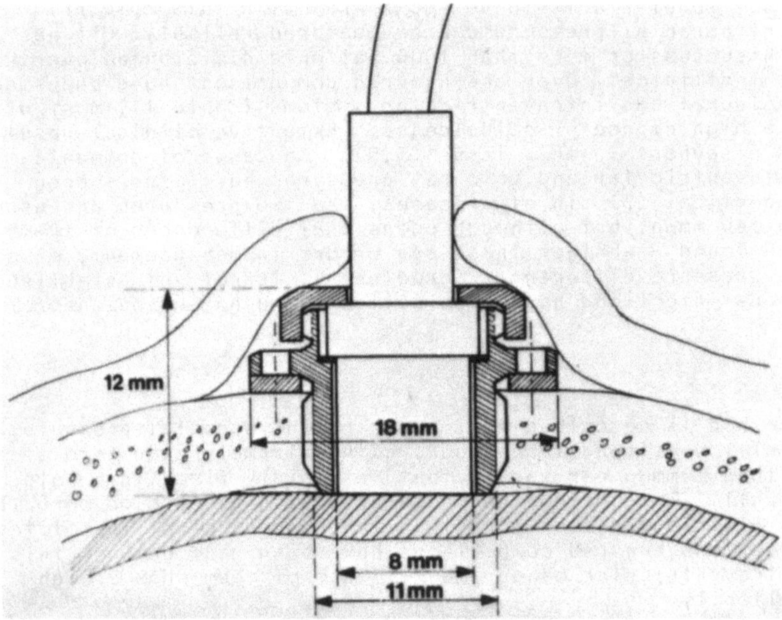

Fig 1. Implanted transducer

A NEWLY DEVISED TRANSDUCER FOR EPIDURAL PRESSURE MEASUREMENT AND ITS CLINICAL USE

H.NAGAI, I.KAMIYA, J.IKEYAMA, AND O.INAGAKI

Epidural measurement of the intracranial pressure is correctly obtained when the transducer is positioned at a coplanar point. However, in practice, the EDP value measured by the conventional types has failed to coincide with the intraventricular pressure. The following possible causes could be estimated: adhesion, ambient temperature and minute irregularities of the dural surface. To eliminate them, we covered the surface of the diffuse type semiconductor strain gauge with silicone rubber of 0.5 mm thickness. This device has two advantages as follows. First, the diaphragm may not be directly affected by changes of the ambient temperature because of the increased heat capacity. Second, pressure on the concavities of the minute structure of the dural surface will be transmitted diffusely and thus stress concentration effect may be diminished. For the artifact, due to adhesion of the transducer with the dural surface, teflon was coated on the silicone rubber.

Two clinical prototypes of the transducer were made as illustrated in Fig I. On the right of Fig I is the transducer for adults and on the left for infants. The former was equipped with a tapered screw to fit the skull configuration and the latter was applied directly to the dura through a small burr hole. The correlation between pressure in the physical model (P-in) and transducer output (P-out) was investigated. As far as the transducer adjusted the coplanar point, the reactive force on the transducer could be minimized in the range from 0 to 800 mm H_2O of P-in. The P-out/P-in slopes obtained with the various examined membranes closely approximated those with hydrostatic pressure. When the device was applied to the dura at an angle of 15 degrees the output deviation of the transducer was within 10 percent of the standard value. This result suggested that the angulation effect was negligible in clinical use.

The transducer output/input curves of animals and humans were similar. The output began to increase when the transducer touched the dura. The pressure attained the ICP level at the depth of the coplanar point. The output revealed a plateau even when the transducer was further advanced in the depth of one or two milimeters in the vicinity of the coplanar point.

This shows that a considerable depth range is permitted in coplanar measurements of a living body with this transducer. Moreover, when the pressure transducer was advanced further so as to contact the brain tissue, the output increased sharply. This is the finding which corresponds to that of SCHETTINI et al. Coplanar EDP measurements showed good repeatability, and the EDP-IVP curves of the patients represented a linear correlation. However, some discrepancies are observed between these two pressures, which might be caused by individual differences and measured sites. Generally speaking, the higher the ICP, the larger the difference between pressures. These discrepancies are mainly attributed to the fact that stress concentration effects could not be entirely eliminated.

Fig 2 shows an example of these cases, demonstrating a continuous record of EDP in a patient with a metastatic brain tumor. The typical plateau waves on a high baseline level were frequently observed, concomitant with deteriorated consciousness and generalized convulsive seizure. After one week irradiation, reduction in frequency of the plateau waves and lowering the baseline pressure were recognized with association of slight clinical improvement. From these results, EDP measurement of our transducer was found to be a safe, reliable and easy-performed method.

Reference

1. Schettini A, McKay L, Majors R, Malig J, Nevis AH (1971) Experimental approach by monitoring surface brain pressure. J Neurosurg 34:38-47

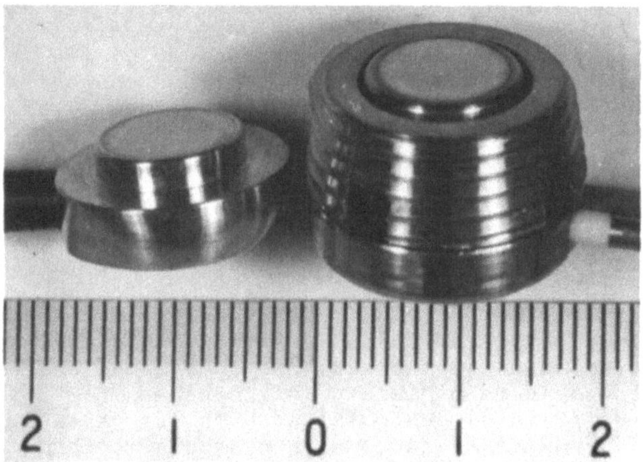

Fig. 1

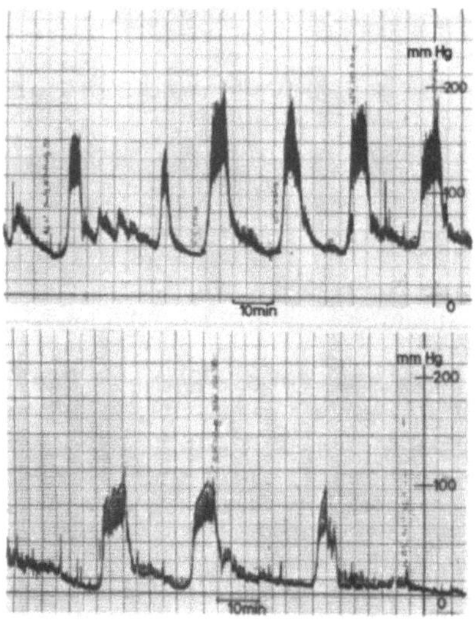

Fig. 2

SPECTRAL ANALYSIS OF THE ICP SIGNAL - PRACTICAL APPLICATION IN COMPUTER-ASSISTED LONG-TERM PATIENT CARE

J. SZWECZYKOWSKI, J. KORSAK-SLIWKA, A. KUNICKI, S. SLIWKA, J. DZIDUSZKO, AND P. DYTKO

Introduction

Modern analysis of the intracranial pressure (ICP) makes it possible to determine the "optimum pressure" (1), the cerebrospinal fluid outflow resistance and the intracranial elastivity (2). Another method consists in analyzing the morphology of the recorded ICP waves (3). This work presents the usage of the power spectral density (PSD) of the ICP signal in long-term patient care.

Material and methods

The studies were performed on patients monitored in the neurosurgical intensive care room. The ICP was measured from one of the lateral ventricles. A total of 225 PSD_{ICP} were obtained and evaluated. An on-line, real-time computer system was used. The system is a modification of an earlier intensive care set-up (4). Briefly, 1024 samples of an ICP signal has been taken at a frequency of 25 c/sec, that gives the time of observation of about 41 sec. The PSD_{ICP} has been obtained by the Fast Fourier Transform method.

Results

In patients without intracranial tightness the most prominent components on the PSD_{ICP} diagram are related to cardiac and respiratory function. Several peaks are usually seen in the PSD_{ICP} plots. The peak, at the left side, at a frequency corresponding to the frequency of the respiration, represents the respiratory pulsations of the ICP. The peak at the frequency corresponding to the frequency of cardiac action, represents the pulse-related pulsations of the ICP (Fig.1a). The others are harmonics. However, when the intracranial volume compensating capacity is decreased, a distinct shift in the relationship between individual components of the PSD_{ICP} is being observed. One may observe the occurence of subrespiratory components that dominate the picture (Fig.1b). The respiratory component becomes relatively low. The changing relationship between the respiratory and the subrespiratory components, according to our observation, constitute one of the early signs of imminent intracranial volume decompensation (5). The PSD_{ICP} proved to be helpful in the evaluation of the ICP corrective procedures such as Furosemide. With the patient who was monitored in the intensive care room after brain tumor surgery, the PSD_{ICP} has been evaluated. Because of the symptoms of intracranial volume decompensation, administration of Furosemide 40 mg i.v. had been decided. Before Furosemide the subrespiratory components dominated the PSD_{ICP} picture (Fig.2). Ten minutes later, after Furosemide application, ICP had begun to stabilize. Thirty minutes post Furosemide - ICP waveform normalized. An hour later one might have observed gradual build up of subrespiratory PSD_{ICP} components which preceeded the occurence of other symptoms of intracranial volume decompensation. Three and a half hours later ICP increased again and, the subrespiratory components again started to dominate in the spectrum.

Discussion

The intracranial volume decompensation might be better diagnosed if there is a possibility to analyze accurately the morphology of the ICP signal as well as other indices such as "optimum" and "opening" pressure, intracranial elastance and CSF outflow resistance. The method helps the physician to decide whether the patient's intracranial system possesses sufficient volume-compensating capacity, or is on the verge of decompensation. The procedure is clinically useful only, when the processed data are presented during the actual measurements and not at a later time.

Summary

A new method that helps to an early diagnosis of intracranial volume decompensation is presented. The method consists in analyzing of the ICP signal in the frequency domain. The changes in the PSD_{ICP} diagram might be detected earlier than other symptoms of intracranial decompensation. This method of quantifying the morphology of the ICP helps the physician to detect earlier the probability of an imminent intracranial decompensation.

References

1. Szewczykowski J, Korsak-Sliwka J, Kunicki A, Dytko P, Sliwka S, Dziduszko J (1976) Computer-assisted determination of optimum ICP levels. In: Beks JWF, Bosch DA, Brock M (eds) Intracranial Pressure III. Springer, Berlin Heidelberg New York, p 295

2. Szewczykowski J, Sliwka S, Kunicki A, Dytko P, Korsak-Sliwka J (1977) A fast method of estimating the elastance of the intracranial system. A practical application in neurosurgery. J Neurosurg 47:19-26

3. Szewczykowski J, Dytko P, Sliwka S, Korsak-SliwkaJ(1979) Computer-assisted analysis of intracranial pressure for clinical applications. In: Anaesthesiologie und Intensivmedizin, Band 116. Springer Berlin Heildelberg New York, p 88

4. Szewczykowski J, Korsak-Sliwka J, Kunicki A, Wliwka S, Dytko P (1975) A computerized neurosurgical intensive care system. Europ J Intensive Care Med 1:189-192

5. Szewczykowski J, Sliwka S, Junicki A, Korsak-Sliwka J, Dytko P (1979) Power spectrum density of the ICP signal as an early sign of the cerebral venous outflow disturbances in neurosurgical patients. In: Gotoh F, Nagai H, Tazaki Y (eds) Cerebral Blood Flow and Metabolism. Munksgaard. Copenhagen, p 396

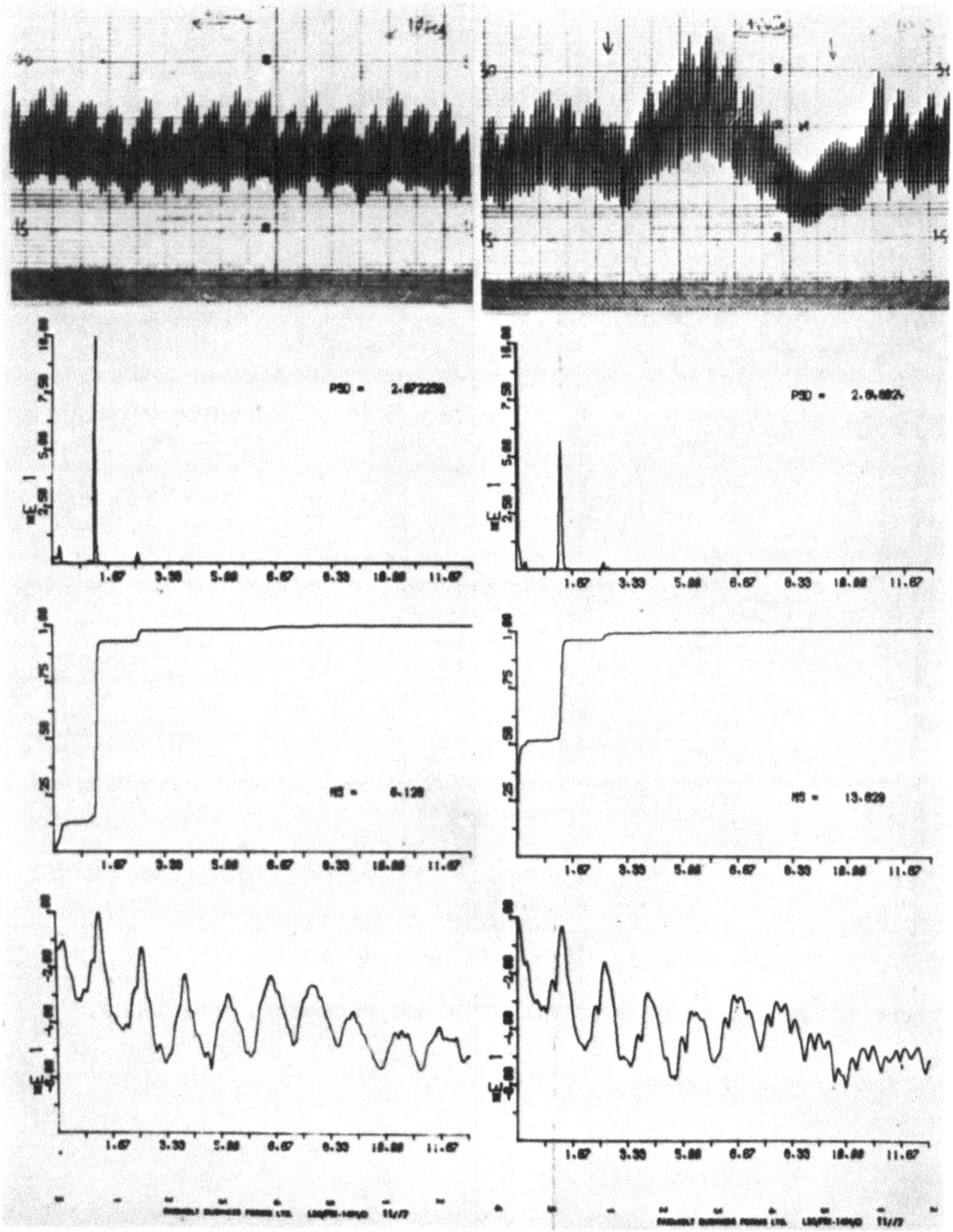

Figure 1

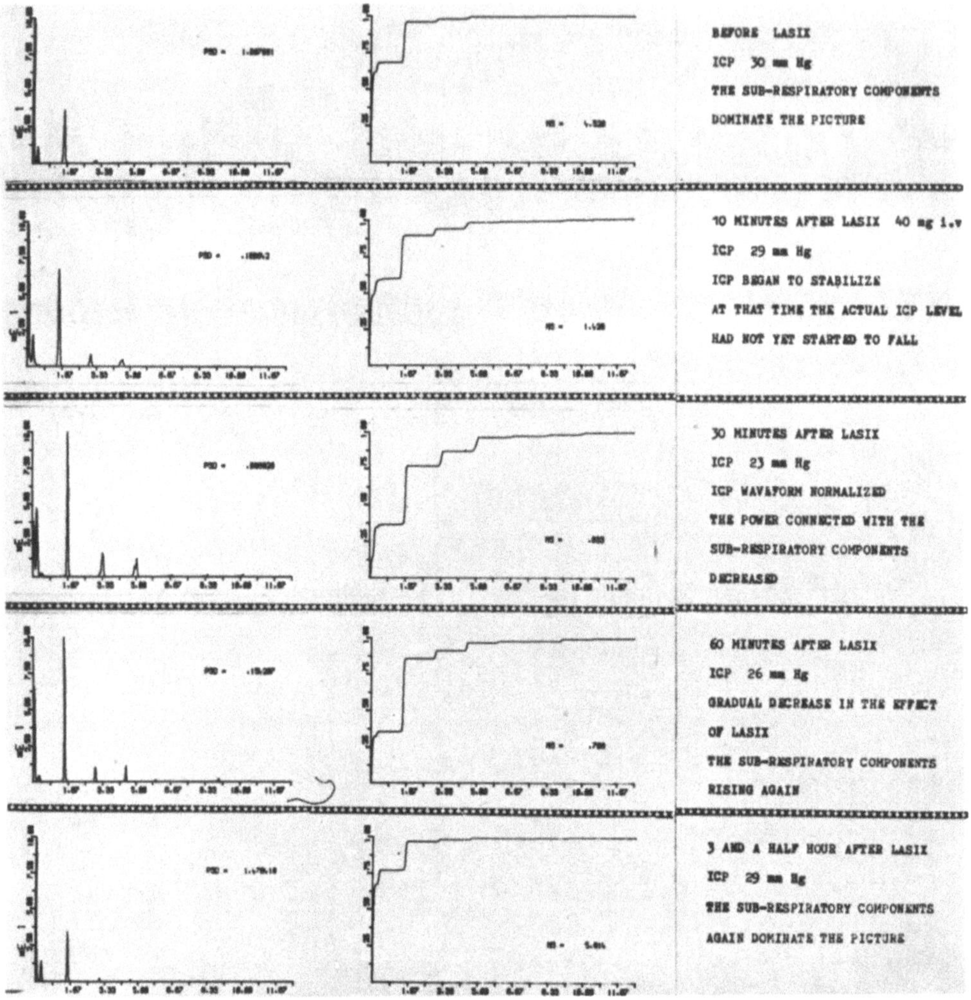

Figure 2. Spectral analysis of the ICP signal before and after lasix.

CHRONIC ICP MONITORING UTILIZING AN IN VIVO CALIBRATING SENSOR

P.R.COOPER, S.MOODY, AND F.SKLAR

Introduction

Multiple techniques are now avialable for the short term monitoring of ICP. The danger of infection and the inconvenience of external connections make their use for long periods of time inappropriate. Disease entities where chronic measurement of ICP would be useful include hydrocephalus, brain tumors and pseudotumor cerebri. A number of devices have been described for use in such situations but drift at uncertain rates from zero point readings render most of these devices unreliable (1,2,3,5). Moreover, the need to do lumbar punctures for calibration would seem to limit their usefulness. In 1978 MEYER et al (4) reported the use of a fully implanted radioisotope activated subdural pressure sensor capable of in vivo calibration in animals. We now report the use of this device (Hittman-Meyer Intracranial Pressure Sensor) for periods ranging up to 14 months in 8 patients with pseudotumor cerebri.

Material and methods

All patients had pseudotumor cerebri and presented with visual symptoms or headaches. All had papilledema or visual loss, elevated LP pressure, and normal CT scans. The mechanism of action of the sensor has previously been described (4). In brief, changes in ICP are transmitted to a working fluid which in turn causes a radioactive source (^{145}Pm) to move in and out of a collimator. Radioactivity recorded at the scalp varies as a function of ICP. A compensating tambour connected to the system is located in the subgaleal space. Digital pressure on this tambour permits in vivo calibration.

Patient monitoring is begun two weeks following implantation. The frequency of ICP monitoring is determined by the activity of the patient's disease, visual signs and symptoms and therapy changes which might affect ICP. All patients had at least one measurement of LP pressure in the post-implantation period. LP and sensor pressures were recorded simultaneously but independently by two observers.

Results

Table I shows the correlation between pressures measured simultaneously by the ICP sensor and LP. LP pressures were varied by removal of cerebrospinal fluid or by infusion and removal of cerebrospinal fluid utilizing a servo-controlled lumbar infusion technique. Correlations of LP and sensor pressure were obtained on 10 occasions in eight patients. In all but one patient there was a statistically significant correlation of pressure obtained by the two methods.

The course of pseudotumor cerebri is a variable one. Our series consisted exclusively of patients with chronic elevations of ICP and it

Table I. Correlation of LP Pressure & ICP Sensor Pressures

Patient	Months following implantation L.P. & sensor correlation obtained	# Points studied	Coefficient of correlation (r)	p Values
HH*	1	8	.862	< .01
HH	5	7	.760	< .05
DO	6	7	.907	< .005
TW	3	4	.874	< .05
AL	1	5	.987	< .002
WA	7	4	.996	< .005
CJ*	1	6	.994	< .001
CJ	2	12	.981	< .001
TWr.	1	11	.989	< .001
SK	1	7	.993	< .001

*These patients studied on two occasions.

is in this group that chronic ICP monitoring can be a valuable management aid. The Hittman-Meyer intracranial pressure sensor is well suited for long term monitoring of intracranial pressure in patients with pseudotumor cerebri. The device is reliable and statistically significant correlations of lumbar puncture and sensor pressure were obtained in seven of eight patients at periods ranging up to 7 months following implantation. Isolated measurements of lumbar puncture pressure from seven to fourteen months following sensor implantation have shown close correlation with ICP as recorded by the sensor.

Because this device allows in vivo calibration, invasive procedures, such as LP, for determining the accuracy and drift of the system may be avoided. This capacity for in vivo calibration has particular relevance to other disease entities such as brain tumors. In these situations accuracy of the device may be assured without the need to resort to LP and risk cerebral herniation. The need to do LP's to correct for inconstant drift is a particular disadvantage of virtually all other previously described systems. At present the length of continuous ICP readings in our patients has been limited to a period of three hours. After this time, the scintilation counter tends to slip over the scalp away from the radioactive source and must be re-positioned to prevent spurious readings. Design modifications currently being tested will allow prolonged periods of continuous ICP monitoring.

References

1. Atkinson JR, Shurtleff DB, Foltz EL (1967) Radio telemetry for the measurement of intracranial pressure. J Neurosurg 27:428-432

2. Brock M, Diefenthaler K (1972) A modified equipment for the continuous telemetric monitoring of epidural or subdural pressure. In: Brock M, Dietz H (eds) Intracranial Pressure. Springer, Berlin Heidelberg New York, p 21

3. Gucer G, Viernstein L (1978) Long-term intracranial pressure recording in the management of pseudotumor cerebri. J Neuorsurg 49:256-263

4. Meyer GA, Millis RM, Budzinski J (1978) Validation of a new technique for measurement of intracranial pressure with a scintillation counter. Neurosurg 2:35-38

5. Olsen ER, Collins CC (1972) Passive radio telemetry for the measurement of intracranial pressure. In:Brock M, Dietz H(eds)Intracranial Pressure. Springer, Berlin Heidelberg New York, p 18

DATA DISPLAY FOR INTRACRANIAL PRESSURE MONITORING

S.D.CORBIN, A.K.REAM, E.V.SCHMIDT, G.D.SILVERBERG, AND T.B.FRYER

Introduction

The epidural, capacitive transducer used in this study (1) is powered inductively through the intact skin. It is attached to the skull with a unique mounting system that prevents edge-loading and insures that the transducer diaphragm is coplanar with the dura. Pressure measurement is isometric; a 50-torr pressure change displaces the diaphragm only 25 μm.

Six transducers were treated in a constant-temperature water bath for periods up to 2 years (2). Units were pressurized to 50 torr at frequent intervals for calibration. They were periodically removed, implanted in dogs, and returned to the water bath to continue stability tests. The two best units had an average drift in baseline of 0.10 torr/day with a standard error of the estimate of y on x, Sy.x = 1.15 torr. The average drift in sensitivity was 0.01%/day with Sy.x = 2.06%.

Acute studies were performed in 5 dogs. The transducer was implanted and the scalp was closed. Cerebrospinal fluid (CSF) pressure was measured independently with a cisternal needle and was varied by means of an epidural balloon or by infusing sterile saline. The correlation coefficient between the epidural pressure and CSF pressure was 0.993 for 142 measurements over a range of 0-90 torr; slope was 1.03. The most stable units were selected for chronic implantation. Results are given in SILVERBERG et al in this symposium.

Monitoring and display: A Hewlett Packard 9845 desktop computer was selected for the clinical monitoring/display station. Continuous sampling was not feasible, so the program was constructed to take a high-speed (10 msec sampling interval) "snapshot" of the intracranial pressure (ICP) for 15 seconds once every minute. Since ICP is a relatively slowly-changing variable, sampling at this rate has not proved to be detrimental.

Before display, the pressure signal is corrected for transducer drift, temperature, and barometric pressure. From the epidural pressure signal, mean pressure, pulse pressure, standard deviation of pulse pressure, and heart rate are calculated. (The standard deviation is used to assess the quality of the recording: excessively large values usually indicate poor coupling with the dura.) If an arterial line is present, mean arterial pressure and cerebral perfusion pressure are also calculated. These values, plus barometric pressure and patient temperature are averaged every 5 minutes and stored.

A standard header has been adopted for all displays. It contains the patient's name and identification number, the date and time of day, and the values of the primary pressure variables (Fig 1). These values are updated every minute, while the graph is updated from the 5-minute average.

The initial graphs presented were mean epidural pressure and the epidural waveform. These were selectable under keyboard control. The waveform display (updated every minute) has proved invaluable in assessing the adequacy of transducer/dura coupling.

The display of mean epidural pressure is typically selected for viewing. This display provides the historical course of the patient's pressure along with the present value. Trends can be observed and therapy initiated as required. A display of pulse pressure has been added, but has not achieved widespread use.

Two formats display the relationship between pulse pressure and epidural pressure: a possible early indicator of intracranial decompensation (3). One plots the ratio of pulse pressure to epidural pressure versus time; the other plots pulse pressure versus epidural pressure.

Summary

A sensitive, stable system for measuring epidural pressure has been developed and is presently undergoing clinical trials. Our monitoring philosophy has been to automate retention of measurements and subsequent calculation, to develop improved graphical summaries, and to evaluate the influence of display concepts on patient management, using a desktop computer with graphics. This experience is being used to design a dedicated clinical monitoring console.

References

1. Fryer TB, Corbin SD, Silverberg GD, Schmidt EV, Ream AK (1978) Telemetry of intracranial pressure. Biotelemetry and Patient Monitoring 5:88-112

2. Ream AK, Silverberg GD, Corbin SD, Schmidt EV, Fryer TB. To be published. The epidural measurement of intracranial pressure. Neurosurgery

3. Szewczykowski J, Dytko P, Kunicki A, Korsak-Sliwka J, Sliwka S, Dziduszko J, Grochowski W, Augustyniak B (1976) A method of estimating intracranial decompensation in man. J Neurosurg 45:155-158

Work was supported in part by NASA NGR 05-020-634.
Work was carried out at Stanford University School of Medicine.

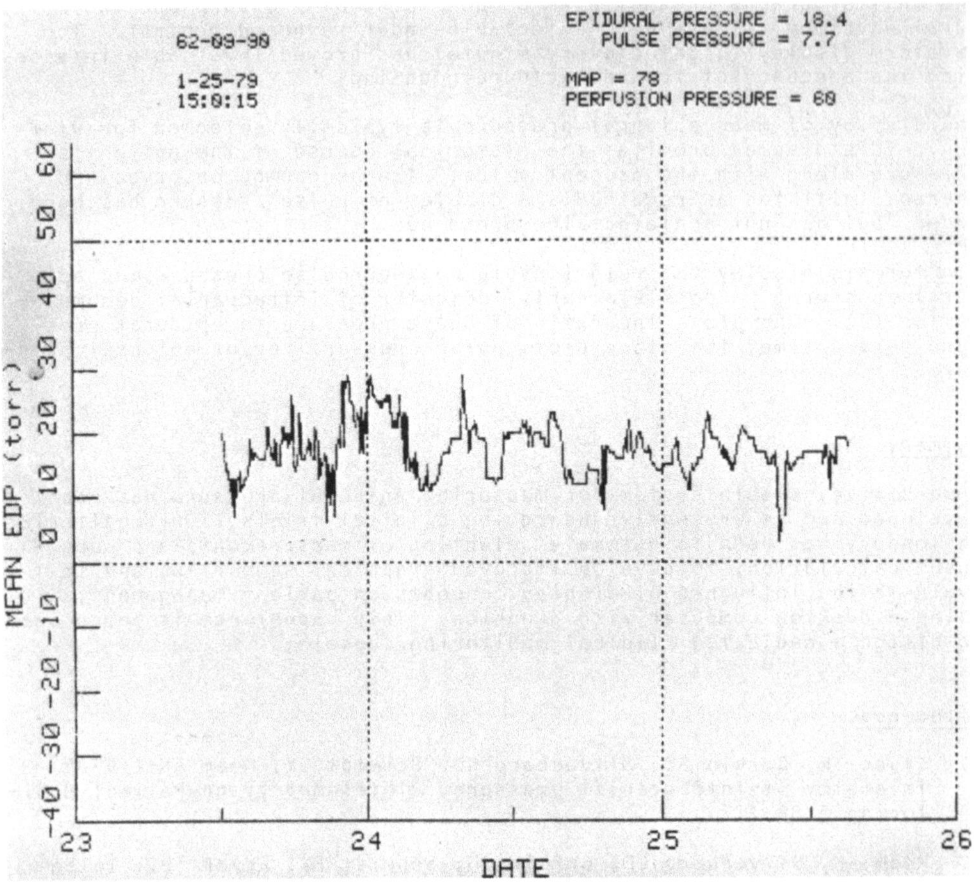

Fig. 1. Typical display of mean epidural pressure. Digital values are updated every minute; graph is updated from 5-minute average. Header is unchanged when alternate displays are selected.

THE INTEGRATION OF ICP WITH OTHER MONITORING SIGNALS ON A SINGLE COMPUTER DATA BASE

J. MASON, D.J. PRICE, AND S. TRIMNELL

Introduction

Continuous on-line computer analysis of ICP following severe head injury results in the isolation of several potentially useful parameters which are not available from conventional chart recordings (1). Unfortunately, these computer records, however complex and precise, are of limited use unless they can be easily correlated with all the factors which might affect the ICP signal. Under the conventional system of medical notes and records, with data being stored on several charts with differing time scales, such correlation is, at best, difficult and time-consuming. We have solved this problem by combining ICP and other analogue signals with all the routine medical and nursing records in a single computer data base coordinated in real time.

Methods

Fig 1 illustrates the basic system configuration. ICP, EEG and end-expired CO_2 signals are input through a multi-channel analogue interface (1). Data collected on patient admission, and results of subsequent diagnostic tests and surgery are input off-line from a small microcomputer on the ward. In our department, over 50 parameters are routinely measured or observed at various frequencies and these either directly affect the ICP or must be included in a data base for completeness. They are grouped as follows:

Physiological data: Conventional methods of measurement are used for arterial BP, pulse rate, temperature and fluid balance. It has been shown that routine automation of BP and pulse rate is more prone to error than simple manual techniques (3).

ICP therapy: This includes drug therapy, CSF drainage and also the timing of tracheo-bronchial toilet, tilting or turning of the patient, and physiotherapy.

Respiratory data: Rate and type of spontaneous respiration, or features of assisted ventilation, arterial blood gas concentrations and details of drug therapy are recorded.

Pupils and conscious level: As the most fundamental strategic monitoring test in a neurosurgical ward is the accurate assessment of the conscious level, we utilize a 0 - 40 scale comprising 12 component parameters (2). Its high sensitivity ensures early recognition of any deterioration and it can be translated to cruder scales for predictive research studies.

Other monitoring tests: These include ICP bolus tests, changes in mid-line shift and brain stem reflex tests.

We have rejected the use of a conventional keyboard as the input device for such a large number of parameters, some of which may be assessed as frequently as every 15 minutes. Instead, we have designed and constructed an interface, for use at the bedside, which is based on the use of separate thumbwheel switches allocated to each parameter. A principal advantage of this approach is that only switches corresponding to parameters which have changed during any 15-minute period need be reset. At any time the switch settings provide a complete display of current patient status. Every 15 minutes, all parameters from the bedside interface are read under program control and integrated with 20 items of ICP data and 10 parameters isolated from the other analogue signals. Other factors are related to program-driven transducer calibration and ICP control, these being carried out by special hardware within the interface. In total there are a maximum of 125 entries to the data base in each 15-minute period and in this way all data is co-ordinated to the central computer clock. Any combination of parameters can be displayed on a selected time axis at a graphics terminal at the nurses' station, and a printed summary is produced every 24 hours, or on request.

Results and discussion

The prototype bedside interface has been installed on the neurosurgical intensive care ward and has been well accepted by medical and nursing staff. The interface is cheap (approximately $600) and simple to construct, and provision has been made for the simultaneous use of up to 7 units. Our impressions are that it is indeed feasible to dispense with almost all hand-written charts and so save significant amounts of nursing time. To attempt to quantitate these advantages, an independent ergonomic study of the system is in progress (4). As a result of the pilot phase of this study a second prototype is under construction, taking advantage of microprocessor technology. This will give added flexibility to the system, enabling it to be used in any centre with a minimum of modification.

Summary

A small computer system has been developed which enables ICP data to be continuously analyzed and integrated with other analogue signals and with medical and nursing data on a co-ordinated data base. A unique bedside interface has been constructed for data entry and is being evaluated. Nursing time is saved and correlation of ICP with other parameters, for example in the evaluation of treatment regimes, becomes a simple and accurate procedure.

References

1. Mason J, Price DJ (1977) Continuous on-line data processing of electroencephalogram and intracranial pressure. Intensive Care Med 3:209

2. Price DJ, Delbridge D, Turner D (1976) Analogue to digital conversion of consciousness. J Neurol Neurosurg Psychiat 39:919

3. Taylor DEM, Whamond JS (1975) Reliability of human and machine measurements in patient monitoring. Europ J Intensive Care Med 1:53

4. Yap L(1979) M.Sc.Dissertation. Loughborough Univ.,to be published

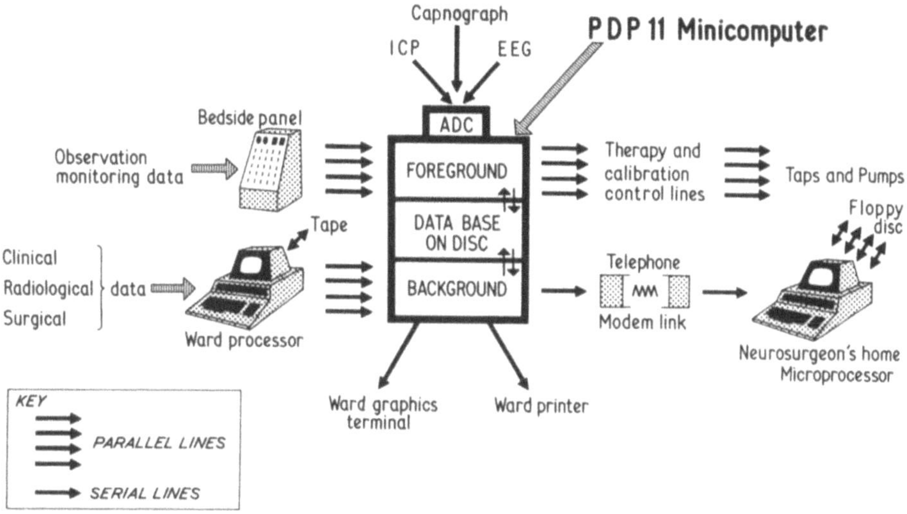

Fig.1. Block diagram of the complete system.

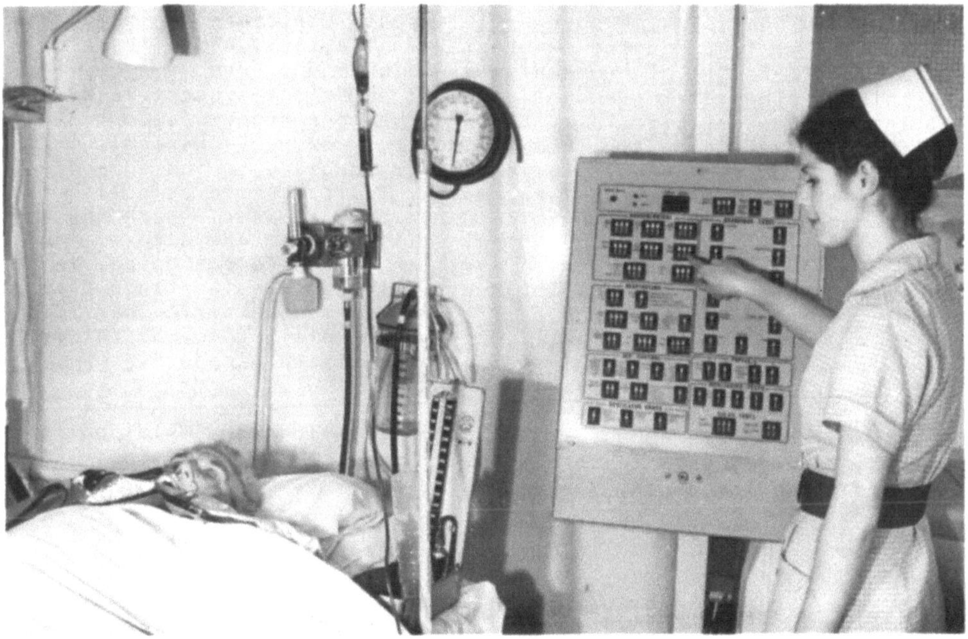

Fig.2. The bedside interface in use in the intensive care area.

LONG TERM STUDY OF ICP WITH IMPLANTED SENSORS IN PATIENTS WITH BRAIN TUMOR

G.A.MEYER, J.A.BUDZINSKI, AND S.GALLANT

Introduction

This report describes the authors' experience[1] with implantation of long-term indwelling H-M[2] intracranial pressure (ICP) sensors in nine patients with brain tumors. The development of the pressure sensor and chronic animal testing have been previously described (1,3,4,5). Our goal was to develop an accurate non-invasive means of obtaining intracranial pressure readings for a minimum of one year.

Material and methods

H-M ICP sensors were installed in nine patients when operated upon for tumor resection. The sensors detect pressure differentials between the sub-dural and the sub-galeal spaces with oil-filled silastic tambours in both spaces which have an interposed miniature spring-loaded piston. The piston, mounted externally on the skull, contains a minute dose (3-5 µCi) of Promethium[145] which moves beneath a collimating shield. The varying amount of gamma emission is quantitated by a scintillation detector in turn connected to a processing circuit permitting read-out directly in mm of Hg or cm of H_2O. Periodic in vivo calibration is made by placing finger pressure on the sub-galeal referencing tambour allowing the read-out instrument to establish the low pressure end of the calibration curve, the slope of which has been previously established in pre-implant calibration. The size of the radiation cone and the in vivo calibration method detection crystal eliminates the need to adjust for scalp thickness in the range of 0-9 mm. Later patients in the series had continuous strip-chart records of ICP made by fixing the 10 oz 1" x 5" detector to the patient's head with a helmet. In most instances, records were made by non-specialized nursing personnel.

Autopsies with complete photographic documentation were obtained on the first five patients in the series. Seven of the nine sensors were available for external and then invasive analysis.

Results

There were no major complications during the total of 70 patient months of experience (Table 1). There was no infection of the transducer site despite 3 prior operations all with prior radiation therapy, one diabetic patient, and post-implant radiation therapy in five cases and chemotherapy in four cases. Only one patient complained of significant pain at the transducer site. This patient, #6, was thought to have bilateral metastatic tumors, but instead had encephalomalacia

[1]Department of Neurosurgery, Med Coll of Wisconsin, Milwaukee, Wisc. Wood VA Med Ctr

[2]Hittman-Meyer ICP sensors manufactured by the Hittman Corp. of Columbia,Maryland

Table 1

	Patient	Age	Sex	Implant	Trans. #	Tumor Type	Tumor Location	Prior Op.	Death or Removal	Autopsy	Months monitored
1.	E.G.	59	F	1/7/76	039	Glioma-IV	L front	-	9/20/76	+	9.5
2.	M.B.	54	M	4/2/76	043	Microgl.	R pariet	-	5/26/77	+	13
3.	L.M.	46	M	5/11/76	040	Glioma-IV	R pariet	2/10/75	10/25/76	+	5.5
4.	R.S.	56	M	6/9/76	044	Glioma-IV	R temp.	-	4/14/77	+	10
5.	R.Si.	63	M	12/17/76	131	Glioma-IV	L front.	8/24/76	4/20/77	+	5
6.	H.G.	60	M	2/18/77	135	C.V.A.&-R Mening.-L	pariet.	-	11/30/77 (Removal)	-	9.5
7.	M.C.	60	M	5/4/77	134	Glioma-III	R front.	12/13/76	10/22/77	-	5.5
8.	M.W.	68	M	2/20/78	555	Glioma-III	R occip.	-	3/29/78	-	1.5
9.	S.B.	76	M	6/7/78	584	Glioma-III	R pariet.	-	3/18/79	partial	9

secondary to infarction on the right and a convexity meningioma on the left. The sensor was monitored during the peri-operative period of meningioma removal confirming normal ICP. He then lost enthusiasm for the study and requested removal of the ICP sensor because of scalp discomfort.

Detailed autopsy study of 5 cases showed no significant unexpected tissue reaction at multiple biopsy sites surrounding the sensor. The silastic sub-dural sensing tambour became encapsulated by a thin (7-10μ)avascular membrane on the arachnoidal side which was slightly thicker and more vascular on the dural side. There was loss of significant amounts of the pressure transmitting fluid (oil) in two cases but, no difference in the tissue reaction could be observed. We found no change in the scalp directly over the window in the collimating shield. The only unexpected tissue change observed was due to ionization of metal from several of the stainless steel retaining screws in three of the early cases. This did not affect the patients or the operation of the sensor adversely. It was found to be due to incomplete "passivation" in manufacture of a small portion of the screws and did not recur in later cases.

Discussion

We believe that this study established that the H-M ICP sensor can be implanted into relatively debilitated brain tumor patients with acceptable morbidity. We thus had the immediate availability of non-invasive, accurate ICP pressure data during radiation therapy, chemotherapy and tumor recurrence. Further, the study indicated that useful data can be acquired by routine ward personnel with a minimum of instruction once the read-out device had been set-up and calibrated. The autopsy studies established the absence of any inherent adverse reaction by histologic methods of analysis at intervals of 3 to 13 months post implantation.

The study also established that the H-M sensor is very accurate and that with certain limitations imposed by the fluid loss from the sensing tambours in the early patients of the series, the sensor can be reliable over the long term. Reliability data are much improved in recent series as documented by COOPER et al (2).

The clinical utility of ICP data has been previously established. We found the pressure data extremely useful in several cases to guide administration of dexamethasone and/or glycerol.

The authors have described the clinical evaluation of the H-M ICP sensor in nine patients with brain tumors. There was no significant morbidity and no complication attributable to the sensor. Ward personnel were able to obtain clinically useful pressure recordings. Modifications made in the manufacture and design of the sensor during the early phases of the program have resulted in an accurate and reliable device for periods of at least one year.

References

1. Bustard TS, Lyon WC, Meyer GA(1974) A nuclear intracranial pressure sensor. IEEE Trans Nuclear Sci NS21(1):697-701

2. Cooper PR, Moody SF, Sklar FH (1979) Long term measurement of ICP using an implanted sensor with in vivo calibration. Neurosurg4:480

3. Meyer GA, Lyon WC, Bustard TS (1974) Chronic in vivo testing of a fully implantable intracranial pressure sensor. IEEE Trans Nucler Sci NS21(1):702-706

4. Meyer GA, Lyon WC, Bustard RS (1975) A new device for long-term intracranial pressure measurement. Child's Brain 1:217-227

5. Meyer GA, Millis RM, Budzinski J (1978) Validation of a new technique for measurement of intracranial pressure with a scintillation counter. Neurosurg 2:35-38

CLINICAL APPLICATION OF TELEMETRIC INTRACRANIAL PRESSURE MONITORING

N.T.ZERVAS, P.H.CHAPMAN, AND E.R.COSMAN

Introduction

An implantable intracranial pressure (ICP) sensor for long-term monitoring of epi- or subdural pressures would be very useful. Others have proposed sensor designs, summarized by ZERVAS et al (2). Their major problems have been: drift of calibration; no calibration check in vivo, and non-standardized calibrations. We first proposed a sensor which overcomes these problems by incorporating an internal stop within the sensor, so that the zero-point can be confirmed in vivo (2). We also proposed a pressure-balancing method to determine the pressure calibration of the device in vivo (2). A single-diaphragm version of this sensor is suited for ventricular fluid ICP monitoring (1), and a two-diaphragm version is designed for epidural measurements. Updated clinical results on the latter are described here.

Material and methods

The two-diaphragm sensor (Fig 1) fits into a ½ inch burrhole and has a length equal to the skull thickness. The inner diaphragm senses the ICP, the outer diaphragm contacts the scalp, and a tuning piston couples the two. When ICP increases, the diaphragms bulge upward, and the tuning piston changes the frequency of the passive resonant circuit in the sensor. The frequency is detected by an antenna and electronics outside the body, and is thus a measure of ICP. A stop of the tuning piston relative to the circuit at the zero pressure position enables in vivo check of zero frequency and pressure calibration versus frequency by pressing on the scalp with a known pressure using an inflated cuff beneath the antenna (Fig 1). By balancing the ICP with a known external pressure one avoids the problem of having to know the sensor calibration before implantation (2). Coplanarity of the diaphragms reduces wedge pressure errors.

The sensors have been implanted in 46 patients since 1975; 29 were epidural, and 17 subdural. Diagnoses included neoplasm, head trauma, hematoma, herpes encephalitis, and pseudotumor. ICP monitoring was done regularly in the early postoperative period and during follow-up visits.

Results

Most sensors worked well for the entire period of follow-up which was as long as 8 months. In several cases the telemetric measurements detected dangerously elevated ICP and aided in treatment to control it. Nine sensors failed within 1 to 4 weeks, mostly due to damage to the sensor on implantation or improper length of the sensor. The inner diaphragm should go beyond the inner table by about 1 mm to contact the dura fully. No infections or unpleasant side effects occurred. Fibrotic reaction to sensor was minimal. In 20 patients telemetric ICP values were checked by lumbar puncture. The results are shown in Fig 2. Accuracy was unaffected by duration of implantation or whether the sensor was epi- or subdural. Scalp edema caused inaccuracies if the sensor was placed within swollen craniotomy sites. Cardiac pulsations were useful in confirming proper function.

Discussion

The ICP sensor has given a reliable indication of ICP over a wide range of pressures for many months of implantation. Its built-in stop at zero pressure and the method of external pressure-balancing enable both the zero-point calibrat-on and the full pressure calibration of the sensor to be determined in vivo, thus overcoming two major problems of other ICP sensor designs. Diaphragm coplanarity and proper placement of the inner diaphragm made epidural measurements appear no less accurate than subdural. Results so far indicate that the system is a practical approach to ICP monitoring.

Summary

A passive, fully implantable radio-telemetric ICP sensor has been developed for epi- or subdural measurements using coupled diaphragms. An internal stop at zero pressure allows in vivo zero calibration. Applying a known pressure to the scalp above the sensor balances, and thus measures, the ICP while also determining the pressure calibration of the sensor in vivo. The sensor has been used in 46 patients and has proved stable and accurate for many months.

References

1. Cosman ER, Zervas NT, Chapman PH, Cosman BJ, Arnold MA (1979) A telemetric pressure sensor for ventricular shunt systems. Surg Neurol 11:287-294

2. Zervas NT, Cosman ER, Cosman BJ (1977) A pressure-balanced radio-telemetry system for the measurement of intracranial pressure. J Neurosurg 47:899-911

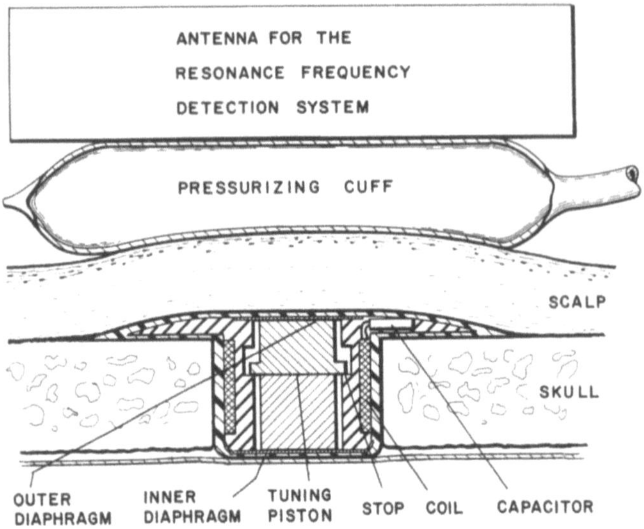

Fig.1. The two-diaphragm pressure sensor (sectional view).

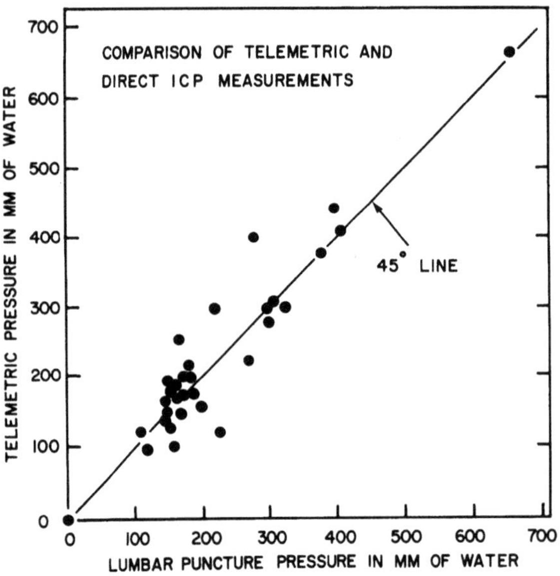

Fig. 2. Comparison of simultaneous measurements of telemetric sensor ICP and lumbar puncture pressure.

Session VIII

CSF FORMATION AND ABSORBTION

Chairman: G.M.Hochwald
Co-chairman: J.Ekstedt

SUMMARY

EDVISSON, LINDVALL and OWMAN have demonstrated that CSF formation may be under nervous control. They have provided both histochemical and ultrastructural evidence for the presence in choroid plexus of adrenergic, cholinergic, and peptidergic nerve fibres that innervate small arterioles and epithelial cells. Fluid secretion by the choroid plexus can be influenced by the effect of adrenalin on both carbonic anhydrase activity of the epithelial cells and choroidal blood flow. They have also shown the presence of alpha and beta adrenergic receptors in the choroid plexus which are accessible to both blood and CSF.

MANN et al determined in rats a decrease in CSF outflow resistance as the CSF pressure increased. This decrease in resistance was extrapolated from their experimental data. The points on the outflow resistance/pressure curves, however, were questioned when they extrapolated their resistance to zero at zero pressure. It was felt that the opposite conclusion was equally valid as resistance could be infinite at zero pressure.

In comparison of two methods to determine CSF outflow resistance, SULLIVAN et al showed that the bolus method progressively underestimated the value of the resistance. However, FRIDEN and EKSTEDT claimed that in more than 100 studies on CSF hydrodynamics in man, with the infusion method, that the elastance/pressure curve always passed initially through a minimum and then increased with increasing CSF pressure. If FRIDEN and EKSTEDT fitted a straight line to the ascending part of their curve it never passed the origin of the elastance and pressure axis. When drawn by SULLIVAN et al, this same curve was assumed to pass through the origin. It was FRIDEN and EKSTEDT's thought that this change in the slope of the line describing the elastance/pressure relationship would be mainly responsible for the discrepancy of the results obtained between the bolus and infusion methods.

LOVE and LESLIE showed that there was a dramatic reduction in the resistance to CSF outflow at CSF pressure exceeding 20 mmHg. They felt that this was due to the induction of alternate CSF absorption mechanisms. It was suggested that one of the possible alternative absorption sites was the arachnoid villi in the spinal subarachnoid space. As to tracer dye entered the ventricles, transependymal absorption was excluded. Under similar conditions EKSTEDT was not able to reproduce these findings in man with CSF infusion maintained at 50 mmHg for two hours.

BROCKLEHURST looked for a correlation between the disappearance of intraventricular injected metrizamide, the presence of B waves, and intraventricular pressure. An effect of intraventricular pressure on metrizamide disappearance was not detected. However, the effect of ventricular size on CSF turnover rate was not considered.

NEUROGENIC CONTROL OF CSF PRODUCTION FROM THE CHOROID PLEXUS

M. Lindvall, L. Edvinsson, and Ch. Owman

The choroid plexus, present in all four ventricles of the mammalian brain, plays an important and probably major role in the production of cerebrospinal fluid (CSF)(4,5,6,7,24,27). That the CSF is formed by an active secretion from the choroid plexus is supported by the morphological structure of the tissue. It is villous, highly vascularized and covered by a single layer of cuboidal cells supplied with various membrane elaborations and numerous mitochondria. The production of CSF is an energy-requiring secretory process involving at least two enzymes, carbonic anhydrase and an ouabain-sensitive sodium-potassium activated ATPase. The first report about nerves in the choroid plexus was published about one hundred years ago (1). Later morphological studies confirmed these observations (3,25), although investigation of the possible involvement of neurogenic mechanisms in the control of CSF formation from the choroid plexus has to a large extent been hampered by the widely held opinion that the choroid plexus is a non-innervated structure. However, the use of modern neurohistochemical techniques has revealed that the plexus is indeed supplied with an extensive system of autonomic nerves (10,18).

Innervation of the Choroid Plexus

Histochemistry of Adrenergic Nerves: Using the highly sensitive specific Falck-Hillarp histofluorescence technique (2) we have shown that the mammalian choroid plexuses receive an ample supply of adrenergic nerves in all ventricles (10,16). The adrenergic fibers form networks around small blood vessels belonging to the arterial and venous systems, and the fluorescent terminals run between the epithelium and the underlying vascular wall, suggesting that both structures are supplied. There is a rather great variation in the innervation density between different animal species (16). Pig and cat plexuses have the largest number of nerves; the innervation density is intermediary in those from baboon, guinea-pig, rat, rabbit and hamster, whereas only few fluorescent nerves are found in cow and mouse plexuses. The total norepinephrine concentration varies between 0.10 and 0.73 ng per mg protein. The amount of nerves is usually in the order third > lateral > fourth ventricular plexuses (16). The adrenergic nerves originate from the superior cervical sympathetic ganglia with the exception of a few fibers in the plexus from the fourth ventricle (seen in rabbits), which obviously arise from lower ganglia. This has been demonstrated histochemically (8,10,19) and by fluorometric measurement of norepinephrine (11) in denervation experiments. Unilateral sympathetic denervation shows ipsilateral supply from the superior cervical ganglia to the lateral plexuses and a mixed contribution to the midline ones (16).

Ontogenetically, the first signs of adrenergic nerves (of the rabbit) appear in the plexus of the third ventricle within the first day after birth. Fluorescent fibers subsequently appear in the choroid plexuses of the lateral ventricles (five days post partum) and the fourth ventricle (two weeks post partum)(22). During the following development nerve fibers grow along blood vessels to form a plexus located between small vessels and the overlying epithelium. The nerve plexus, characterized by varicose axon terminals, is fully developed at three weeks post partum, and maturation is then established by an increase in the number of terminals within the network of axons. There is a good agreement between the development of the fluorescent nerves and histochemically visible adrenergic innervation on one hand, and the tissue level of norepinephrine in the various choroid plexuses on the other. In view of available information on the development of the sympathetic nervous system and secretory functions in choroid plexus it may be assumed that a first step in a functioning neurogenic influence on the rabbit choroid plexus becomes established within the first three weeks after birth (22).

Histochemistry of Cholinergic Nerves: The mammalian choroid plexus is also supplied with cholinergic nerves (18), which have been visualized by the histochemical cholinesterase technique following inhibition of pseudocholinesterase (13,14). The plexuses of all ventricles receive acetylcholinesterase-containing nerves, which are associated not only with the choroidal blood vessels but also with the plexus epithelial cells in the same manner as nerves belonging to the adrenergic system. The plexus of the third ventricle is usually best supplied with cholinergic fibers, whereas that of the fourth ventricle contains hardly any stained nerves at all. The most well-developed cholinergic innervation is found in plexus tissue from pig and cat: baboon, cow, rabbit, guinea-pig and rat have an intermediary nerve density, while the mouse and dog plexuses, on the other hand, receive comparatively few cholinergic nerve fibers.

Immunohistochemistry of Peptidergic Nerves: It has been shown that vasoactive intestinal polypeptide (VIP), a potent hypotensive and dilatory agent, is present in a system of nerves which innervate brain vessels in much the same manner as the autonomic fibers (15). Immunofluorescence studies have revealed that this type of peptidergic nerves also supplies the choroid plexus. Thus, a moderate number of VIP-immunoreactive delicate nerve fibers with a perivascular orientation has been found in choroid plexuses from pig. The corresponding concentration of VIP measured chemically is approximately 10 pmol/g. VIP nerves are few in plexuses from cow, cat and rabbit and rare in plexuses from mouse and rat. Isolated twigs are occasionally seen to run between the wall of small blood vessels and the overlying plexus epithelium(17). Pure porcine VIP produces relaxation of isolated bovine anterior choroidal artery in vivo (17).

Ultrastructure of Innervation: Electron microscopy of cats and rabbits shows numerous nonmyelinated nerves running in relation to the wall of small arterioles and to the base of plexus epithelial cells(8). Thick bundles of axons enclosed by Schwann cells, and a thin collagenous investment are found in preparations taken near the border of attachment of the plexuses, where they accompany small arterioles. Further out in the plexus tissue, toward the free border, the axons are collected in bundles of smaller size and are located contiguous to the wall of small arterioles as well as to the base of epithelial cells. Near the fringes of the plexus tufts the nerve terminals run singly and are devoid of their neurilemmal sheath (8).

The adrenergic nature of one population of the nerve terminals has been secured by the presence of electron-dense synaptic vesicles after injection of the "false adrenergic transmitter" 5-hydroxydopamine. An approximately equal number of terminals contains electron-lucent synaptic vesicles: they are interpreted as the cholinergic terminals visualized at the light-microscopic level by the cholinesterase technique. Both types of nerve terminals come as close as 20 nm to epithelial cells, where they are located either contiguous to the base of the cell or cellular processes, between adjacent cells, or within a cellular invagination. The distance between the nerve endings and the smooth muscle cells of the arterioles is in the order of 90 nm, which is characteristic of a functioning autonomic innervation of blood vessels (8). The VIP-containing nerves have so far not been identified at the electron microscopic level.

Sympathetic Influence on Choroid Plexus Function

The structural observations have suggested that the innervation of the choroid plexus may influence functions through an effect on its vascular bed and its secretory epithelium.

Adrenergic Receptors in Plexus Vessels: The anterior choroidal artery of cow was used as a model vessel in the pharmacological analysis of vascular smooth muscle receptors in vitro (9). A weak contractile effect was obtained by epinephrine, norepinephrine, phenylephrine, and isoproterenol in the mentioned order of potency. The reversible α-receptor antagonist, phentolamine, inhibited the contraction, supporting the presence of contractile α-adrenergic receptors. Histamine, prostaglandin F_{2a}, and saturated potassium chloride all produced strong contractions of the artery (9).

The β-adrenergic receptor function was tested on vessels previously given an active tone by prostaglandin F_{2a}. The potency of the sympathomimetic relaxation was in the order isoproterenol > norepinephrine > epinephrine > terbutaline. The β-receptor nature of the relaxation was confirmed in terms of the competitive inhibition of the isoproterenol-induced effect achieved by propranolol. Relaxation was also obtained by adenosine and cyclic AMP (9).

Sympathetic Effects on Carbonic Anhydrase Activity: More direct evidence for a true functioning relationship between the sympathetic nerves and the secretory epithelium of the plexus was obtained in quantitative determinations of carbonic anhydrase activity of blood-free rabbit plexus by measuring the formation of $^{14}CO_2$ from $NaH^{14}CO_3$ in the presence of a plexus homogenate (8). The activity of the enzyme which is essential for the production of CSF, was twice as high in the plexus of the fourth ventricle compared to that of the lateral ventricles. As expected, treatment of the animals with acetazolamide markedly reduced the enzyme activity in both plexus regions. Cervical sympathectomy (1 week postoperatively) or injection with reserpine significantly increased the activity (as measured in the lateral plexuses) by 125-150%. These findings thus indicate that the sympathetic innervation has an inhibitory action on carbonic anhydrase activity and hence probably on CSF production.

Measurement of Bulk CSF Production on Rabbit: In order to obtain a direct measure of the nervous influence on the rate of CSF production, the ventriculo-cisternal perfusion technique of PAPPENHEIMER and collaborators (12,26), utilizing radioactive inulin (12), was applied to experiments on rabbits (19,20,21,23). According to this technique, the rate of bulk CSF production is determined on the basis of radioactive dilution (12).

The measurements are carried out on rabbits. The animal is anesthetized, tracheotomized and artifically ventilated, resting prone in a specially made hammock with its head fixed in a metal frame.

Artificial CSF, containing inulin-^{14}C-carboxylic acid (1μCi/100ml), is infused through an inflow probe into the right lateral ventricle and drained at the same rate (30μl/min) through a needle placed in the cisterna magna, the outflow being collected at 5-min intervals. Infusion pressure is continuously recorded on a Grass polygraph via the inflow cannula and a Statham pressure transducer. Arterial blood gases and systemic blood pressure are followed during the whole experiment. Body temperature of the animal is maintained normal with a heating blanket and is checked by a rectal thermometer. Radioactivity of the effluent and samples from the infusate are measured by liquid scintillation spectometry. Since diffusion of inulin from the ventricular system is negligible, it follows that any dilution of inulin during the passage through the ventricles results from newly formed, inulin-free fluid at a rate equal to the rate of inflow times the difference between the inulin concentrations in the inflow and outflow, divided by the concentration in the outflow (12). The mean production rate of CSF in the untreated rabbit was found to be 10,8-11,3μl/min(19,21).

<u>Sympathetic Nerve-Induced Reduction of Bulk CSF Production:</u> Electrical stimulation intermittently of the sympathetic trunks in the neck during 1 - 2 hrs reduced the rate of CSF formation by a mean of 32% compared to the control situation before stimulation (19). After cessation of stimulation, the production rate returned approximately halfway towards normal during a 1-hour observation period (19).

On the other hand, bilateral excision of the superior cervical ganglia (which produces extensive sympathetic denervation of the choroid plexuses) resulted in a 33% increase in bulk CSF production as compared to an unoperated control group (19). The results are in agreement with the enhanced carbonic anhydrase activity of the plexus following sympathectomy (8).

In view of the finding that the sympathetic nerve terminals in the choroid plexus have a close relation both to the secretory epithelium and to the smooth muscle cells of the arterioles, indicating a true innervation of both components (8), the effects of sympathetic nerve stimulation or denervation may be the result of a direct action on the secretory cells, of changes in plexus blood flow through a vascular response, or both.

Adrenergic Receptor Mechanisms Mediating Sympathetic Effects on the Rate of CSF Production: The type of adrenergic receptors involved in the nerve-induced sympathetic effects (19) were studied by analyzing the quantitative changes in the CSF production rate in the presence of various doses of different agonists, with or without specific antagonists (21). The drugs were either administered in the ventriculocisternal perfusion system or intravenously, with the intention to sort out systemic side-effects and to interpret results with regard to the involvement of epithelial or vascular receptors in the plexus tissus.

Intraventricular perfusion of norephinephrine (10^{-11} - 10^{-3}M) in increasing doses caused a dose-related reduction in the CSF production (21). The log dose-response curve seemed to comprise two phases with a transition around 10^{-7}M. A maximal inhibition was seen at a concentration of 10^{-3}M. The norepinephrine-induced reduction in CSF formation rate was counteracted both by the a-receptor antagonist, phentolamine (10^{-6}M), and by the β-receptor inhibitor, propranolon (10^{-6}M): in the presence of the latter antagonist, production was even slightly increased (21). The results of the blocking experiments suggest that both a- and β-adrenergic receptors are involved. Of the two components in the dose-response curve for norepinephrine, it is possible that the fall in the CSF production seen at low concentrations primarily represents a β-receptor mediated effect on the secretory epithelium, while that occurring at higher concentration reflects an added a-receptor mediated local vasoconstriction (cf.9), affecting the perfusion of blood through the plexus tissue.

Also i.v. infusions of norepinephrine (5.5-55µg/kg/min) gave a dose-dependent reduction in the rate of CSF formation (21) but, as expected, systemic side-effects were marked. Phentolamine, whether given intraventricularly (10^{-6}M) or i.v. (1 mg/kg), as well as intraventricular perfusion of propranolol (10^{-6}M), counteracted the norepinephrine-induced decrease in the production, though the effect of propranolol was weak. On the other hand, there was a potentiation of the reducing norepinephrine effect when propranolol was injected iv (1 mg/kg).

In an attempt to differentiate that component of the inhibition of CSF formation mediated by the epithelial β-receptors from the vascular a-effect, the ventricular system was perfused with the specific β-receptor stimulating drug, H80/62, which primarily activates the β_1-type receptors, and terbutaline, which mainly stimulates the β_2-type receptors. The CSF production was reduced in a dose-dependent manner by H80/62, while terbutaline had no significant effect. Intravenous infusion of either H80/62 or terbutaline had little or no effect on the production rate (21). Thus, the β-receptor induced decrease of the production is presumed to represent a direct inhibitory action on the plexus epithelium, primarily supplied with the β_1-subtype of adreno-ceptors.

Monoamine Oxidase in the Choroid Plexus: The presence of monoamine oxidase (MAO) in the choroid plexuses from all brain ventricles of rabbit was established radiometrically (23). Histochemical staining of MAO revealed the enzyme to be present primarily in the secretory epithelium. The mode of inhibition by the selective inhibitors, clorgyline and deprenyl, showed that type A and B MAO are present in approximately euqal portions in the plexus. Intraventricular administration of nialamide markedly reduced CSF production measured by ^{14}C-inulin dilution during ventriculocisternal perfusion. The niala-effect was significantly diminished after sympathetic denervation of the plexus, indicating that also neuronal MAO is present in the plexus: it probably represents a small fraction of the total MAO A activity in the tissue. In addition, nialamide tended to potentiate the reduction in CSF formation obtained by intraventricular norepinephrine (23).

Cholinergic Influence on CSF Formation

Intraventricular administration of the parasympathomimetic agonist, carbamylcholine, resulted in a dose-related reduction in the CSF formation by as much as 55% at a concentration of 10^{-3}M(20). At 10^{-9}M(the lowest given dose) there was even a tendency to a slightly enhanced production. Infusion of acetylcholine (10^{-5}M) in the presence of the cholinesterase inhibitor, neostigmine (10^{-5}), reduced the formation rate of CSF with about the same amount as an equimolar dose of carbamylcholine. The cholinergic receptors seem to be of the muscarinic type, since the effect of carbamylcholine was completely blocked by atropine, while hexamethonium was without effect on the carbamylcholine response (20).

The site of action of the parasympathomimetic agents is still not known. It is possible that the effects mainly involve the secretory epithelium of the choroid plexus rather than its vascular system:

carbamylcholine, in contrast to norepinephrine, has little or no vasomotor effect on isolated small choroidal arteries (9), and, if anything, it should be expected that the cholinergic agents would increase plexus blood flow and thus not provide a lowered CSF formation.

Summary

The choroid plexus receives a well-developed adrenergic and cholinergic innervation to both epithelium and vascular smooth muscle cells. A sympathetic inhibitory effect on the plexus epithelium was indicated in determinations of carbonic anhydrase activity. Pharmacological in vitro analysis showed the choroidal arteries to possess both vasoconstrictory a-adrenergic receptors and vasodilatory β-adrenoceptors. Electrical stimulation of the sympathetic trunks in the neck resulted in a 32% reduction in the net rate of CSF production, while sympathectomy gave a pronounced increase (33% above control) in the CSF formation. From pharmacological in vivo experiments it is suggested that the sympathomimetic reduction in the rate of CSF formation is the result of a combined β-receptor mediated inhibition of the secretion from the plexus epithelium and a reduced blood flow in the choroid plexus tissue resulting from stimulation of the vascular a-receptors. The CSF production rate was also reduced by cholinomimetic agents, an effect that implicates the presence of the muscarinic type of cholinergic receptors in the choroid plexus.

References

1. Benedikt M (1874) Über die Innervation des Plexus Choroideus Inferior. Virch Arch Path Anat 59:395-400

2. Bjorklund A, Falck B, Owman CH (1972) Fluorescence microscopic and microspectrofluorometric techniques for the cellular localization and characterization of biogenic amines. In: Berson SA (ed) Methods of Investigative and Diagnostic Endocrinology; Rall JE, Kopin IJ (eds) The Thyroid and Biogenic Amines, Vol I. North Holland Publ Co, Amsterdam, p 318

3. Crosby EC, Humphrey T, Laner EW (1962) Correlative Anatomy of the Nervous System. Macmillan, New York

4. Cserr HF (1971) Physiology of the choroid plexus. Physiol Rev 51:273-311

5. Cserr HF (1975) Physiology of the choroid plexus. In: Netsky MG, Shuangshoti S (eds) The Choroid Plexus in Health and Disease. John Wright and Sons Ltd, Bristol, p 175

6. Davson H (1967) Physiology of the Cerebrospinal Fluid. Little, Brown, Boston

7. Dohrmann GJ (1970) The choroid plexus: a historical review. Brain Res 18:197-218

8. Edvinsson L, Hakanson R, Lindvall M, Owman CH, Svensson KG(1975) Ultrastructural and biochemical evidence for a sympathetic neural influence on the choroid plexus. Exp Neurol 48:241-251

9. Edvinsson J, Lindvall M (1978) Autonomic vascular innervation and vasomotor reactivity in the choroid plexus.Exp Neurol 62:394-404

10. Edvinsson L, Nielsen KC, Owman CH, West KA (1974) Adrenergic innervation of the mammalian choroid plexus. Amer J Anat 139:299-308

11. Edvinsson L, Owman CH, Rosengren E, West KA (1972) Concentration of noradrenaline in pial vessels, choroid plexus, and iris during two weeks after sympathetic ganglionectomy or decentralization. Acta Physiol Scand 85:201-206

12. Heisey SR, Held D. Pappenheimer JR (1962) Bulk flow and diffusion in the cerebrospinal fluid system of the goat. Am J Physiol 203: 775-781

13. Holmstedt B (1957) A modification of the thiocholine method for the determination of cholinesterase. II Histochemical application. Acta Physiol Scand 40:331-337

14. Koelle GB (1963) Cytological distributions and physiological functions of cholinesterases. In: Koelle GB (ed) Cholinesterases and Anticholinesterase Agents, Handbuch der experimentellen Pharmakologie, Suppl 15. Springer, Berlin, p 187

15. Larsson LI, Edvinsson L, Fahrenkrug J, Hakanson R, Owman CH, Schaffalitzky de Muckadel OB, Sundler F (1976) Immunohistochemical localization of a vasodilatory peptide (VIP) in cerebrovascular nerves. Brain Res 113:400-404

16. Lindvall M (1979) Fluorescence histochemical study on regional differences in the sympathetic nerve supply of the choroid plexus from various laboratory animals. Cell Tiss Res 198 (in press)

17. Lindvall M, Alumets J, Edvinsson L, Fahrenkrug J, Hakanson R, Hanko J, Owman CH, Schaffalitzky de Muckadell OB, Sundler F (1978) Peptidergic (VIP) nerves in the mammalian choroid plexus. Neuroscience Letters 9:77-82

18. Lindvall M, Edvinsson L, Owman CH (1977) Histochemical study on regional differences in the cholinergic nerve supply of the choroid plexus from various laboratory animals. Exp Neurol 55:152-159

19. Lindvall M, Edvinsson L, Owman CH (1978) Sympathetic nervous control of cerebrospinal fluid production from the choroid plexus. Science 201:176-178

20. Lindvall M, Edvinsson L, Owman CH (1978) Reduced cerebrospinal fluid formation through cholinergic mechanisms. Neurosci Letters 10:311-316

21. Lindvall M, Edvinsson L, Owman CH (to be published) Effect of sympathomimetic drugs and corresponding receptor antagonists on the rate of cerebrospinal fluid production. Exp Neurol 64

22. Lindvall M, Owman CH (1978) Early development of noradrenaline-containing sympathetic nerves in the choroid plexus system of the rabbit. Cell Tiss Res 192:195-203

23. Lindvall M, Owman CH (to be published) Evidence for the presence of two types of monoamine oxidase in rabbit choroid plexus and their role in breakdown of amines influencing cerebrospinal fluid formation. J Neurochem

24. Milhorat TH(1975) The third circulation revisited.J Neurosurg 42: 628-645

25. Millen JW, Wollam DHM (1962)The Anatomy of the Cerebrospinal Fluid Oxford University Press, New York

26. Pappenheimer JR, Heisey SR, Jordan EE, Downer J(1962) Perfusion of the cerebral ventricular system in unanesthetized goats. Am J Physiol 203:763-774

27. Pollay M (1975) Formation of cerebrospinal fluid. Relation of studies of isolated choroid plexus to the standing gradient hypothesis. J Neurosurg 42:665-673

This work supported by the Swedish Medical Research Council (grant No. 04X-732).

CHANGES IN RESISTANCE TO CEREBROSPINAL FLUID ABSORPTION DURING PROLONG INFUSION STUDIES

J.A. LOVE AND R.A. LESLIE

Introduction

Cerebrospinal fluid (CSF) outflow resistance is an important factor in regulating intracranial pressure (ICP). Normally this resistance is considered as residing in the arachnoid villae (4), the structures principally concerned with the return of CSF to the blood (7). The outflow resistance is thought to remain constant over a wide range of intracranial pressures (4,6,10). There is some evidence that CSF may be absorbed by routes other than the arachnoid villae, e.g. across the ventricular ependyma (8,9).

The present study was designed to investigate the possibility that such alternate systems do exist and can facilitate significantly the absorption of CSF. It was postulated that if alternate absorptive mechanisms exist and if they can be activated, then there should be a decrease in CSF outflow resistance. This would be seen as a change in the slope of a pressure-flow curve derived from steady state infusion data.

Methods

Cats were anesthetized with sodium pentobarbital (30 mg/kg), intubated, paralyzed with gallamine hydrochloride (5mg/kg), and ventilated to normal blood gases. Arterial and central venous pressures were monitored. The cats were held in a stereotaxic frame and an infusion cannula was inserted into the cisterna magna through the atlanto-occipital membrane. A Harvard infusion pump was used to infuse artificial CSF and the ICP was measured at the hub of the cannula. A correction for the pressure drop across the cannula was made for each infusion rate. At the termination of each experiment, Evans' Blue was added to the CSF to check for leaks in the system and the infusion pump was recalibrated.

Four infusion rates were employed, namely 17, 35, 69 and 170 µl/min. After the subarachnoid space was catheterized the preparation was allowed to stabilize for 30 min. Infusions were started at the lowest rate, increased sequentially to the highest and reduced to the lowest again before being finally stopped. A period of time was allowed to elapse before the experiment was repeated. The infusion rate was changed only after the ICP had been steady (± 1 mmHg) for at least 30 min. For a number of animals the infusion rates were applied in a random order to determine if the steady state for a particular infusion rate was independent of the previous infusion rates. Animals with unstable arterial or central venous pressures were excluded from the series as were any in which the pressure difference between systemic arterial pressure and ICP was less than 50 mmHg at any time during the experiment.

Results

Fig I shows the course of a typical experiment. With the start of infusion after a period of stabilization, ICP rose and became steady with each increase in infusion rate up to 69 μl/min. At 170 μl/min the ICP rose to a peak, remained steady for one to ten minutes and then started a slow fall. The steady state was reached after 3-4 hours. Steady state ICP was measured for the lower infusion rates and the infusion was terminated. ICP values for each infusion rate before and after facilitation are shown in Table I.

While the ICP remained below 20-22 mmHg on the initial infusions there was no evidence of facilitation. This was the case when the infusion rate was 69 μl/min or less. However, when the ICP exceeded 24 mmHg, as it always did when the 170 μl/min infusion rate was used, the peak ICP was followed by a slow fall to a steady state pressure, considerably below the peak. If the period of stabilization after the infusion terminated was less than 90 minutes, then when the experiment was repeated, the values of ICP at each infusion rate were similar to those obtained after facilitation had occurred.

After correcting for the pressure drops across the infusion cannula, the ICP was plotted against each infusion rate as shown in Fig 2. The slope of each curve was measured to determine the outflow resistance. Before facilitation the outflow resistance was 127 mmHg/ml/min. After facilitation the outflow resistance was 63 mmHg/ml/min. Using the formula $\frac{1}{R} = \frac{1}{R_1} + \frac{1}{R_2}$, the outflow resistance of the alternate absorption mechanisms can be calculated to be 125 mmHg/ml/min.

At autopsy it was observed that Evans' Blue was never found in the fourth ventricle even when the dye was added at the peak of facilitation using the maximum infusion rates.

Discussion

For the purpose of these experiments the following assumptions have been made: 1) that the pressure in the large venous sinuses does not change over the range of ICP described above, 2) that intrinsic production of CSF remains constant over the same ICP ranges, 3) that at steady state, ICP absorption of CSF equals the addition of CSF to the CSF spaces.

From the results above we conclude that there is a mechanism for reducing the outflow resistance to the CSF absorption and the mechanism is activated in normal cats when the ICP exceeds 20-22 mmHg. Furthermore, this facilitated absorption continues to occur down to normal values of ICP.

There are several possible explanations for the decrease in resistance. If the assumption that venous sinus pressures remain constant is wrong, then it is possible that a change in the pressure gradient between subarachnoid space and venous sinuses could explain the apparent decrease in resistance. Studies in our laboratory and others (4) have shown that the venous sinus pressure changes little during slow changes in ICP in the ranges described above in normal cats.

The change in outflow resistance could occur at the arachnoid villae if the physical size of conducting channels were altered. JAMES et

Table 1. Average ICP with standard deviation for each infusion rate before and after facilitation. The range of ICP is given in brackets.

	INTRACRANIAL PRESSURE mm Hg	
INFUSION RATE	BEFORE FACILITATION	AFTER FACILITATION
17 ul/min	9.5±1.6 (7.5-11.5)	5.8±1.7 (4.0-8.5)
35 ul/min	13.1±1.4 (11.2-15.0)	6.8±2.1 (5.0-10.0)
69 ul/min	17.2±2.1 (14.5-20.5)	8.4±2.0 (6.5-11.5)
170 ul/min	30.2±2.6 (24.0-35.0)	14.8±3.2 (11.0-20.0)

al (5) have shown that this probably does not occur but further work is required in this area.

Alternate absorptive sites for CSF have been described in animals and man under normal and abnormal conditions (7,8,9). The evidence supporting these alternates has been inconclusive in most cases but transependymal absorption seems to occur in some cases of hydrocephalus(8,9). The present studies do not allow us to define the alternate absorption mechanisms anatomically, but we can measure some of their characteristics. We know that they have different opening and closing pressures and that when fully invoked, their outflow resistance is similar to that of the arachnoid villae. This means that with normal production, the alternate mechanisms could absorb CSF at normal ICP.

The failure of dye to enter the fourth ventricle from the subarachnoid space while facilitation is in progress suggests that transependymal absorption does not represent the major alternate mechanism.

Different opening and closing pressures are characteristic of arterioles and bronchioles. Recent work by CSERR et al (3) has shown that bulk flow of interstitial fluid occurs and while a proportion of this fluid ends up in the CSF either through the ventricle wall or through the pia, some at least enters the perivascular spaces. These spaces are thought to connect with lymphatics in the neck and have been called prelymphatics by one group of workers (2). BRADBURY (1) has shown that up to 19% of radioisotope-labelled albumin injected into the cerebral ventricles can be recovered from lymphatics in the neck of normal cats. It is interesting to speculate that the facilitation described above is due primarily to the opening of prelymphatics and consequent increased absorption of CSF by this route.

References

1. Bradbury MWB (1978) Porportion of cerebrospinal fluid draining into jugular lymphatic trunks of the cat. J Physiol 276:67P-68P

2. Casley-Smith, Foldi-Borcsok E, Foldi M (1976) The prelymphatic pathways of the brain as revealed by cervical lymphatic obstruction and the passage of particles. Br J exp Path 57:179-188

3. Cserr HF, Cooper DN, Milhorat TH (1977) Flow of Cerebral interstitial fluid as indicated by the removal of extracellular markers from rat caudate nucleus. In: Bito LZ, Davson H, FenstermacherJD (eds) Ocular and Cerebrospinal Fluids. Exp Eye Res Suppl 25: 461-473

4. Davson H, Hollingsworth G, Segal MB (1970) The mechanism of drainage of the cerebrospinal fluid. Brain 93:665-678

5. James AE,Jr, McComb JG, Christian J, Davson H (1976) The effect of cerebrospinal fluid pressure on the size of drainage pathways. Neurol 26:659-663

6. Marmarou A, Shulman K, LaMorgese J (1975) Compartmental analysis of compliance and outflow resistance of the cerebrospinal fluid system. J Neurosurg 43:523-534

7. Milhorat TH (1972) Hydrocephalus and the cerebrospinal fluid. Williams and Wilkins Co, Baltimore

8. Sahar A, Hochwald GM, Ransohoff J (1969) Alternate pathway for cerebrospinal fluid absorption in animals with experimental obstructive hydrocephalus. Exp Neurol 25:200-206

9. Strecker EP, Ursual Scheffel J, Kelly ET, James AE (1973) Cerebrospinal fluid absorption in communicating hydrocephalus. Neurol 23:854-864

10. Sullivan HG, Miller JD, Griffith RL, Engr D, Carter W, Rucker S (1979) Bolus versus steady state infusion for determination of CSF outflow resistance. Ann Neurol 5:228-238

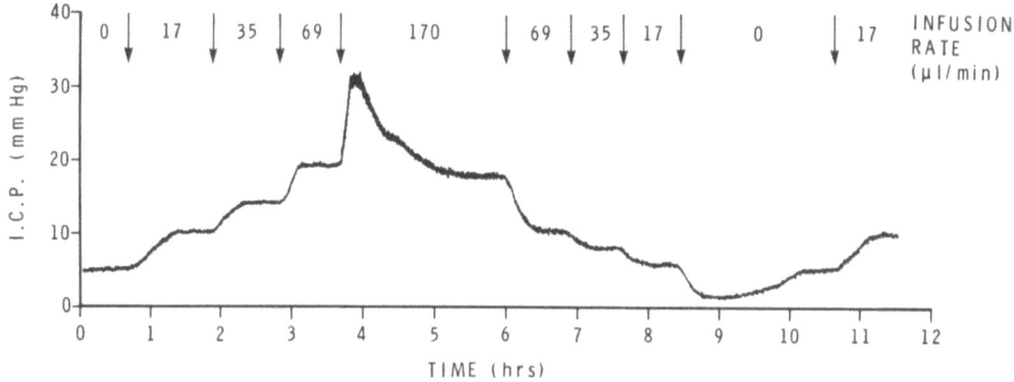

Fig.1. A diagramatic respresntation of a typical experiment to show the time course and the changes in ICP as the infusion rates are changed.

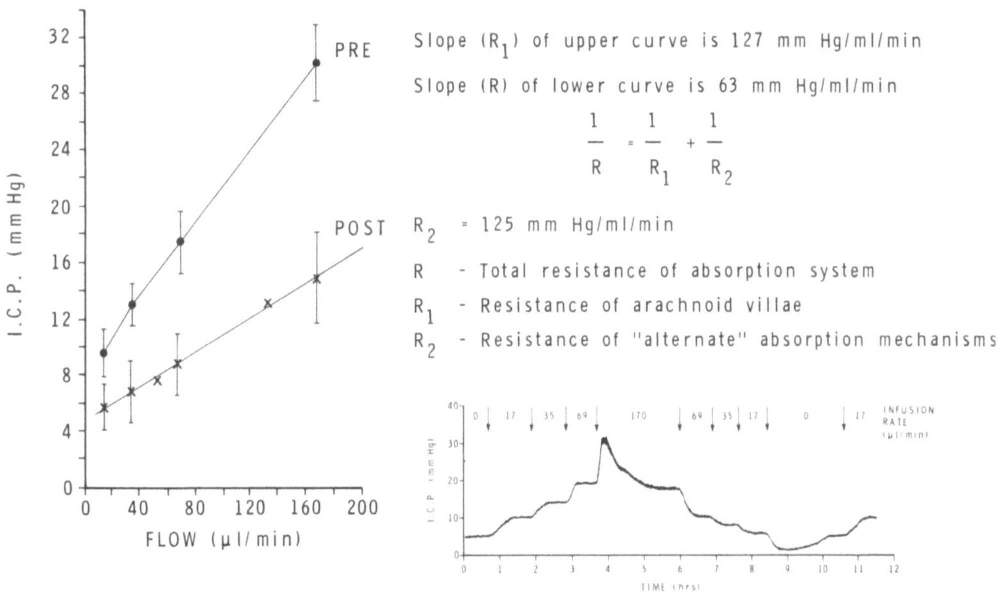

Fig.2. Graph of ICP against infusion rate before (pre) and after(post) facilitation.

LUMBAR SAC INFUSION TEST REVISITED

G.GESSEY, P.BAKER, A.WHITE, AND J.L.FIRTH

Introduction

Despite CAT, differentiation between cerebral atrophy and Low Pressure Hydrocephalus (LPHC) due to CSF resorption block (CSFRB), and within the Benign Intracranial Hypertension (BICHT) sub-groups, remains imperfect (1). Prolonged passive ICP observation may clarify (2), but the apparently simple Lumbar Sac Infusion Test (LSIT) has experienced variable acceptance (7). The requirement for a simple, active, short-term and easily repeatable stress test of the CSF circulation remains. The LSIT was re-assessed.

Material and methods

Of 80 initial cases, the first 27 proved a heterogenous group in which many significant variables were identified (Fig 1) before standardization and reproducibility were achieved. The latter 53 cases, referred as BICHT (19), CAT "Atrophy" (17) and quentionably-"active" hydrocephaly with a known etiology (17), provided 73 studies with 165 perfusions, one incomplete test and one "dry tap".

Under local anesthesia and at least ten days from previous puncture, a sitting, single-pass L4/5 lumbar puncture with an 18 FG needle is made and the patient rolled to a comfortable left lateral decubitus with straightened legs to achieve a horizontal, sagittal-plane baseline. Normal saline is infused at 1.0, 1.5 and 3.0 ml/min, using a Scientific and Research Instruments Ltd (SRI) three-speed constant-rate infusion pump,linked via a three-way tap to an AKER's transducer, a Simonsen and Weel trolley (analogue, digital and CRT pressure, ECG, rate) and a Philips three-channel analogue writer recording mmHg, mm CSF and end-tidal CO_2. Test accuracy of this closed, undamped system is ± 0.1 mmHg. With a running log, the Opening Pressure (OP) is noted and infusion undertaken to establish plateau or an arbitrary safety ceiling of 40 mmHg (550 mmCSF). The lumbar sac pressure (LSP) is allowed to settle to a stable Resting Pressure (RP) after each run. The procedure takes a little over an hour in a quiet, darkened room. There was no infection or clinical complication. One adeolescent female became agitated, she and two others reporting transient sacral paresthesia.

Discussion

RP and infusion responses are tabulated (Table Ia). Four major groups emerged (Table Ib). Analogue records followed seven familiar patterns (Table Ic). OP was inconstant but despite earlier misgivings of the 'Blow-through' phenomenon (step-wise decrease in RP following each infusion), RP proved a repeatable steady state. Leakage (indicated by a spontaneous decline in RP or an established plateau) occurred once. Drift followed inadequate equipment warm-up time. Normal pre-test patient hydration was essential to achieve steady states or the

Table I. LSIT FINDINGS

1a Resting Pressure/Infusion Response : Number of studies

Resting Pressure: Base Line HSP (mm CSF)	SCT (mm Hg)	Infusion Rate				
		3.0	Plateau	Steady-state above Ceiling		
		1.5	Plateau	Plateau	Steady-state above Ceiling	
		1.0	Plateau	Plateau	Plateau	Steady-state above Ceiling
		'Dangerous'		1	2	9
350	20					
		'High'	3	8	12	8
200	10					
		Elevated (arguable)	4	3	8	5
120	4					
		'Normal'	5	2	2	1

HSP Horizontal Sagittal Plane (mmCSF)
SCT Superior Convexity Tangent (mmHg)
1.'Dry Tap' 1.Incomplete Studies = 75

1b Major Groups

Resting Pressure	Infusion Response: Tolerant	Intolerant
High	Pressure dependent	Stress Intolerant
Low	Normal	Rate sensitive

1c Common Analogue Patterns

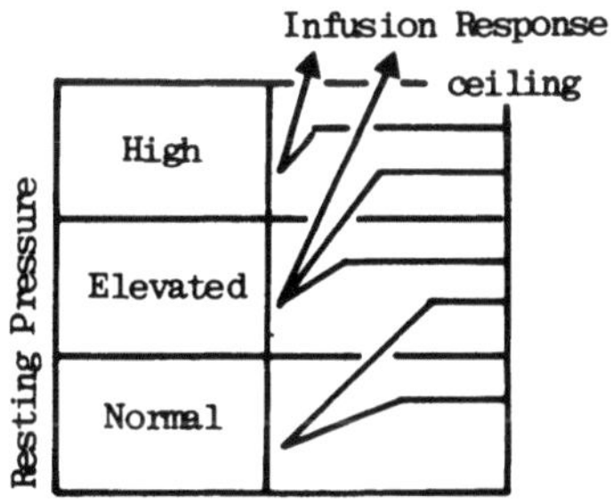

ceiling without large-volume infusion. Less than 18 FG needles produced a 'kick up' artifact on initiating high flows. Suspect system harmonics were traced to the variable positional effects of miniscule bubbles, damping when close to the patient but allowing a 'water-hammer ('ringing')' effect when adjacent to the transducer (5). Absolutely-constant infusion rates were not delivered by commercially-available pumps: SRI produced a reliable model to order. Presumed cortical venous collapse, leading to spontaneous exacerbation of induced high LSP, was encountered twice and promptly aborted without sequelae by hyper-ventilation. There was no suggestion of two resorptive systems (6) - rather the inter-relation of critical opening pressures for CSF resorption with variable available resorptive populations. Waves reflected patient torpor rather than pathology. The parenchymal swelling ("swollen brain") BICHT group could not be differentiated with confidence from minor, focal venous outflow obstruction without a dynamic isotope scan. The effect of major sinus occlusions on both venous and CSF outflow was evident in the "stress intolerant" group, where response to treatment was monitored by serial studies.

Simple in concept, LSIT is complex in execution. Interpretation is incomplete and subject to many labile variables (7,4). Slopes mimic pressure-volume curves, perfusion indices are convenient (3) but both lack precision. Resting pressure and analogue patterns are immediately available, quantifiable, comparable, repeatable and useful - though pattern recognition depends on clinical experience and has yet to be proved in a large series. Matching with CAT and dynamic isotope scan provides an investigatory triad which indicates intracranial compartmental status and outlines the two major intracranial circulations. CAT "atrophy" is uncertain without LSIT normality whilst venous outflow pattern aids BICHT differentiation.

Summary

Once standardized, LSIT defined RP and stress response - both central to management in suspect CSF circulatory abnormality and BICHT. Further identified variables are likely to have contributed to confusion in the past. With its compliemntary investigations LSIT warrants wider application.

References

1. Black PM, Sweet WH (1977) Normal pressure hydrocephalus - idiopathic type selection of patients for shunt procedures. In: Wullenweber R et al (eds) Lumbar Disc Adult Hydrocephalus. Springer Berlin Heidelberg New York, p 106

2. Hartman A, Alberti E (1977) Cerebral blood flow and cerebrospinal fluid pressure in patients with communicating hydrocephalus. In: Wullenweber R et al (eds) Lumbar Disc Adult Hydrocephalus. Springer Berlin Heidelberg New York, p 144

3. Martins AN (1973) Resistance to drainage of cerebrospinal fluid: clinical measurement and significance. J Neurol Neurosurg Psychiat 36:313-318

4. Trotter JL, Luzecky M, Siegel BA, Gado M (1974) Cerebrospinal fluid infusion test: identification of artifacts and correlation with cisternography and pneumoencephalography. Neurol 24:181-186

5. Schmidt-Anderson P, Holt DW, Baldwin A (1978) Personal Communications

6. Sokolowski SJ (1976) Bolus injection test for measurement of cerebrospinal fluid absorption. J Neurol Sci 28:491-504

7. Sprung Ch, Collman H, Fuchs EC, Suwito S, Duisberg R (1977) Pre- and post-operative evaluation of hydrocephalus using the infusion test. In: Wullenweber R et al (eds) Lumbar Disc Adult Hydrocephalus. Springer, Berlin Heidelberg New York, p 161

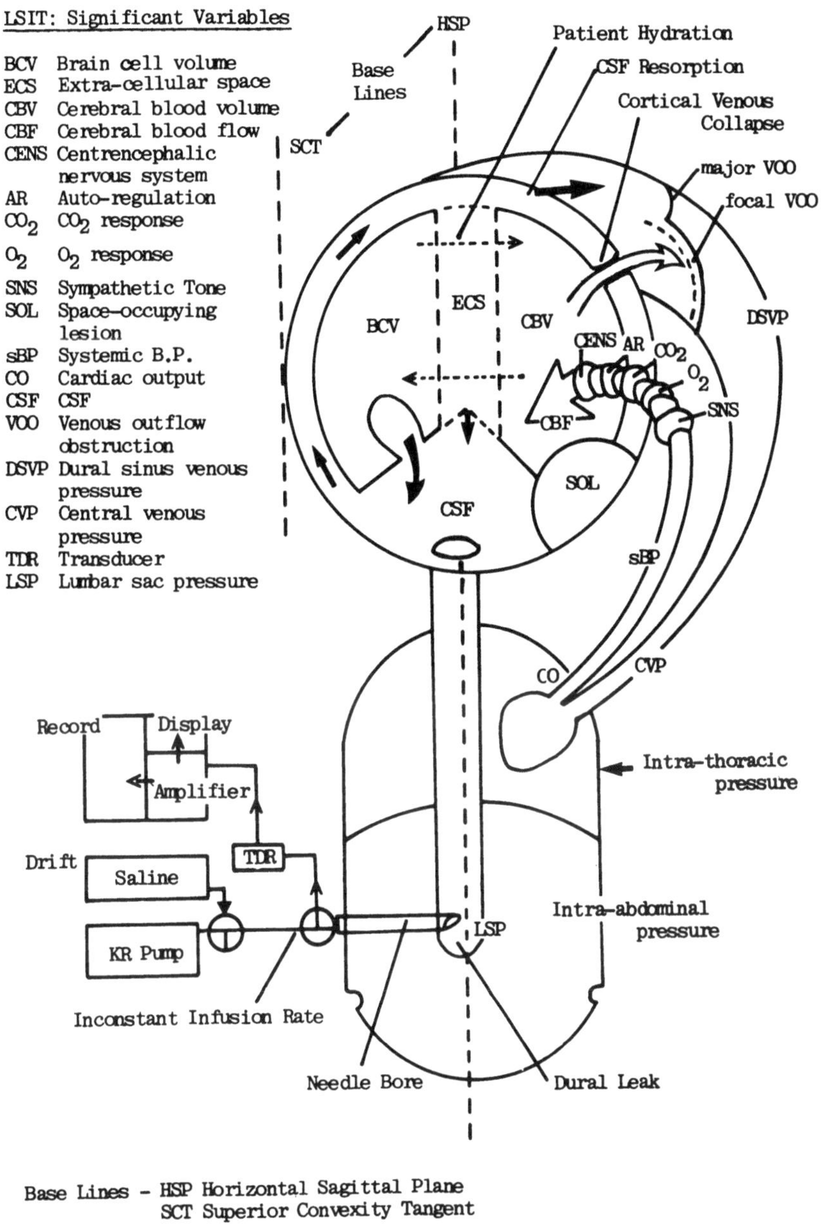

Fig. 1. Significant Variables.

COMPARISON OF CSF OUTFLOW RESISTANCE DETERMINED BY BOLUS AND STEADY-STATE TECHNIQUES

H.G.SULLIVAN, R.L.GRIFFITH, AND J.D.MILLER

Introduction

CSF outflow resistance R_{csf} may be calculated from bolus injections into the CSF space and this method has been employed to evaluate R_{csf} in man. The bolus technique is appealing because measurements of R_{csf} can be easily made in patients undergoing ventriculography, shunt insertion, or ICP monitoring: however, the bolus technique has not been compared with other, more standard methods of determinations of R_{csf}. This comparison affords not only the opportunity for judging the validity of bolus determinations of CSF outflow resistance but, perhaps more importantly, also allows one to test the validity of an unproven assumption utilized in developing the bolus method. The unproven assumption is that the same CSF P/V relationship holds for both rapid and slow changes in CSF volume.

Material and methods

Eighteen mongrel cats were anesthetized with i.v. Brevital, paralyzed with a continuous infusion of succinylcholine, and maintained on controlled ventilation. A 21G needle was placed stereotaxically into the anterior horn of each lateral ventricle. One of these needles was used to measure ICP and the other was used for either constant rate (Harvard Pump) or bolus infusions of Ringer's lactate into the CSF space. In each animal a set of three intraventricular bolus injections was paired with a single slow infusion. Three or four such pairings were made for each animal. All boluses were 0.3 ml while constant rate infusions varied 0.04 to 0.40 ml/min. The maximum pressure plateau due to constant infusion was adjusted for each animal so that it was approximately equal to the peak CSF pressure after a bolus of 0.3 ml. Thus, R_{csf} by bolus and steady-state methods were compared over nearly the same pressure range. For each animal a value of CSF outflow resistance (R_B) was computed for each bolus intraventricular injection and the mean value of R_B was compared with the value of CSF outflow resistance (R_S) from the slow infusion data. The theory behind the bolus and slow infusion methods for CSF outflow resistance calculation has been previously published (1).

Results

R_S varied from 74 to 293 mmHg/ml min^{-1} while R_B varied from 56 to 161 mmHg/ml min^{-1}. In all but 3 cats R_B was less than R_S. The three exceptions were at relatively low values of R_{csf} and the underestimate of R_S by R_B grew as R_{csf} increased so that, at high R_{csf}, R_B was only about half as large as R_S.

Discussion

The discrepancy between R_B and R_S suggests that the CSF P/V relationship known to be valid for bolus changes in CSF volume is not valid when CSF volume change is less rapid. We hypothesize that tissue relaxation - a fundamental property of brain as a viscoelastic material (2) - has produced the discrepancy noted between R_B and R_S. The bolus method assumed that P_{csf} decay after intraventricular bolus injection is due only to CSF absorption. Our data suggest that after bolus intraventricular loading P_{csf} decays not only as a result of CSF absorption but also as a result of tissue relaxation.

References

1. Sullivan HG, Miller JD, Griffith RL, Carter W, Rucker S (1979) Bolus versus steady-state infusion for determination of CSF Outflow resistance. Ann Neurol 5:228-238

2. Schettini A, Walsh EK (1973) Pressure relaxation of the intracranial system in vivo. Am J Physiol 225:513-517

Work supported by NIH grants #1 RO1 NS 14309-01; # 7 RO1 NS 15995-01.

THE CORRELATION OF OVERNIGHT VENTRICULAR FLUID PRESSURE RECORDING WITH SERIAL METRIZAMIDE VENTRICULOGRAPHY IN HYDROCEPHALUS

G.BROCKLEHURST

Introduction

The reports of SYMON and DORSCH (2,3) emphasized the value of overnight recordings of intracranial pressure in the elucidation of chronic hydrocephalus. Our initial experience in the use of this technique suggested that the appearance of A-waves and B-waves of increased magnitude were important findings, in addition to elevation of mean intracranial pressure. We have extended overnight ventricular fluid pressure (VFP) recordings to the investigation of a wide range of patients with suspected abnormalities of cerebro-spinal fluid (CBF) dynamics. More recently, following the introduction of the CAT scanner, we have extended conventional (static) metrizamide ventriculography to the study of the elimination of the contrast medium from the ventricular system, and termed this technique Serial Metrizamide Ventriculography (SMV) (I). This communication presents the results of the two types of investigation, and studies the possible correlation between them.

Material and methods

A number of patients with symptoms and signs indicating possible pathology in the CSF system have received an intraventricular injection of 3.75 grams of metrizamide (Amipaque) diluted with 8.9 mls of solvent through a Number 6 FG umbilical catheter which had been previously inserted into the right lateral ventricle through a twist-drill hole, performed under a general anesthetic. Conventional ventriculography was performed to define the anatomical situation, and 24 hours after the insertion of the metrizamide a serial CAT scan of the lateral ventricles was performed. The mean density and standard deviation (in Housfield units) for a selected area of the lateral ventricles was recorded (I). Overnight VFP recordings were made through the same catheter, using a Gaeltec 3EA (type A) pressure transducer placed at the level of the intraventricular foramen. The VFP was recorded on a Devices MI9 recorder calibrated from 0 to 50 mmHg for pressure, and recording at a rate of 50 divisions per ten minutes. The pressure recordings have been analyzed in terms of mean pressure throughout 20 minutes taken at least eight hours after the onset of recording. For each recording the absence or presence of A-waves, B-waves and zero drift was noted.

The clinical condition of each patient has been analyzed on a point system described in the accompanying table. Correlations between the clinical condition, VFP recordings and SMV have been explored by graph analysis.

Results

Fig. I shows the overnight VFP recording in 25 patients plotted against

TABLE. CLINICAL GRADING

Headache/Vomiting Papilledema Midline tumor A-waves	3 points each
Congenital malformation of CSF compartments Trauma or operation Meningitis Subarachnoid hemorrhage B-waves > 5mm	2 points each
Dementia or drowsiness Incontinence Ataxia	1 point each
Cerebral contusion Infarction	Deduct one point each

the clinical grade, as defined above. A similar plot of the 24 hour SMV against the clinical grade for 30 patients was made and appeared entirely haphazard (not illustrated). The VFP and SMV results in 22 patients who had both forms of investigations are plotted against each other in Fig 2.

Discussion

Fig 1 suggests a correlation between VFP and clinical grade, the higher the score of clinical grade the higher the mean VFP. However, the table shows that the clinical grade is not only weighted towards clinical features and conditions well known to be associated with raised intracranial pressure, but it includes also A-waves and B-waves observed in the records. In general, gross symptoms of raised intracranial pressure, and obviously obstructing tumors are associated with grossly raised mean pressure and A-waves. Perhaps more importantly, mean VFP records just above or below 10 mmHg are associated with B-waves and such clinical causes of chronic hydrocephalus as subarachnoid hemorrhage and trauma. Patients without such features, or with associated evidence of severe brain destruction from cerebral contusion or infarction, have lower pressures. The SMV is clearly delayed in those patients with grossly raised pressure and an obvious block of the ventricular system by a midline tumor. It also appears to be delayed in patients with ventricular dilatation and loss of cerebral tissue from cerebral contusion, infarction and previous long-standing hydrocephalus, or idiopathic cerebral atrophy. On the other hand, serial metrizamide ventriculography in patients with a grossly raised pressure but an undistorted ventricular system (such as in a benign intracranial hypertension) is relatively rapid.

Conclusion

In the results so far obtained, overnight VFP recording does not correlate with serial metrizamide ventriculography. The former, particularly when observed for the absence or presence of A-waves and B-waves is the most useful investigation for the detection of chronic hydrocephalus which will benefit from shunting procedures.

In a group of patients with various abnormalities in CSF dynamics, investigations have been performed using overnight VFP recordings, and SMV. The VFP recordings show some correlation with the clinical conditions as graded on an arbitrary scale, and is confirmed as a useful investigation for the elucidation of chronic hydrocephalus in particular. SMV, as experienced in 30 patients does not correlate with either clinical grading, or the VFP recordings. This latter investigation may indicate delayed clearance caused by loss of cerebral tissue from various pathologies.

<u>References</u>

1. Bockelehurst G (1978) Serial Metrizamide ventriculography - a preliminary communication. Z Kinderchir 24:336-340

2. Symon L, Dorsch NWC, Stephens RJ (1972) Pressure waves in so-called low-pressure hydrocephalus. Lancet II:1291-1292

3. Symon L, Dorsch NWC (1975) Use of long term pressure measurement to assess hydrocephalic patients prior to shunt surgery. J Neurosurg 42:258-273

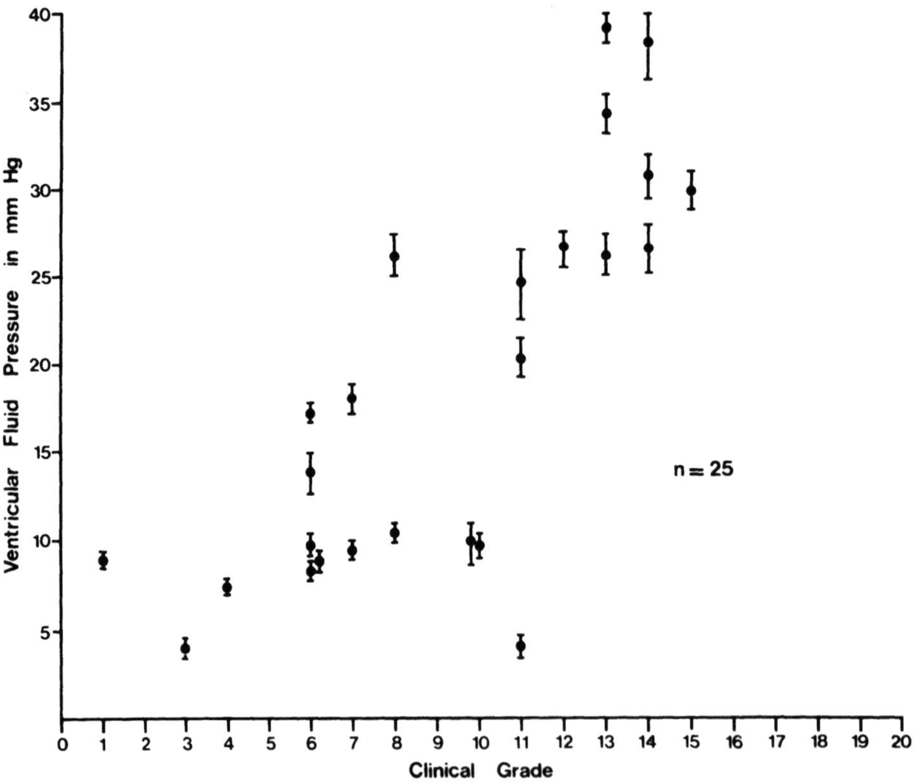

Fig. 1. VFP (overnight record of mean pressure throughout 20 min) plotted against the clinical grading of CSF abnormality as defined in table. A positive correlation is suggested.

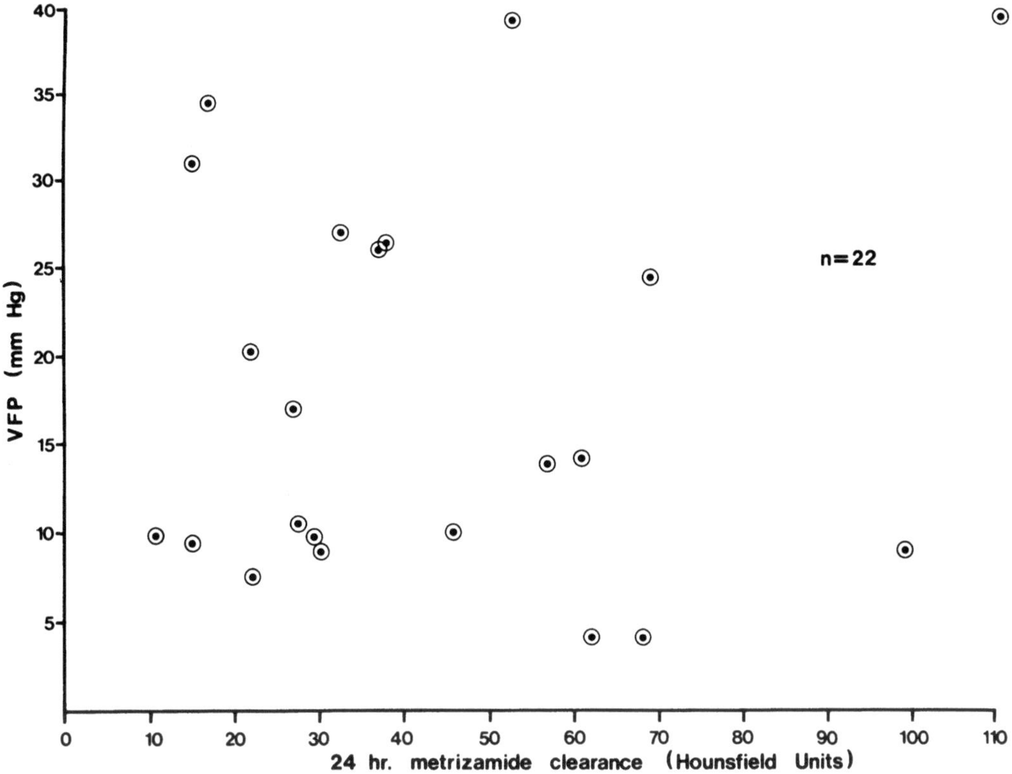

Fig.2. VFP plotted against SMV (mean and standard deviation of X-ray density of lateral ventricles in Hounsfield Units). The distribution appears to be haphazard.

DIFFERENTIAL EFFECTS OF PENTOBARBITAL, KETAMINE HYDROCHLORIDE, AND ENFLURANE ANESTHESIA ON CSF FORMATION RATE AND OUTFLOW RESISTANCE IN THE RAT

J.D.MANN, S.L.COOKSON, AND E.S.MANN

Introduction

Administration of general anesthesia can lead to profound changes in intracranial fluid dynamics and pressure, in part through effects on cardiac function, blood pressure and cerebrovascular reactivity. In this study, we have examined the effects of three anesthetic agents on two other components of intracranial pressure regulation in the rat, CSF reabsorption at the arachnoid villi, and rate of CSF formation.

Methods

Adult albino Sprague Dawley rats were anesthetized with one of the following agents: pentobarbital 40 mg/kg, i.p; ketamine hydrochloride, 40 mg/kg/hr, i.v.; or enflurane 2.5% in oxygen. Animals were paralyzed with pancuronium and artifically ventilated; body temperature was maintained at 37°C and blood pressure, EKG and CSF pressure were monitored continuously. pCO_2 was maintained in the range of 37 to 42 torr. Manometric infusions were performed through a 20 gauge spinal needle stereotaxically placed in the subarachnoid space at the cisterna magna. Artificial CSF was infused at multiple rates, between 5.0 and 20 µl/min. in each animal, and continued until steady state pressures were achieved for each infusion rate. Pressure responses to infusion were monitored and recorded continuously.

Our previously described mathematical model of CSF dynamics was used to determine outflow resistance and CSF formation rate (3,6). Equations for this model are: $Q = I/M \cdot e^{P/P_R}$, and $R = MP \cdot e^{-P/P_R}$, where Q is the rate of infusion in µl/minute, R is resistance to CSF outflow at the arachnoid villi, P is steady state CSF pressure, and M and P_R are species specific equation coefficients.

Results

Resting CSF pressure was significantly higher in the ketamine and enflurane animals compared to the pentobarbital group (Table I). In contrast, arterial blood pressure was well maintained for both ketamine and pentobarbital animals, while rats anesthetized with enflurane exhibited the expected fall in MABP. Maximum CSF outflow resistance was increased more than two-fold in enflurane and ketamine treated rats compared to those given pentobarbital. Outflow resistance at resting pressure for ketamine was 50% greater than for enflurane and 3-fold greater than for pentobarbital. Calculated CSF formation rate was not significantly different between the ketamine and pentobarbital animals. However, enflurane animals exhibited a significant two-fold increase in rate of CSF production.

Comparison of equation coefficients revealed a marked increase in the pressure at which outflow resistance is maximal (P_R) for enflurane,

Table 1. Tabulation of observed and calculated physiologic variables and equation coefficients for the three anesthetics studied.

	Resting CSF Pressure (mm H_2O)	MABP[1] (mm Hg)	Maximum CSF Outflow Resistance (mm H_2O/ul/min)	CSF Outflow Resistance at Resting Pressure	CSF Formation Rate (ul/min)	Equation Coefficients 1/M	P_R
Pentobarbital (n = 13)	35 ± 19 SD	106 ± 10 SD	10.2 ± 1.97 SD	8.41 ± 1.37 SD	4.62 ± 1.87 SD	3.36 ± .42 SEM	97 ± 3.6 SEM
Ketamine Hydrochloride (n = 16)	85 * ± 9	110 ± 8	27.4 ** ± 5.64	25.7 ** ± 5.24	3.29 ± 1.24	1.63 ** ± .23	120 * ± 6.2
Enflurane (n = 14)	130 ** ± 19	78 ** ± 13	23.7 ** ± 3.48	18.4 ± 4.95	7.30 ** ± 1.52	3.95 ± .38	255 ** ± 14.7

Significance compared to pentobarbital:

* $p < .01$,
** $p < .001$.

[1] Mean Arterial Blood Pressure.

and a drop in I/M for ketamine. The net effects of these variations are shown in Figures 1 and 2. The semi-log plots in Fig 1 illustrate the smaller CSF pressure responses for all infusion rates in the pentobarbital animals compared to the other two groups. While rats given enflurane exhibited smaller pressure increments than ketamine treated animals at low infusion rates, this effect was reversed at flows above 10 μl/min and at pressures above 200 mm H_2O. Examination of the outflow resistance profiles for each agent (Fig 2) reveals a marked elevation in outflow resistance for both ketamine and enflurane compared to pentobarbital. Ketamine produces an increase in outflow resistance at lower pressures, which then rapidly falls off as higher pressures and flows are reached, while enflurane produces an increase in outflow resistance which is maintained at both high and low pressures.

Discussion

Major findings which emerged from this study are: 1) the increased rate of CSF production in the enflurance anesthetized animals; and 2) the increase in CSF outflow resistance which occurs with both ketamine and enflurane compared to pentobarbital.

The possibility of increased CSF production with enflurane was suggested by MYERS and SHAPIRO when they found a striking increase in choroid plexus glucose utilization in the enflurane anesthetized rat (8). CSF production by choroid plexus has recently been shown to be influenced by the autonomic nervous system, in that sympathetic denervation of the plexus enhances production while sympathetic stimulation suppresses the rate of CSF formation (5). Hence, the reduction in sympathetic tone which accompanies enflurane anesthesia, and which is reflected in a decreased MABP, may trigger an increase in CSF production when this agent is administered. Ketamine, which generally increases sympathetic tone, was associated with the lowest calculated rate of CSF formation of the three groups, while animals given pentobarbital at doses which did not significantly depress MABP, had an intermediate rate of production.

The biologic mechanisms resulting in increased CSF outflow resistance observed with ketamine and enflurane have not been defined. CSF outflow at the arachnoid villi is governed in part by pressure dependent pinocyte (low pressure), vacuole and large transcellular pore (high pressure) formation in endothelial cells covering arachnoid villi in the major venous sinuses (1). Hence, membrane fluidity, or the property of a membrane which allows it to deform in response to pressure, may be critical in CSF reabsorption. Additionally, endothelial cell pinocytosis may be dependent on a number of metabolic factors, including calcium, circulating hormones, cofactors and vasopressin.

In terms of the proposed cellular mechanisms for CSF reabsorption, ketamine has been shown to decrease membrane fluidity, probably as a result of changes in membrane protein configuration (2). If pressure deformation of endothelial cell membrane is important in pinocyte and/or vacuole formation, membrane stiffening in response to ketamine would result in an increase in the pressure required for pinocyte formation, and thus an increase in resistance to reabsorption of CSF as found in our experiment. Additionally, ketamine displacement of calcium from the membrane (9) would result in impaired fusion of pinocytes to the cell surface membrane and reduced exocytosis of CSF containing vacuoles and pinocytes on the venous surface of endothelial cells covering arachnoid villi.

The response to ketamine may be a graded one in that outflow resistance drops relatively rapidly at higher pressures and flows compared to enflurane, suggesting that mechanisms involved in large vacuole and/or transcellular pore formation may be less affected by ketamine than pinocyte formation.

The possible mechanisms for enflurane induced changes in outflow resistance are less clear. Enflurane, like pentobarbital, is reported to increase membrane fluidity and thus should result in enhanced transport of CSF by pinocytosis (2). However, it has also been reported that enflurane increases cerebral blood flow (7). A resulting rise in sagittal sinus pressure would tend to impede CSF reabsorption. Increased CSF production observed with enflurane would also contribute to an apparent rise in outflow resistance. Enflurane depression of endothelial cell metabolism might also account for the observed increase in outflow resistance, and a similar effect on cardiac function would result in an elevation in intracranial venous sinus pressure, slowing CSF reabsorption as observed in our experiment.

Low resting CSF pressures with a normal formation rate suggests enhanced CSF reabsorption in pentobarbital treated animals. This may be related to a direct effect of pentobarbital on membrane formation and distribution (4), or may be a secondary effect related to changes in regional cerebral blood flow, the release of vasopressin, or other as yet undefined factors.

We conclude that both ketamine and enflurane have major, potentially adverse, effects on mechanisms which regulate intracranial pressure, including CSF formation and reabsorption, and that these agents may be contraindicated in situations where control of intracranial pressure is important.

Summary

A comparison of the effects of pentobarbital, ketamine and enflurane on the rate of CSF Production and resistance to CSF reabsorption in rats is reported. A significant increase in CSF formation rate was found with enflurane, while use of either enflurane or ketamine resulted in increased resistance to CSF reabsorption compared to pentobarbital. Results are in part consistent with previously reported effects of these agents on membrane function, and have important implications in terms of choice of anesthesia in situations where intracranial pressure buffering mechanisms are compromised.

References

1. Butler AB, Mann JD, Bass NH (1977) Vesicular transport of peroxidase across the endothelium of the rat arachnoid villus. Anat Rec 187:543

2. Familiari M (1977) Meccanismo d'azione della ketamine a livello di membrana. Minerva Anest 43:435-448

3. Johnson RN, Maffeo CJ, Mann JD, Butler AB, Bass NH (1978) Intracranial pressure regulation: A comparative model of cerebrospinal fluid systems. T -I -T J Life Sci 8:79-92

4. Jones DG, Devon RM (1978) An ultrastructural study into the effects of pentobarbitone on synaptic organization.BrainRes 147:47-63

5. Lindvall M, Edvinsson L, Owman C (1978) Sympathetic nervous control of cerebrospinal fluid production from the choroid plexus. Science 201:176-178

6. Mann JD, Butler AB, Rosenthal JE, Maffeo CJ, Johnson RN, Bass NH (1978) Regulation of intracranial pressure in rat, dog, and man. Ann Neurol 3:156-165

7. Michenfelder JD, Cucchiara RF (1974) Canine cerebral oxygen consumption during enflurane anesthesia and its modification during induced seizures. Anesthesiol 40:575-580

8. Myers RR, Shapiro HM (1978) Paradoxical effect of enflurance on choroid plexus metabolism; Clinical implications. In: Abstracts of Scientific Papers, American Society of Anesthesiologists Ann Meeting

9. Seeman P (1972) The membrane actions of anesthetics and tranquilizers. Pharmacol Rev 24:583-655

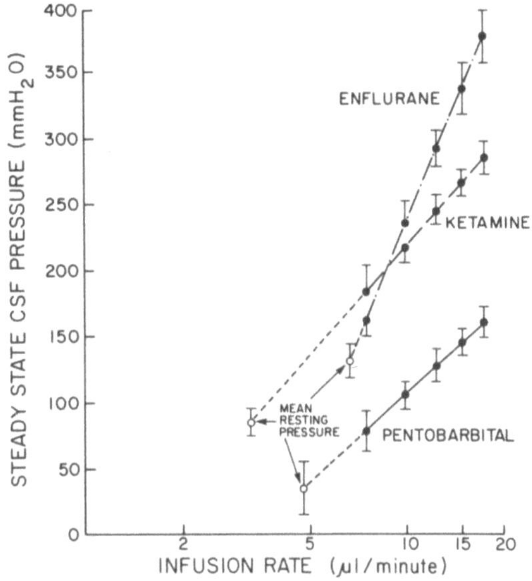

Fig. I. Steady state CSF pressure vs infusion rate for three anesthetic agents in the rat. Extrapolation of steady state values to resting pressure gives an estimate of rate of CSF formation.

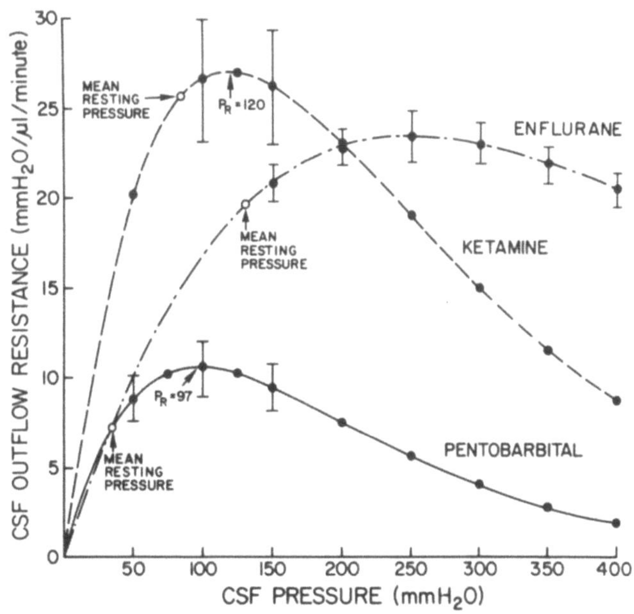

Fig.2. CSF outflow resistance (resistance to absorption) vs intracranial pressure. Outflow resistance profiles are non-linear for all three agents.

CEREBROSPINAL FLUID FORMATION RATE IN COLD INDUCED BRAIN EDEMA

G.M.HOCHWALD AND K.G.GO

Introduction

Cold induced brain edema fluid is thought to propagate through the white matter from the site of the lesion. In the severe cold lesion brain edema model, a large increase in white matter content occurs with hours, and edema fluid can be isolated (1). The edema fluid is driven through white matter by blood pressure and causes tissue pressure gradients to extend from the lesion to normal tissue along the edema pathway (2). As both labelled substances within edema and components of edema fluid are found in the ventricular CSF (2), clearance of edema fluid by CSF flow is thought to occur. This model was used to determine whether severe cerebral edema alters CSF formation. To eliminate individual variation, CSF formation was measured in the same animal by ventriculocisternal perfusion both before and after a cold lesion. In addition, brain water content and arterial blood pressure were measured.

Materials and methods

Pentobarbital anesthetized and paralyzed adult mongrel cats were artificially ventilated. End-tidal CO_2 was monitored, and body temperature controlled. Anesthesia was maintained with nitrous oxide-oxygen mixture. Arterial blood pressure was recorded, and prior to the cold injury 10ml of 0.5% Evans blue was injected intravenously. A 19-G needle was stereotaxically placed into the cerebral ventricle. A 19-G needle was also inserted into the cisterna magna. To avoid excessive ICP following the cold lesion, a large part of the skull overlying cerebral hemispheres was removed. Ventriculocisternal perfusion was performed at a rate of 6 ml/hr (3) and ventricular pressure was measured with a pressure transducer. The perfusion fluid was a mock CSF (3) containing 50 mg of bovine serum albumin, and ^{125}I-serum albumin as the non-diffusible indicator substance. During steady state perfusion (3), i.e., about 2-1/2 hours after the start of the perfusion, a cold injury was made to the parietal region of one cerebral hemisphere by holding a cryogenic probe (-30°) of 13 mm diameter against the dura for 5 minutes. The perfusion was continued until steady state was again attained. The cat was then killed and the brain removed. The extent of the lesion was assessed by examining brain slices for extravasation of intravenously injected Evans blue dye, and by comparing water content of edematous and contralateral hemisphere after drying tissue to constant weight. CSF formation rate was calculated as previously described (3).

Results

Only those cats were included in these studies who had cold induced brain lesions extending from pial to ventricular surfaces as judged by Evans blue staining. After cold injury perfusate was also stained with Evans blue. Table I shows the effects of a cold lesion on CSF formation, intraventricular pressure, arterial pressure and cerebral water content. CSF formation measured in 7 cats before cold injury was 21.6 ± 1.1 µl/min (mean ± SE). After lesion, formation rate was 17.5 ± 1.3 µl/min. When results from individual cats were compared, an 18.1% decrease in CSF formation was calculated (P<0.001 Wilcoxon signed rank test).

The mean arterial pressure measured before the cold injury was 159.9± 8.6 mmHg, and after it was 155.9 ± 10.5 mmHg. The decrease in pressure was not statistically significant (P<0.05). As a result of the cold lesion there was a significant increase in mean ventricular pressure which rose from 2.0 ± 0.8 to 15.6 ± 3.6 mmHg (P>0.001). This resulted in a decrease in cerebral perfusion pressure of 9.9 ± 2.0% (P<0.02). In the edematous hemisphere cortical and subcortical white matter was 85.7 ± 1% and 79.7 ± 1.4% respectively. In the contralateral control hemisphere cortical and subcortical white matter content was 80.6 ± 1.4% and 68.3 ± 2.5% respectively. The increase in water content of the lesion side was significant (P<0.01).

Discussion

In contrast to other organs, the brain does not have a lymphatic system. Brain edema fluid must therefore be cleared either by the blood or by CSF. The results of REULEN et al (2) indicate that bulk flow is the primary means responsible for flow of edema fluid through the extracellular space, and that clearance of cold injury induced edema fluid into ventricular CSF is the result of the hydrostatic pressure gradient between the edematous brain and CSF. However, they did not measure CSF formation rate. Under the conditions of our experiments the cold lesion causes a small but consistent decrease in CSF formation. The lesion also causes a marked increase in brain water content, an increase in pressure, and a decrease in cerebral perfusion pressure. Previous studies (3) on the effects of cold injury showed no significant changes in CSF formation rate. No attempt was made in those studies to estimate the extent of the cold lesion.

The means by which the rate of CSF formation is decreased by a cold lesion was not persued in these studies. Previous studies have shown that 4-5 hours of ventriculocisternal perfusion alone does not result in a measurable decrease in CSF formation (3). A significant fraction of the total CSF production is derived from extrachoroidal sources. The effect of a cold lesion on CSF production may then be due to the partial inhibition of fluid flow from this source. The possible mechanisms responsible for this decrease in flow include: a) a decrease in cerebral blood flow and capillary filtration rate, b) a decrease in cerebral perfusion pressure, c) an interruption of the extracellular fluid pathway.

References

1. Gazendam J, Go KG, VanZanten W(to be published) Composition of isolated edema fluid in cold-induced brain edema. J Neurosurg
2. Reulen HJ, Tsuyuma M, Tack A, Fenske AR,Prioliau GR(1978) Clearance of edema fluid into cerebrospinal fluid.J Neurosurg 48:754-764
3. Hochwald GM, Marlin AE, Wald A. Malhan C (1976) Movement of water between blood, brain and CSF in cerebral edema. In: Pappius HM, Feindel W(eds) Dynamics of Brain Edema. Springer, Berlin Heidelberg New York, p 129

TABLE I

EFFECTS OF CEREBRAL COLD LESION ON CSF FORMATION (Vcsf), INTRAVENTRICULAR PRESSURE (Vp), ARTERIAL PRESSURE (Ap), CEREBRAL PERFUSION (Cpp), AND CEREBRAL WATER CONTENT (%H_2O)[1].

n	Vcsf (ul/min) Before	Vcsf (ul/min) After	Vp (mm Hg) Before	Vp (mm Hg) After	Ap (min Hg) Before	Ap (min Hg) After	Cpp (mm Hg)[2] Before	Cpp (mm Hg)[2] After	%H_2O WM[3] Control	%H_2O WM[3] Lesion	%H_2O C_x[4] Control	%H_2O C_x[4] Lesion
7	21.6 ±1.1	17.5 ±1.2	2.0 ±0.8	15.6 ±3.6	159.9 ±8.7	155.9 ±10.5	157.9 ±8.9	140.3 ±9.2	68.3 ±2.5	80.6 ±1.4	79.7 ±1.4	85.7 ±1.1

1) All values are mean ± SE, calculated from measurements made before and after a cold lesion to the cerebrum of n=7 cats. The differences between before and after values in each category is statistically significant (see results).
2) Difference between arterial and intraventricular pressure.
3) WM, white matter.
4) Cx, cerebral cortex.

CORTICAL BULK FLOW IN NORMAL AND HYPOSMOLAR EDEMA

R.O.DUNKER

Introduction

In an earlier report we described a series of experiments in which we measured the migration of horseradish peroxidase (HRP) through the interhemispheric cortical extracellular space of adult rabbits (1). The pattern of migration suggested that the cerebral extracellular space (ECS) volume was quite heterogeneous and that in the deeper cortical laminae the diffusing HRP was entrained in a bulk flow of ECS fluid flowing toward the white matter. It would follow from this theory of cortical bulk flow that an increased production of cortical ECS fluid would increase the centripetal bulk flow and thereby increase the rate of migration of HRP into the deeper cortical laminae. PATBERG (4) and HOCHWALD(2) have demonstrated an increased production of cortical ECS fluid in hyposmolar edema. We have measured the migration of HRP through the cerebral cortex of normal and water intoxicated rabbits to test our theory of cortical bulk flow.

Materials and methods

Two groups of four adult New Zealand rabbits weighing 2.7 - 4.2 kg were anesthetized with i.v. pentobarbitol (56 mg/kg) or Halothane anesthesia. The animals were placed in a sphinx position with a tracheostomy and arterial and venous catheters in place. A 30-gauge needle was advanced through the dura at the bregma to lie within the interhemispheric fissure. A 20-gauge needle was advanced into the cisterna magna transcutaneously for venting CSF and thereby maintain CSF pressure constant at atmospheric pressure.

In the water intoxication group of animals sterile water (94 ml/kg) was administered intravenously over one hour. Thirty minutes later a 5% solution of HRP was infused into the interhemispheric subarachnoid space at a constant rate (1). The experiments were terminated by transcardiac vascular perfusion with a glutaraldehyde-paraformaldehyde fixation solution. The control group of animals were treated in an identical manner as the water intoxication group except that no sterile water was administered and the 60 min HRP infusion was begun shortly after the animals had been prepared for infusion.

Within one hour of fixation coronal sections (30 µm) of the brain through the infusion site were incubated in diaminobenzidine-hydrogen peroxide (DAB-H_2O_2), and the maximum depth of penetration of the least optically detectable concentration of HRP-DAB-H_2O_2 reaction production perpendicular to the pial surface was ascertained with an optical micrometer.

Results

Femoral arterial pressure was monitored in each animal and did not vary more than 20 torr from animal to animal nor more than 10 torr from beginning to end of each experiment. Serum osmolarity was measured in the water intoxicated animals throughout the experimental protocol (Table 1).

Table 1. Course of serum osmolarity in water intoxicated rabbits

	Initial determination	Time after i.v. water administration immediate	30 minutes	90 minutes
serum osmolarity in milliosmoles	302±1 (3)	258±2 (2)	268±4 (3)	266±2 (2)

The maximum depth of penetration (mdp) of HRP after 60 minutes of exposure in the control animals was 0.96 mm from the pial surface. Diffusion kinetics predicted a maximum depth of diffusion of 0.71 mm at 60 minutes. A diffusion profile for water intoxicated animals had predicted a mdp of HRP to be 0.70 mm at 60 minutes (this diffusion profile was constructed from data from a large group of water intoxicated rabbits in which cerebral bulk flow had ceased). The mdp of HRP measured in the water intoxicated group was 1.24 mm (Table 2).

Table 2. Maximum depth of penetration of HRP at 60 minutes exposure

	estimated mdp	measured mdp
control rabbits	0.71 mm	0.96 mm
water intoxicated rabbits	0.70 mm	1.24 mm $p<0.001$

Discussion

If at least part of the cortical ECS fluid is formed within the cerebral cortex in accordance with Starling's laws, then one would expect that lowering the plasma oncotic pressure while maintaining intracranial pressure constant would increase the quantity of cortical ECS fluid formed. Neither VAN HARREVELD (5) nor OPPELT (3) have demonstrated any change in the extracellular space volume of the cortex following water intoxication. Therefore, if cortical bulk exists normally, an increase in ECS fluid production such as observed by PATBERG (4) and HOCHWALD (2) should result in an increased rate of ECS fluid bulk flow.

In our experimental design the maximum deviation of experimental data from estimated diffusion occurs at 60 minutes. The mdp of HRP in the control rabbits falls outside 99% tolerance limits for diffusion kinetics and this suggests that normally there is a centripetal bulk flow with a velocity of at least 8.3×10^{-3} mm/min (difference between estimated and measured mdp divided by the time HRP migration could be influenced by bulk flow or 30 minutes). The bulk flow velocity in water intoxicated rabbits was found to be 2.2 times greater than in controls.

Bulk flow velocity is proportional to ECS fluid production, and the increase we observed agrees nicely with the increased ECS fluid production reported by HOCHWALD (2) in similar water intoxication experiments in cats. The different time course of increased ECS fluid production in his experiments and ours probably reflects the differences in experimental design.

References

1. Dunker RO, Harris AB, Jenkins DP (1976) Kinetics of horseradish peroxidase migration through cerebral cortex. Brain Res 118:199-217

2. Hochwald GM, Wald A. Malhan C (1976) Sink action of cerebrospinal fluid volume flow. Arch Neurol 33:339-344

3. Oppelt WW, Patlak CS, Rall DR (1964) Extracellular space in brain exposed to hypo- or hypertonic environments. Clin Res 12:197

4. Patberg WR, Go KG, Teelkan AW (1977) Isolation of edema fluid in cold-induced cerebral edema for the study of colloid osmotic pressure, lactate dehydrogenase activity, and electrolytes. Exp Neurol 54:141-147

5. VanHarreveld A, Collewign H, Malhotra SK (1966) Water, electrolytes and extracellular space in hydrated and dehydrated brains. Am J Physiol 210:251-256

Session IX

HYDROCEPHALUS

Chairman: H.D.Portnoy
Co-chairman: P.Janny

SUMMARY

It was brought out in the discussion on valves that the spring-ball valve of HAKIM had a tendency to overdrain when the patient was standing. Changing to a higher pressure valve did not alter this because of the hydrostatic pressure generated by the distal catheter. PORTNOY indicated that this problem was readily corrected by placing an antisiphon device immediately at the outlet of the valve. He also warned that the antisiphon device should not be used with the high pressure slit valves. This will result in inadequate shunting since the slit valves, when working properly, are gauged to overdrain when the patient is standing to compensate for the underdrainage occurring when the patient is supine.

CHAPMAN was asked regarding calibration of the shunt pressure sensor. He indicated it could be calibrated in vivo, thus obviating any problems with drift as a result of temperature and barometric changes.

JAMES brought out that many so-called arrested hydrocephalics insidiously deteriorate over the years, and stressed the necessity of watching the group closely. PORTNOY recommended shunt revision for children with an I.Q. under 80, or in which the I.Q. was deteriorating as evidenced by progressive difficulty in school or a decreasing I.Q. on repeated testing. After 6-12 months many of these children increase their I.Q. by 10-15 points.

In response to a question by LANGFITT, GJERRIS indicated that none of his patients with increased sulci on CT improved. It was also brought out in the discussion that some patients with increased sulci also have an absorption defect and may partially improve after shunting.

Several authors indicated that in the patients reviewed, the presence of B waves during at least 5-10% of a day was associated with a high rate of successful shunts. The question as to what qualified as a B wave ensued. TEASDALE defined the B wave as a periodic change in the ICP of at least 10mmHg at 1-2 cpm. BROCK indicated that the B waves had two forms, and were related to respiration. In addition to the usual form he has noted a more prominent B wave frequently associated with snoring. He felt that those patients demonstrating the larger form of the B wave were particularly good candidates for shunting. It was also pointed out that the B waves were related to REM sleep.

Several comments were made regarding the various tests used to distinguish between NPH and cerebral atrophy. TEASDALE noted that his group had difficulty in carrying out CBF studies because these patients would not hold still. EKSTEDT pointed out that a low conductance to the outflow of CSF did not necessarily have a good outcome following a shunt unless the resting pressure was also high. GJERRIS noted that in a small series of patients there was good correlation between B waves and the sum of the conduction and compliance values, but neither value separately. He felt that this sum was also predictive of a good result when found to be low. GJERRIS noted that all except four of his patients who had improved following a shunt had some decrease in ventricle size.

CROCKARD reminded the session that a test removal of CSF with subsequent transient clinical improvement was a good indication that the patient would improve after a shunt. He also noted that improvement following a shunt may not be clinically evident for several months and that better ways of psychometric testing are necessary.

HYDRODYNAMIC PROPERTIES OF CSF SHUNT SYSTEMS

J. EKSTEDT AND H. FRIDÉN

Introduction

A cerebrospinal fluid shunt is intended to lower the intracranial pressure. It should work in parallel with the physiological CSF outflow pathways. Very little has been done, so far, to analyze the hydrodynamics of the CSF in the individual patient, the hydrodynamics of the shunt implanted in such a patient, and the hydrodynamics of the combined patient-shunt system. This paper is part of a more extended study of shunts and deals mainly with the variability of the shunt properties.

Method

A modification of the apparatus used for hydrodynamic studies in man by EKSTEDT (1) was used. The experimental set-up is shown in Fig. 1. The shunt valve was kept in a water bath at 37°C. Pressure across the valve could be varied by varying the air pressure to a weighed bottle containing perfusion fluid. When almost empty, the weighed bottle was automatically refilled from a container via a millipore filter. Thus, the apparatus could be working automatically for days without supervision. Inlet pressure was measured with a transducer which was the input to a regulator circuit so that the pressure either could be kept constant or varied according to a preset function. Flow through the shunt was recorded by measuring the weight of the bottle and electronically differentiating the weight with a time constant of 5 s. The inlet pressure and flow signals were fed to an XY-recorder and to a continuously running multichannel recorder. Distilled water was used as perfusion fluid. Small air bubbles appeared to be a considerable problem by obstructing the valves. This was partly overcome by boiling the perfusion water for 10 minutes under vacuum. The water was then kept in a container at 90°C until used. It was also necessary to de-aereate the shunt itself. For a period of 24 hours before the experiment each shunt was continuously perfused with de-aereated water at a rate of about $10 mm^3/s$.

The experiments were always performed with the pressures and flows within the limits to be expected to occur when the shunt is inserted in the patient. Two main types of tests were used: In the first, short term, the perfusion pressure was continuously increased at a rate of 0.3 kPa/min until the flow through the shunt amounted to $20 mm^3/s$ and then decreased again at the same rate to a pressure of -0.25 kPa. The cycle was repeated at least 5 times. The second, long term, used two pressure levels which alternated every 15 minutes and lasted several days. At least 10 of each of the shunt systems commercially available in Sweden have been tested (HOLTER, PUDENZ, DENVER, AMES, RAIMONDI, Multi purpose-HEYER SCHULTE, HAKIM, H-V Lumbar Valve - CORDIS). Totally about 80 slit valves and 100 spring loaded ball valves have been tested.

Results

There was a striking similarity in hydrodynamic properties between all shunt systems which base their resistance and valve action on one or several slits in a silicone material. The other shunt system, using a spring-loaded ball in a conical opening (HAKIM and H-V Lumbar) behaved in a different way to the others.

The following principal findings were made:

A. Slit valves

1. When slowly increasing and decreasing pressure: The valves had no defined opening or closing pressure. Flow started at zero pressure and increased progressively with increasing pressure. Sometimes the shunt could remain shut during the lower pressure range and then suddenly pop open. Even in those cases the flow followed the typical curve when returning to low pressures.
2. Flushing the valve, i.e. forcing 10 ml of water through it within a time period of a few seconds, always resulted in considerably increased flow characteristics. Nevertheless, the flow curves rapidly shifted towards lower flows.
3. Even when not flushing the valve an extended experiment always resulted in a decrease of flow with time.
4. In the constant pressure long-term experiments there was always a decrease of the flow commencing soon after the start of the experiment and sometimes decreasing to zero during the following 5-15 hours. A short pressure increase for a few seconds usually restored some flow but the flow soon decreased again (Figure 2).

B. Spring-loaded ball valves

1. When slowly increasing and decreasing the perfusion pressure there was always a well-defined opening pressure below which there was no flow and above which the flow increased linearly with pressure.
2. Flushing of the device did not alter the pressure/flow characteristics.
3. Repeated experiments with increasing and decreasing pressure did not result in impaired flow characteristics.
4. In the constant pressure long-term experiments there could be some changes of flow with time but of much less magnitude than for the slit valves (Figure 3).

Discussion

Several hydrodynamic investigations on the hydrodynamic properties of shunt systems have been published (2-9). The question of variability of the properties in one and the same shunt at different occasions and with time do not seem to have been taken into account. The reason for the observed variability in the slit valves may be explained in different ways. When flushing the device, i.e. forcing a big volume of fluid through the slits in a very short time, the modulus of elasticity of the silicone is probably exceeded, resulting in deformation of the material which, however, will return to normal within a couple of hours. When flow through the valve is low the sides of the slit will adhere to each other, starting with the corners but within tens of hours involving the whole of the slit. A sudden pressure increase of flushing will open up the adhesed sides for a while but the adherence process will repeat itself. These slow changes in the material makes it very difficult to define what properties these devices will have when inserted in the CSF pathways. Sudden pressure increases as when coughing, sneezing or straining may change the properties for hours towards higher flow and thus cause unintended variations in the intracranial pressure. What may happen with the properties when the shunt has been working for years is not known.

Summary

The hydrodynamic properties of CSF shunt systems have been investigated with special attention to long term in vitro behavior. Systems based on slits in a silicone tube proved to have highly variable properties with the flow tending to decrease with time. This was not the case with the spring-loaded ball systems. It may be difficult to predict the long-term behavior of an inserted shunt system from an acute in vitro experiment.

References

1. Ekstedt J (1976) Studies in CSF hydrodynamics in man.Method of constant pressure CSF infusion. J Neurol Neurosurg Psych 40:105-119

2. Forrest DM (1962) Flow characteristics of the Spitz-Holter valve. Dev Med Child Neurol 4:295-297

3. Fox JL, McCullough DC, Green RC (1972) Cerebrospinal fluid shunts: an experimental comparison of flow rates and pressure values in various commercial systems. J Neurosurg 37:700-705

4. Fox JL, McCullough DC, Green RC (1973) Effect of cerebrospinal sluid shunts on intracranial pressure and on cerebrospinal fluid dynamics. J Neurol Neurosurg Psychiat 36:302-312

5. Hakim S (1973) Hydraulic and mechanical mis-matching of valve shunts used in the treatment of hydrocephalus: the need for a servo-valve shunt. Dev Med Child Neurol 15:646-653

6. Hakim S, Duran Dela Roche F, Burton JD (1973) A critical analysis of valve shunts used in the treatment of hydrocephalus. Dev Med Child Neurol 15:230-255

7. Portnoy HD, Schulte RR, Fox JL, Croissant PD, Tripp I (1973) Anti-siphon and reversible occlusion valves for shunting in hydrocephalus and preventing post-shunt subdural hematomas. J Neurosurg 38:729-738

8. Singh G, Anthony M, Marino LL, Zachary RB (1975) A study of the indian valve for ventriculo-atrial shunts in the treatment of hydrocephalus. Dev Med Child Neurol Suppl 35 to Vol 17:85-88

9. VanDerVeer PH (1972) Hydrodynamics of Holter ventriculo-atrial shunt systems under various conditions. Dev Med Child Neurol Suppl 27 to Vol 14:132-139

Work supported by grant No. B79-04X-04125-06 from Swedish Medical Research Council.

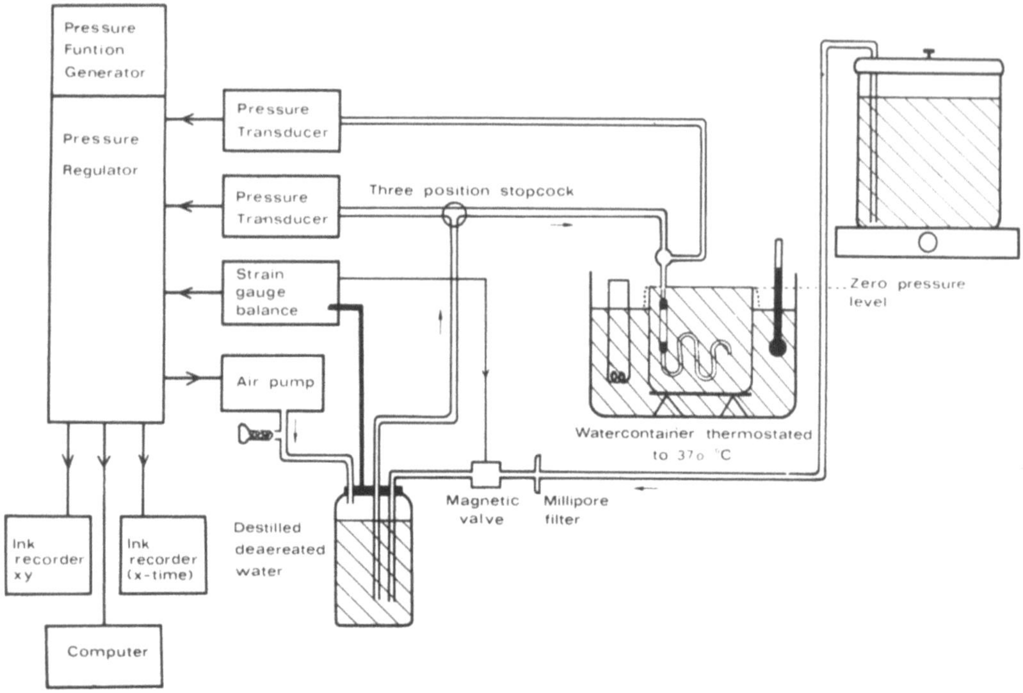

Figure I.
The experimental set up. The shunt is in a water bath in which it is continuously weighed. The perfusion pressure is regulated by varying the air pressure in the bottle with an air pump controlled by the pressure transducer at the inlet of the shunt device. The weighed bottle is automatically refilled when empty.

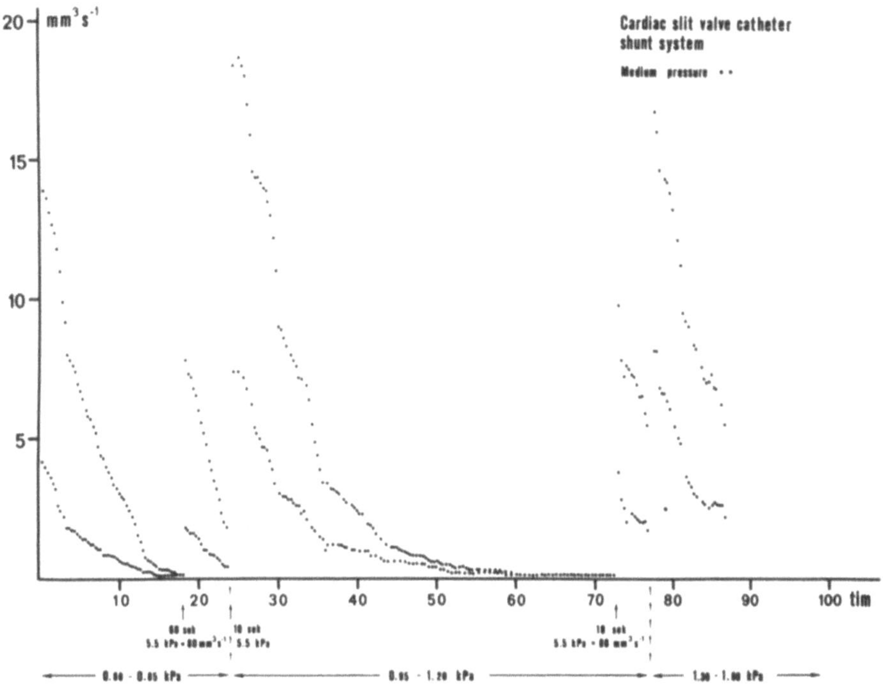

Figure 2.
A long-term experiment with a slit-valve. Two pressure levels have been used, alternating every 15 minutes. The flow decreases continuously towards zero, but can be temporarily increased by increasing the perfusion pressure for some seconds. During the 100 hour experiment the pressure levels have been increased as indicated in the figure.

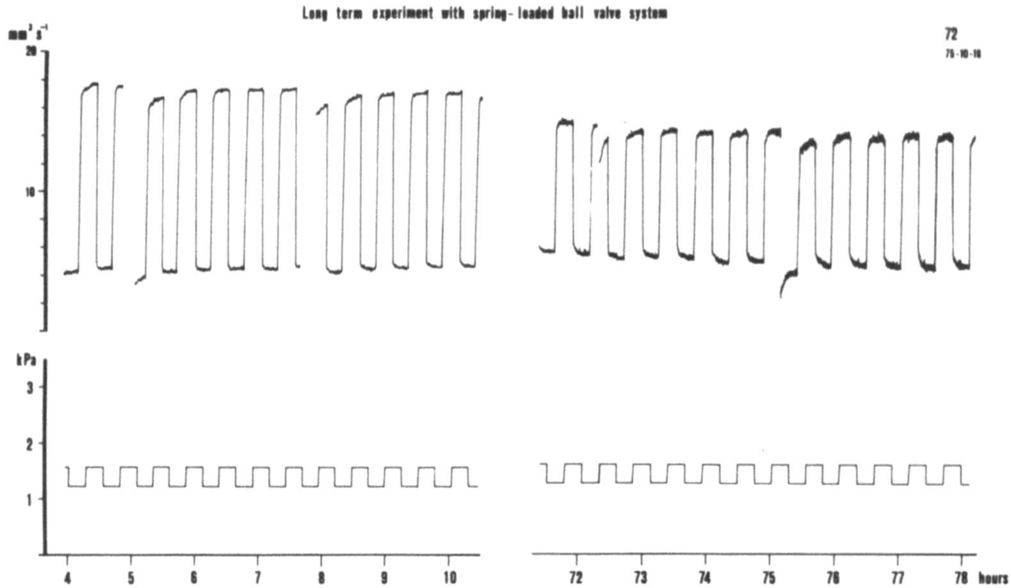

Figure 3.
A long-term experiment with a spring-loaded ball valve. The pressure has been alternated between pressure 1.2 and 1.6 kPa every 15 minutes throughout a 72 hour period. The flow values at the end of this period are close to the values at the beginning of the experiment.

A DEVICE FOR TELEMETRIC PRESSURE MEASUREMENT IN SHUNT SYSTEMS

P.H.Chapman, N.T.Zervas, and E.R.Cosman

Introduction

The ability to easily determine ventricular pressure in a shunt-treated hydrocephalic patient would allow an immediate check of shunt function and valve regulating characteristics. Ideally any pressure monitoring system should be accurate and stable over prolonged periods, capable of continuous recording with rapid response, and non-invasive. The device we shall describe fulfills these criteria. Several telemetric intracranial pressure (ICP) monitoring devices have been devised. The principal difficulty has been drift of sensitivity and zero baseline with time. The first system to overcome these problems was that of ZERVAS and COSMAN (2). Using the same measurement principle, the sensor described here is used in shunt systems (1).

Methods

The telesensor (Figure 1) is placed in-line, proximal to the shunt valve, to monitor ventricular pressure. It consists of a chamber with a flexible wall that bulges upward against the scalp when the ICP increases. The bulge causes a change in the resonant frequency of a circuit inside, which is detected by electrodes outside the body and which is a measure of ICP. A stop in the sensor allows zero-point and pressure calibration to be measured in vivo. Manipulations such as position change, straining, or abdominal or jugular compression will be reflected as ICP changes at the sensor. Proximal catheter obstruction will obviate these changes and will, in addition, obliterate the usual cardiac and respiratory oscillations. Distal obstruction will be reflected not only as elevated ICP but also as loss of pressure regulating capacity of the valve system when manipulations such as jugular compression are carried out. The telesensor has been employed in twelve ventriculoperitoneal and three ventriculoatrial shunts (Figure 2) as well as three closed ventricular pressure monitoring systems (Figure 2). The hydrocephalus was due to tumor in six, congenital five, subarachnoid hemorrhage two, trauma one, and idiopathic normal pressure two. Patient ages ranged from two to seventy years.

Results

To date there have been two instances of sensor inaccuracy: one was due to an overlying scalp condition at three months and another to circuit failure at six months. All other devices have continued to give accurate stable recordings for up to eighteen months. Pressure readings have been corroborated by either lumbar or reservoir punctures. Three cases of ventricular catheter obstruction have been detected using the telesensor. In addition, it was most helpful in verifying proper shunt function in three cases where serious question existed. There was no morbidity related to its use.

Discussion

In any sizable population of shunted patients the question of shunt patency arises with frustrating regularity. A common maneuver employed in addressing this problem involves needling the system for pressure/flow measurement or for contrast/isotope injection. Otherwise one depends on palpation of the valve assembly. The disadvantages of either approach are familiar to anyone dealing with the problem frequently. A reliable accurate non-invasive technique is desirable. The telesensor has been used in a substantial number of patients with prolonged follow-up. During this time it has been useful not only in detecting shunt malfunction but also in confirming proper shunt function in circumstances where serious question has arisen. It also has allowed us to study the in vivo characteristics of various shunt assemblies. Finally, the closed ventricular pressure monitoring system (Figure 2) represents a useful alternative to other telemetric devices where access to the ventricular system is desirable.

Summary

A radio frequency telemetric pressure measuring device based on the grid-dip principle has been developed for in-line use with shunt systems or a closed ventricular pressure monitor. Its design eliminates the problem of baseline drift, and the operating characteristics are stable for prolonged periods of in vivo use. It has been employed in eighteen patients for periods up to eighteen months. The telesensor has proven useful in detecting malfunction as well as confirming proper function in shunts in which it has been used.

References

1. Cosman ER, Zervas NT, Chapman PH, Cosman BJ, Arnold MA (1979) A telemetric pressure sensor for ventricular shunt systems. Surg Neurol 11:287-294

2. Zervas NT, Cosman ER, Cosman BJ (1977) A pressure-balanced radiotelemetry system for the measurement of intracranial pressure. J Neurosurg 47:899-911

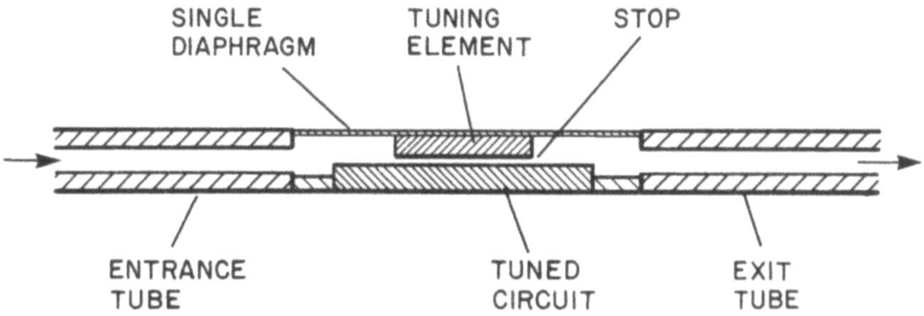

Figure 1.
The single diaphragm ICP telesensor (sectional view).

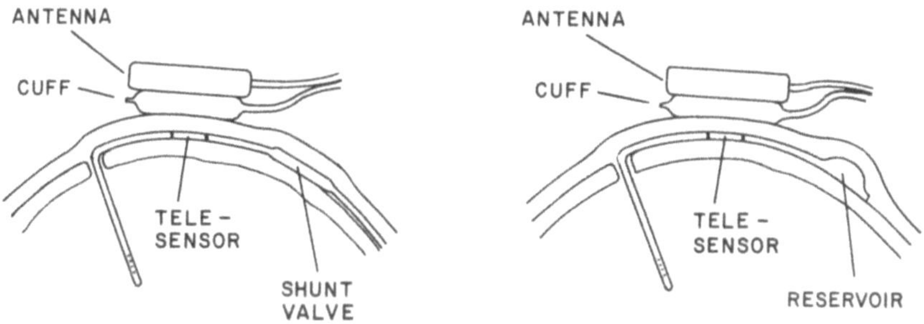

Figure 2.
On the left, the sensor is placed in-line with and proximal to a ventricular shunt valve to monitor shunt function. On the right, the sensor is coupled between a ventricular catheter and reservoir to monitor ventricular fluid pressure only. The air cuff provides pressure to balance, and thus measure the ICP, and the antenna detects the radio frequency of the sensor's passive circuit.

INTRACRANIAL PRESSURE CHANGES IN "ARRESTED" HYDROCEPHALUS

M. Blesser, G. Coltheart, I. Johnston, and J. Wright

Introduction

Spontaneous arrest of hydrocephalus has been reported as occurring in up to 27% of previously shunted patients (1). The dilemma facing the clinician is whether or not the absence of the usual clinical features of intracranial hypertension (ICHT) can be relied upon as indicating non-progression of hydrocephalus. The present study examines this question using continuous intracranial pressure (ICP) monitoring in 10 patients.

The age range was from 2-14 years with 6 male patients and 4 female patients. All patients were thought to have a non-functioning shunt on clinical grounds for up to 8 years prior to investigation. In 9 patients failure of shunt function was confirmed operatively. In the other patient, with a lumbar-peritoneal shunt, confirmation was by isotope study. In no case was there clinical evidence of raised ICP nor had there been any documented progression of neurological deficit.

Methods

ICP was monitored continuously for 24-72 hours via a lateral ventricular catheter, a Statham P50 pressure transducer and a Gilson paper chart recorder. Two patients were monitored twice.

Isotope ventriculography was carried out in 6 patients using Technetium $99m^{DTPA}$. Scans were done up to 24 hours from injection. Additional assessments included clinical examination, psychometric testing, CT scanning and ventriculography.

Results

ICP - All 10 patients showed abnormal tracings. In 2, ICP levels were not thought to be high enough to warrant treatment. Both were monitored on a second occasion - 1 showing quite marked abnormalities, and 1, again, only minor changes.

Baseline ICP levels were below 20mmHg. Nine patients showed 'A' waves, 'B' waves or both. All showed frequent low amplitude 1/minute waves. Peak pressures ranged from 30-70mmHg. In all cases, the main abnormalities were seen during sleep. In no case were there symptoms associated with the pressure waves.

Isotope ventriculography in all 6 patients studied was markedly abnormal. In only 1 was there slight movement of isotope into the subarachnoid space after 24 hours. One patient showed activity in stomach and salivary glands at 24 hours despite complete absence of movement into the subarachnoid space. All patients had moderate to marked ventricular enlargement on ventriculography or CT scanning. Psychometric assessment was carried out before and at the time of investigation in 6 patients. Three patients showed an unequivocal fall (up to 18 points) while 1 showed a marginal reduction. In 1 patient the fall was reversed on retesting one year after replacement of the shunt.

The 9 patients with significant ICHT had their shunts re-established. Seven of these had subjective evidence of improvement (i.e., in the opinion of the patient, parents or teachers) and 3 also had objective evidence in the form of psychometric testing or developmental assessment. The other 2 patients showed no changes.

Summary

The present study highlights the dangers inherent in the diagnosis of "arrested" hydrocephalus and suggests that the incidence of "arrest" in previously shunted patients is low. It is clear from this, and other studies (2) that the absence of the usual clinical signs and symptoms of ICP cannot be taken as sufficient evidence of arrest of hydrocephalus. Marked ICHT may be present in children with large ventricles despite the absence of these signs and may be accompanied by insidious deterioration of intellectual function. Continuous ICP monitoring clearly has an important role to play in assessing patients with so-called "arrested" hydrocephalus, particularly when used in conjunction with isotope studies and psychometric testing.

References

1. Holtzer GJ, de Lange SA (1973) Shunt independent arrest of hydrocephalus. J Neurosurg 39:698-701

2. di Rocco C, Caldarelli M, Maira G, Rossi GF (1977) The study of CSF dynamics in apparently arrested hydrocephalus in children. Child's Brain 3:359-374

PREDICTING THE RESULTS OF VENTRICULAR SHUNTING IN NORMAL PRESSURE HYDROCEPHALUS BY LUMBO-VENTRICULAR PERFUSION TEST

F.GJERRIS, S.E.BØRGESEN, AND S.C.SØRENSEN

Introduction

The syndrome of normal pressure hydrocephalus (NPH) i.e. progressing dementia, gait disturbances and urinary incontinence is now a widely accepted clinical entity. Following the first optimistic reports about the effect of shunting (1) a number of recent reports have been discouraging (6, 10, 12). The sometimes disappointing results of shunting makes it desirable with a test, which can predict the results of shunting.

The purpose of the present study was to examine the predictive value of a lumbo-ventricular perfusion test for measuring conductance to CSF-outflow (C_{out}).

Methods

Fifty patients who fulfilled the common clinical criteria for NPH were studied prospectively. All patients had hydrocephalus on CT-scan (Evans ratio exceeding .30). Intraventricular pressure (IVP) was measured continuously for 24 hours with the transducer placed at the level of the foramen of Monro. Then the lumbo-ventricular perfusion test was performed (2). In this test the volume of CSF absorbed (V_{out}) is measured during stepwise steady state elevations of IVP. The conductance to outflow is calculated as the slope of the line relating V_{out} to IVP. Two patients developed non-bacterial meningitis following ICP measurement and perfusion test. The symptoms subsided within a few days during treatment with antibiotics.

Results

In all patients mean IVP was less than 13mmHg. The C_{out} values showed a wide range (.013-.520 ml/min x mmHg). The regression lines were always straight with an r-value above .95. The patients were divided in two groups with a dividing point of C_{out} .125 ml/min x mmHg. Patients with C_{out} values above this were not shunted, but all patients with C_{out} values below received a ventriculoatrial shunt (HAKIM, medium). All patients who had received a shunt were seen again in the outpatient clinic three and six months after the operation. They were examined clinically and by CT scan. The results are shown in the table.

In 28 of the 40 patients who received a shunt the condition improved clinically. Dividing the 40 shunted patients into two groups from the C_{out} values, it appears that none of the eleven patients with C_{out} values between .075 and .125 ml/min x mmHg showed any evidence of clinical improvement after shunting. In contrast, 28 of the 29 patients with C_{out} values below .075 showed clinical improvement, although in five of the patients the improvement lasted for less than three months. In 32 of the 40 patients who received a shunt the ventricular system

Patient number	Age	Sex	Etiology	C_{out}	Shunt	Clinical course
1	54	M	Trauma ?	0.057	+	Trans
2	59	F	SAH	0.040	+	+
3	66	M	Men.	0.013	+	+
4	49	F	Unknown	0.133	None	-
5	62	M	Unknown	0.045	+	Trans
6	60	M	Trauma	0.060	+	+
7	47	M	Unknown	0.119	+	None
8	48	M	Tumour	0.055	+	+
9	65	M	Unknown	0.070	+	Trans
10	60	M	SAH	0.071	+	Trans
11	56	M	Unknown	0.058	+	+
12	21	M	Cong.?	0.157	None	-
13	53	M	Trauma	0.086	+	None
14	61	M	SAH	0.044	+	+
15	60	M	Unknown	0.113	+	None
16	57	M	Unknown	0.055	+	+
17	65	F	Unknown	0.390	None	-
18	53	M	Unknown	0.410	None	-
19	67	F	Tumour	0.126	None	-
20	52	M	Unknown	0.112	+	None
21	59	F	Trauma	0.068	+	+
22	56	M	Unknown	0.025	+	+
23	48	M	Trauma	0.056	+	+
24	69	M	Unknown	0.035	+	+
25	69	M	Men.	0.032	+	+
26	50	F	Unknown	0.066	+	+
27	66	M	Men.	0.098	+	None
28	54	F	Unknown	0.051	+	+
29	44	M	Trauma	0.098	+	None
30	63	M	Unknown	0.026	+	Trans
31	73	M	Unknown	0.024	+	+
32	65	F	Men, cong.?	0.149	None	-
33	61	F	Unknown	0.116	+	None
34	71	M	Unknown	0.094	+	None
35	53	M	SAH	0.074	+	+
36	49	F	Unknown	0.062	+	+
37	57	M	Men.	0.062	+	None
38	71	F	SAH	0.043	+	+
39	58	F	Unknown	0.073	+	+
40	68	F	Unknown	0.132	None	-
41	39	M	Unknown	0.058	+	+
42	59	M	Unknown	0.177	None	-
43	47	F	SAH	0.033	+	+
44	62	M	Unknown	0.098	+	None
45	60	F	Unknown	0.511	None	-
46	47	F	SAH	0.019	+	+
47	71	M	Unknown	0.083	+	None
48	56	M	Apoplex.	0.108	+	None
49	69	M	Unknown	0.061	+	+
50	59	F	SAH	0.126	None	-

Age, sex, etiology and clinical course in patients with NPH correlated to conductance to CSF-outflow. The known etiologies are: subarachnoid hemorrhage (SAH), meningitis (Men), tumor, cranial trauma and congenital (Cong). Unknown indicates that the history gave no suspicion of an etiology. In the column clinical course plus (+) indicates permanent improvement and "Trans" only transient improvement (less than three months). Only patients with C_{out} values below .126ml/min x mmHg were shunted.

diminished on CT scan. Three patients got subdural hematoma. In one of these patients the subdural hematoma was further complicated with a severe cerebral infarction, and this patient belongs to the group with a severe resorption defect. Two patients with subdural hematoma were among the 11 patients with C_{out} values between .075 and .125 ml/min x mmHg. Three of the five patients who had a transient improvement had an unknown etiology to NPH. The patient from the low group of C_{out} values, who did not improve after shunting, was in a vegetative clinical state before the operation.

Discussion

The results indicate that this method has a high predictive value regarding the effect of shunting in patients with NPH. In patients who improved, the improvement was always within the first three months after the operation, similar to the findings by MAGNAES (10). We have been assuming that C_{out} values above .125 ml/min x mmHg must be considered normal values (3), and we have therefore only shunted patients with C_{out} values below this value. It appears that we have chosen too high a value as the lower limit of the normal range, because none of the 11 patients with C_{out} values between .075 and .125 ml/min x mmHg improved after shunting. It is thus apparent that if one chooses .075 ml/min x mmHg as the lower limit of the normal range for C_{out}, we can exclude most of the patients who will not benefit from shunting. Isotope cisternography or ventriculography do not have such a high predictive value (9). In studies where methods comparable to ours have been used in patients with NPH, the number of patients studied have been too few to evaluate the predictive value of these tests (4,8,11).

It must be emphasized that a decrease in ventricular size on CT following shunting does not correlate with an improvement in clinical conditions. It must also be pointed out that in 5 of the patients the improvement lasted less than three months. In three of these patients the etiology was unknown. The method has some risks, but considering the complication rate of shunting (5,7), we feel it is important to be able to exclude the patients who may not benefit from a shunt.

Summary

The conductance to outflow of CSF (C_{out}) measured by lumboventricular perfusion-test has been compared to the results of shunting in 50 patients with NPH. Only 40 patients with values of C_{out} below .126 ml/min x mmHg were shunted. None of 11 patients with C_{out} between .125 and .075 improved after shunting. Twenty-eight of 29 patients with C_{out} below .075 showed various degrees of improvement. It is thus possible to predict the result of shunting therapy in NPH by measurement of C_{out} by lumbo-ventricular perfusion test.

References

1. Adams RD, Fisher CM, Hakim S, Ojeman RG, Sweet WH (1965) Symptomatic occult hydrocephalus with "normal" cerebrospinal fluid pressure. New Eng J Med 273:117-126

2. Borgensen SE, Gjerris F, Sorensen SC (1978) The resistance to cerebrospinal fluid absorption in humans. Acta Neurol Scand 57:88-96

3. Ekstedt J (1978) CSF hydrodynamic studies in man. 2 normal hydrodynamic variables related to CSF pressure and flow. J Neurol Neurosurg Psychiat 41:345-353

4. Edstedt J, Friden H (1976) CSF hydrodynamics especially in the adult hydrocephalus syndrome. In: Beks JWF, Bosch DA, Brock M (eds) Intracranial Pressure III. Springer, Berlin Heidelberg New York, p 177.

5. Faulhauer K, Schmitz P (1978) Overdrainage phenomena in shunt treated hydrocephalus. Acta Neurochir 45:89-101

6. Hughes CP, Siegel A, Coxe WS, Gado MH, Grubb RL, Coleman RE, Berg L (1978) Adult idiopathic communicating hydrocephalus with and without shunting. J. Neurol Neurosurg Psychiat 41:961-971

7. Illingworth RD (1970) Subdural haematoma after the treatment of chronic hydrocephalus by ventriculocaval shunts. J Neurol Neurosurg Psychiat 33:95

8. Janny P, Flori B, Jouan JP, Janny L (1975) CSF resistance to flow as an aid to diagnosis of normal pressure hydrocephalus. In: Lundberg N, Ponten U, Brock M (eds) Intracranial Pressure II. Springer, Berlin Heidelberg New York, p 512

9. Jensen F, Jensen FT (1979) Acquired hydrocephalus. I. A clinical analysis of 160 patients studied for hydrocephalus. Acta Neuochir 46:119-133

10. Magnaes B (1978) Communicating hydrocephalus in adults. Neuro28: 478-484

11. Philippon J, George B, Levante A, Thurel C, Visot A, Cophignon J (1976) Subarachnoid infusion test. Its value in the prognosis of shunted normal pressure hydrocephalus. In: Beks JWF, Bosch DA, Brock M (eds) Intracranial Pressure III. Springer, Berlin Heidelberg New York, p 193

12. Stein SC, Langfitt TW (1974) Normal pressure hydrocephalus. Predicting the results of cerebrospinal fluid shunting. J Neurosurg 41:463-470

INTRAVENTRICULAR PRESSURE WAVES - THE BEST PREDICTIVE TEST FOR SHUNTING IN NORMAL PRESSURE HYDROCEPHALUS

J.D.PICKARD, G.TEASDALE, M.MATHESON, K.LINDSAY, S.GALBRAITH, D.WYPER, AND P.MACPHERSON

Introduction

The response to shunting in patients with NPH is difficult to predict. We have reviewed 26 patients presenting with symptoms and signs of NPH, to compare the results of pre-operative tests with the outcome of surgery.

Methods

Twenty-six patients with presumed NPH have been shunted: 18 patients with a preceding cause and 8 patients without. Dementia was present in 85%, gait disturbance in 90% and incontinence in 71%.

Pre-Operative Tests: CT scans were assessed independently, both for degree and distribution of ventriculomegaly and for evidence of cerebral atrophy. Intraventricular pressure (23 patients) was recorded continuously for 24-48 hours and analyzed in respect of baseline ICP and occurrence of B waves (1 per minute waves). No lower limit was placed on the height of a wave but, when present, these occupied more than 5% of the recording time. The VPR was also assessed. CSF infusion test (14 patients): The change in ICP with intraventricular infusion of mock CSF (1 ml/min) for 20-30 minutes (until ICP plateaued) was determined. The threshold for abnormality was taken as 13mmHg/ml/min (4). Ventricular isotope clearance (19 patients): 50uC ^{99m}Tc-DTPA was injected isovolumetrically into the ventricles and the rate of clearance determined with a gamma camera. The 95% upper fiducial limit of normality for the $t_{\frac{1}{2}}$ was taken as 10 hours (1). CBF studies (7 patients): The CBF response to hypercapnia was assessed using the inhalational ^{133}Xe method before and after ICP was lowered to 2-3mmHg by drainage.

Results

1. Clinical response to shunting (low pressure VP or VA shunts)

In the secondary group 7 made complete recoveries, 5 usefully improved and 6 were unchanged. One idiopathic patient made a complete recovery, 3 improved, 3 were unchanged and 1 was made worse by shunting. When present, dementia improved in 55% of patients, gait in 72% and incontinence in 67%. There were no complications attributable to the pre-operative tests but there was 1 shunt infection, 1 subdural haematoma and 7 patients required 12 revisions; 3 patients died later.

Correlation with Pre-Operative Tests

The presence or absence of B waves provided the best predictive test (Table 1). The baseline ICP differed in the two groups: responders 12.5 $\pm$ 6 SD mmHg and non-responders 7.5 $\pm$ 2mmHg ($p<0.02$). Patients who did not respond to shunting had a mean ICP below 15mmHg. The VPR is of limited value in hydrocephalus: 2.4 $\pm$ 2.3mmHg/ml and 1.6 $\pm$ 0.9mmHg/ml respectively. CBF studies were successful in only half the patients

Table 1. Correlation of Response to Shunting in NPH with Pre-Operative Tests

Pre-Operative Test	Idiopathic		Secondary		Response to Shunting
	Abnormal	Normal	Abnormal	Normal	
ICP B waves	3	0	10	0	Improved
	0	4	1	5	No change
Infusion Test	3	0	5	0	Improved
	3	1	2	0	No change
Isotope Clearance	2	1	4	4	Improved
	2	1	2	3	No change

because of inability to cooperate with the inhalation procedure and there was little correlation between the change in either baseline CBF or CBF CO_2 response after CSF drainage and outcome. Of 6 patients with sulcal widening on pre-operative scan, 2 improved with shunting. Of 8 patients with fourth ventricle enlargement, 6 improved with shunting.

Discussion and Conclusion

The level of intracranial pressure and the presence or absence of waves do not in themselves indicate the nature of the underlying abnormality but do provide a reliable indication of the potential of a patient with normal hydrocephalus to recover after shunting (2,5). Conversely, isotope clearance and CSF infusion tests demonstrate an abnormality but are not such reliable predictors in the individual patient. It is perhaps misleading to define rigidly a limiting height for waves (3); patients with waves of 2-3mmHg responded well to shunting. A visual review of a record of the level of intracranial pressure during continuous monitoring provided the best test.

References

1. Cabanes J, Vazquez R (1977) Quantitative radioisotope ventriculography: a comparative study. Surg Neurol 8:209-215

2. Chawla JC, Hulme A, Cooper R (1974) Intracranial pressure in patients with dementia and communicating hydrocephalus. J Neurosurg 40: 376-380

3. Crockard HA, Hanlon K, Duda EE, Mullan JF (1977) Hydrocephalus as a cause of dementia: evaluation by computerised tomography and intracranial pressure monitoring. J Neurol Neurosurg Psychiat 40:736-740

4. Martins AN (1973) Resistance to drainage of cerebrospinal fluid: clinical measurement and significance. J Neurol Neurosurg Psychiat 36:313-318

5. Symon L, Dorsch NWC (1975) Use of long-term intracranial pressure measurement to assess hydrocephalus patients prior to shunt surgery. J Neurosurg 42:258-273

ICP, CAT SCANS AND PSYCHOMETRIC ASSESSMENT IN DEMENTIA: A PROSPECTIVE ANALYSIS

A. CROCKARD, H. MCKEE, K. JOSHI, AND I. ALLEN

Introduction

At the last ICP symposium we suggested certain guide lines to select which demented patients would benefit from a shunt operation. These were: 1) Ventricular dilatation in the absence of widened cortical sulci on CAT scan; 2) ICP monitoring for 48 hours which showed either raised intracranial pressure (> 10mmHg) or significant 'B' waves (at least 10mm high) present for 10% of the time (1,2). Since that time we have been carying out a prospective psychometric assessment of demented patients treated according to these criteria.

Methods and Materials

31 patients (17 males, 14 females) have been assessed during the last three years using EMI Scanner and extra dural pressure monitoring (Gaeltec). Full psychiatric and psychometric assessments were carried out by one of us (MCKEE), and the tests video taped and scored independently. All patients had identical psychometric tests before ICP monitoring and six monthly thereafter up to three years: the study continues. The tests included the Wechsler Adult Intelligence Score (WAIS) where applicable, the Geriatric Mental State, Bender Gestalt Digit Copying, Inglis Paired Associated Learning tests and Behavioral Rating Score. A ventriculo-atrial shunt was inserted in 9 patients and brain biopsy performed at the site of insertion: 3 had changes consistent with Alzheimer's disease.

Results

A) CAT Scans: With increasing experience, the exact measurements described by HUCKMAN et al (4) were not used, but no patient with large sulci had pressure waves. Serial studies revealed brain stem or post fossa tumors in three patients; these were excluded from the study.
B) ICP: The mean monitoring time for the whole group was 52 $\pm$ 3.6 hours. The criteria for shunting was strictly observed and using them, 9 patients had significant 'B' wave activity and were considered to have normal pressure hydrocephalus (the NPH group). The mean percentage "wave time" for them was 28.2 $\pm$ 7.8%, i.e. a quarter of the time monitored. Seven other patients had either persistently raised ICP or demonstrated significant pathology on subsequent CAT scans and although they had shunt operations, they were excluded from this study. Fifteen patients had normal ICP and no 'B' waves and were designated the Atrophy group, they had some "ripples" especially during REM sleep, but nothing significant by our criteria.
C) Psychometry: The standard intelligence test (WAIS) did not prove to be useful in our study as many of our patients could not be scored on it; instead, the Geriatric Mental State Test was used on all patients. This test evaluates orientation, memory, concentration and general knowledge. Results have been expressed as a percentage of original score (Figure 1).

The Atrophy group showed a 65.3 ± 43.1% deterioration and this downward trend continued so that at one year the group was 116.2 ± 78.2% worse and at two 122.3 ±85.3%. There was a wide scatter of results. Seven patients showed little change but in the other eight the deterioration was marked.

The NPH group surprisingly had a poor performance at six months (14 ± 10.3% worse) but one year after shunting there was a uniform improvement (30 ± 10.6%) which was maintained at two years (51.5 ± 13.2%), unlike the Atrophy group there was little scatter in results. The psychological tests (Bender, Gestalt, etc) demonstrated the same phenomenon (Figure 1); both groups were worse at six months but at one year the groups were widely separated with a progressive downhill course in those with Atrophy, while the NPH group maintained the improvement noted at one year. Both groups were significantly different from each other at one year ($p<0.01$), but neither group altered significantly from their control performance.

The Behavioral Rating Score provides an assessment of the patients' social graces and ability to look after themselves. There was a significant difference between both groups at one year and the NPH group showed a marked improvement in social behavior compared to their original performance (Table 1).

Discussion

This prospective study has provided some interesting results, but it has left many questions unanswered. We have merely confined ourselves to the question of whether or not, in some cases, intermittently raised ICP plays a part in the production of the dementia. Many workers have shown the inevitable downhill progress of patients with dementia with a dilated ventricular system and cortical atrophy, and our results in 15 "Atrophy" patients and normal ICP would be in agreement with this work.

The group who had episodic raised ICP (NPH) are interesting in that as a group they improved following shunting, or at least did not deteriorate at the same rate at which others of a similar age in the Atrophy group had done. What was surprising was that the group did not show the immediate improvement following shunting which we had expected. The group, in fact, was worse six months after the insertion of the shunt, and this is unlike those with raised ICP following subarachnoid hemorrhage or head injury in whom we have noted periventricular lucencies (GRANHOLM) (3). The fact that both groups are statistically significant in all the tests at one year would suggest that those who had shunt inserted, or who were selected for shunting, differed from the group with normal ICP. To prove that the deterioration in this group was due to hydrocephalus, or at least raised ICP, would require a study of such patients, observed but not shunted. We did not consider this to be ethical in view of our initial findings. The delayed improvement in the NPH group may be due to slow recovery of the limbic system after relief of the pressure, but the exact mechanism is uncertain. The presence of Alzheimer's disease and normal pressure hydrocephalus is well known and the primary brain disease may be a further cause for the patient's deterioration. Nevertheless, in our cases only one showed gross deterioration and it is reasonable to suppose that the removal of one factor, i.e. raised ICP, may have slowed down the rate of deterioration.

Table 1. Dementia Study: behavioural score

	pre.	1 yr.	
ATROPHY (15)	8.2 (1.2)	12.3 (1.7)	
			$P < 0.02$ (ATROPHY 1 yr. vs N.P.H. 1 yr.)
N.P.H. (9)	11.7 (2.0)	4.5 (1.9)	
	$P < 0.05$ (N.P.H. pre. vs 1 yr.)		

The group mean scores (with standard error) for the Behavioral Rating Score are shown; high numbers indicate poor performance. Note the marked improvement in social skills of the NPH group one year after shunting; the Atrophy group deteriorated.

Conclusion

Using previously described criteria, it is possible to identify which demented patients will benefit from a shunting procedure. Prospective psychometric assessments have shown that, following a shunt, those with "normal pressure" hydrocephalus are significantly better one year later than those without evidence of raised ICP. The improvement may be delayed and the reason for this is unclear. Normal pressure hydrocephalus and Alzheimer's disease may both contribute to the dementia in some cases; treatment of one factor may slow the deterioration.

References

1. Crockard HA, Hanlon K, Duda EE, Mullan JF (1976) Evaluation of hydrocephalus as a cause of dementia. In: Beks JW, Bosch D, Brock M (eds) Intracranial Pressure III. Springer, Berlin Heidelberg New York, p. 177

2. Crockard HA, Hanlon K, Duda EE, Mullan JF (1977) Hydrocephalus as a cause of dementia: evaluation by computerised tomography and intracranial pressure monitoring. J Neurol Neurosurg Psychiat 40:736-740

3. Granholm L (1976) An explanation of the reversible memory defect hydrocephalus. In: Beks JW, Bosch D, Brock M (eds) Intracranial Pressure III. Springer, Berlin Heidelberg New York, p. 176

4. Huckman MS, Fox J, Topel J (1975) The validity of criteria for evaluation of cerebral atrophy by computerised tomography. Radiol 116:85-92

Supported by research grants from the Royal Victoria Hospital, Belfast.

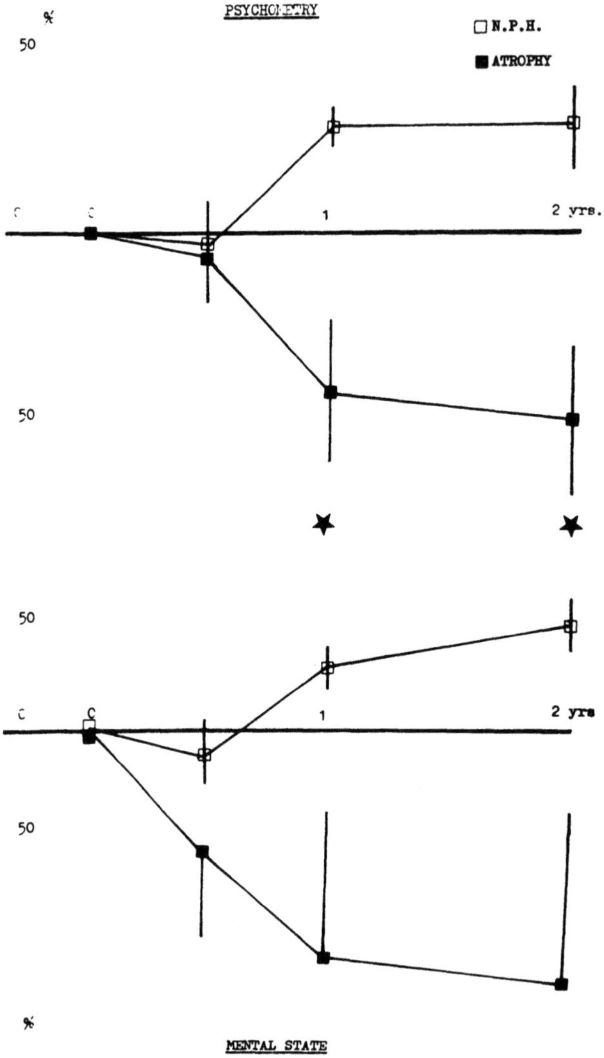

Figure I.
The results of the psychological tests and the Geriatric Mental State for both groups over two years is demonstrated. The data is expressed as percent of original scores, and the group means and standard errors displayed. Note how both groups differ at one year and the trend continues at two years. It is possible to identify patients who will benefit from shunting.

LONG-TERM INTRAVENTRICULAR PRESSURE MEASUREMENT IN CHRONIC COMMUNICATING HYDROCEPHALUS

E. LAMAS, R.D. LOBATO, AND J. ESPARZA

Introduction

The analysis of the CSF dynamics may be used to differentiate hydrocephalus "ex vacuo", a passive event, from active communicating hydrocephalus in which neurological function deteriorates. In fact with continuous recording of intraventricular pressure (IVP), it is possible to detect the influence that certain physiological parameters may exert on CSF pressure in patients with altered CSF dynamics, (1,7). By rapidly injecting controlled amounts of saline into the CSF circulation the state of the CSF pressure/volume relationships in patients with active and "ex vacuo" hydrocephalus can be estimated (4). Also by infusing fluid at a constant rate the state of the reserve in CSF reabsorptive capacity in both groups of patients may be determined (2,3,5). The validity of the foregoing procedures in selecting adult hydrocephalic patients for shunt therapy is controversial at the present time.

In this paper we present the findings with the preoperative analysis of CSF hydrodynamics in 32 adult hydrocephalic patients treated with external shunts.

Materials and Methods

Thirty-two patients, 19 men and 13 women, of ages ranging from 33 to 70 years have been studied. All of them had some degree of neurological disturbance when communicating hydrocephalus was demonstrated by neuroradiological means.

IVP was continuously measured during at least 24 hours by the method described by LUNDBERG. Factors liable to induce artifacts in the recordings were carefully avoided. Recordings were analyzed either manually or by means of an automatic analyzer. Single or repeated estimations of the CSF pressure/volume relationships were achieved by ventricular and/or lumbar routes in 22 patients using a rapid bolus injection technique (4). Constant infusion tests (CIT) were performed by ventricular and/or lumbar routes in 31 patients. In most cases sterile normal saline at room temperature was used as a perfusate. Infusion rates were 0.76 and 2ml/min in 20 and 31 cases respectively. The CIT was performed in such a way that a closed system for infusion and continuous pressure recording were obtained. Infusion was started when a stable opening pressure was present and stopped either when pressure reached a steady-state longer than 8 min or when pressure rose above 52mmHg. The resistance to CSF reabsorption was caluclated when pressure reached a steady-state in accordance with equation RESISTANCE = $\frac{\Delta \text{CSF Pressure}}{\Delta \text{Flow}}$. In some cases the CIT was used to verify shunt competence. No complications occurred as a result of these studies.

Results

Cases with positive shunt response: Hydrocephalus followed the occurrence of primary subarachnoid hemorrhage in six patients of this group (cases 1-6 in Table 1). Two patients presented posttraumatic hydrocephalus (cases 7,8). In case 9 hydrocephalus followed the removal of a posterior fossa meningioma. In cases 10 and 11 ventricular enlargement was concomitant with brain and cisternal infestation by cysticercus. In the remaining patients (cases 12-16) hydrocephalus was of unknown origin. Mild dementia was present in 13 patients of this group. Gait disturbance was as frequent as dementia. Three patients were akinetic and mute. Duration of symptoms was 6.4 months in average. All patients in this group had abnormal IVP recordings. Although pressure remained within normal limits most of the time, episodic abnormal increases occurred (Figure 1). Thirteen patients had small plateau waves (A waves) characterized by sudden pressure rises 8 to 34mmHg in amplitude and 4 to 12 min in duration. Fifteen patients had B waves appearing in a continuous rhythmic form for long periods of time. Both plateau and B-wave activity most often occurred during sleep. IVP oscillated between -10 and 37mmHg in this group of patients. The mean lowest and highest resting pressures were 5.7 and 28.3mmHg respectively. The mean IVP ranged from 4.58 to 17.95mmHg, and the mean IVP for the whole group was 12.74 $\pm$ 3.3 mmHg (SD). CIT were performed in all patients (Figure 2). Resistance to CSF reabsorption was abnormal in all cases except in cases 13 and 16. In five instances resistance could not be calculated because a steady-state in pressure was not reached. Neither the route (lumbar or ventricular) nor the rate of infusion (0.76 or 2ml/min) gave significant differences in the results. The compliance of the CSF compartments oscillated between 0.35 and 0.72, the mean value for the group being 0.50 $\pm$ 0.12.

Cases with negative shunt response: Hydrocephalus followed the occurrence of severe head injuries in six patients of this group (cases 4-9 in Table 1). In another six patients (cases 10-15) the origin of the ventricular enlargement was unknown. In case 16 hydrocephalus appeared following the repair of a ruptured intracranial aneurysm. Three patients had Alzheimer's disease proved by biopsy. All patients in this group had mild or severe dementia. Four patients were bed-bound. All patients in this group had flat IVP recordings (Figure 1). The pressure profile was regular and there were not significant differences between diurnal and nocturnal recordings. Only two patients showed short rhythmic B-wave activity. Isolated B waves occurred in another five cases. IVP was below zero level for long periods of time in seven patients. IVP oscillated between -10 and 20mmHg. The mean lowest and highest resting pressures were -2.25 and 12.43mmHg respectively. The mean IVP ranged from -6.51 to 8.97mmHg, and the mean for the group was 5.09 $\pm$ 2.47 mmHg (SD). CIT were performed in 15 patients of this group (Figure 2). The resistance to CSF reabsorption was normal in all patients except two (Table 1). The compliance of the CSF compartments oscillated between 0.49 and 2.20, the mean value for the group being 1.07 $\pm$ 0.43.

Discussion

There was a poor correlation between the response to CSF shunting and the clinical presentation in this series; 68% of the patients improved with shunts and 43% of those not improved presented the syndrome of the so-called normal pressure hydrocephalus.

According to our findings there are significant differences in the IVP recordings of adult hydrocephalic patients showing positive or negative response to CSF diversion. The pressure profile was irregular in pati-

Table 1

CASES IMPROVED BY CSF SHUNTING

Case nº	Age sex	Resting pressure range low (mmHg)	Resting pressure range high (mmHg)	Mean IVP (mmHg)	Abnormal waves	CIT Resistance (mmH_2O/ml.min)	Compliance
1	47 F	5	35	10.12	B waves	Abnormal(V) 357	-
2	44 F	-5	16	8.22	A waves	Abnormal(V) -	-
3	64 F	3	27	12.57	A and B waves	Abnormal(V) 447	-
4	61 M	3	22	9.81	A and B waves	Abnormal(V) -	-
5	70 M	12	32	17.52	A and B waves	Abnormal(V-L) -	0.42
6	50 M	8	30	14.36	A and B waves	Abnormal(V) 410	0.41
7	57 M	9	34	16.75	A and B waves	Abnormal(V) 400	-
8	42 M	4	35	12.08	A and B waves	Abnormal(V) 334	0.42
9	59 F	-2	22	14.10	B waves	Abnormal(V) 288	0.35
10	52 F	6	30	10.65	A and B waves	Abnormal(V-L) -	0.56
11	51 F	12	37	14.43	A and B waves	Abnormal (L) -	0.39
12	54 F	6	32	13.60	A and B waves	Abnormal(V) 413	-
13	66 F	6	25	13.51	A and B waves	Normal (L) 108	0.65
14	62 M	10	35	17.95	A and B waves	Abnormal(V-L) 419	0.52
15	63 F	8	27	13.61	A and B waves	Abnormal (V-L) 565	0.72
16	53 M	-10	15	4.58	B waves	Normal (V) 167	0.63

CASES NOT IMPROVED BY CSF SHUNTING

Case nº	Age sex	Resting pressure range low (mmHg)	Resting pressure range high (mmHg)	Mean IVP (mmHg)	Abnormal waves	CIT Resistance (mmH_2O/ml.min)	Compliance
1	52 F	-1	5	1.58	Erratic B waves	Normal (V) 100	0.91
2	64 M	7	20	7.63	Rhythmic B waves	Normal (V) 122	0.49
3	63 F	1	12	7.57	-	-	-
4	60 M	-4	14	7.52	-	Normal (V) 196	1.09
5	33 M	-1	10	2.52	Rhythmic B waves	Normal (V) 176	1.08
6	35 M	-2	14	6.22	-	Abnormal(V) 272	-
7	47 M	-10	6	-6.51	-	Normal (V) 98	-
8	62 M	-5	15	2.72	Erratic B waves	Normal (V) 156	2.20
9	61 M	-5	16	2.81	-	Normal (V) 170	0.89
10	59 M	4	14	7.65	Erratic B waves	Normal (V-L) 201	0.97
11	52 F	4	12	4.71	-	Abnormal (V) -	1.01
12	60 M	-1	7	5.32	-	Normal (V) 170	1.62
13	52 F	6	17	8.97	-	Normal (V) 142	0.62
14	53 M	4	10	4.92	-	Normal (L) 130	0.78
15	52 M	-2	12	4.39	Erratic B waves	Normal (L) 197	1.21
16	62 M	0	15	6.48	-	Normal (V) 190	-

ents improved by shunts and flat in those not improved. The mean IVP was usually higher in the former than in the latter type of patient, the difference being statistically significant ($p<0.001$). On the other hand, all patients showing positive response to CSF shunting had plateau waves and/or profuse B-wave activity. Although the mean IVP was significantly different in these groups of patients, there is not a definite pattern of pressure which clearly separates one type of patient from the other. It is the irregular versus the flat pressure profile and the presence or absence of pathological waves which helps in the prognostic evaluation. Moreover, the higher the mean IVP found, the higher the probability that a positive response to shunt therapy will be obtained. On the basis of the IVP monitoring it would be possible to predict the response to CSF shunting in about 93% of our patients.

Many reports confirm the prognostic validity of the CIT (2,3,5) in order to select hydrocephalic patients for surgery, but others question its value (6). The resistance to CSF reabsorption calculated by means of the CIT was significantly different ($p<0.001$) in patients improved by shunts than in those not improved. In our experience resistance measured by this method has been considerably higher than resistance estimated by means of bolus techniques (4). Considering the results with the CIT it would be possible to predict the response to CSF shunting in about 87.5% of our patients.

The compliance values found in patients improved and not improved by shunts were significantly different ($p<0.02$). Six patients with hydrocephalus "ex vacuo" showed abnormal values.

Summary

The findings with continuous IVP monitoring and the CIT in 32 adult hydrocephalic patients undergoing shunt therapy are presented. A good correlation has been found between the state of CSF dynamics and the final response to CSF external diversion.

References

1. Chawla JC, Hulme A, Cooper R (1974) Intracranial pressure in patients with dementia and communicating hydrocephalus. J Neurosurg 40: 376-380

2. Janny P, Flori B, Georget AM (1975) La resistance a l,ecoulement du liquide cephalorachidien dans l,hydrocephalie a pression normale. Rev Neurol 131:211-215

3. Magnaes B (1978) Communicating hydrocephalus in adults. Neurology 28:478-484

4. Marmarou A, Shulman K, LaMorgese J (1975) Compartmental analysis of compliance and outflow resistance of the cerebrospinal fluid system. J Neurosurg 43:523-534

5. Philippon J, George B, Levante A, Thurel C, Visot A, Copignon J (1976) Subarachnoid infusion test. Its value in the prognosis of shunted normal pressure hydrocephalus. In: Beks JWF, Bosch DA, Brock M (eds) Intracranial Pressure III. Springer, Berlin Heidelberg New York, p. 193

6. Stein SC, Langfitt TH (1974) Normal pressure hydrocephalus. Predicting the results of cerebrospinal fluid shunting. J Neurosurg 41:463-470

7. Symon L, Dorsch NWC (1975) Use of long-term intracranial pressure measurement to assess hydrocephalic patients prior to shunt therapy. J Neurosurg 42:258-273

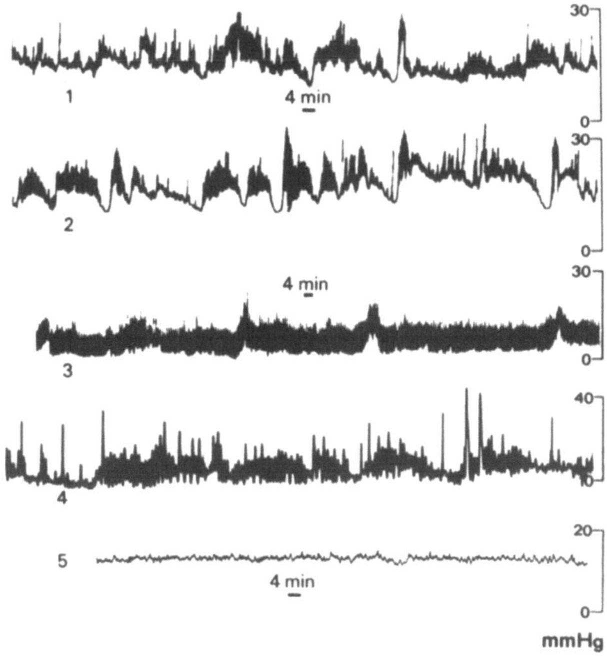

Figure 1.
Preoperative recordings of IVP in patients with positive responses to CSF shunting (1,2,3,4); the irregularity of the profile recording, the small plateau waves and the profuse B wave activity may be clearly appreciated. Recording No. 5 was obtained in a patient with negative response to CSF shunting. The profile of the recording is regular and there are not abnormal waves.

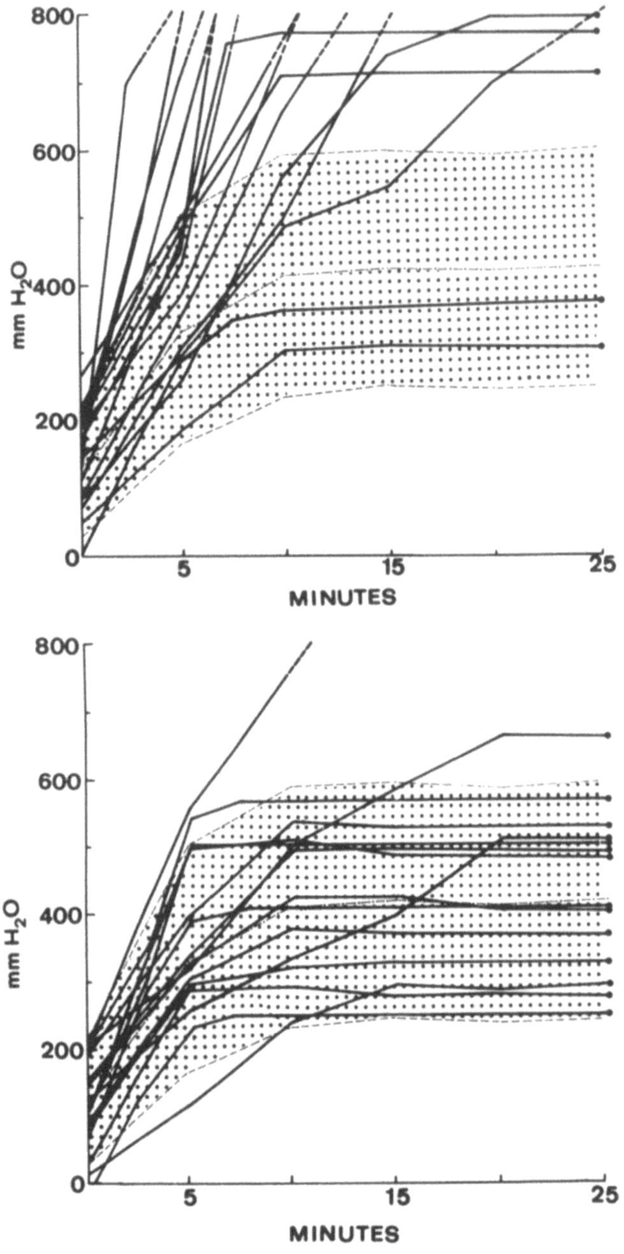

Figure 2.
Representation of the results of the CIT performed with a 2ml/min infusion rate in a pressure-time diagram. Cases showing positive shunt response are represented in the upper part and cases with negative response to CSF shunting in the lower part. As may be appreciated there are two false normal results and two false abnormal results.

INTRAVENTRICULAR PRESSURE MONITORING AND CSF DYNAMICS IN NON-TUMOR AQUEDUCTAL STENOSIS

R.D.LOBATO, E.LAMAS, J.ESPARZA, J.M.PORTILLO, AND J.J.RIVAS

Introduction

There are not systematic studies of the CSF hydrodynamics in adult patients suffering non-neoplastic obstruction of the aqueduct. In this work we analyze intraventricular pressure (IVP) and CSF Pressure/Volume relationships in 17 juvenile and adult patients affected by non-tumor aqueductal stenosis. The degree of hydrocephalus and the site of the aqueductal stricture was demonstrated in all these cases by means of pneumoventriculography. Some patients had CT scans.

Methods

IVP was preoperatively measured for periods ranging from 1 to 6 days according to the method described by LUNDBERG. Constant infusion tests (CIT) were performed in 13 patients infusing 0.76 and 2ml/min of normal saline by ventricular and lumbar routes respectively. Infusion was stopped either when pressure reached a steady-state longer than 8 min or when it rose above 52mmHg. Resistance to CSF reabsorption was calculated according to the equation: Resistance = $\frac{\Delta CSF\ Pressure}{\Delta flow}$. CSF P/V relationships were estimated by rapidly injecting variable amounts of saline solution at the level of ventricular and lumbar compartments in 11 patients. Ten patients in this series received external CSF shunts and the remainder were treated with supraoptic ventriculostomy. Sixteen patients had postoperative CSF pressure recordings. CIT and estimations of the CSF P/V relationships were also performed in 9 patients postoperatively.

Results

IVP levels and the results obtained with CIT are listed in Table I. Cases 1-6 presented with long clinical histories consisting of headaches, personality changes and gait disturbances. Although mean IVP was normal in all these patients, transitory abnormal rises in pressure over the base line occurred (Figure I). Cases 7-17 presented with symptoms and signs of severe intracranial hypertension. In these patients IVP was above normal limits during all the recording time (Figure I). In the cases in which CSF pressure was simultaneously measured at ventricular and lumbar levels there were not significant pressure gradients.

CSF reabsorption estimated by means of the CIT was considerably reduced in all patients (Table I). As could be expected, reabsorption was lower at the level of the isolated ventricular compartment than by lumbar route.

CSF compliance as defined by MARMAROU et al (2) was abnormal in all cases being always lower when estimated at ventricular level than when estimated at lumbar level. Mean ventricular compliance in this series

Table 1

Case nº	Age Sex	PREOPERATIVE Mean IVP (mmHg)	CIT, Resistance (mmH$_2$O/ml.min) Lumb.	Ventric.	POSTOPERATIVE Mean CSF Pressure (mmHg)	CIT, Resistance (mmH$_2$O/ml.min) Lumbar (2)
1	68M	14.5±3.1	-		-	-
2	65M	17.0±3.8	A(2)	A(0.76)	3.1±0.8 (L)	N, 180
3	45M	17.8±2.7	-		-	-
4	71F	6.5±3.8	A(2) 200	A(0.76)	2.9±1.7 (L)	-
*5	47M	7.4±2.2	A(2) 392	A(0.76)	1.9±0.5 (V)	-
6	48F	11.3±3.2	A(2) 421	A(0.76)	3.4±1.5 (L)	N, 174
7	24F	28.8±4.5	-		5.4±2 (L)	-
8	23F	35.1±7.1	-		7.7±0.9 (L)	-
9	14F	22.6±2.5	A(2)	A(0.76)	6.2±1 (V)	N, 96
*10	12M	29.4±5	A(2)	A(0.76)	9.1±0.7 (V)	-
*11	13M	29.5±4.7	A(2)	A(0.76)	12.3±0.9 (V)	N, 68
*12	12M	32.6±5.7	A(2)	-	10.7±0.2 (V)	N, 47
13	10M	29.2±5.6	A(2)	-	4.1±1.3 (V)	-
*14	19M	46.8±7.2	A(2)	-	14.1±1.3 (V)	-
15	15M	28.3±6.8	A(0.76) 303	A(0.76) 394	4.6±1 (L)	N, 34
*16	11M	28.4±5	A(2)	-	9.8±1.2 (V)	-
*17	22F	21.1±5.9	A(0.76)	A(0.76)	10.1±1.2 (V)	N, 26

A and N= abnormal and normal respectively. L and V= lumbar and ventrioular respectively.

*** Cases treated with supraoptio ventriculostomy.**

was 0.37 ± 0.1 and mean lumbar compliance was 0.50 ± 0.1. Ventricular compliance was smaller with greater degrees of hydrocephalus.

Postoperatively CSF pressure was normalized in all patients but the profile of the pressure recording was different in cases treated with external shunts than in those treated with supraoptic ventriculostomies. Following this operative procedure IVP fell to normal levels in periods ranging from 1 day to 3 weeks, and all patients so treated showed extremely low resistance to CSF reabsorption and high CSF compliance values postoperatively.

Discussion

Some patients with non-tumor aqueductal stenosis present clinically with symptoms and signs of severe intracranial hypertension and, as has been shown here, they have high actual IVP levels. Other patients present with chronic clinical courses, showing actual IVP levels similar to these found in patients with chronic communicating hydrocephalus.

Nevertheless, all patients with chronic non-communicating hydrocephalus studied in this series have had episodes of severe intracranial hypertension at the beginning of their clinical evolution.

In our experience CSF compliance is similar when estimated at lumbar and ventricular levels in patients with communicating hydrocephalus, while it is significantly lower at ventricular than at lumbar levels in patients affected by aqueductal stenosis. The mean preoperative ventricular compliance in our series of patients with chronic communicating hydrocephalus was considerably greater than the mean ventricular compliance in the present series (0.50 ± 0.12 and 0.37 ± 0.1 respectively), the difference being statistically significant ($p<0.001$). LIM et al (1) reported similar findings in the laboratory and probably the explanation is that in the presence of aqueductal blocks compliance measured by ventricular route is that of the supratentorial compartment, while in cases of communicating hydrocephalus compliance measured also includes the spinal sac and the posterior fossa.

The normalization of the CIT observed in this study, either after external CSF derivations or following a successful supraoptic ventriculostomy, indicates that patients had competent subarachnoid pathways and that the obstruction of these pathways seen preoperatively is more functional than anatomical in origin. This hypothesis has been previously formulated by other authors (3,4). In our opinion the CIT may be used (after a temporary ventricular drainage) in order to determine what patients with aqueductal stenosis have free subarachnoid pathways and consequently are good candidates for internal CSF derivative procedures such as supraoptic ventriculostomy or Torkildsen operation.

References

1. Lim ST, Potts DG, Deonarine V, Deck MDF (1973) Ventricular compliance in dogs with and without aqueductal obstruction. J Neurosurg 39:463-473

2. Marmarou A, Shulman K, LaMorgese J (1975) Compartmental analysis of compliance and outflow resistance of the cerebrospinal fluid system. J Neurosurg 43:523-534

3. Milhorat TH, Hammock MK, Chandra RS (1971) The subarachnoid space in congenital obstructive hydrocephalus. Part 2. Microscopic findings. J Neurosurg 35:7-15

4. Williams B (1973) Is aqueduct stenosis a result of hydrocephalus? Brain 96:399-412

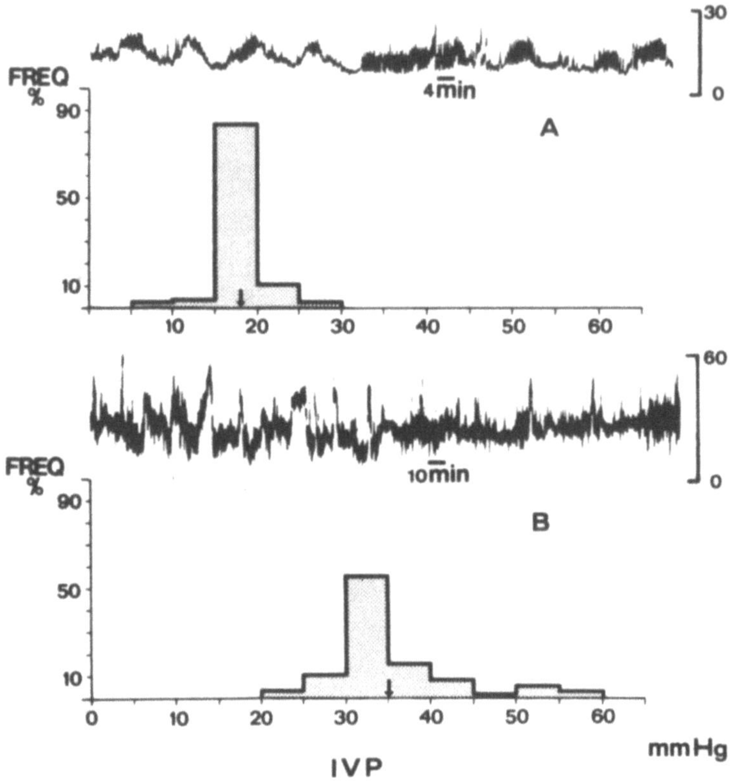

Figure 1.
In the upper part are the IVP recordings and the 24 hour pressure-frequency hystogram obtained in an adult patient showing chronic hydrocephalus secondary to aqueductal stenosis (A). In the lower part are the IVP recordings and the 24 hour pressure-frequency hystogram obtained in a juvenile patient presenting with subacute intracranial hypertension secondary to aqueductal obstruction.

QUANTITATIVE DETERMINATION OF CSF-FLOW IN DIAGNOSIS OF CSF-RESORPTION DISORDERS

R.W.OBERBAUER, W.D.SAGER, L.AUER, AND G.F.FUEGER

Introduction

Whereas in acute hydrocephalus problems in diagnosis are rather usual, adequate treatment of chronic cases appears much more difficult (7). Bare detection of enlarged ventricles and ICP measurements turned out to be often insufficient. Thus, CSF-dynamic studies gained more and more importance.

Among different methods, isotope clearance has proved to be a quite useful procedure (3). The decrease of radioactivity in the ventricles allows a qualitative judgement of CSF-resorption, indication for CSF-drainages still remained difficult and often subject to personal feelings of the physician.

Methods

20u Cu of radioactive isotopes (iodine 131-hippurane) are instilled into the ventricles. The decrease of radioactivity in the ventricles is measured and the diminution-rate/h determined.

Using computerized tomography, an adequate calculation of the ventricle volume can be performed because of different density of brain tissue and CSF-spaces (5). All picture-elements with attenuation values of CSF are counted in two different ways: 1) by encircling of all CSF-spaces with the rollerball or joystick; 2) by automatic counting of picture-elements with predetermined values of CSF-absorption. Both methods have been used simultaneously and proved correct results.

Relating ventricular volume to decrease of radioactivity leads to the actual CSF-FLOW from the ventricles (4).

Results

Our indications for CSF-FLOW measurements have been cases with posttraumatic hydrocephalus, hydrocephalus in posterior fossa tumors after surgery, chronic hydrocephalus with unknown reason and infants with myelomeningoceles and hydrocephalus. 34 patients from 3 weeks to 51 years of age have been examined in the described way, the CSF-FLOW was ranging between 1.3ml/h and 35.3ml/h.

Comparing the CSF-FLOW values with the clinical results, the method turned out to be quite reliable. All patients with flow-values below 10ml/h showed marked clinical and CAT-scan improvement after shunt surgery. Two posttraumatic cases and one after posterior fossa tumor removal with CSF-FLOW values between 20 and 30 ml/h did not show any changes after the shunting procedure, neither in CAT-scan nor clinically. In addition, clear information about function of implanted shunts can be obtained.

Discussion

According to numerous experimental studies (1,2,6), CSF-FLOW values for humans have been estimated between 500-900cc daily and seen to confirm our results of sufficient CSF-FLOW. At the present stage of this study, it would be too early to give a determined threshold-value for normal and pathological CSF-FLOW values. Basically, the comparison of clinical outcome, CAT-scan controls and CSF-FLOW values proved the reliability of this method. Necessarily, the method requires access to the ventricles. Thus, the range of application has been limited to cases of chronic hydrocephalus, in which the possible necessity of a shunting procedure could not be ruled out by common examinations satisfactorily.

References

1. Cutler RWP, Page L, Galilich J, Watters GV (1968) Formation and absorption of cerebrospinal fluid in man. Brain 91:707-720

2. Davson H (1967) Physiology of the cerebrospinal fluid. J Churchill, London

3. Knoetgen I, Fueger GF, Gell G (1973) 131-J-Hippuran in prognose und behandlung des kindlichen hydrocephalus. In: Urban, Schwarzenberg (eds) Radioaktive Isotope in Klinik und Forschung. 10, München Berlin Wien

4. Oberbauer RW, Fueger GF, Sager WD, Auer L (1979) Quantitative Liquorflußbestimmungen zur Diagnostik von Liquorresorptionsstorungen. In press

5. Sager WD (1978) Der Gehirn-Liquorraum-Index. Ein Parameter zur Diagnose des Hydrocephalus mit Hilfe der Computertomographie. Rontgen-Bl. 31, Georg Thieme Verlag, Stuttgart, S. 67-74

6. Sweet WH, Brownell GL, Scoll JA, Bowsher DR, Benda P, Stickley EE (1954) The formation, flow and absorption of cerebrospinal fluid; newer concepts based on studies with isotopes. Proc Ass Res Nerv Dis 34:101-159

7. Wood JM, et al (1974) Normal pressure hydrocephalus: diagnosis and patient selection for shunt surgery. Neurol 24:517

THE PATHOPHYSIOLOGY OF INTRACRANIAL HYPERTENSION/HYPOTENSION

D.A.ROTTENBERG

The pathophysiological basis of various disease states associated with altered intracranial pressure (ICP) relationships is best understood with reference to 4 model parameters (1-3); dural sinus venous pressure, P_d, cerebrospinal fluid (CSF) absorption resistance, R_a, CSF formation rate, I_f, and the pressure-volume index, PVI, a measure of cerebrospinal compliance. As illustrated in Table 1, chronic elevations of CSF pressure (CSFP) result from an increase in P_d, an increase in R_a or an increase in I_f; similarly, prolonged reductions in CSFP result from a decrease in P_d, a decrease in R_a or a decrease in I_f. The magnitude and time course of acute elevations in CSFP prodcued by pathological fluctuations in cerebral blood volume (plateau waves, acute subarachnoid hemorrhage) are determined by i) the effective cerebrospinal compliance (PVI), which, in turn, depends upon the elasticity of the craniospinal venous bed, the viscoelastic properties of the cerebral parenchyma and the presence or absence of pathological compartmentalization (e.g. herniation), and ii) R_a. With reference to the known effects of antihypertensive agents/therapies on the 4 primary model parameters (Table 2), serial determinations of P_d, R_a, I_f and PVI in neurological and neurosurgical patients undergoing ICP monitoring--accomplished by bolus and/or graded injections of mock CSF directly into the ventricular system--should provide objective criteria for the selection of specific treatment modalities. In hydrocephalic patients with ventriculo-systemic shunts incorporating subcutaneous reservoirs and percutaneous reversible occlusion valves, "shunt open" vs "shunt closed" measurements of CSF flow resistance permit an assessment of shunt patency and function (3).

References

1. Marmarou A (1973) A theoretical and experimental evaluation of the cerebrospinal fluid system. Ph.D. Thesis. Drexel University

2. Marmarou A, Shulman K, L'aMorgese J (1975) Compartmental analysis of compliance and outflow resistance of the cerebrospinal fluid system. J Neurosurg 43:523-534

3. Rottenberg DA, Posner JB (1979) Intracranial Pressure. In: Cottrell JE, Turndorf H (eds) Anesthesia and Neurosurgery. C.V. Mosby, In press

TABLE 1. SOME CAUSES OF ALTERED INTRACRANIAL PRESSURE

Perturbation	Proximate Cause	Clinical Examples
Increased P_d	Sinus compression/ occlusion	Sagittal sinus thrombosis Otitic hydrocephalus Brain tumors
	Increased sinus blood flow	CO_2 retention Arteriovenous malformations
	Increased peripheral venous pressure	Internal jugular vein occlusion Superior vena cava syndrome Congestive heart failure
Decreased P_d	Decreased sinus blood flow	Dehydration Shock Hyperventilation
	Decreased peripheral venous pressure	Dehydration
Increased R_a	Ventricular outflow obstruction	Brain tumors Aqueductal stenosis
	Obliteration of the cisternal and/or convexity subarachnoid space	Meningitis Extra/subdural masses Cerebral edema
	Plugging of the arachnoid villi	Subarachnoid hemorrhage Infectious polyneuritis Spinal cord tumors
Decreased R_a	Diversion of CSF from the ventriculo-subarachnoid space	External ventricular drainage Ventriculosystemic shunts Lumbar-puncture headache Dural tears and CSF fistulae
Increased I_f	Increased choroidal CSF formation	Choroid plexus papilloma
	Increased extrachoroidal CSF formation	Hypo-osmolality Cerebral edema
Decreased I_f	Choroidal "atrophy"	? Chronic hydrocephalus
	Decreased extrachoroidal CSF formation	Hyperosmolality ? Dehydration

TABLE 2. EFFECTS OF VARIOUS ANTIHYPERTENSIVE TREATMENT MODALITIES

	P_d	I_d	R_a	PVI
Systemic Diuretics	0	↓	0	0
Hypertonic Solutions	?↑	↓	0	↑
Corticosteroids	0	↓	?↑	↑
Acetazolamide	0	↓↓	0	0
Barbiturates	?↓	0	0	0
Controlled Hyperventilation	?↓	↓	0	0
Hypothermia	↓	↓	0	0
CSF Diversion	?↓	0	↓↓	?↑
Surgical Decompression	↓	0	↓	↑

Symbols: Major effect, ↑↑ or ↓↓; minor or secondary effect, ↑ or ↓; questionable effect, ?↑ or ?↓; no information, 0.

OUTFLOW POSSIBILITIES OF VENTRICULOLYMPHATIC SHUNT

J. VAJDA, I. NYARY, M. HORVATH, AND E. PASZTOR

Introduction

Since some preliminary speculations have shown that a ventriculolymphatic shunt might have, at least theoretically, many advantages over other more conventional methods, a project was initiated in our department as early as in the sixties (1), to validate this conjecture. Using the ventriculolymphatic shunt to convert CSF flow, one need only a connecting tube and the valve. Also a major source for infection can be ommited, and, because the catheter-tip will not immerse into blood less thrombo-embolic complications can be expected (6).

Material and Methods

13 patients presented with hydrocephalus or various etiologies (occlusion of aqueduct, axial tumor, normal pressure hydrocephalus, etc) and considered for shunt operation were selected out of a larger group. Ventriculolymphatic shunt was performed following the description of KEMPE et al (2). On the day preceding surgery, a catheter was placed into the right lateral ventricle and intracranial pressure (ICP) was assessed by measurement of ventricular fluid pressure (VFP). The intracranial volume-pressure relationship was tested pre- and postoperatively by intraventricular bolus injections of 1-4ml mock CSF besides overelinight VFP recording. Figure 1 shows a series of VFP responses elicited by increasing volume load to the CSF space. The last diastolic value of VFP at the inspiration right before the volume-injection was designated as P_o, corresponding value immediately after injection as P_+. Since in most patients presented with decreased intracranial compliance, subsequent to immediate pressure increase due to the volume-load, a further, prolonged ICP elevation occurred (Figure 1, panel A), on the top of these waves P_{max} was also defined. Volume pressure response (VPF) and pressure volume index (PVI) were calculated for both P_+ and P_{max} using standard equations (3,5).

Surgical procedure consists of dissection of the thoracic duct, isolation of its terminal part adjacent to the internal jugular or subclavian vein. After ligating the duct a few cm below its termination and insetting a sylastic tube into this secluded part a few simple maneuvers were undertaken to assess outflow characteristics and make opening-pressure-estimation. A slight suction on the tube caused the duct to collapse and no reflow of blood occurred from the vein due to lymphatic-jugular valve. Filling the tube with saline, on the elevation of its end even a few cm-H_2O pressure head was enough to produce pooling in the system and initialize flow toward the vein. We have observed that this type of outflow required a very low opening pressure--a condition most favorable in cases of normal pressure hydrocephalus, since the valve was governed by ventilation and became patent at each inspiration due to negative intracaval pressure. The artificially increased end-tidal pressure stopped the flow. Thus in cases of low VFP, passage of fluid also becomes periodical with ventilation and the drained volume depends on the size of that saccular pool formed from the terminal part of thoracic duct, so the syphon-effect of some shunts can be avoided. On the other hand at higher VFP a steady flow can be expected through the permanently opened lymphatic-jugular valve.

Results

Figure 1 demonstrates a typical run of induced VFP responses in a patient presented with hydrocephalus concomitant to a spinal cyst. Repeated bolus injections of increasing volumes have produced an immediate elevation of VFP and also elicited a response that very often precipitated in a B-wave like pressure increase (panel A). After a ventriculolymphatic shunt was established, VFP responses to the same or even greater volume load became significantly diminished. The substantial change in intracranial volume-pressure relationship that occurred due to converting CSF from the intracranial space can be seen Figure 2. Plotted preoperative values of ΔV against log P (both for P_+ and P_{max}) fit excellently to a straight line. On the other hand, corresponding data obtained after shunt operation could be fitted to a more complex exponential equation. Table 1 comprises calculated PVI in 9 patients. Mean PVI_+ calculated from P_+ was 11.4 ± 1.71ml and PVI_{max} was 8.39 ± 1.32ml before operation, the difference being not significant. A significant increase in PVI as compared to PVI_{max}, indicating increased intracranial compliance occurred postoperatively. Since secondary B waves almost never appeared after shunting, only one PVI was calculated.

Discussion

In this small series of patients we were able to demonstrate by intraoperative observations some favorable characteristics of a ventriculolymphatic shunt. Effectiveness of this shunt in increasing intracranial compliance (in terms of increased PVI) can be compared with that of the more conventional ventriculoatrial shunt (4). Beneficiary effects can also be measured on the improved postoperative state of patients. However, promising acute postoperative results were overshadowed by the occlusion of connecting tube at the site of thoracic duct occasionally, due to extensive fibrosis. In order to keep ventriculolymphatic shunts patent for long run further investigations are warranted, for example application of autologous superficial vein suturing to thoracic duct.

References

1. Gatai C, Foldi M (1961) The treatment of hydrocephalus by ventriculo-lymphatic anastomosis. Neurochirurgia 4:57-64
2. Kempe LG (1977) Ventriculolymphatic shunt. J Neurosurg 47;86-95
3. Marmarou A, Shulman K, LaMorgese J (1975) Compartmental analysis of compliance and outflow resistance of the CSF system. J Neurosurg 43:523-534
4. Sullivan HG, Becker DP, Miller JD (1978) Choice of a shunt system for the therapy of surgical hydrocephalus. J Neurosurg Sci 22:205-220
5. Sullivan HG, Miller JC, Griffith RL, Becker DP (1978) CSF pressure-volume dynamics in neurosurgical patients: a preliminary evaluation in six patients. Surg Neurol 9:47-54

6. Vajda J, Horvath M, Nyary I (1979) Ventriculolymphatic shunt and decompensated intracranial volume-pressure relationship. Acta Neurochir Suppl 28:521-525

▷

Figure 1.
Tracings of VFP before (panel A) and after (panel B) ventriculolymphatic shunt operation. Interposed numbers indicate the amount of fluid injected into ventricle. Arrowhead marks where patient complained about discomfort.

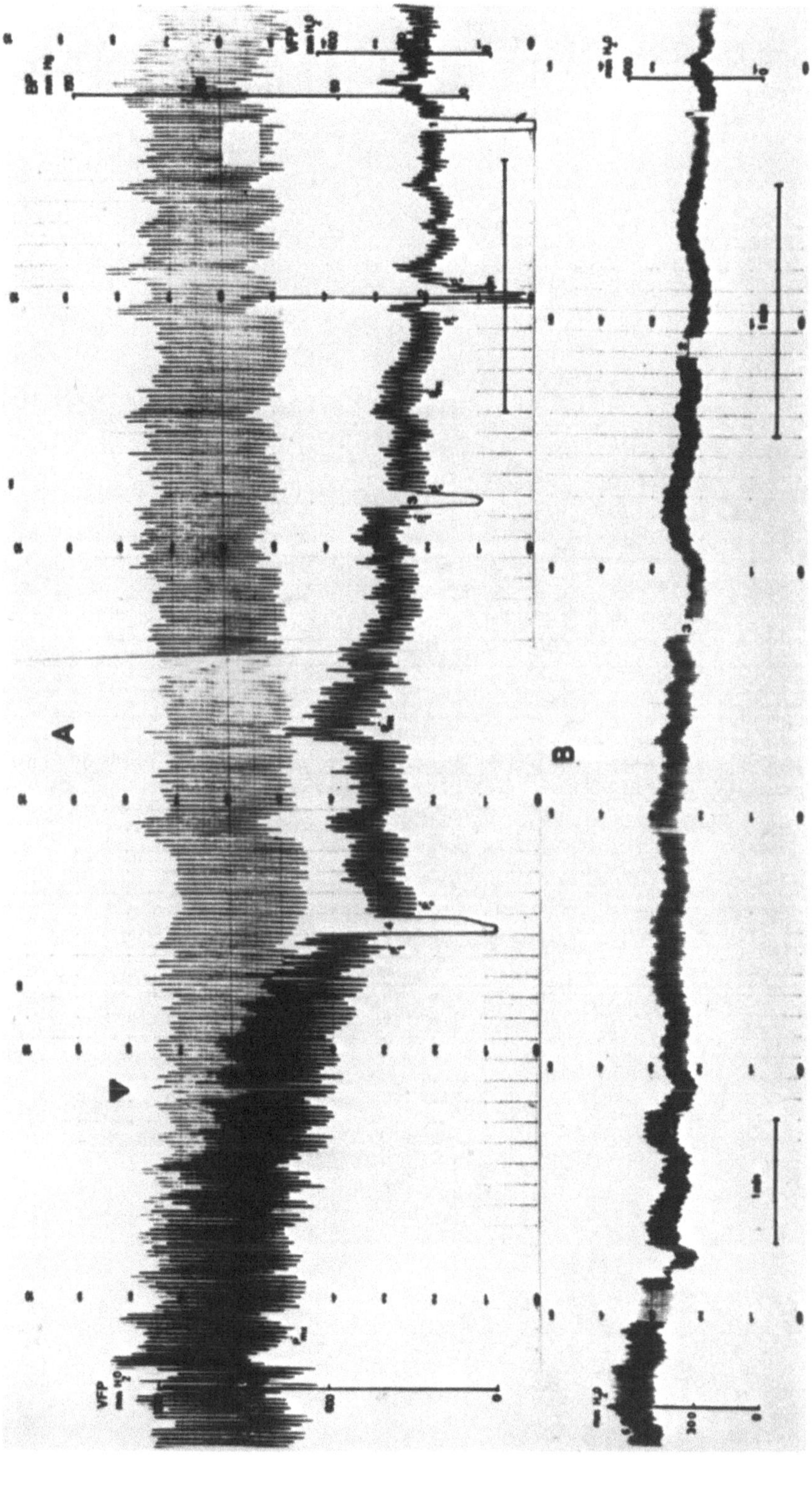
A
B
VFP

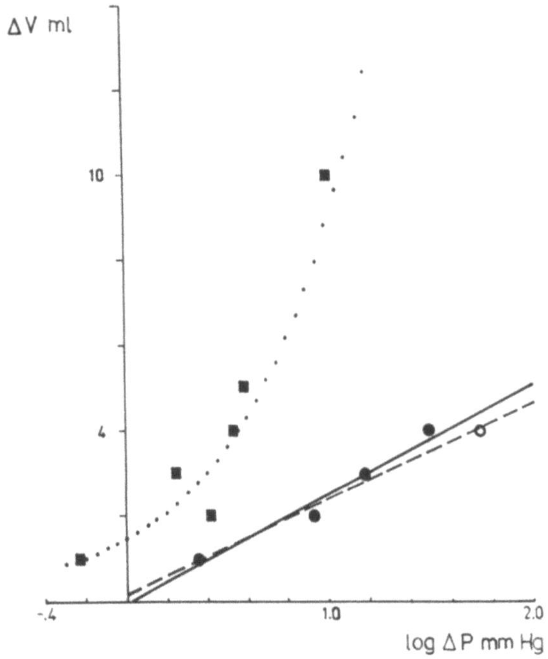

Figure 2.
Intracranial volume-pressure relationships before and after shunting in patient No. 4. Dots and circles represent preoperative data calculated from P_{+} and P_{max} values, continuous and broken lines fit their respective linear regression. (Correlation coefficients: $r_{+} = 0.9831$, $r_{max} = 0.9896$). Quadrangles are postoperative values, dotted line fits the curve ($V = a \times 10^{b \times \log P}$; $r = 0.9537$).

PLATEAU WAVES: PRODUCTION IN THE RAT AND SIMULATION BY MEANS OF A MECHANICAL MODEL

H. ARNOLD AND R. LAAS

Introduction

The pressure increase of plateau waves (PW) is due to augmented cerebral blood volume (CBV) (4,7,8). Precapillary regulatory phenomena have been proposed as causative; we believe that this is incompatible with the size and the steepness of the pressure increase. We wish to demonstrate in a mechanical model and in experiments in the rat that an inhibition of venous drainage occurs due to a valve mechanism and that this model readily explains PW.

Materials and Methods

a. Mechanical model (simulation of intracranial circulations): A motor pump ("heart") propels water ("blood") through a collapsible tube ("intracerebral and leptomeningeal veins") which traverses a rigid container ("skull") filled with water ("cerebrospinal fluid", CSF). The distal portion of the collapsible tube is suspended in straight fashion to simulate the distal segments of the bridging veins that are fixed to dura matter and prone to compression. Pressure in the outlet tube ("sinus") and internal container pressure ("intracranial pressure", ICP) can be varied hydrostatically by means of vertical tubes. Container pressure is recorded by electronical means. If the vertical tube of the container (VTC) is occluded pressure variations of the outlet are fully transmitted into the container. If the container pressure is elevated previously to a critical level further increase of container pressure by outlet pressure elevation over a defined threshold cannot be reversed any more by decrease of the outlet pressure. By contraries, container pressure rises steeply and assumes a higher level which permits a new equilibrium between flow and pressure. Beyond the threshold any further distension ("CBF-increase") of the collapsible tube induces a compression of its distal segment suspended in straight fashion. At the obtained pressure plateau only a sufficient decline in pump performance ("decline of CBF") leads to a progressive drop of container pressure that is at first gradual and then precipitous (Figures 1 and 2).

b. Animal experiments: The only known model for the production of PW involves the occlusion of spinal compensatory pathways in cats with kaolin induced hydrocephalus (10). An attempt to adapt that model to the rat did not yield sufficient results. A systematic search for other methods in rats with and without hydrocephalus has produced the following experimental design in animals without hydrocephalus: Three electrodes for electroencephalography (EEG) were inserted and a cannula was placed in the lateral ventricle. Four days later the aqueduct was occluded via cisterna magna and the fourth ventricle by silicone paste, a piece of muscle and an acrylic polymer. CSF drainage was permitted via the ventricular cannula. Two days later catheters were placed into the extracranial part of the transverse sinus and the femoral artery. Subsequently, parenchymatous absorption of CSF was blocked by fractional instillation of homologous blood plasma (0.2ml) into the lateral ventricles. The following parameters were recorded in the alert animal: ICP, systemic arterial pressure (SAP), transverse sinus pressure, EEG.

Results

ICP rose regularly within 1-2 hours after plasma instillation to a level of 30-40mmHg. At this pressure level, occasionally PW occurred spontaneously. Furthermore, PW could be elicited by sudden pressure increase resulting from injection into the transverse sinus or by sudden tactile or acoustic stimulation (Figure 3). The EEG revealed slow wave activity when the pressure was high. Changes in SAP did not influence the appearance and the course of PW.

Discussion

Our results conform to all criteria that have been established for PW, i.e. rapid rise and prompt or gradual decline (3,4,8), CBV increase during the plateau (8), maximal CBV at the end of the plateau (8), reduction in CBF during the plateau and slowing of the EEG (2), and no influence of SAP changes on PW appearances and disappearance (3,4,7,8).

Valvular function of the bridging veins near their sinus entry points is assured under physiological and pathophysiological conditions (1,5,6,9). From our findings it is concluded that the sudden ICP increase of PW is initiated by a sudden extracranially induced venous pressure elevation. Following release of an extracranially induced venous congestion a transient increase of the pressure difference between the leptomeningeal veins and the sinus is established. If the ICP is above a defined threshold and the intracranial compliance is critically reduced this pressure gradient causes an occlusion of the compressible segment of the bridging veins thus inducing an intracranial venous congestion concomitant with a further rapid increase of ICP.

The findings of RISBERG et al (8) suggest that the venous outflow obstruction must not be a global one, but may be limited to a single or several venous drainage areas. Thus the intraindividual variation in PW may be explained.

References

1. Hacker H, Huhner G (1972) Due Bruckenvenen. Radiologe 12:45-48

2. Ingvar DH, Lundberg N (1961) Paroxysmal symptoms in intracranial hypertension, studied with ventricular fluid pressure recording and EEG. Brain 84:446-459

3. Lundberg N (1960) Continuous recording and control of ventricular fluid pressure in neurosurgical practice. Acta Psychiat Neurol Scand 36:Suppl 146

4. Matsuda M, Yonada S, Handa H, Gotoh H (1979) Cerebral hemodynamic changes during plateau waves in brain tumor patients. J Neurosurg 50:483-488

5. Miller JD, Stanek A, Langfitt TW (1973) Cerebral blood flow regulation during experimental brain compression. J Neurosurg 39:186-196

6. Nakagawa Y, Tsuru M, Yada K (1974) Site and mechanism for compression of the venous system during experimental intracranial hypertension. J Neurosurg 41:427-434

7. Nornes H, Magnaes B, Aaslid R (1975) Observations in intracranial pressure plateau waves. In: Lundberg N, Ponten U, Brock M (eds) Intracranial Pressure II. Springer, Berlin Heidelberg New York p. 421

8. Risberg J, Lundberg N, Ingvar DH (1969) Regional cerebral blood volume during acute transient rises of the intracranial pressure (plateau waves). J Neurosurg 31:303-310

9. Shulman K (1965) Small artery and vein pressures in the subarachnoid space of the dog. J Surg Res 5:56-61

10. Wald A, Hochwald M (1977) An animal model for the production of intracranial pressure plateau waves. Ann Neurol 1:486-488

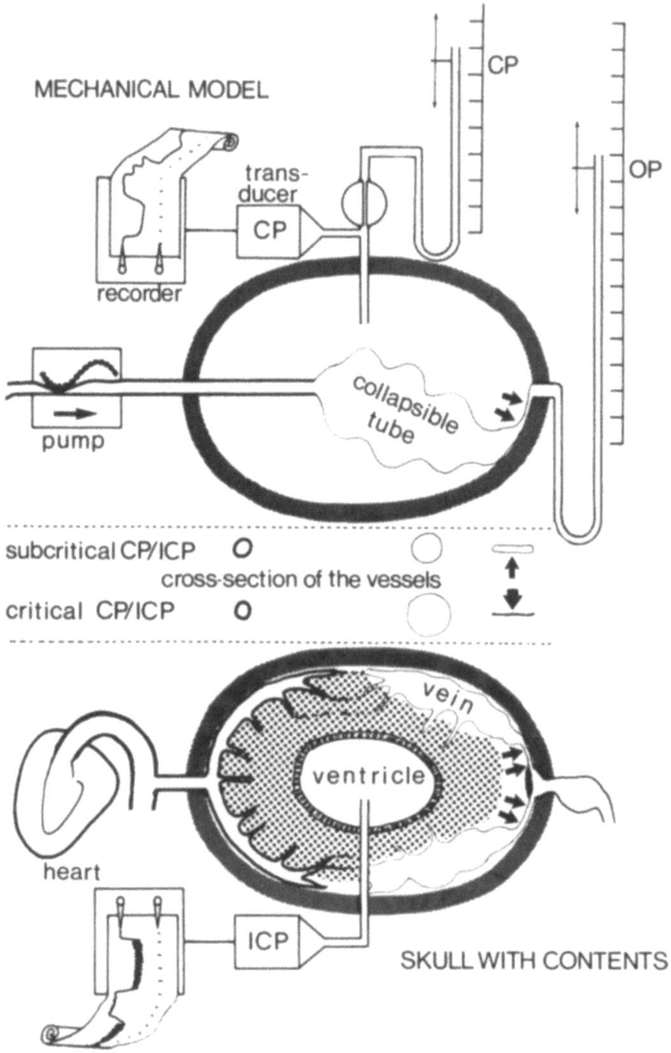

Figure 1.

Schematic drawing of a mechanical model for simulation of plateau waves and of the analogous intracranial situation.
CP: container pressure, ICP: intracranial pressure
OP: outlet pressure
->: compressible segment of the callapsible tube and the bridging veins, respectively.

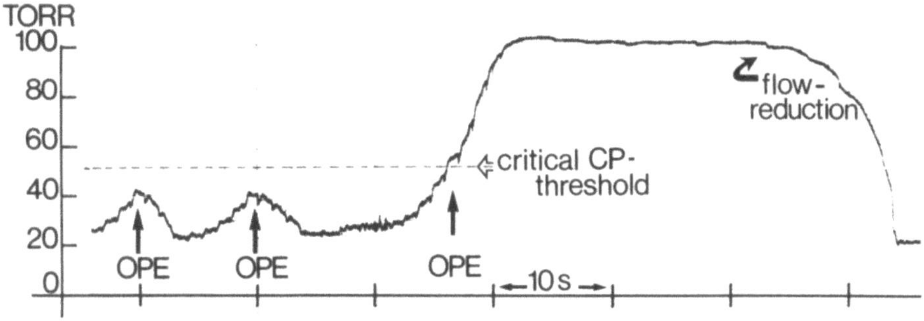

Figure 2:
Course of container pressure. OPE: outlet pressure elevation.

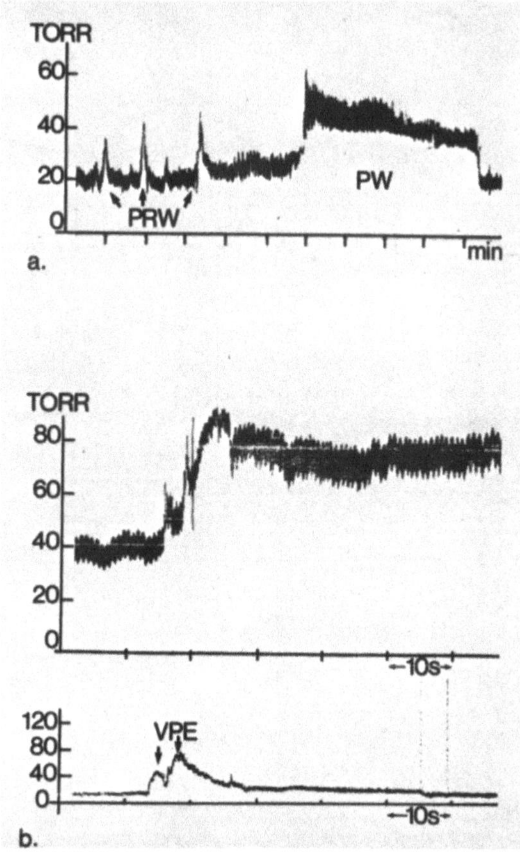

Figure 3.
a. Spontaneous plateau wave (PW) and precursor waves (PRW).
b. Plateau wave elicited by venous pressure elevation (VPE).

Session X

CLINICAL ASPECTS OF ICP MONITORING

Chairman: T.W. Langfitt
Co-chairman: N. Lundberg

SUMMARY

Recordings of ICP in benign intracranial hypertension in an attempt to understand the pathogenesis of this perplexing condition remain inconclusive. Clearly a defect in resorption of CSF can be demonstrated, but the lack of ventricular dilatation goes unexplained. KARSAKIS demonstrated that Vitamin A deficiency in rats results in a reversible intracranial alteration of arachnoid villi, causing a syndrome similar to benign intracranial hypertension. This work followed the case of an infant with a malabsorption syndrome in whom ICP responded to Vitamin A therapy. Such an observation, and others, during the course of the Symposium emphasized the important issue that the resistance to CSF absorption might occur in response to a variety of systemic "toxins" and not solely from particulate matter obstruction of arachnoid villi. In the Reye Syndrome considerable experience in ICP monitoring now suggests that fewer children are dying of raised pressure than from fluid depletion into a third space with a fall of cerebral perfusion pressure. Acute pancreatitis occurred in four of MENEZES' patients. This complication may reflect differing virulence of the primary agent.

During this Session and others, phasic phenomena that raise ICP have been addressed. Seizures, decerebrate rigidity, certain nursing maneuvers, and REM sleep are such episodes. The finding of pressure elevations and B-waves with REM sleep is likely due to an increase in cerebral blood volume related to a decrease in vasomotor tone. This important hypothesis needs further correlative data between basic chronological mechanism controlling both sleep cycles and brain vascular tone.

BENIGN INTRACRANIAL HYPERTENSION: A CLINICAL EVALUATION OF THE CSF ABSORPTION MECHANISMS

P. JANNY, J. CHAZAL, A.M. GEORGET, AND G. COLNET

Introduction

Benign intracranial hypertension (BICH) has been variously ascribed to increased cerebral blood volume (6) cerebral edema (9), or inflation of the CSF compartment (1). Johnston specially developed the third hypothesis (3,4), and assuming that CSF absorption follows the POISEUILLE'S law, he supposed a reduced CSF absorption syndrome that could result from either abolition of the pressure difference between CSF and the sagittal sinus (SS), or elevation of the resistance to flow across the arachnoid villi.

JOHNSTON himself provided an experimental confirmation of his theory (3), and MARTINS (5) in a paper on the measurement and significance of resistance to drainage, incidentally studied without detail five cases of BICH. A large clinical verification is still needed.

Methods

Fifteen patients suffering from verified BICH were investigated according to a program including:

1. A continuous ICP monitoring course of at least 24 hours.
2. A simultaneous recording of the pressure in the ventricle (IVP) and in the sagittal sinus (SSP) in which a catheter was inserted.
3. A measurement of the flow resistance (FR) according to a previously reported procedure (3) based on the KATZMAN and HUSSEY's constant infusion manometric test.
4. A checking of dural sinus patency by means of direct sinography and/or phlebography.
5. A conventional isotope cisternography, using ^{111}In.DTPA injected by lumbar route.

Results

The patients studied fall into two main groups according to Tables 1 and 2. In a first group, made up of 6 patients, the IVP-SSP difference was zero or even reversed; the resistance to flow was normal or slightly elevated; the sinuses were to some extent obstructed; and the isotope cisternography was normal.

In a second group, comprising also six patients, we found a very high resistance to flow, a normal pressure gradient, and patent sinuses. The cisternographies were normal in two patients, and slightly delayed in two others.

Finally, three patients could not be classified into either group, because of normal or contradictory results.

Table 1. CSF absorption factors in 6 cases of BICH with sinuses pathology

Patients No.	History	Gradient IVP - SSP	Flow resistance mm Hg/ml/mn	Sinuses	Radioisot. cisterno
1	Otitis	- 18	20	Obstructed	
3		0	8	Obstructed	Normal
7	a.v.a.	- 40	26	Patent	Normal
9	Oral contracept.	- 2	12	Obstructed	
14	Ear infection	0	23	Obstructed	Normal
15	Head injury	1	12	Obstructed	Normal

Mean gradient: -10 mm Hg. Mean flow resistance: 17 mm Hg/ml/mn.
Sinuses: constantly abnormal.

Table 2. CSF absorption factors in 6 cases of BICH without sinuses pathology

Patients No.	History	Gradient IVP - SSP mm Hg	Flow resistance mm Hg/ml/mn	Sinuses	Radioisot. cisterno
2	Perhexiline maleate	+ 25	70	Patent	
4			30	Patent	Delayed
8	Head injury	+ 15	60	Patent	Delayed
10	Head injury		100	Patent	
11	Chronic meningitis	+ 18	92	Patent	Normal
12		+ 9	60	Patent	Normal

Mean gradient: +17 mm Hg. Mean flow resistance: 70 mm Hg/ml/mn.
Sinuses: patent.

Discussion

In the first group of patients, the principal feature is obviously the abolition, or even the reverse of the pressure gradient between CSF and SS. The abnormalities constantly met with in the sinuses, as well as the etiological factors involved in the history, easily account for this fact, which, in accordance with the Poiseuilles' law, prevent any resorption of CSF into the SS. However, the normal cisternographies denote a normal flow of CSF, and strongly suggest that CSF is absorbed into other sites of exit, the flow resistance of which is significantly higher than that of the usual ones: 17 instead of 10 mmHg/ml/mn (2).

In the second group of patients, it appears that a considerable increase of the resistance to flow is the main cause of the high ICP. The arachnoid villi seem therefore to be involved in those cases, although no evidence of it can be supplied, since the etiological factors are not helpful, and the pathological information concerning the villi is lacking. The isotope cisternographies were also most often normal in this group, and we think that the CSF flow is maintained in those patients as the result of the elevation of the ICP and, consequently, of the pressure difference between CSF and SS: mean gradient: 17 mmHg instead of 5 - 7 in normal individuals.

In spite of the three patients who could not be classified in either group (probably because of artifacts in the measurements), we feel that our results are in good general agreement with those of JOHNSTON and MARTINS.

However, our interpretation is at variance with JOHNSTON's as regards the consequence of the impairment of the CSF absorption. JOHNSTON, using two observations from BERCAW (1), and on his own experiments on dogs (3), considers that a delayed isotope cisternography is a constant feature indicating a reduced CSF absorption. On the contrary, isotope cisternography was normal in 6 of 8 patients of ours, and we think that CSF flow is most often preserved in BICH. The reason for this is probably the high ICP iself, which forces the CSF either to be reabsorbed into other ways than the obstructed sinuses, or to overcome the elevated resistance of the arachnoid villi. In accordance with this conclusion, is the opinion widely accepted that the secretion rate is largely independent from the pressure (7), even though it is eventually reduced by it (8). Furthermore, JOHNSTON, himself, measuring the CSF formation rate by indirect calculation, found values within normal range.

Summary

Fifteen patients suffering from Benign Intracranial Hypertension of various causes were investigated by measuring the CSF resistance to flow, and the pressure difference between the CSF and the sagittal sinus. An isotopic cisternography was also obtained, and the patency of the dural sinuses was checked by sinusography and/or phlebography.

In 12, the results confirm a defect in the resorption mechanism, the nature of which proved to be venous in 6, and eventually linked to impairment of subarachnoid villi in 6 others. Three patients could not be classified.

Isotope cisternography was normal in 6 of 8 patients, and slightly or clearly delayed in 2. The flow of CSF seems therefore often normal in BICH, and the reason for this is discussed.

References

1. Bercaw BL, Greer M (1970) Transport of intratehcal 13/RISA in benign intracranial hypertension. Neurol (Minneap) 20:787-390

2. Jannp P, Godeneche P, Flori B, Raynaud EJ (1973) La resistance a l'ecoulement du L.C.R.Methode en mesure et application clinique. Rev Neurol 128:161-170

3. Johnston I (1973) The reduced CSF absorption syndrome: A reappraisal of benign intracranial hypertension and related condition. Lancet II:418-420

4. Johnston I, Patterson A (1974) Benign intracranial hypertension. II CSF pressure and circulation. Brain 97:301-312

5. Martins AN (1973) Resistance to drainage of cerebrospinal fluid: clinical measurement and signficance. J Neurol Neurosurg Psych 36:313-318

6. Mathew NT, Meyer JS, Ott EO (1975) Increased cerebral blood volume in benign intracranial hypertension. Neurol 25:646-649

7. Pappenheimer JR, Heisey SR, Jordan EF, Downer J de C (1962) Perfusion of the cerebral ventricular system in unanesthetized goat. Am J Physiol 203:763

8. Sahar R, Hochwald GM, Ransohoff J (1970) Experimental hydrocephalus. Cerebrospinal fluid formation and ventricular size as a function of intra-ventricular pressure. J Neurol Sci 11:81-88

9. Sahs AL, Joynt RJ (1956) Brain swelling of unknown cause. Nuerol 6:791-803

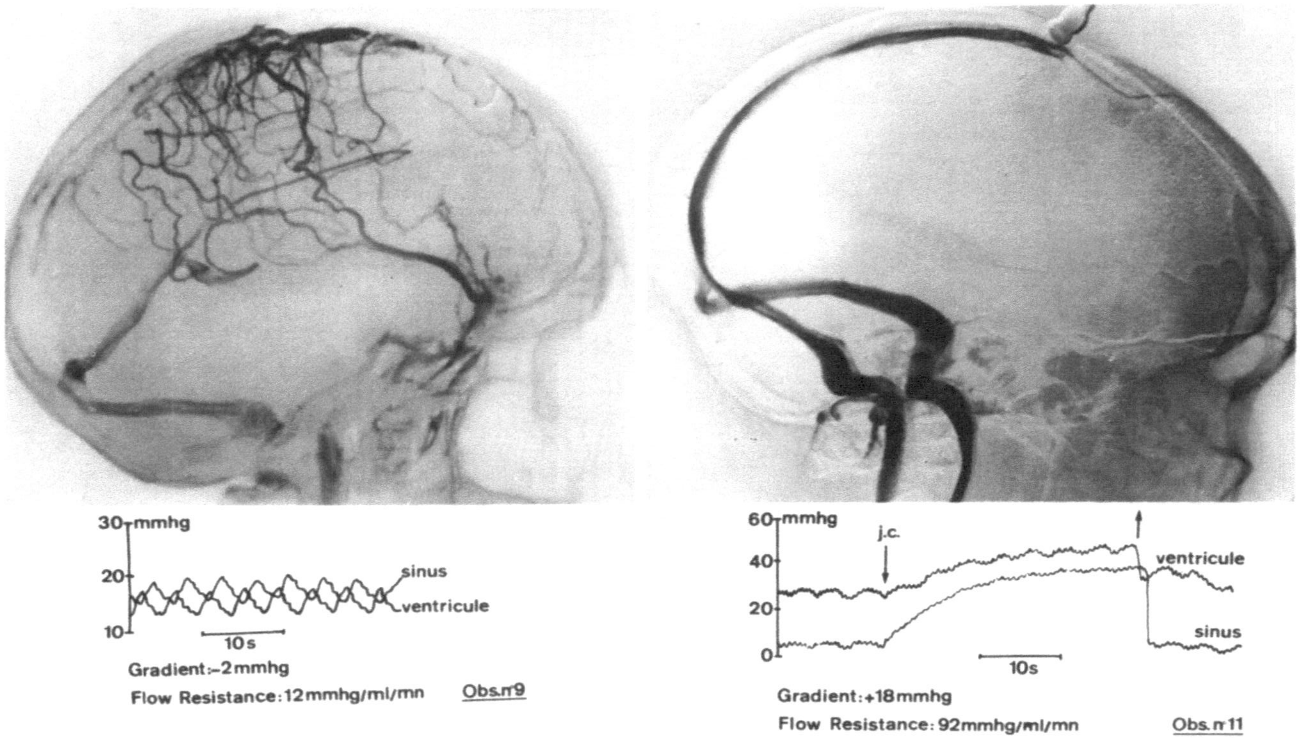

Fig I. Left: Obs No 9. Oral contraceptive history. The IVP-SSP difference is reversed; the RF is slightly elevated; the blood circulation is severely impaired in the sinuses.

Right:Obs No II. Chronic meningitis. The IVP-SSP difference is moderately elevated; the RF is considerably increased; the circulation is normal in the sinuses.

BENIGN INTRACRANIAL HYPERTENSION SECONDARY TO VITAMIN A DEFICIENCY IN RAT AND MAN: REVERSIBLE COLLAGENOUS OBSTRUCTION OF CSF OUTFLOW BY METABOLICALLY DERANGED FIBROBLASTS

E.J.KASARSKIS, C.J.MAFFEO, K.VAN LANDINGHAM, R.N.JOHNSON, A.B.BUTLER, AND N.H.BASS

Pseudotumor cerebri or benign intracranial hypertension can result from impaired outflow of newly-formed cerebrospinal fluid (CSF) from functionally deranged arachnoid villi. An infant with a fat malabsorption syndrome accompanied by deficiency of circulating retinol developed sustained intracranial hypertension that responded to Vitamin A (Vit A) replacement. Simulation of this condition in the rat revealed the reversible pathophysiological mechanism for decreased CSF outflow.

An 8 month old male infant was admitted to the University of Virginia Hospital for evaluation of increased intracranial pressure and failure to thrive. He was the full-term, 3.6 Kg (50th percentile) product of an uncomplicated pregnancy and was delivered without forceps to a 25 year old Caucasian female. The infant's development was apparently normal until four months of age when he presented with failure of body growth secondary to a fat malabsorption syndrome. During the subsequent 4 months, he continued to lose weight, and motor milestones, previously attained, were lost. He became emaciated and irritable, with head circumference measuring 45 cm (50th percentile) despite body weight less than 5 S.D. below the mean (4.8 kg) (Fig IA). In addition to clinically evident rickets and hepatomegaly, his cranial sutures were widely separated and fontanels bulging. He had a right esotropia, poor grasp and rooting reflexes, did not sit unsupported, but recognized his mother and followed objects brought past his midline.

A CT scan demonstrated normal ventricular size without a mass lesion (Fig IB) and serial lumbar punctures revealed acellular, sterile, clear CSF under opening pressures of 250 mmH_2O. Deficiency of the fat-soluble vitamins was documented, but despite replacement therapy with clinical and laboratory normalization of vitamins D, E and K, his intracranial hypertension did not resolve. Finally, after 8 weeks of Vit A by intravenous therapy, serum retinol rose, associated with normalization of intracranial pressure and head size (Fig IA).

The mechanism for intracranial hypertension induced by Vit A deficiency was studied in adult male rats fed diets devoid of the vitamin from the time of weaning. Rats were severely Vit A deficient on the basis of their characteristic clinical appearance and absence of retinol in liver and serum. Intracranial pressure was measured at the cisterna magna in Vit A deficient and pair-fed control rats ventilated to maintain normal blood gasses. In severely deficient rats, there was a three-fold elevation of intracranial pressure, and as in our Vit A deficient patient, ventricular size was normal.

Measurements of CSF dynamics were performed by means of a graded series of low volume, constant rate infusion of artificial CSF into the spinal subarachnoid space and CSF outflow resistance was calculated according to our previously-described mathematical model (1,2). In Vit A deficient rats, the resistance to outflow at the arachnoid villus was increased twelve-fold compared to pair-fed controls(Fig2A). Detailed ultrastructural study of arachnoid villi demonstrated extensive accumulation of collagen in the subarachnoid space(Fig 2B). Four weeks of Vit A replacement therapy normalized arachnoid villus ultrastructural pathology, CSF outflow resistance, and intracranial pressure, in association with return of serum retinol to normal levels.

Vitamin A has several distinct biochemical and physiological functions (3,4) and affects the pathway of cytodifferentiation of epithelia. In the intracranial compartment, Vit A deficiency causes a reversible metabolic derangement of arachnoidal cells leading to an extensive deposition of collagen in the subarachnoid space. The fibrous collagen meshwork forms a high resistance, partial barrier to CSF outflow placed in series with the physiological, pressure-sensitive outflow resistance at the arachnoid villus endothelial cell. Via A resupplementation corrects the underlying metabolic abnormality of arachnoid cells causing regression of the collagen barrier, restoration of physiological pressure regulation at the arachnoid villus, and normalization of intracranial pressure.

References

1. Mann JD, Butler AB, Rosenthal JE, Maffeo CJ, Johnson RN, Bass NH (1978) Regulation of intracranial pressure in rat, dog and man. Ann Neurol 3:156-165

2. Johnson RN, Maffeo CJ, Mann JD, Butler AB, Bass NH (1978) Intracranial pressure regulation: A comparative model of cerebrospinal fluid systems. T.I.T.J. Life Sci 8:97-92

3. Wolf G (1977) Retinol-linked sugars in glycoprotein synthesis. Nutr Rev 35:97-100

4. Wolf G, DeLuca L. (1970) Recent studies on some metabolic functions of vitamin A. In: DeLuca HF, Suttie JW (eds) The Fat-Soluble Vitamins. Univ of Wisconsin Press. Madison, p 257

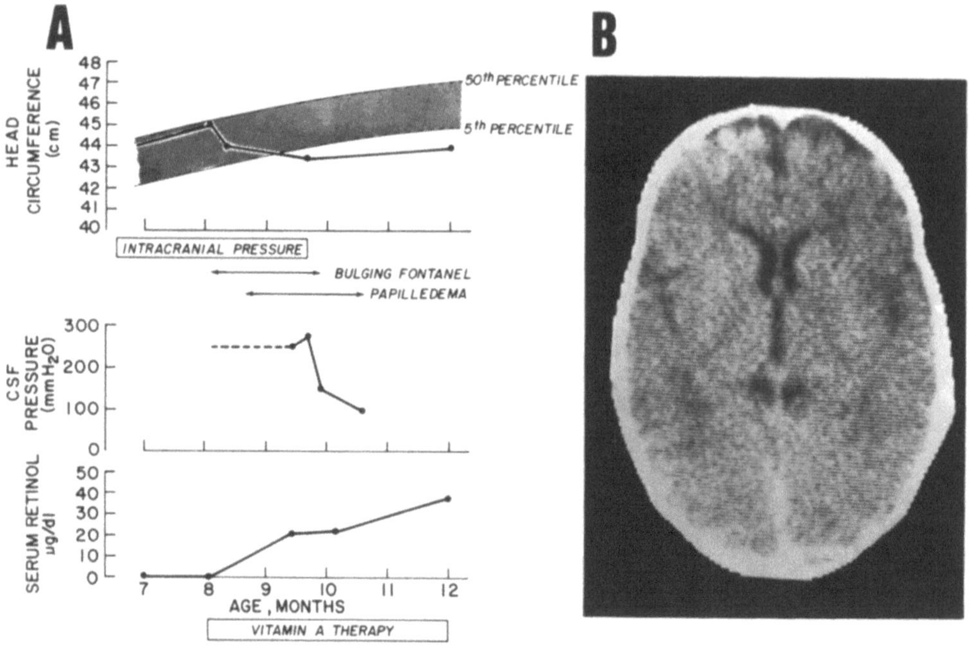

Fig 1A. Intracranial hypertension in an 8 month old vitamin A deficient male infant and its clinical resolution during intravenous replacement therapy with retinol. Note the head circumference was disproportionately increased with respect to body weight which was less than 5 S.D. below the mean. Normalization of head circumference and intracranial pressure was associated with increasing levels of serum retinol. Fig 1B. A CAT scan with contrast enhancement at 8 months of age demonstrated normal ventricular size, absence of mass lesion, and minimal atrophy of right frontal pole. These radiographic findings were unchanged following normalization of intracranial pressure by vitamin A therapy.

Fig 2A. Intracranial hypertension in vitamin A deficient rats: Relationship of CSF outflow resistance and steady state pressure during a graded series of low volume, constant rate infusions of artificial CSF into the lumbar subarachnoid space. Elevated outflow resistance in deficient rats approached normal levels following treatment with vitamin A. Arrows indicate the pressure at maximal resistance P_R (2). Fig 2B. Electromicrographs of arachnoid villi of pair-fed controls (left), vitamin A deficient (center), and vitamin A deficient rats following replacement therapy (right). Note the extensive deposition of collagen in the subarachnoid space proximal to the arachnoid villus in the superior sagittal sinus (SSS) of vitamin A deficient rats and the dissolution of collagen following 4 weeks of replacement therapy.

A

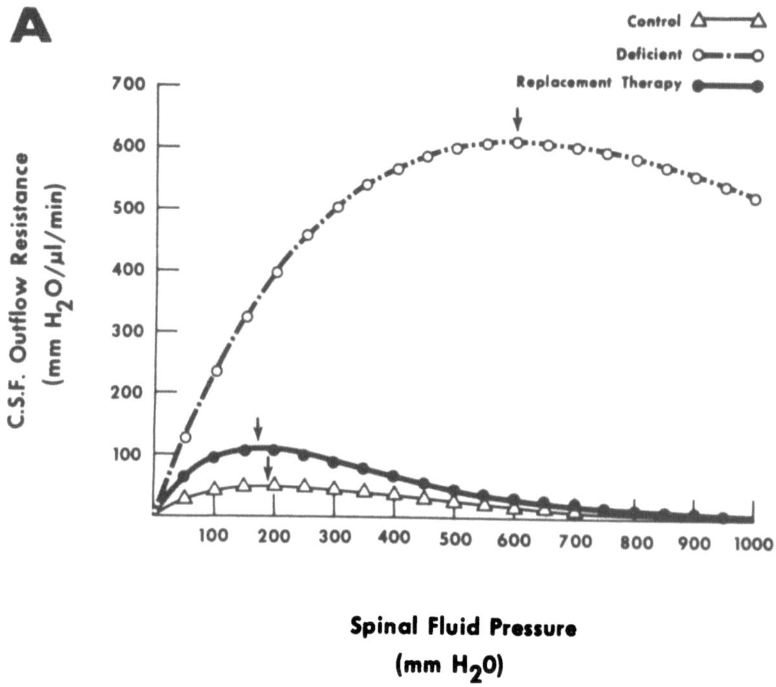

Control
Deficient
Replacement Therapy
C.S.F. Outflow Resistance
(mm $H_2O/\mu l/min$)
700
600
500
400
300
200
100
100
200
300
400
500
600
700
800
900
1000
Spinal Fluid Pressure
(mm H_2O)

B

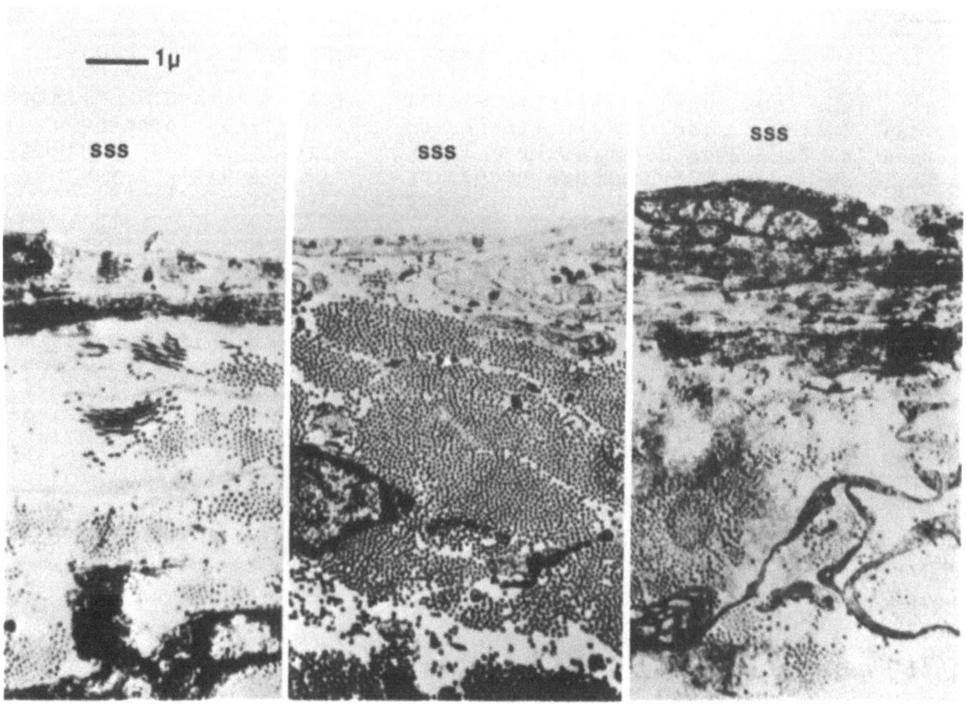

1μ
SSS
SSS
SSS

BENIGN INTRACRANIAL HYPERTENSION: THERAPEUTICAL APPROACH AND PATHOPHYSIOLOGICAL IMPLICATIONS

S. MINGRINO, M. SCANARINI, AND D. D'AVELLA

Introduction

Benign intracranial hypertension (BIH) or pseudotumor cerebri is a syndrome of intracranial hypertension without clinical and neuroradiological signs of focal lesions, with normal ventricular system and normal CSF composition. The aim of the present study was to test the effect of Escin and of cortisone in the treatment of BIH by recording CSF pressure. Escin is a triterpenic pentacyclic glycoside similar to saponine which has proved effective in reducing intracranial hypertension (1,2).

Material and methods

This work regards a group of 13 adult patients that have been studied in the last three years. All had presented with a clinical syndrome of BIH including headache, vomiting and papilledema, sixth nerve palsy in 9 cases, visual impairment in one.

Neuroradiologic studies including CT scan and carotid angiogram disclosed negative findings in 11 cases and a slight ventricular dilatation in two. Constant-infusion test (IT) (infusion rate 0.76 ml/min) was done in four cases. All patients were administered intravenous Escin while recording CSF pressure; in 6 the effect of dexamethasone was also tested by CSF pressure recording. Only one patient was treated by CSF shunt. Renal function was controlled in all patients before and after Escin treatment.

Results

In ten patients i.v. Escin lowered CSF pressure within 10 minutes from infusion (Fig 1). In 4 cases infusion of the drug brought the normalization of the previously altered ICP (Fig 2). In 2 of these Escin-responding patients intravenous administration of 10 mg of dexamethasone did not modify CSF pressure. In the patients who responded to Escin, chronic treatment with Escin (20 mg every 8 hrs for 3 days) was carried out, after which CSF pressure was controlled by subarachnoid continuous monitoring. In 9 patients normal values were recorded (Fig 1).

These patients continued oral treatment with the same dosage of the drug for 20-30 days. All showed subjective improvement of their symptoms, normalization of the fundus and disappearance of the paresis of the VI cranial nerve in cases where it was present. At one year follow-up, these patients were cured and no one to date has presented recurrence of the syndrome. The tenth patient, who had presented with a severe symptomatology of intracranial hypertension and very high CSF pressure (50 mmHg), did not responde to chronic treatment with Escin nor with chronic dexamethasone therapy. Since this patient presented improvement of visual acuity and other symptoms after CSF external drainage, a CSF shunt was carried out, which normalized the intracranial pressure and brought to clinical remission.

Three cases, which did not respond to the three day treatment with Escin, were favorably treated by cortisone (4 mg dexamethasone every 6 hrs) for a week with normalization of CSF pressure and improvement of clinical symptomatology. These patients continued oral treatment with reduced doses of cortisone for about a month. Only one patient treated with Escin presented at four days a transitory and slight impairment of the renal function, which reversed after a week with normalization of laboratory findings. This patient had tuberculosis of the kidney five years before.

Discussion

Escin is an important and useful drug in the treatment of BIH. Seventy percent of our patients were normalized and remained under control. We do not know if the same patients could have been cured by dexamethasone, as the lack of ICP modification to a single 10 mg dose in two cases cannot be taken as a reliable test.

Three patients without any particular clinical feature, did not respond to Escin but were cured by cortisone. According to JOHNSTON(3,4) cortisone is not useful in most cases of BIH and MATHEW (5) considers it contraindicated. In agreement with others (6,7) we have found cortisone useful in many cases of BIH. Besides the small group of patients presented here, we have experience of a larger group of cases favorably treated but evaluated on a clinical basis only.

It is inviting to explain Escin responsiveness or not as due to diverse pathogenetic mechanisms underlying BIH. The hypothesis suggested for BIH, when sinus thrombosis or arteriovenous fistula are excluded, are: 1) JOHNSTON (3,4) thinks that BIH is due to CSF reabsorption derangement; 2) GREER (8) and SUGAR (9) believe BIH is caused by an alteration of the blood-brain barrier that translates essentially into an alteration in the membrane transport mechanisms (Fig 3).

Escin should be more effective in cases where disturbance of reabsorption play a major role. In our experience, in fact, Escin is able to treat alteration of CSF absorption, such as those arising after SAH or after intracranial surgery, whereas cortisone has proved completely ineffective. The drug, being a glycoside similar to saponine, with surface active properties, may act at the level of the arachnoid villi facilitating CSF reabsorption. Still the action of Escin is not definitely known. It does not act with a mechanism similar to that of osmotic agents, since diuresis, plasma osmolarity and electrolyte changes are not observed during treatment. That Escin may in some way influence CSF reabsorption is also supported by the normalization of the response to infusion test (IT) previously altered in four cases of our series. Cortisone's therapeutic action is also not completely known, it is thought to stabilize cellular membrane and to reduce CSF production (11), but not to increase CSF reabsorption. Thus cortisone should be more useful in cases with alteration of the blood-brain barrier.

The only case treated by shunt presented a particularly severe syndrome of intracranial hypertension and very high ICP. Although there was an initial improvement after Escin, ICP did not normalize after three days treatment nor improve with cortisone. This patient should perhaps be included in a third group of cases with yet a different pathogenetic mechanism. Escin has proved to be a safe drug. The only contraindication to high dose administration is the pre-existence of kidney dysfunction.

Summary

In the treatment of pseudotumor cerebri or benign intracranial hypertension (BIH) we have adopted the following steps in treatment. First, the patients are administered parenteral Escin (20mgx3) for three days. If CSF pressure normalizes, then oral Escin is continued for a month. Nine cases (70%) were definitely cured after a year follow-up. If Escin is not useful, then dexamethasone is given (4mgx4) for three days. Three patients (23%) were definitely relieved of their syndrome and CSF pressure became normal. Only one patient, presenting with a severe intracranial hypertension and visual impairment, did not improve with Escin and cortisone and was cured by CSF shunt.

References

1. Mingrino S, Scanarini M (1977) Effetto dell'escina sull'edema cerebrale. Min Anest 43:1

2. Hemmer R, Diezemann E (1962) Attivita dell'escina, saponina dell'ippocastano, sulla pressione del liquor. Archiv f. Psychiat u Ztschr Neurol 407:203-204

3. Johnston J (1973) Reduced CSF absorption syndrome. Lancet 25: 418-420

4. Johnston J, Paterson A (1975) Intracranial pressure monitoring in patients with benign intracranial hypertension. In: Lundberg N, Ponten U, Brock M (eds) Intracranial Pressure II. Springer, Berlin Heidelberg New York, p 500

5. Mathew NT, Stirling MJ, Ott EO (1975) Increased cerebral blood volute in benign intracranial hypertension. Neurol 25:646-649

6. Mingrino S, Scanarini M (1978) Treatement of pseudo-tumoral encephalopathy. Acta Neurochirurg 44:257-258

7. Mingrino S, Scanarini M, d'Avella D (to be published) Treatment of benign intracranial hypertension. J Neurosurg

8. Greer M (1963) Benign intracranial hypertension: II Following corticosteroid therapy. Neurol 13:439-441

9. Sugar O (1953) Central Neurological complications of hyperparathyroidism. Arch Neurol Psych 70:80107

10. Welch K, Friedmann V (1960) The cerebrospinal fluid valves. Brain 83:454-469

11. Weiss MH, Nulsen FE (1970) The effect of glucocorticoids on CSF flow in dogs. J Neurosurg 32:452-458

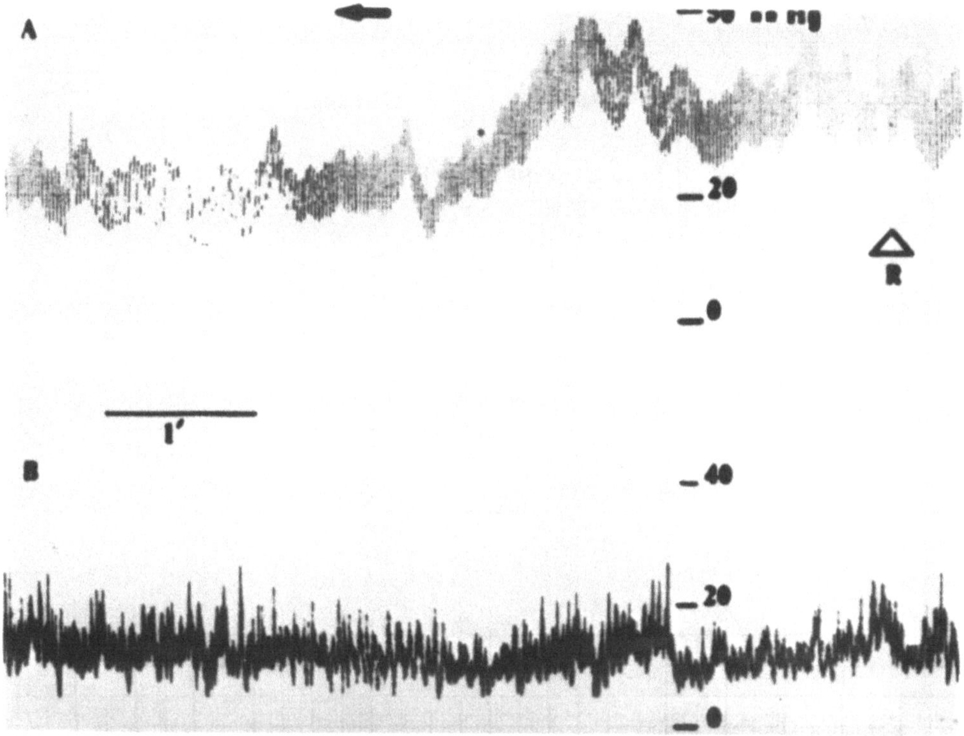

Fig. I. A) the acute hypotensive effect of high dose of intravenous Escin (R=50 mg) on CSF pressure, Case n 2.

B) Normal CSF pressure after chronic treatment with Escin (20 mg every 8 hrs for three days). Case n 2.

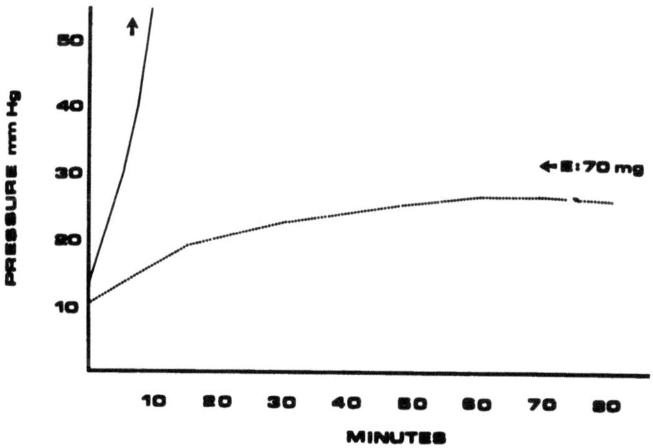

Fig. 2. Pressure response to infusion of saline at 0.76 ml per min before and after Escin 70 mg. Case 6

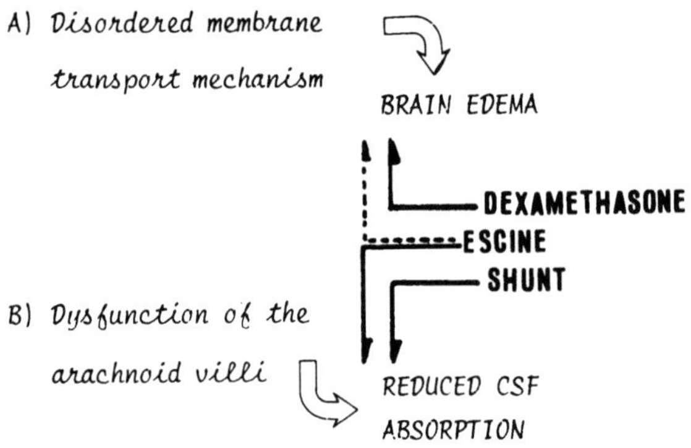

Fig. 3. Picture showing correlation between the different pathogenetic mechanisms underlying BIH and the different type of treatment.

ICP MONITORING IN BENIGN INTRACRANIAL HYPERTENSION

F. VILA, E. FERRER, AND F. ISAMAAT

Introduction

The purpose of our work has been to follow up the ICP in a group of patients with benign intracranial hypertension from admission to discharge. Patients were studied to normalization of the clinical symptoms and until a double control of ICP had been recorded.

Material and method

We have had the chance to study 17 patients with benign intracranial hypertension (BIH). In 13 of them we made intraventricular recordings, through reservoirs implanted at the moment of their admittance to the hospital, as well as daily, during their stay in our department, and after they had been discharged, every two weeks. In the last of four patients, after diagnoses were made using the CT scan recordings were undertaken through the subarachnoid lumbar space, first weekly, and after discharge, fortnightly. All of these recordings were made under basal metabolic conditions. During 1 or 2 hours, analysis of frequencies were carried out and histograms were drawn (Fig 1). We placed special emphasis on the mode (most frequent class of pressure) and range (number of classes that appeared during the recording). In this way, we were able to draw a chart (Fig 2) for each of our patients. The mode is shown as a continuous line; the range representing the stability of the recording by the shadowed area. Regarding treatment, Dexamethasone was given in 13 of our patients; four of them were treated with Diamox also; two received only Diamox and two pregnant patients were given no drugs at all.

Results

All our patients showed at the onset of the symptoms an unstable ICP (mode greater than 20 - 25 mmHg, and range greater than 3 classes of pressure) (2). The V/P ratio was altered in all 5 cases studied. In 14 patients ICP normalization preceded fundi normalization. Dexamethasone stabilized the ICP line in 12 of our 13 patients; however in 5 of them, the withdrawal of corticoid therapy produced a rebound effect even though it was discontinued gradually. The two pregnant patients, who were not treated at all, had a satisfactory follow up like the other patients. They did not at any time show evidence of residual visual sequela. Such sequelae are reported in the range of 2 to 8% (1,4,6).

Discussion

Based on our investigation, in 17 patients, it appears that ICP and its clinical course follow, in most of our patients (14 out of 17), three evolutive phases:

Phase I Increased ICP (mode greater than 20 - 25 mmHg), unstable pressure (range greater than 3 classes of pressure) and V/P ratio altered. Papilledema, visual symptoms and headaches characterize the clinical syndrome.

Phase II Stable pressure (range less than 3 classes of pressure), ICP still high, clinical syndrome outlined by no visual symptoms and fundus begins being normal.

Phase III-Normal ICP

It seems that Dexamethasone is useful in Phase I of BIH course, based on its stabilizing action on ICP. The rebound effect makes control of ICP necessary. On the other hand, Diamox did not appear to improve, neither in the range nor in the mode, the favorable effects of Dexamethasone already obtained.

Summary

It seems that ICP follows a characteristic course, which can be altered by its different pathogenic factors. However, drugs especially those with stabilizing effect, can modify the course as well. The control of ICP behavior seems to be mandatory in making the diagnosis (6) and in a rational management of an illness which is called "Benign" (3) but is followed by a range of 2 to 8% of residual visual sequelae.

References

1. Boddie MG, Banna M, Bradley WG (1974) Benign intracranial hypertension. A survey of the clinical and radiological features and long-term prognosis. Brain 97:301-313

2. Dandy WE (1937) Intracranial pressure without brain tumor. Ann Surg 106:492-513

3. Foley J (1955) Benign form of intracranial hypertension: "toxic" and "otitic" hydrocephalus. Brain 78:1-41

4. Greer M. Benign intracranial hypertension. Handbook of Clin Neurosurg 16

5. Gucer G, Viernstein L (1978) Long-term intracranial pressure recording in the management of pseudotumor cerebri. J Neurosurg 49: 256-264

6. Johnston I, Paterson A (1974) Benign intracranial hypertension: I.Diagnosis and prognosis; II.CSF pressure and circulation. Brain 97:273-301

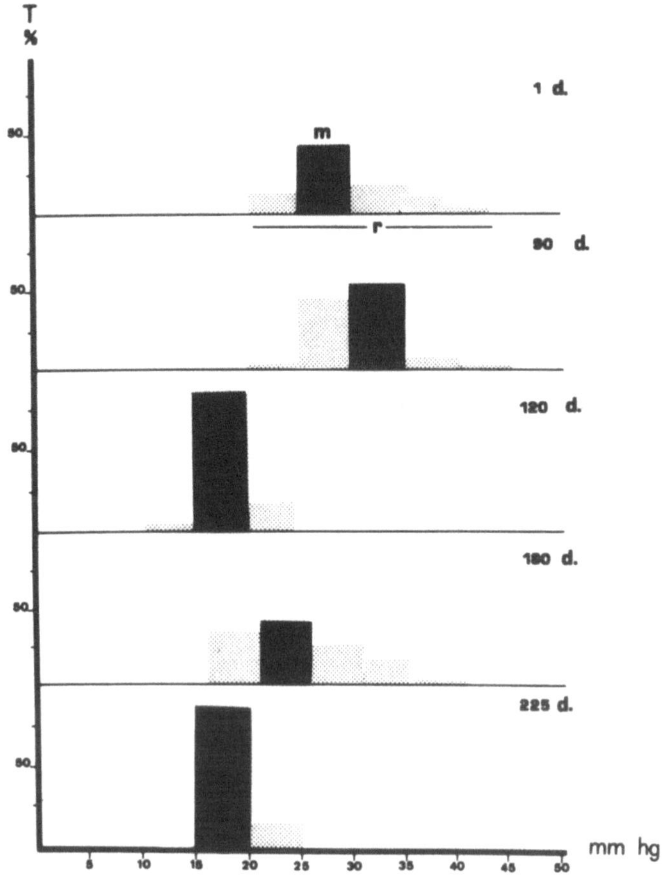

Fig.1. Different histograms in a patient with benign intracranial hypertension. m = mode, r = range.

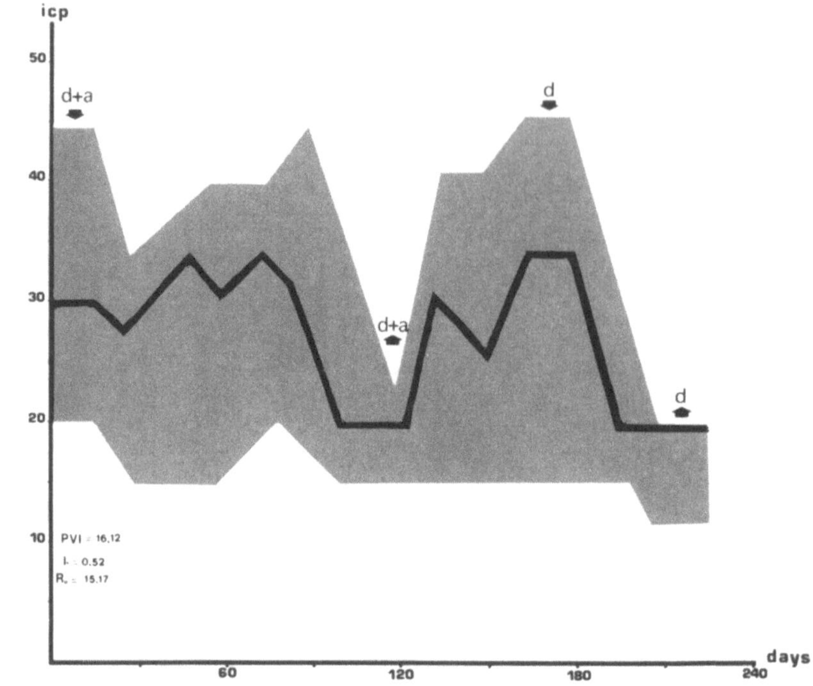

Fig. 2. With all the histograms we made this figure. The shadow corresponds to range and the continuous line to mode.
d = Dexamethasone, a = Acetazolamide (Diamox).

EXPERIENCE IN MANAGEMENT OF CRITICAL PATIENTS WITH REYE-JOHNSON SYNDROME

A. MENEZES, W.E. BELL, G.P. KEALEY, E. CHAVES-CARBALLO, AND T. YAMADA

Introduction

REYE-JOHNSON syndrome is a common acute childhood neurological disorder consisting of rapidly progressive encephalopathy and fatty degeneration of certain visceral organs. The mortality rate or severe neurological sequelae is variously reported between 50% and 80% or more in patients with stage III-IV of the disease (1,2,3). Our experience with 14 severe cases is analyzed.

Materials and method

Fourteen children in clinical stage IV {I-V (3)} and electroencephalographic (EEG) grade IV {I-V (1)} or worse were treated in a prospective study (2) between April 1976 and April 1978. The protocol consisted of controlled hyperventilation ($PaCO_2$ 20-25 torr), fluid restriction and hypothermia to 31-32°C. In all cases the EEG, subarachnoid (screw) intracranial pressure (ICP), cardiac output and arterial blood gases were constantly monitored. Mannitol was utilized to normalize ICP above 15-18 mmHg. The pulmonary artery wedge pressure was maintained between 3-5 torr. Barbiturate coma (5) was reserved for intracranial hypertension despite the above protocol. An initial loading dose of 7-9 mg/kg pentobarbital was followed by 2-3 mg/kg/hr. If the cardiac output (thermodilution technique) was less than 60% of normal or mean arterial blood pressure below 70 mmHg, the next dose of barbiturate was withheld. Therapy was terminated when the EEG pattern improved to grade II-III (Fig 1) and/or if ICP remained below 15 mmHg for 48 hours when pentobarbital therapy was utilized (2,4,5).

Results (Table I)

Eleven children made a complete recovery and 3 died. Intracranial hypertension under this protocol occurred in 3 patients necessitating barbiturate therapy (5) and all 3 recovered. A relapse was documented in 2 children who recovered. Pancreatitis occurred in 4 children, 3 of whom died. Acute renal failure was seen in 1 child, cardiomyopathy 1, autoimmune response with coagulopathy 1, and in 2 patients a GUILLAIN-BARRE picture presented during recovery.

Discussion

This series deals with children in state IV-V of the disease. Seventy-nine percent survived without neurological sequelae at the end of one year. Until now, fatal outcomes have been attributed to uncontrollable raised ICP. With our protocol using hypothermia, ICP refractory to therapy occurred in only 3 patients who responded to barbiturate coma and survived. The fatal cases in our series manifested rather sudden systemic hypotension indicative of fluid loss into a "third space"

Table 1. Results of treatment of severe reye's syndrome

Case	Age (Yrs)	Sex	Initial Clinical Stage	Initial EEG Grade	Admission Blood NH_3	Admission Mean ICP	Complications	Barbiturate Therapy (Hours)	Results
1	8	M	IV	V	150	7	Renal failure	-	Recovered
2	14	F	IV	IV	184	5	-	-	Recovered
3	2	M	V	V	764	4	Severe hypoglycemia on admission; pancreatitis	-	Died
4	6	M	IV	IV	348	3	-	-	Recovered
5	6	M	IV	IV	509	9	-	-	Recovered
6	10	F	IV-V	IV	194	10	-	-	Recovered
7	5½	F	V	V	367	9	Renal failure, pancreatitis	-	Died
8	13	M	V	IV	380	11	Pleural effusion, G.I. bleeding	90	Recovered
9	6	M	IV	IV	480	20	Guillain-Barre syndrome	142	Recovered (delayed)
10	14	M	IV	IV	210	26	Pancreatitis, relapse, cardiomyopathy, Guillain-Barre syndrome	96	Recovered
11	16	M	IV	IV	244	10	-	-	Recovered
12	2½	M	IV-V	IV	860	3	Severe hypoglycemia on admission; pancreatitis	-	Died
13	2	M	IV	IV	90	4	-	-	Recovered
14	8	F	IV	IV	380	20	-	-	Recovered

with loss of cerebral perfusion pressure. These patients had pancreatitis and expired within 48 hours of admission. Acute pancreatitis was seen in 4 cases, 1 of whom was successfully treated. Severe hypoglycemia encountered in the younger age group usually had a fatal outcome. In comclusion: (a) Fatal outcomes were not a direct result of intracranial hypertension under this protocol. (b) Acute pancreatitis should be considered as part of the disease process and can be lethal. (c) Extreme hypoglycemia with blood amonia above 500 was prognostically unfavorable. (d) "Barbiturate coma" has a definite role in management of severe REYE-JOHNSON syndrome.

Summary

Seventy-nine percent recovery was obtained in severe REYE-JOHNSON syndrome with control of ICP. The protocol described has proven that hypothermia and barbiturates are effective in treating elevated ICP in this syndrome.

References

1. Aoki Y, Lombroso CT (1973) Prognostic value of electroencephalography in Reye's syndrome. Neurol 23:333-343

2. Boutros A, Hoyt J, Menezes A, Bell W (1977) Management of Reye's syndrome. A rational approach to a complex problem. Crit Care Med 5:234-238

3. Lovejoy FH, Smith AL, Bresnan MJ, Wood JN, Victor DI, Adams PC (1974) Clinical staging in Reye's Syndrome. Amer J Dis Child 128: 36-41

4. Marshall LF, Shapiro HM, Rauscher A, Kaufman NM (1978) Pentobarbital therapy for intracranial hypertension in metabolic coma. Crit Care Med 6:1-5

5. Shapiro HM, Wyte SR, Loeser J (1974) Barbiturate-augmented hypothermia for reduction of persistent intracranial hypertension. J Neurosurg 40:90-100

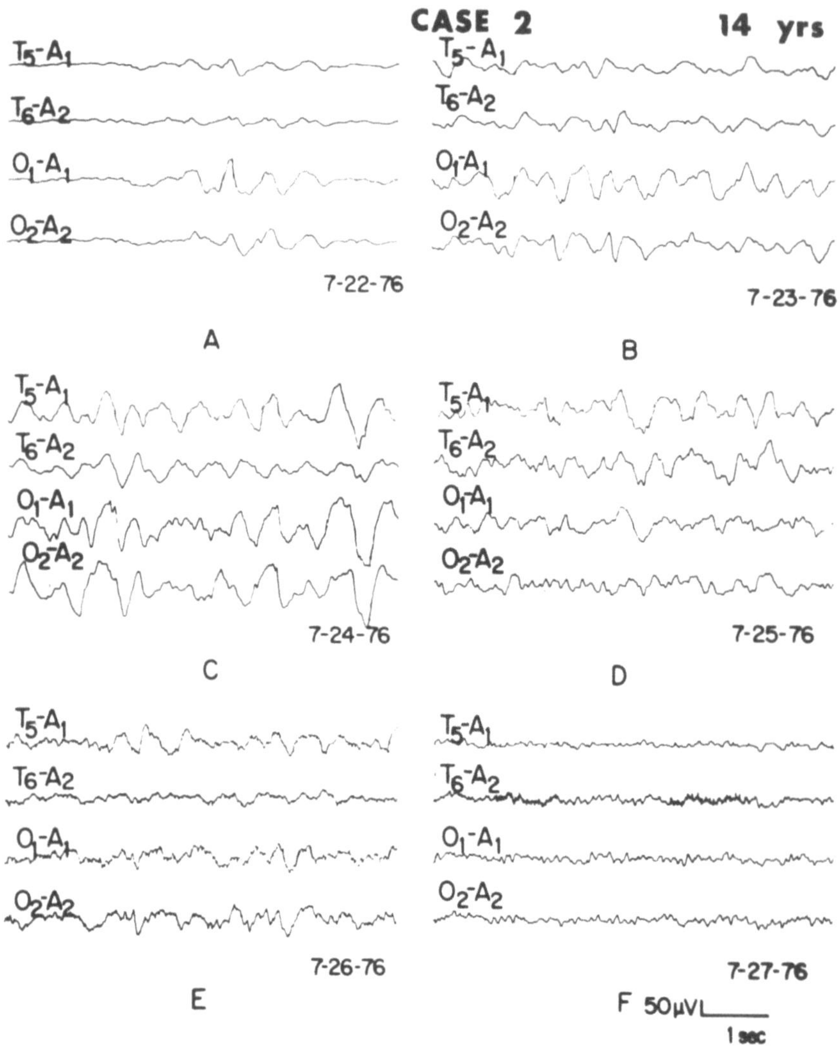

Fig I. Progressive improvement in the electroencephalograms from Grade IV/V on admission to normal - during therapy.

INTRACRANIAL HYPERTENSION IN PATIENTS WITH REYE SYNDROME

H.G.SULLIVAN, E.C.MEYER, W.F.BERMAN, AND J.J.MICKELL

ICP monitoring and treatment of intracranial hypertension has become an accepted adjunctive therapy in patients with Reye Syndrome. We report 8 such patients who were treated during the two previous years with intensive supportive therapy, intracranial pressure monitoring, and measures aimed at prevention and control of intracranial hypertension (ICHT). We are impressed with the variability of ICHT in patients of similar clinical grade and with the possible importance of considering the severity of ICHT along with other factors in evaluating outcome in patients with Reye Syndrome.

Patient Management: Patients at the lower level of Lovejoy clinical stage II or worse were considered candidates for ICP monitoring and intensive supportive therapy. After receiving pentobarbital (3mg/kg i.v.), hyperventilation with 100% O_2 and pancuronium (0.1 mg/kg), all patients in this group underwent endotracheal intubation. Each patient was then placed on controlled ventilation adjusted to maintain $PaCO_2$ between 25-85 mmHg. Fresh frozen plasma (15-20 ml/kg) was given to correct clotting abnormalities and each patient underwent CT scan, lumbar puncture, liver biopsy, ventricular catheter placement for ICP monitoring, and placement of CVP or Swan Ganz catheter. There were three levels of therapy for prevention of increases in ICP and for management of ICP elevations (Table I).

Table I. Reye's Syndrome - Treatment of Elevated ICP

ICP Tx Level	Maintenance TX	TX ↑ ICP
I	Controlled RSP Normothermia	Bag HV* CSF Drainage
II	Level I	Level I + Mannitol
III	Level I + ↓T° and Barb	Level II

* Hyperventilation.

Failure of therapy at a given level constituted the rationale for therapy at the next higher level. Ventilation was adjusted to maintain PCO_2 between 25-28 mmHg. When mannitol therapy was required, we employed initial small doses (0.25 gm/kg) progressing to larger doses (2 gm/kg) as necessary to control elevated ICP. Current mg loading dose is wt(kg) x 8 over 30 min and sustaining dose is wt(kg) x 0.75 per hour as required to keep ICP low and as allowed by cardiovascular function.

Patient Data and Results: With one exception all patients deteriorated to clinical stage IV or worse. Admission CT scan showed only small midline ventricles without evidence of mass effect and CSF from lumbar puncture was normal in all eight patients. ICP monitoring was initiated between 1 to 16 hours after admission and all but two patients had sustained elevations of ICP exceeding 20 mmHg. Of the two patients who did not have elevated ICP, one remained at clinical stage II while the other declined precipitously from clinical stage II to clinical state IV. In this latter patient, ICP monitoring was initiated after mannitol had been given on clinical grounds; however, the patient did not improve with mannitol and ICP was 18 mm or less during the 2 days of monitoring. Two patients had massive elevations of ICP exceeding 130 mmHg and one of these survived. Of the remaining four patients with ICP > 20 mmHg maximum ICP varied between 36 to 70 mmHg. None of the six patients with ICP >20 mmHg could be controlled with CSF drainage and bag hyperventilation alone (level I). However, the combination of these measures was often successful in aborting elevations of CIP and we hypothesize that CSF drainage and additional hyperventilation allowed us to minimize the use of mannitol, hypothermia and barbiturates. No patient was treated successfully with only small dose mannitol infusion, and it was not our feeling that small dose therapy decreased the total mannitol dose. Four of the six patients with raised ICP required hypothermia and/or barbiturates (level III); two of these patients expired, both related to uncontrolled elevations of ICP; one of the other level III patients was moderately to severely disabled, and only one patient in this group was in the good to excellent category. There was no mortality or permanent morbidity at treatment levels I and II. Table II relates outcome to ICP treatment level, worst clinical stage and maximum sustained ICP elevation.

Table II. Reye's Syndrome Results of Therapy

ICP Tx Level	No PTS	Worst Clinical Stage	Max ICP (mmHg)	Outcome*
I	2	II, IV	12,18	GE, GE
II	2	IV, IV	36,50	GE, GE
III	4	IV,V,IV,IV	40,130,130,70	GE,D,MS,D

*GE= Good to Excellent; MS =Moderately to Severely Disabled; D= Dead.

Discussion

Our series illustrates the following three well known points: 1) ICP in Reye Syndrome patients is a very unstable parameter and large plateau waves may occur, frequently without accompanying clinical signs; 2) not all patients with severe encephalopathy have elevated ICP; and 3) among those with severe encephalopathy and elevated ICP, there is considerable variation as to the magnitude of ICP elevation. Our data suggest that the severity of intracranial hypertension is an important factor in determining outcome in patients with Reye Syndrome. We propose that therapy for elevated ICP in Reye Syndrome should be based on a treatment plan where less dangerous measures precede those with more significant complications and where failure of therapy at a given level constitutes the reason for instituting treatment at the next level. We also suggest that the treatment level required to control elevated ICP could be used to classify patients as to the severity of intracranial hypertension. In order to obtain enough data for meaningful analyses of factors effecting outcome in Reye Syndrome, a multicenter cooperative study will be required. Each center in the study must use the same management protocol. Such a study would establish the data base which is needed to evaluate both new and old therapies for intracranial hypertension in Reye Syndrome.

THE EFFECT OF DECEREBRATE RIGIDITY ON ICP AS MODIFIED BY BRAIN ELASTANCE

S.A.TSEMENTZIS, F.J.GILLINGHAM, A.GORDON, AND E.R.HITCHCOCK

Introduction

Decerebrate rigidity (DR), as a potential mecahnical factor in raising and maintaining the raised ICP, and the brain elastance, as a possible modulator of this effect have been measured in head-injured patients. These were correlated with the level of ICP during DR with a view to clarifying some of the problems posed by these difficult cases.

Material and methods

Thirteen head injuries with DR were selected for study as having well developed rigidity, as assessed clinically. Ten were studied as soon as possible after surgery and a period of mechanical ventilation(IPPV) in order to stabilize the blood gas tensions. When instrumentation had been set up and several measurements of muscle tone, ICP, systemic arterial (SAP) and intrathoracic (ITP) pressures had been obtained, the relaxant was allowed to wear off. DR soon developed and the measurements were repeated over a period of 20 - 30 min. If during this period technically satisfactory data had not been obtained, the patient was reparalyzed and the procedure was repeated the following day. As DR spontaneously waxed and waned, we had the opportunity to study its effect on ICP, ITP, and SAP. The other three cases who suffered from post-traumatic hydrocephalus, still exhibited severe DR 3-4 wks after injury. These were not paralyzed and were examined repeatedly to study the effects of diazepam and chlorpromazine (CPM) on DR and ICP.

Rigidity: A printed circuit motor was used to apply alternating torques of logarithmically varying frequency to the wrist(6,7). The torque, angular displacement and velocity, and surface electromyographic (EMG) data from flexor and extensor muscles were all graphically displayed.
ICP: was continuously measured from the lateral ventricle by a Bell & Howell pressure transducer.
Brain Elastance (E'): The ventricular pressure/volume (P/V) ratios were calculated at 10 min intervals; the pressure was continuously recorded while the ventricular CSF volume was rapidly changed by ±1.0 ml (5).
Other parameters: The SAP was recorded either directly from the radial artery or intermittently (every 5-10 min) by a sphygnomanometer. The ITP was measured by a balloon catheter in the distal oesophagus(4). Arterial gas tensions and acid-base balance were repeatedly measured before, during and immediately after the spasms. The EEG was recorded in several cases.

Results

1) The wrist was forced to oscillate in phase with applied sinusoidal torques. Resonance of the joint was recognized when the amplitude of its movement was greatest. The resonant frequency (RF) at which this

occurred was measured from the "envelope" of the angular velocity trace: the greater the RF the greater the rigidity and vice versa.

The mean RF of a fully relaxed normal subject's wrist is 2.3±0.2 Hz. When partially stiff the RF ranged between 4.8 - 6.0 Hz and maximal stiffening of the wrist raised it to 10.3±1.3 Hz (6). Accordingly, two groups could be distinguished in this study:
Group 1: The mean FR was 9.1±1.5 Hz while during spontaneous relaxation it was reduced to 2.9±0.6 Hz; these patients showed severe DR.
Group 2: The mean RF was 5.3±0.8 Hz while during spontaneous relaxation it was reduced to 2.4±0.3 Hz; these patients showed only moderate DR.

Muscle paralysis decreased the mean RF to 1.8±0.2 Hz; diazepam reduced it to 2.1 Hz and CPM to 2.3 Hz. The difference in the mean RF of the groups 1 and 2 during DR, spontaneous relaxation, and muscle paralysis were highly significant, significant and not significant respectively.

II) Elastance: This is considered to be normal if successive measurements of V/P ratios differ by less than 2 mmHg (5). We distinguished, thus, Group A (normal), Group B (increased) and Group C (decreased).

III) Changes in ICP during DR: Summarized data are shown in Table 1. It appeared from this work that the two main determinants of the magnitude of the ICP rise were brain elastance and muscle hypertonicity. The relationship between these parameters is graphically displayed in Fig 1a. In each elastance group the rise of ICP from rest to spasm was plotted against values of DR. The relative influence of rigidity, resting ICP level, and elastance was studied by multiple regression analysis. The resting ICP did not significantly influence the rise when the other two factors were taken into account. The effect of elastance was highly significant (F-63.23 with 2 and 9 d.f); that of rigidity was significant (t=2.42 with 9 d.f) and there was no significant difference in the slope between the lines (F=1.60 with 2 and 7 d.f). The fitted parallel lines are shown in Fig 1b.

The intracranial hypertension of DR was always reduced after the administration of muscle relaxants; the deeper the relaxation the quicker and more lasting was the reduction. Both diazepam and CPM returned the ICP rise to its previous level but although the spasms were reduced in number and severity they were entirely abolished.

IV) Associated phenomena during DR: 1) Cardiovascular: A significant tachycardia (mean 140±20 was always present. A very variable elevation of both the systolic and diastolic blood pressure was seen; some cases showed virtually no change. During DR both pressures might be greatly increased, particularly the former (average 156±22/90±19 mmHg respectively); only in Group A were rises in the systolic SAP significant. These rises coincided with the onset of DR, lasted as long as it did and were restored to previous levels immediately it ended.
2) Respiration and ITP: Pulmonay hyperventilation occurred. The ITP was the first parameter to alter (Fig 1). The mean ITP was increased significantly from -3 mmHg to 27 mmHg; this rise was proportional to the DR and was statistically greater in group 1 than that in group 2 (t-3.82, P<0.01). 3) Arterial gas tensions and acid-base balance during or immediately after a spasm did not differ significantly from those seen during relaxation. 4) EEG: This was comparable with that of a comatose patient and showed no epileptic features.

Table 1. Mean increases in ICP, ITP, SAP, and pulse rate (PR) during decerebrate spasms under conditions of normal (A), increased (B), and decreased (C) brain elastance (E')

E'	$\bar{x}$ ICP	$\bar{x}$ ITP	$\bar{x}$ SAP		$\bar{x}$ PR
			SYST.	DIAST.	
	mmHg				Beats/min.
A	13.3***	25.6***	20.8*	9.8	32.6*
B	41.9***	28.6***	25.6	13.0	31.2*
C	2.0	26.0***	12.4	4.5	20.2**

Student's t -test: (***) P $<$.01 , (**) P $<$0.025 , (*) P $<$0.05.

Discussion

Systemic hypertension alone does not increase the ICP, but in some head injuries extreme and sustained intracranial hypertension may accompany it. This has been attributed to an increase in blood volume due to loss of autoregulation and cerebral vasodilatation (2). Evidence of intact vasomotor tone is offered by a) intracranial hypertension showed no constant relationship to the systemic, and b) all rises in SAP were concomitant with or followed the rises in ICP and both returned to their previous values when DR passed off. Blood gas tensions were normal and could have no effect on the ICP. Fits were not observed during DR. The rapidity of the events makes it unlikely that the ICP rises could result from either edema or dys-equilibrium in CSF dynamics.

An increase in the craniospinal venous blood volume can cause a rise in ICP partly from dynamic obstruction of the superior vena cava and partly from compression of the valveless trunkal veins by a rise in ITP and intraabdominal pressure. As these veins directly communicate with the spinal epi- and subdural venous plexuses the volume of the craniospinal venous bed increased and the CSF pressure is, therefore, increased; this CSF pressure rise is a volumetric displacement effect (1). It was evident that a) the increase in ICP was proportional to the increase in ITP, b) the waveform of the ITP was phase-locked with that of the ICP, c) a rise in ITP preceeded that in the ICP. Since these increases in ICP are volumetric displacement phenomena their magnitude is effectively determined by the brain elastance. The SAP rise may contribute to the overall effect since raising the SAP from 23 to 200 mmHg produced a 5-fold increase in elastance (3).

It, thus, appears that intracranial hypertension results from muscle rigidity and that the magnitude of this effect is directly related to the cerebral elastance.

References

1. Bowsher D(1953) The CSF pressure. B M J 1:863-865

2. Langfitt TW, Marshal WJS, Kassell NF, Schutta HS (1968) The pathophysiology of brain swelling produced by mechanical trauma and hypertension. Internatl Symp in "CSF" and "CBF", Lund. Scand J Clin Lab Invest Suppl 102 XIV:B

3. Lofgren J (1973) Effects of variations in arterial pressure and arterial carbon dioxide tension on the cerebrospinal fluid pressure-volume relationships. Acta Neurol Scand 49:586-589

4. Milic-Emili J, Mead J, Turner JM (1964) Topography of oesophageal pressure as a function of posture in man. J Appl Physiol 19:212-219

5. Miller jD, Garibi J (1972) Intracranial volume-pressure relationships during continuous monitoring of ventricular fluid pressure. In: Brock M, Dietz H (eds) Intracranial Pressure. Springer, Berlin Heidelberg New york, p 270

6. Tsementzis SA, Gillingham FJ, Gordon A, Lakie MD (to be published) Two methods of measuring muscle tone applied in patients with decerebrate rigidity. J Neurol Neurosurg Psychiat

7. WalshEG(1974)A torque-induced motion analyzer.J Physiol 244:14-15

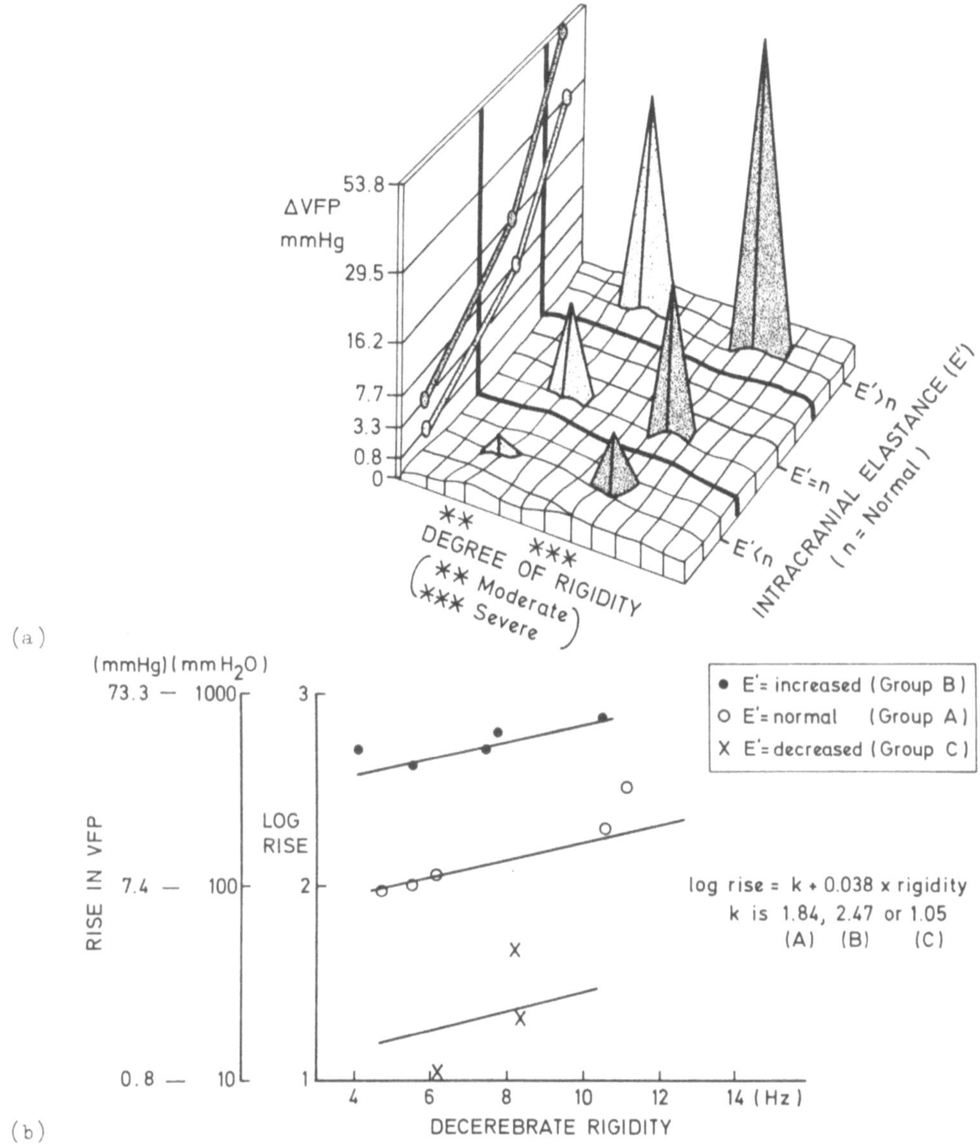

Fig I. a) A three dimentional representation of the changes in ventricular fluid pressure (VFP) during moderate and severe degrees of decerebrate rigidity and under conditions of altered cerebral elastance. The continuous fluctuations of the VFP are expressed by the wavy base. Heavily dotted peaks show VFP rises during severe (xxx) and lightly dotted peaks show VFP rises during moder-te (xx) decerebrate rigidity for each elastance group (E'). The peaks are projected onto a vertical, calibrated board. It is apparent that the greater the rigidity and elastance the greater the rise in VFP.
b) The diagram shows the rise in VFP from rest to spasm plotted against decerebrate rigidity in three groups of patients (A,B, and C) with differing cerebral elastance (E'). A logarithmic scale is used for the VFP to equalize the variability within each group. (k: constant).

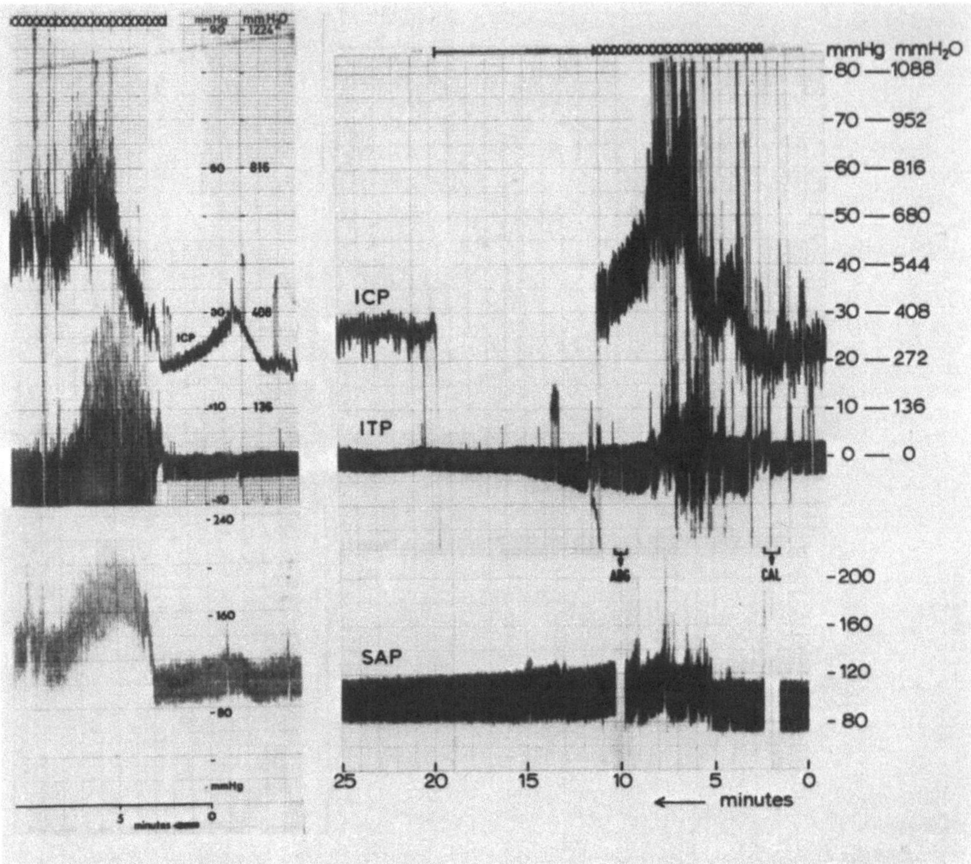

Fig 2. Continuous recording of the intracranial, intrathoracic and arterial blood pressures during onset of decerebrate spasms (xxxxxx). Despite the slow chart recording it is evident that the ITP rises first and is followed by the ICP. (ABG: sample for arterial gas tensions CAL: Calibration of the ICP and ITP pressures).

RELATIONSHIP OF NURSE/PATIENT ACTIVITY AND ICP VARIATION

P.H.MITCHELL, N.K.MAUSS, J.OZUNA, AND H.LIPE

Introduction

Activities such a turning, bathing, and toileting are essential to bed-fast patient care. Aside from anecdotal observation, few studies indicate how consistently such activity is associated with elevation in ICP. This paper reports two studies intended to determine what routine bedside activities consistently influence ICP.

Study I: Eight patients with pressure-regulated ventriculostomy drainage were observed continuously for 24 hours. Incidence and duration of ventricular fluid drainage (VFD) was graphed on a time axis with activity initiated by patient or nursing/medical staff. CHI square with Yates correction for continuity was used to determine the significance of the correlation of all activity with VFD in each individual. Ratio of VFD incidence for specific activities to total incidence of the activity was calculated for each subject.
Results: Incidence of VFD for all activities combined was significantly greater than expected on the basis of time spent in activity for all individuals ($p<.001$). VFD was associated with turning and emotionally charged conversation in 6 of 8 subjects over 80 percent of the time. Six activities were frequently associated with VFD in individuals (Table 1) and 3 activities were never associated with VFD unless they occurred simultaneously with an independently associated activity.

Study II: In 18 subjects with pressure-regulated ventriculostomy drainage, ICP was measured at 15 second intervals before and after each of 8 selected activities. Mean ICP of the last minute preceding the activity was compared to the first and fifth minute after. ICP was measured by an open-bore manometer attached to the external ventriculostomy system. Values were corrected for position of the intraventricular cannula relative to manometer zero and for the degree of head elevation. Although the internal diameter of both the cannula and manometer were equal to those which O'CONNELL (3) found accurate at slow rates of oscillation, the values must be considered relative, rather than absolute ICP.
Results: All subjects increased mean ICP on at least one of four turns; 88 percent increased mean ICP on half the turns. Group mean ICP was increased on all turns at one and five minutes after turn except for the supine to left lateral turn (See Table 2). There were no differences in change in mean ICP between the subarachnoid hemorrhage (SAH) group (n=12) and those with posterior fossa lesions (PF, n=4) except for the supine to left lateral turn, in which the SAH group had a mean decrease in ICP while the PF group showed a mean increase. Passive range of motion (PROM) resulted in a slight mean increase in ICP at both one and five minutes with no difference in SAH and PF groups. Head rotation right (HRR) and left (HRL) produced large mean increase, with slightly greater increase and less variability on HRR. Cumulative increase in ICP was seen with closely spaced activities (15 minutes apart) with the baseline of each

TABLE 1. Patient/Nurse Activities Frequently or Never Associated with VFD in 8 subjects (Adapted from Mithcell, P. and Mauss, N.: Nurs. Res. 27, 440, 1978)

ACTIVITY	N	RATIO VFD/TOTAL INCIDENCE OF ACTIVITY	PERCENT(group)
Turning	5	19/23	83
Conversation About Condition	6	21/24	88
Conversaton About Discomfort	2	10/11	91
Suctioning	2	3/ 5	60
Suctioning	1*	0/19	0
Coughing	3	14/20	70
On-Off Bedpan	2	11/16	69
Chewing	2	18/20	90
Snoring	1	24/38	63

Passive range of motion, tubing manipulation, bathing } in all subjects was not associated with VFD unless simultaneous with one of the above activities.

*VFD did not occurr in any suctionings of the subject who was hyperinflated prior to suction.

TABLE 2. ICP Variation with 8 selected Activites in 18 Subjects

ACTIVITY	MEAN ICP (CM H_2O)			RANGE OF CHANGE IN MEAN ICP from 5th min. pre to:	
	5th min. pre-	1st min. post-	5th min. post-	1st min. post	5th min. post.
PROM-arm extension	16.2 ± 2.3	16.5 ± 2.5	17.5 ± 2.9	- 3.6 to 9.2	- 5.4 to 19.1
PROM-hip flexion	17.0 ± 2.6	17.0 ± 2.8	18.2 ± 2.9	- 6.8 to 5.0	- 3.7 to 8.0
SUPINE to R lateral	17.8 ± 2.8	19.0 ± 3.3	19.6 ± 3.7	-13.2 to 17.7	-13.2 to 23.6
R lateral to supine	14.5 ± 2.5	15.3 ± 2.1	15.4 ± 2.3	- 8.2 to 7.8	-10.8 to 9.0
Supine to L lateral	15.5 ± 1.4	14.3 ± 2.1	15.5 ± 2.1	-12.7 to 15.0	- 8.1 to 14.7
L lateral to supine	10.9 ± 1.7	14.0 ± 1.5	14.7 ± 1.5	- 6.7 to 12.7	- 6.6 to 10.6
Head R (N=5)	12.0 ± 0.5	16.3 ± 4.2	15.3 ± 4.2	- 3.7 to 18.3	- 5.0 to 17.4
Head L (N=5)	15.7 ± 7.0	20.6 ± 7.7	19.3 ± 7.7	- 0.3 to 10.4	- 0.5 to 9.2

activity assuming similar values to the pressure at the fifth minute after the preceding activity. This effect was not present with activities one hour apart. As seen in Table 2, changes in mean ICP for the group are small, but larger changes are evident for individuals. During turns, change in individual ICP ranged from -13 to +24cm H_2O, with one-third to one-half the subjects increasing more than 5cm H_2O on each turn.

Discussion

Although the changes in mean ICP for the group are small, they were sufficient in many individuals to pose danger to neuronal function had the pressures not been vented. The magnitude of the relative ICP assumes more significance when one considers the damping effect of the manometer method of measurement. The true increases could be expected to be as much as twice the measured ICP (3). The drop in ICP seen in the SAH group on turning to left lateral is also clinically significant. Within the first days after SAH reabsorption of CSF is impaired (5), thus increasing the importance of the capacitance function of the spinal dural sac. Slight forward neck flexion in the supine position may be sufficient to impede free flow of CSF and possibly impede posterior collateral venous drainage. Turning to the lateral position could then open pathways for drainage into spinal CSF space. Presumably the subjects with PF lesions had partial or complete obstruction of these pathways. The absence of a beneficial effect for SAH subjects on the right lateral position is puzzling. However, the supine to right lateral turn closely followed two PROM activities and the cumulative effect of closely spaced activities may have obscured any beneficial effect. Head rotation findings are in agreement with others (1,4).

The larger increases on HRR may be a function of cumulative increase since HRR followed HRL by 15 minutes. HULME and COOPER'S unexplained difference in frequency of ICP increase with head right versus head left may be a result of the same effect (1). Closely spaced nursing activities, regardless of nature, may be a factor in steadily increasing ICP in patients with no compensatory reserve. Since head and body were turned as a unit and manual holding of a subject's head did not alter ICP response, we cannot agree with SHALIT and UMANSKY that head rotation is a major factor in increased ICP with turning (4). MAGNAES' finding of blood pressure and CSF filling waves with rapid changes from lateral to sitting posture may be relevant (2). While turning from side to side does not involve the postural changes he induced, the motion is nonetheless rapid and may not be compensated for well in persons with high volume-pressure relationships. Only simultaneous SAP and ICP recording during turning will confirm this speculation.

Summary

A pilot study identified nursing care activities associated with increased ICP. Subsequently, the relative ICP of 18 subjects with intracranial hypertension was measured before and after turning to four positions, PROM to arm and hip and head rotation. All subjects increased ICP on at least one turn with 88 percent increasing at least half the time. Subjects with SAH had decreased ICP in left lateral position, perhaps as a function of spinal sac capacitance. Head rotation right and left produced large mean increase in ICP while PROM was oe negligible consequences in most subjects. A cumulative increase in ICP was noted when activities were spaced 15 minutes apart.

References

1. Hulme A, Cooper R (1976) The effects of head position and jugular vein compression on intracranial pressure. In: Beks J et al(eds) Intracranial Pressure III. Springer, Berlin Heidelberg New York, p 259

2. Magnaes B(1976) Body position and cerebrospinal fluid pressure, part I. J Neurosurg 14:687-697

3. O'Connell J (1943) The vascular factor in intracranial pressure and the maintenance of the cerebrospinal fluid circulation. Brain 61:204-228

4. Shalit MN, Umansky F (1977) Effect of routine bedside procedures on intracranial pressure. Israel J Med Sci 13:881-886

5. Sundbarg G, Ponten U (1976) ICP and CSF absorption impairment after subarachnoid hemorrhage. In: Beks J, Bosch DA, Brock M(eds) Intracranial Pressure III. Springer, Berlin Heidelberg New York, p 139

PATHOLOGICAL INTRACRANIAL PRESSURE WAVES IN ARNOLD CHIARI MALFORMATIONS

J.P.CASTEL, J.F.DARTIGUES, AND M.VANDENDRIESSCHE

Introduction

In adults, ARNOLD-CHIARI malformations (A-CM) are incidentally associated with clinical signs of intracranial hypertension. However, some cases of papilledema (1,3) and some others with clinical signs of "paroxysmal intracranial hypertension" (3,13) have been recently reported. In almost all these cases, the ventricular size was not enlarged (1,3,12,13). So the CSF pathways might be clinically and radiologically presupposed normal, implicating that the mean CSF pressure is also normal. Therefore, concerning the late clinical evolution of these malformations, a certain controversy remains on the hydrodynamic effect of the tonsillar herniation (4,6,7,8,14) that clearly defines A-CM, we studied the CSF dynamics of adult patients suffering from A-CM with or without associated hydromyelia.

Methods

Eighteen patients were selected on clinical and radiological grounds, and classified according to the surgical findings. A-CM were associated with basilar impression (6 cases) or hydrosyringomyelia (12cases) as reported in Table I. The age of patients averaged 42.6 years ranging from 18 to 65. Except two cases in which lateral ventricles were "slightly" enlarged, the ventricular size judged on ventriculography was accepted to be in the normal range.

Before ventriculography was performed, the intraventricular CSF pressure was conventionally recorded with an extracorporal transducer for 6-8 hours. The modal pressure curve was provided by a multichannel annalyzer. The CSF dynamics were tested with an intraventricular incremental CSF injection. Pressure-volume index (PVI) compliance and outflow resistance were calculated according to MARMAROU'S mathematical model (11). For six patients, the CSF pressure was also recorded in the sitting position.

Results

1) In the supine position, the modal value of the intraventricular CSF pressure was always normal, setting between 6 and 10 mmHg. Except in one case, pathological intracranial pressure waves averaging 20 mmHg were always present as transient and irregular moderate spontaneous variations of the resting ICP (See Table I). They could be compared to the well-known B or C vasomotor waves (See Fig 2). The PVI was lower than 10 ml in 8 cases. Compliance and outflow resistance (except in one case) were within the normal range (See Fig 1).

2) In the sitting position, the absolute ICP level could not be accurately measured. However all relative variations were obviously considered as valuable. In all patients, the pathological ICP waves

Table I. No relationship could be found between the anatomo-clinical Arnold-Chiari syndrome and the importance of the pathological ICP waves (BI = basilar impression; A-C = Arnold-Chairi; S-syringomyelia)

	PATHOLOGICAL ICP WAVES				
	0	+	++	+++	
A-C		2	1		3
A-C + S	1	3	3	2	9
BI + A-C		1	1	1	3
BI + A-C + S			2	1	3
TOTAL	1	6	7	4	18

were always clearly enhanced, exceeding 35 mmHg in 3 cases. Likewise, the amplitude of the systolic CSF pulse wave has always largely increased. PVI and compliance were significantly decreased if compared to their value calculated in the supine position. The outflow resistance could only be calculated in 2 cases and was abnormally high (Fig 2).

Discussion

A-CM is a herniation of the hindbrain downwards through the foramen magnum. WILLIAMS (14) and DU BOULAY (4) considered that the malformative tonsillar herniation may potentially act as a ball-valve, creating pressure-gradients between the cranial and the spinal cavity. The first effect of this anatomical malposition is that cranial and spinal compliance are pathologically separated; according to MARMAROU'S experimental study (10), the spinal compliance could be estimated as 32% of the total craniospinal compliance. The second effect of the hindbrain herniation is supposed to be a reduction of the CSF outflow capacity.

In our clinical study, when CSF dynamics were tested in the supine position, only 8 patients of 18 had a slightly reduced PVI (between 6.5 and 10 ml). However, the compliance calculated (11) at the modal CSF pressure value was within the accepted normal range. The outflow resistance was never higher than 10 mmHg/ml/min, except in one case. We can conlude that whatever the severity or the duration of the neurological signs may be, pathological ICP waves are almost always present at various degress in all A-CM. Nevertheless, we suggest that our methodology of compliance and outflow resistance testing might be likely considered as inadequate to demonstrate a transient ball-valve-like effect. It is proposed that these ICP waves are of vasomotor origin, owing to a mechanical neuronal disturbance of the herniated hindbrain.

In the sitting position, the ICP waves were always enhanced, sometimes unexpectedly higher than 35 mmHg. When reducing the arterial pCO_2 by hyperpnea, the vasomotor waves disappeared quite completely. The theoretical reduced craniospinal compliance was confirmed either by the reduced PVI and compliance, or by the constant increased amplitude of the systolic CSF pulse wave.

Our findings reinforce GARDNER'S hydrodynamic theory (7,8) on the late development of a "communicating" syringomyelia accompanying an A-CM, as has been found in experimental studies (2,4,9). We also suggest that whatever hydrodynamics may be (4,5,6,8,14), in A-CM, the CSF pressure is always disordered above the craniospinal block resulting from the tonsilar herniation. These CSF pressure disorders may be due either to pathological vasomotor waves, or to a reduced intracranial compliance or to an increased CSF outflow resistance, present at various degrees and with various additive effects. The standing position always enhanced this pathological situation.

Summary

In the supine position, intraventricular CSF pressure dynamics were studied on 18 selected patients suffering from A-CM. Hydromyelia was present in 12 cases. There was no ventricular enlargement. Pathological intracranial pressure waves were observed in all cases except one. No relationship could be found between ICP findings and the severity or the duration of the neurological syndrome. These ICP waves were increased and compliance or outflow resistance were affected by the sitting position. Furthermore the standing position always enhances the CSF pressure disorders accompanying this dysraphic state.

References

1. Banerji NK, Millar JHD (1974) CHIARI Malformation presenting in adult life. Its relationship to syringomyelia. Brain 97:157-168

2. Becker DP, Wilson JA, Watson GN (1972) The spinal cord central canal: response to experimental hydrocephalus and canal occlusion. J Neurosurg 36:416-424

3. Caetano Debarros M, Farias W, Ataide L, Lins S (1968) Basilar impression and Arnold Chairi malformation. A study of 66 cases. J Neurol Neurosurg Psychia 31:596-605

4. DuBoulay G, Shah SH, Currie JC, Logue V (1974) The mechanism of hydromyelia in Chiari type I malformations. Brit J Radiol 47: 579-587

5. Ellertson A, Greitz T (1969) Myelocystographic and fluorescein studies to demonstrate communication between intramedullary cysts and CSF space. Acta Neurol Scand 45:418-430

6. Ellertson AB, Greitz T (1970) The distending force in the production of communicating syringomyelia. Lancet 1:1234

7. Gardner WJ (1975) The dysraphic states from syringomyelia to anencephaly. Excerpta Medica, Amsterdam

8. Gardner WJ, McMurry FG (1976) "Non communicating" syringomyelia: a non-existent entity. Surg Neurol 6:251-256

9. Hall PV, Muller J, Campbell RL (1975) Experimental hydrosyringomyelia, ischemic myelopathy, and syringomyelia. J Neurosurg 43: 464-470

10. Marmarou A, Shulman K, LaMorgese J (1975) Compartmental analysis of compliance and outflow resistance of the CSF system. J Neurosurg 43:523-534

11. Marmarou A, Shulman K, Rosende RM (1978) A non-linear analysis of the CSF system and intracranial pressure dynamics. J Neurosurg 48:332-344

12. Rhoton AL (1976) Microsurgery of Arnold Chiari malformation in adults with and without hydromyelia. J Neurosurg 45:473-483

13. Saez RJ, Onofrio BM, Yanagihara T (1976) Experience with Arnold Chiari malformation, 1960 to1970. J Neurosurg 45:416-422

14. Williams B(1972) The valvular action of the Arnold-Chairi malformation. In: Brock M, Dietz H (eds) Intracranial Pressure. Springer Berlin Heidelberg New York, p 338

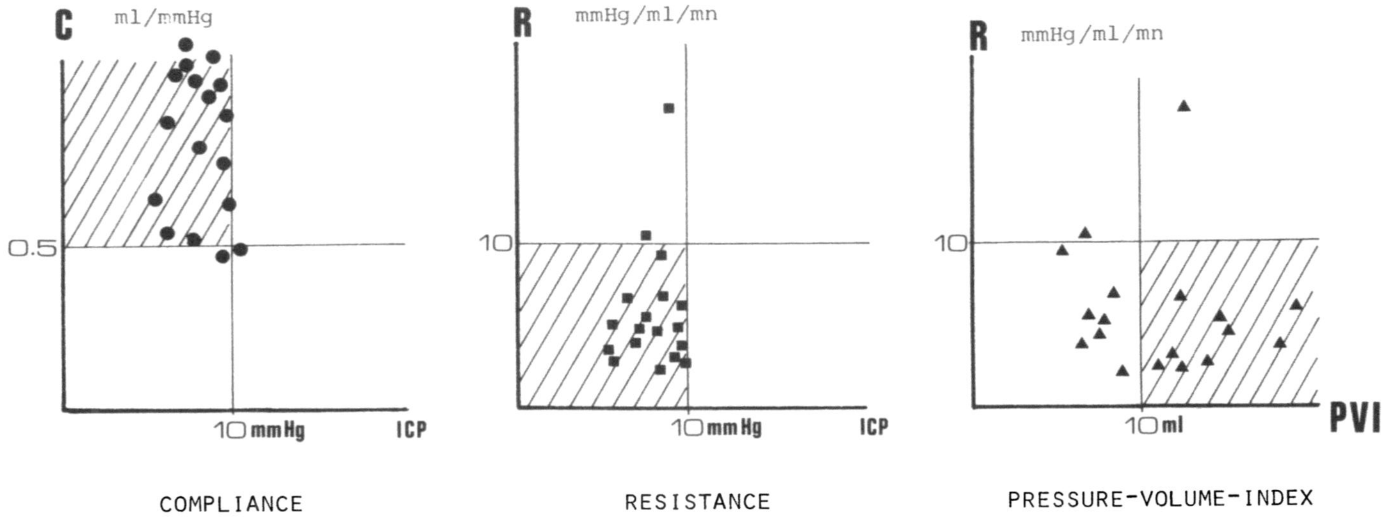

Fig. 1. Left and center: compliance and outflow resistance (in ordinate) are plotted against modal ICP value (in abscissa). The accepted normal range is shown by the shadowed area.
Right: outflow resistance is plotted against PVI (in abscissa) 8 patients over 18 had a slightly reduced PVI.

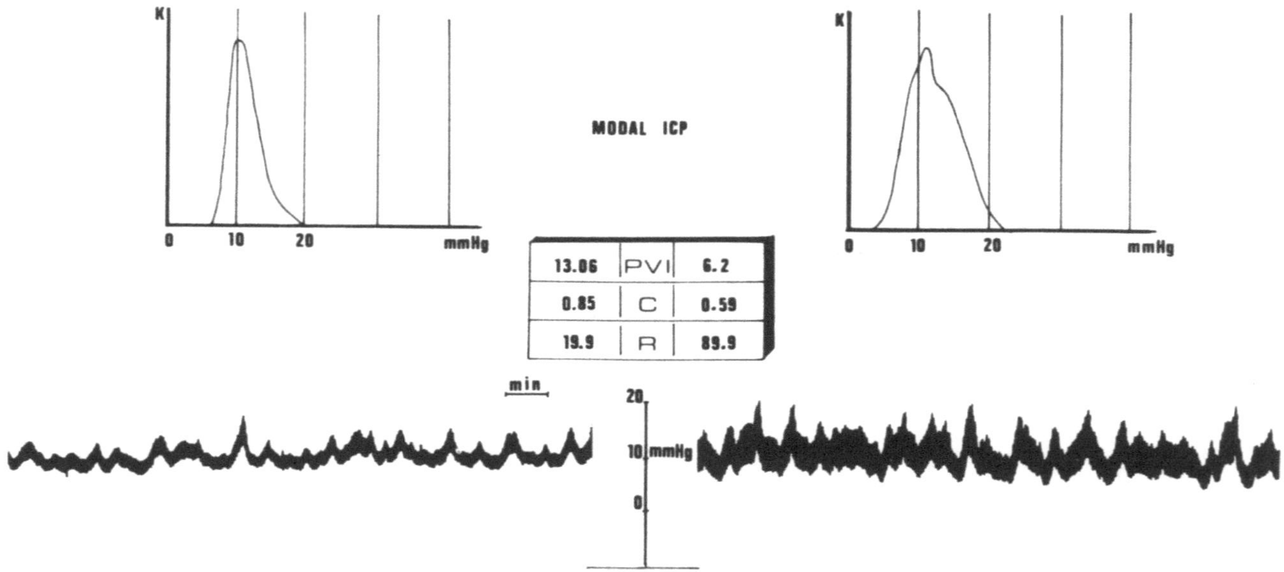

Fig. 2. Left: in the supine position, the modal ICP curve (upper left) and the conventional ICP recording (lower left) of a patient suffering from Arnold-Chiari malformation associated with hydromyelia. Right: the same patient's recordings in the sitting position. Note the modified values of the PVI, compliance or outflow resistance, and the amplified pathological ICP waves.

CONTINUOUS RECORDING OF ICP IN THE NORMAL MONKEY

G.GUCER AND L.J.VIERNSTEIN

Introduction

Continuous 24-hour monitoring of intracranial pressure (ICP) is being used to an increasing extent for the management of neurological patients. The telemetry procedures for making these recordings are comparatively new, and there is considerable interest in determining the significance of ICP wave phenomena observed. Since insufficient information exists concerning the temporal behavior of ICP in the normal mammal, we have undertaken to study the ICP profile in normal undrugged monkeys during sleep and wakefulness.

Methods

Seven monkeys from the primate colony were acclimated to a primate chair for approximately one week. An intracranial pressure sensing device was implanted epidurally in the burr-hole and secured in place with skull screws and covered with acrylic cement. At the same time EEG and EMG electrodes were implanted in the skull and neck muscles respectively. Throughout the night EEG, EMG and intracranial pressure were recorded as the monkey passed through his normal sleep cycles. Each monkey had two days of baseline intracranial pressure recording in addition to EEG and EMG recordings.

Four of the monkeys had an indwelling arterial catheter placed in the brachial artery for recording the systemic blood pressure. The catheter was connected to a Statham pressure transducer for the continuous recording of blood pressure. Heparin was used in the catheter to prevent blockage. The recordings were made with a Grass model 6 EEG machine operating at a chart speed of 1.5 mm/sec.

Results

Intracranial pressure in all seven monkeys was steady during wakefulness except for transient changes caused by movements, heart beat and respiration (Fig 2). The intracranial pressure showed no significant variation during slow wave sleep except for small pressure changes secondary to heart pulsation and respiration (Fig 3). However, intracranial pressure rose duing all episodes of desynchronized (REM) sleep to an average pressure level of 169 ± 4.6mm H_2O (n=168) above the levels found in other sleep states. At the end of the REM sleep period the ICP returns abruptly to the original level (Fig 1). Desynchronized sleep episodes were defined as periods in the sleep cycle in which the amplitude of the EEG potentials had low values and EMG activity decreased markedly. The ICP during the onset of REM sleep rose gradually over a period of 1/2 to 1 minute then reached a more or less constant level of pressure lasting between 2 and 12 minutes. The cessation of the ICP wave was abrupt. The pressure returned to the original ICP in 5 to 10 seconds coinciding with the end of the

REM sleep epoch (Fig 1). The ICP wave and REM sleep lasted an average of 7 ± 0.8 minutes (n=170) during which time the systemic blood pressure decreased by an average of 17 ± 1.2 mmHg (n=37). The ICP waves and the concurrent REM sleep states occurred at an average of 9 ± 1.2 times per night (n=137). Bilateral sympathectomy in four monkeys had no significant effect on the properties of the REM sleep or the ICP wave phenomenon.

Discussion

The results of our study support the belief that raised ICP during REM sleep is a normal physiological occurrence. The raised ICP is in the form of a pressure wave having the shape and characteristics of the A-wave described by LUNDBERG (2), but differs in magnitude. The rapid changes in pressure in the ICP wave that occurs during REM sleep suggests the effect is caused by vascular changes. In a number of neurological disease states the ICP is initially high thus using up much of the reserve compliance of the brain. Therefore, a small rise in blood volume when the reserve is exhausted will cause a large increase in the ICP. Under these circumstances, during REM sleep the patient who has little ICP reserve could have, rather than two to three times normal ICP, a level of 5 to 10 times normal pressure, that is thepathological A-wave or plateau wave. In such cases, the conditions for cerebrovascular decompression (3) exist in which these dangerous levels of ICP can depress nervous function.

The results of our studies indicate that, in neurological patients, continuous recordings during the sleep states may be useful for assessing the patient's ICP reserve. A rise in ICP should be expected during REM sleep; the magnitude of this rise will be a measure of the intracranial compensatory reserve left to the patient. More studies with the use of 24-hour ICP recordings in patients are required to establish what levels of ICP waves in REM sleep are to be considered normal, and what levels are indicative of pathology.

Summary

Twenty-four hour recordings of ICP by telemetry were performed in seven normal monkeys. During wakefulness and all stages of sleep except desynchronized sleep the ICP record showed small variations in pressure. However, during desynchronized sleep the mean ICP rose 170% above the ICP levels in the other states of sleep and the cardiac pulsation pressure increased by a factor of three. These ICP waves occurring during desynchronized sleep resemble the plateau waves described by LUNDBERG, but are of smaller magnitude and appear to be a normal characteristic of sleep in the macaque monkey.

References

1. Walker AE, Viernstein LJ, Chubbuck JG (1977) Intracranial pressure monitoring in neurosurgery. In: Fleming DG, Ko WH, Neuman MR(eds) Indwelling and Implantable Pressure Transducers. CRC Press,Ohio

2. Lundberg N (1960) Continuous recording and control of ventricular fluid pressure in neurosurgical practice. Acta phychiat scand Suppl 149, 36

3. LangfittTW, Kassell NF, Weinstein JD(1965)Cerebral blood flow with intracranial hypertension. Neurol 15:761-773

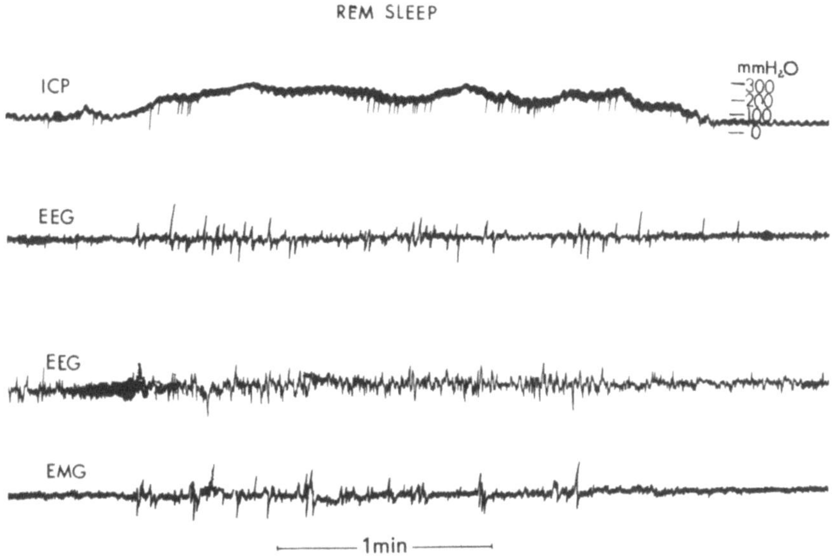

Fig. I. Recordings of ICP, frontal EEG activity, occipital EEG activity, and temporalis electromyogram during REM sleep. The EEG showed dysynchronized activity with pontogeniculate occpital waves. REM artifacts can be seen in the EMG record. Note the 3 min plateau wave as the ICP rises to a level of 300 mm H_2O. The pulse pressure from the heartbeat becomes about three times larger than that observed in the other sleep states. The downgoing pulses on the ICP record are artifacts.

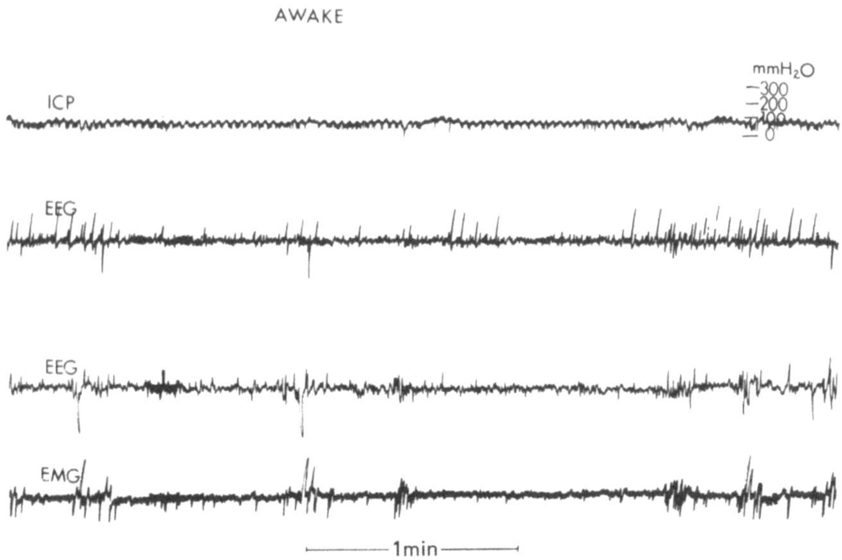

Fig. 2. Recordings of the same parameters as in Fig I in the awake undrugged monkey. Note that ICP was at a level of 90 mmH_2O with smaller variations in pressure due to the heartbeat and respiration.

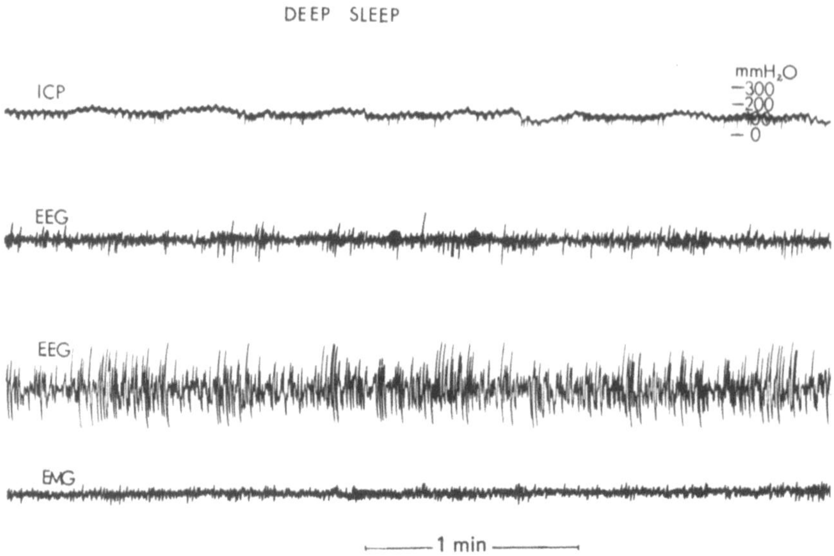

Fig.3. Recordings from the same monkey of the same parameters as in Figures 1 and 2 taken during deep sleep. No movement artifacts appear in the EMG, and the EEG's show large amplitude waves characteristics of deep sleep. ICP showed small variations about a pressure level of 100 mmH_2O.

THE RESULTS OF ICP AND EEG MONITORING OF SLEEP IN CASES OF PATIENTS WITH SUPRATENTORIAL BRAIN TUMORS

K.MOSZYNISKI, B.DARWAJ, H.KOZNIEWSKA, T.CZOCHRA, K.SMYK, AND W.LEWELT

Introduction

The rise of intracranial pressure during sleep has been observed (1,2,3) This phenomena is explained by lowering of electric resistance and capacity of oxygen in the brain. In this way vasomotor mechanisms determine the change of cerebrospinal fluid pressure. Such a situation is especially significant during REM sleep.

Material and methods

The patients studied were five men and one woman, ranging in age from 38 to 59 years. They were operated on for supratentorial brain tumors. This paper concerns the analysis of the polygraphic recording of sleep with simultaneous measurements of ICP, before, and on the third day after the removal of the brain tumors (Table 1).

All patients were conscious. The measurements of the pressure of cerebrospinal fluid in the ventricular system were carried out by LUNDGERG'S method (6). The cannula was inserted in the frontal horn of the lateral ventricle on the opposite side to the space-occupying lesion. The recording of ICP was done by a pressure transducer (Max Sievert) while the registration was carried on by Spidomax H. To get the polygraphic picture of sleep we used the RECHSTCHAFFEN and KALES method (8), recording two electro-oculograms (EOG); one offtake of EEG with constant time 0.3 and one offtake of EMG from submandibular muscle with constant time 0.1. In the analysis of sleep and while drawing hypnograms the stage of REM sleep and the stage of NREM sleep were taken under consideration. Wakefulness (W), the first and the second stages of sleep were treated in isolation but the third and the fourth stages of sleep were treated together. The results of polygraphic records of sleep were compared with ICP in the identical time units (5 minutes). Finally, the hypnograms and the diagrams of mean ICP were sketched for all cases.

Results

In the comparison between sleep recording before and after the removal of space occupying lesions, it was found that the number of awakenings rose after the operation and this caused a decrease of NREM sleep. In the 3rd day after the operation both the REM sleep and its density rose while the total sleep time did not change (Table 2). In the evaluation of ICP before and after the removal of brain tumors no changes in steady state levels were found. Before surgery, the mean ICP of NREM sleep, from the first to the fourth stage was higher than the mean ICP before sleep. ICP rose higher during awakening. The highest values of ICP, almost four times higher were noticed during REM sleep. After the operations the amplitude of ICP during REM sleep and awakenings decreased.This decrease was not observed in NREM sleep (Table 3).

Table 1

No.	Age	Diagnosis
1	44	Meningioma of the left parietal region
2	52	Reticulosarcoma of the right parietal region
3	55	Glioblastoma of the right occipital region
4	38	Intracerebral hematoma of the right temporal region
5	59	Astrocytoma of the right frontal region
6	49	Parasagittal meningioma of the left parietal region

Table 2. The parameters of the patients' sleep before and after operation

		TOTAL SLEEP TIME (MIN)	AWAKENINGS	NREM SLEEP		REM SLEEP	REM DENSITY
				STAGE 1+2	STAGE 2+3		
			% OF SLEEP TIME				
BEFORE OPERATION	MEAN	368.6	8.9	53.1	26,4	11.6	0.005
	STAND. DEVIAT	46.7	8.5	8.5	10.1	4.9	0.008
3rd DAY AFTER OPERATION	MEAN	417.2	26,3	40,4	14,8	18,5	0,028
	STAND DEVIAT	90,9	15,1	6,8	24.5	11,6	0,038

Table 3. The mean value of ICP before and after operation

		ICP in mm Hg			
		BEFORE ASLEEPING	NREM STAGE	REM STAGE	STAGE OF AWAKENINGS
BEFORE OPERATION	MEAN	14,2	18.3	53.3	30.8
	STAND. DEVIAT.	1.9	2.3	5.5	7.3
3rd DAY AFTER OPERATION	MEAN	13.3	20.0	36,6	19,2
	STAND. DEVIAT.	5,5	6,2	5,3	6.7

Discussion

The results of our investigation correspond with the papers of ROSSI (9) SYMON (10) MUNARI (7) which dealt with patients with normal and high pressure hydrocephalus. The rise of ICP during REM sleep and the lowering during NREM sleep were observed. Analyzing the polygraphic sleep records we discovered that following the third postoperative day, the number of awakenings, the periods of REM sleep and its density rose. We may associate the increase of awakenings with pain stimuli caused by the operation procedure. The increase of REM sleep and its density may be interpreted as the reactions of the renewal of sleep after the operation. This removal from the eleventh to the fourteenth day is close to normal in all parameters of sleep, except for the density of REM sleep.

Conclusions

1) All stages of REM sleep are associated with a rise of ICP in patients before and after removal of brain tumors. The increase in the amplitude of ICP is higher before operation.
2) During the third and fourth stage of NREM sleep ICP decreases in comparison with REM sleep.
3) The results of the polygraphic recording of sleep show that after removal of a space-occupying lesion, the number of REM sleep periods, their density and the number of awakenings rise, while the total sleep time is not changed.

Summary

In six cases (age 38-59 years) EEG monitoring of sleep and ICP were carried out before and one the third day after removal of the brain tumor. The comparison of polygraphic records of nocturnal sleep with parallel measurements of intraventricular pressure show all REM sleep phases associated with a rise in intraventricular pressure, while during the 3rd and 4th stage of sleep (NREM) the intraventricular pressure was always lower. In the remaining 1st and 2nd stages of NREM sleep and during the episode of nocturnal awakening no associations were found. The amplitude of ICP was higher before the operation.

References

1. Cooper R, Hulme A (1966) Intracranial pressure and related phenomena during sleep. J Neurosurg Psych 29:564-567

2. Cooper R, Hulme A (1967) Changes intracranial pressure cortical impedance and oxygen availability associated with changes in the EEG during sleep. Electroenceph Clin Neurophysiol 22:393-397

3. Cooper R, Hulme A (1969) Changes of the EEG, intracranial pressure and their variables during sleep in patients with intracranial lesions. Electroenceph Clin Neurophysiol 27:12-22

4. Darwaj B, Moszynski K (1977) Porownanie wynikow badania poligraficznego snu z zapisem cisnienia plynu mozgowo-rdzeniowego u chorych po usunieciu przyczyny nadamiotowego ucisku mozgu. Neur Neurochir Pol 5:573-579

5. Darwaj B, Czochra T (1979) Ocena wynikow badania poligraficznego snu nocnego u chorych z guzami nadnamiotowymi mozgu w okresie przed i pooperacyjnym. Neur Neurochir Pol 1:75-80

6. Lundberg N (1960) Continuous recording and control of ventricular fluid pressure in neurosurgical practice. Acta Psychiatr Scand 36, supply 149

7. Munari C, Calbucci F (1976) Organisation du somneil et variations de la pression intracranienne cher les malades ayant une hydrocephalic a pression normale. Rev EEG Neurophysiol 6:497-501

8. Rechtschaffen A, Kales A (1968) A manual of standardized terminology techniques and scoring system for sleep stages of human subjects. Public Health Service, U.S. Govt Printing Office

9. Rossi GP (1975) Intracranial pressure during sleep in man. Sleep. Bazylea

10. Symon L. Op.cit. ROSSI (9)

(a)

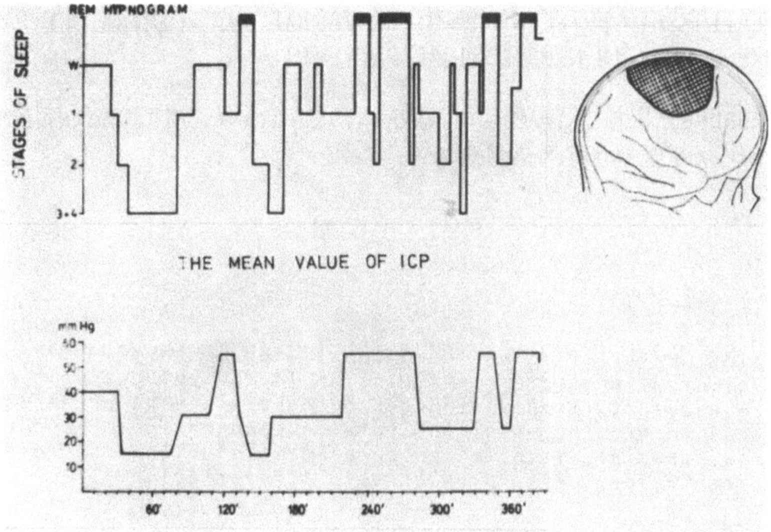

(b)

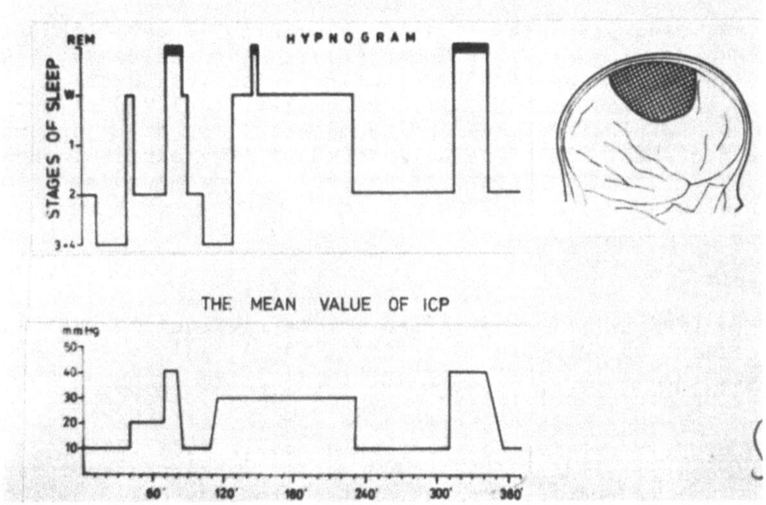

Fig.1. Case No. 2. a Reticulosarcoma of the right parietal region before operation. b Third day after operation.

RELATIONSHIP BETWEEN RAPID ICP VARIATION, RESPIRATORY PATTERN AND WAKEFULNESS IN NEUROLOGICAL PATIENTS

M.FURUSE, H.KUCHIWAKI, T.NAKAYA, K.TOYAMA, M.TERAOKA, M.HASUO, A.IKEYAMA, AND N.KAGEYAMA

Introduction

Rapid ICP variation has been considered to have important implications in clinical pressure monitoring while the pathogenesis of such pressure waves still remains under discussion. The present study was designed to examine relations between changes in ICP and related phenomena, special attention being paid to studying the role of changes in respiratory pattern upon rapid ICP variation.

Material and method

Thirty-five patients of various pathologic conditions, including 22 with brain tumors, 9 with cerebrovascular accidents, 3 with normal pressure hydrocephalus and I with benign intracranial hypertension, were subjected to analysis. Parameters included epidural pressure (EDP), respiratory movement by means of impedance pneumograph (RESP), body movement (BM), eye ball movement (EM) and EEG. Besides the polygraphic recording, state of wakefulness was checked from bedside observation.

Results

Rapid ICP variations of A and B type waves of LUNDBERG'S classification were observed in 28 patients (80%). Plateau-like waves (A type) predominated in basal pressure levels from 20 to 40 mmHg, whereas B-type pressure oscillation occurred in a wide pressure range from 5 to 70 mmHg. The occurrence of ICP variation of both A and B types was closely related to changes in respiratory pattern. The initial pressure rise in plateau wave usually corresponded to a suppressed movement of respiration, while the pressure fall was accompanied by hyperpnea and/or tachypnea. Pressure changes of B-type were related more closely to changes in respiratory pattern (Fig I). In the majority of cases, pressure elevation coincided with a phase of respiratory suppresssion and pressure reduction with hyperpneic phase or periodic respiration. On occasion (less than 5% in incidence), ICP elevation synchronized with hyperpneic movements and sudden drop in ICP accounted for large sigh-like movements.

Long-term polygraphic observations demonstrated a close correlation between ICP changes and wakefulness. The occurrence of rapid ICP variations as well as changes in respiratory movement appeared coincident with depressed state of wakefulness of the patients (Fig 2).

Discussion

The occurrence of rapid ICP variations were closely related with changes in respiratory pattern (2). This accords well with the data obtained in experimentally induced pressure waves (3). Regarding pathogenesis of the coincident alterations, two explanations are possible: namely ICP oscillation caused by changes in respiration and both ICP and respiratory changes due to dysfunction in a central regulatory mechanism. No significant difference was noticed in the values of blood gas analysis, carried out in some cases. Brain stem dysfunction may affect simultaneous fluctuations in ICP and respiratory movement. In our study these coincidental changes appeared apparently dominant during sleep. Under the pathologic conditions, depressed wakefulness may effect brain stem function, accompanying the alterations in sensitivity of respiratory centers.

Recently, existence of two different types of B-wave have been mentioned by BROCK (1). He divided such waves into typical B-wave and "ramp wave" with progressive pressure rise, followed by abrupt fall. The present observations disclose that both types of B-wave appear in close relation to sleep and that corresponding respiratory patterns are quite different. "Ramp waves" augment with shallow respiratory movement and fall rapidly with much larger sigh-like breathing. "Ramp-type" B-wave may occur mainly related to an upper airway obstruction, causing an elevation in systemic venous pressure.

References

1. Brock M (1977) Klinik and Therapie des intermittierend normotensiven Hydrocephalus. Radiolode 17:460-465

2. Furuse M, Ikeyama A, Mabe H et al(1979) Relationship between rapid variations in intracranial pressure and changes in respiratory pattern during postoperative monitoring. Neurol Med Chir (Tokyo) 19:9-16

3. Kuchiwaki H, Furuse M, Makaya T et al (1979) Intracranial dynamics associated with experimentally induced pressure waves. In this symposium.

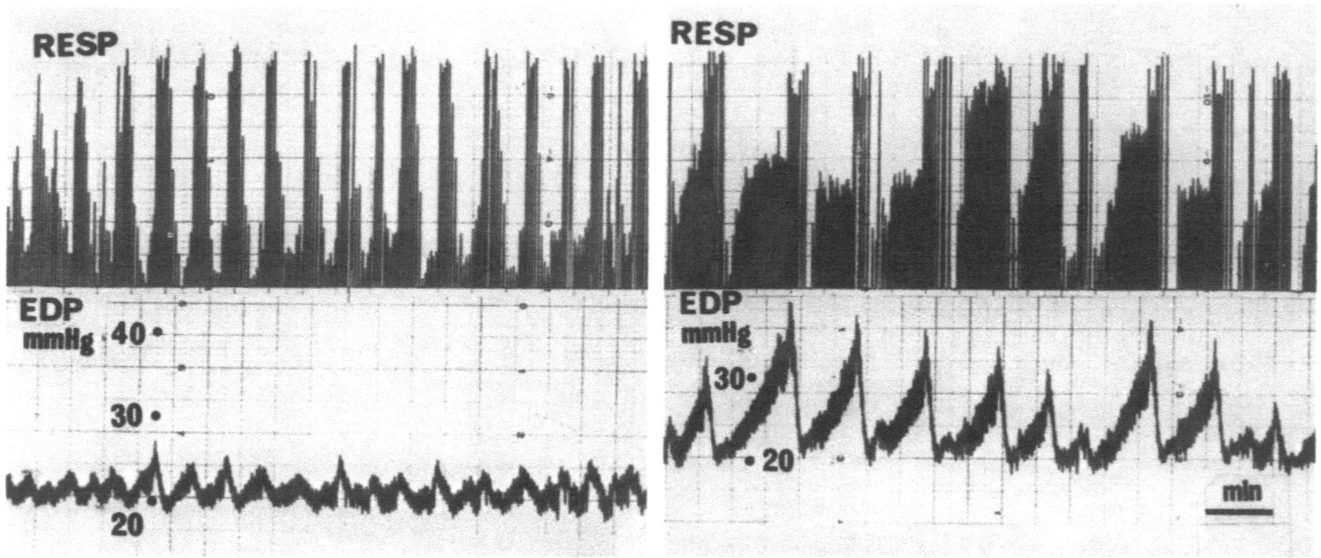

Fig. 1. Two different types of B-wave observed in a patient during sleep. Note the phase difference between respiratory movements and EDP changes.

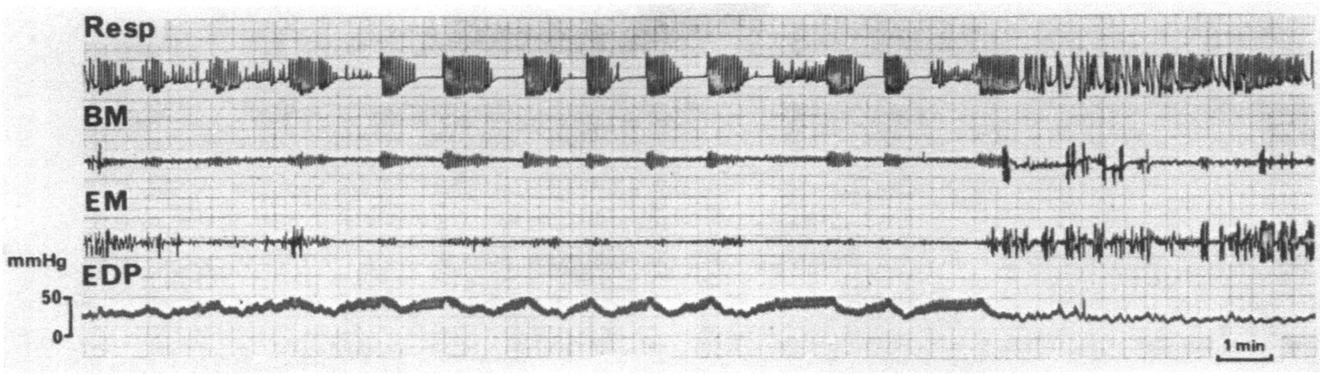

Fig. 2. Polygraph showing rhythmic oscillations of EDP and respiration. These obcillations disappear coincident with awakening of patient.

SELECTION OF PATIENTS FOR INTRACRANIAL PRESSURE MONITORING AND CONTROL

G.W.KINDT AND J.HOPKINS

Introduction

Intracranial pressure (ICP) monitoring is not used, and is occasionally criticized, by some neurosurgeons because they believe the invasiveness of the monitoring procedure is too great in comparison to the value of the information obtained. Perhaps the most valid criticism concerns the monitoring of patients who develop no ICP elevations. This report summarizes our experience in attempting to select patients for monitoring who were likely to have elevations of ICP.

Materials and methods

The general goal for the institution of ICP monitoring was to monitor those patients in whom ICP spikes or elevations were expected regardless of diagnoses. The method used for obtaining ICP measurements involved no special equipment and consisted of placing a twist drill hole at the hairline under local anesthesia. An intraventricular catheter was then inserted, or a stopcock of the appropriate size was plugged into the skull for subdural monitoring (3).

The data were reviewed from both the adult neurosurgical intensive care unit (Neuro ICU) and the Mott Children's Hospital. A computerized monitoring system was installed in the Neuro ICU in February 1976, which can record and process several physiologic parameters and observations from each patient (4). Graphs of ICP vs time can be obtained by the touch of a button. Standard monitoring equipment was used in the Mott Children's Hospital (2). Particular attention was directed toward the data obtained from the children with Reyes Syndrome.

Results

During the 40 month period since the computerized monitoring system has been installed at the main hospital Neuro ICU, 1014 patients have been treated, 947 of whom survived and 67 expired. The diagnosis of a cranial lesion was present in 799 and 104 of these had their ICP monitored. Of those who had their ICP monitored, 93 (89%) had spikes of 20 mmHg or higher requiring some type of therapy.

The experience at Mott Children's Hospital with Reyes Syndrome consisted of 68 patients of whom 46 survived and 22 expired (2). Twenty-nine of the patients with Reyes Syndrome were Stage III or worse and had their ICP monitored. Of those monitored, 25 (85%) had ICP spikes of 20 mmHg or higher requiring therapy directed at the elevated ICP.

Discussion

Ideally, only those patients who have or develop increased ICP should have their pressures monitored and controlled, and those without ICP elevations should not be subjected to invasive monitoring. Our experience using the diagnosis and clinical evaluation as the basis for choosing patients for ICP monitoring appears quite satisfactory. Review of the records revealed that an uncomplicated program was followed

Prior to instigating ICP monitoring, urgent measures were first accomplished. Wherever possible, the diagnosis of the cause of the increased ICP was obtained. Hypertonic agents, such as mannitol or urea, were promptly administered and any intracranial mass present was excised. Cerebrospinal fluid was withdrawn when appropriate and blood gases were controlled.

After any of these necessary emergency measures were completed, the ICP was monitored in those patients in whom elevations were expected. the CT scan would often show shifts or edema. The presence of an appropriate coma level and particularly the history of any deterioration in level of consciousness in the absence of an intracranial mass resulted in ICP monitoring. The most common diagnoses noted in patients who were monitored were, head trauma (not operated as well as those that had a hematoma removed), post operative brain tumors, spontaneous intracranial hemorrhage (intracerebral and subarachnoid), Reyes Syndrome, cerebral infarction, and hydrocephalus. Other conditions monitored less frequently included: meningitis, post anoxic encephalopathy, hepatic encephalopathy, mushroom poisoning (1), Herpes encephalitis, and meningeal malignancies.

The patients with Reyes Syndrome had their ICP monitored according to a protocol (2) after agreement that ICP control was a valuable adjunct in therapy (5). The point at which invasive monitoring was usually begun was Stage III. Some general criteria used were: no response to voice commands, EEG Grade III or worse, decorticate or decerebrate posturing, unequal or slowly reactive pupils, serum ammonia 300µg% and rising.

All patients who had their ICP monitored also had the ICP promptly controlled to a level below 20 mmHg and preferably below 15 mmHg(1). Pressure monitoring and control were usually abandoned in those cases in which signs of brain death persisted despite the reduction in ICP. However, in those patients who had a potential for survival, ICP elevations were treated vigorously and rapidly with a sense of urgency similar to that displayed when sudden hypoxia or hypotension occurred. Standard methods of controlling ICP were used, including: cerebrospinal fluid drainage, hypertonic agents, hyperventilation, hypothermia, barbiturates and steroids.

Summary

Our experience with monitoring ICP was reviewed with the goal of determining if an excessive number of invasive monitoring procedures were performed. In general, all patients were monitored if the attending physicians thought they were likely to have ICP elevations or spikes. Of the adult patients monitored 89% had pressure elevations observed in excess of 20 mmHg and 86% of the children with Reyes Syndrome monitored exhibited similar elevations. In many of these patients, the control of ICP appeared critical in their eventual outcome.

References

1. Chandler WF, Kindt GW (1976) Monitoring and control of intracranial pressure in non-traumatic encephalopathies. Surg Neurol 5: 311-314

2. Engle WD, Baublis JV, Duff TE, Rosenberg NM, Tucker RP, Kindt GW, Kelsch RC, Weeks R (1979) In: Crocker JFS (ed) Reyes Syndrome II Grune and Stratton, New York, p 195

3. Gosch HH, Kindt GW (1972) Subdural monitoring of acute increased intracranial pressure. Surg Forum 23:405-406

4. Kindt GW, Schneider RC (1977) Computerized monitoring in a neurosurgical intensive care unit. Neurosurg 1:68

5. Kindt GW, Waldman J, Kohl S, Baublis J, Tucker RP (1975) Monitoring and control of intracranial pressure in Reyes Syndrome. JAMA 231:822-825

Session XI

ANESTHESIA AND INTRACRANIAL PRESSURE

Chairman: M.S.Albin
Co-chairman: C.Alexander

SUMMARY

This session addressed itself to a wide variety of subjects relating to anesthesia and the action of anesthetics. The development of ICP monitoring and the more recent perfection of techniques relating to CSF/tissue dynamics has added another dimension to the evaluation of anesthetic effects, clinical management and therapeutic responses.

The papers of SCHETTINI and MANN and coworkers (another session) indicated a broadening of appreciation of the effects of anesthetic agents, that multifaceted complexities are involved; that protean responses occur (over and above CBF and $CMRO_2$) affecting CSF formation and outflow resistance, brain pressure depth ratios and brain impedance. Along similar lines, STEVENAERT and colleagues noted experimentally that both halothane (H) and enflurane (E) reduced cerebral perfusion pressure with H > E. CUNITZ and GAAB concluded that both diazepam and etomidate are useful drugs in the ICU or anesthesia environment because of the ability to lower ICP. COLLICE et al evaluated ICP responses in patients with severe head injury and determined that althesin, like thiopental, was effective in reducing intracranial hypertension.

Both intubation and chest physiotherapy can pose problems of increasing ICP in patients with mass intracranial lesions and severe head injuries. BEDFORD and coworkers indicated the efficacy of pretreatment with intravenous lidocaine (1.5 mg/kg after thiopental induction) in attenuating an ICP rise during intubation and MOSS et al concluded that N_2O increased ICP during chest physiotherapy and that althesin and thiopental may modify such increases. Again, these series of papers validate the importance of routine ICP monitoring in the ICU and operating theater in patients with intracranial hypertension.

LIDOCAINE PREVENTS INCREASED ICP AFTER ENDOTRACHEAL INTUBATION

R.F. Bedford, H.R. Winn, G. Tyson, T.S. Park, and J.A. Jane

Introduction

Intracranial pressure (ICP) may increase precipitously when patients with brain tumors undergo endotracheal intubation, presumably as a result of increased arterial pressure and cerebral blood flow (2,4). Recent studies suggest that pretreatment with intravenous lidocaine blunts the increase in arterial blood pressure associated with endotracheal intubation (1), but, to date, there has been no description of the effects of this therapy on ICP. This study examines the efficacy of intravenous lidocaine pre-treatment in modifying the ICP changes associated with laryngoscopy and endotracheal intubation during general anesthesia.

Material and methods

All patients (2) had brain tumors estimated to be larger than 2 cm in diameter by CAT-scan. All were receiving steroid therapy and were scheduled for elective craniotomy. Informed consent for the study was obtained from both the patients and their nearest relative on the evening prior to operation. Pre-medication consisted of intramuscular morphine 0.1 mg/kg, diazepam 0.1 mg/kg and atropine 0.4 mg one hour before arrival in the operating suite. A subarachnoid pressure screw (6), arterial and central venous catheters were placed using local anesthesia (2-chloroprocaine with 1:200,000 epinephrine) and pressures were continuously transduced and recorded. Once a constant level of ICP and vascular pressures was observed, blood samples were drawn for control arterial blood gas and lidocaine levels. The protocol called for examining ICP response to laryngoscopy and endotracheal intubation in 2 groups of 10 patients each: one group received IV lidocaine (1½ mg/kg) at the time of anesthetic induction, and the other group received an identical volume of IV saline solution. The medications were given in double-blind fashion and in random sequence. The two groups proved to be similar with respect to distribution of tumor types and patient age (49 years ± 6 SE for the lidocaine group versus 55 years ± 6SE for the saline group). General anesthesia was induced with thiopental (3 mg/kg), 50 percent nitrous oxide in oxygen, and a continuous IV infusion of 0.1 percent succinylcholine solution. Ventilation was controlled to maintain a constant end-tidal CO_2 fraction (Beckman LB2) and laryngoscopy was initiated exactly 2 minutes after anesthetic induction. Endotracheal intubation was always accomplished within 20 seconds and the resulting changes in intracranial, arterial and venous pressures were monitored over the next 5 minutes while end-tidal CO_2 was held constant. Arterial blood gas and lidocaine values were repeated within 30 seconds of intubation.

Results

Table I summarizes our over-all observations. Both groups of patients were similar with regard to control values for ICP, vascular

Table 1. Variables measured before and after laryngoscopy and endotracheal intubation in patients pretreated with either lidocaine or saline

	LIDOCAINE				SALINE			
Time from Laryngoscopy (seconds)	Control	-60	+30	+60	Control	-60	+30	+60
ICP (torr)	13.4±2.5	8.0±0.9**	14.1±2.6	12.6±2.0†	15.0±4.2	10.2±2.4*	26.2±4.8*	23.2±3.8*
MAP (torr)	97±5	89±5	123±9	117±8.4	95±5	90±3	139±5**	131±9*
$PaCO_2$ (torr)	33.7±1.2		32.3±1.6		35.7±2.1		32.6±2.7	
Blood Lidocaine (μg/ml)	0.6±0.1		3.2±0.6*		0.6±0.1		0.7±0.1	

All Values: Mean ± SE

†P < .05 versus saline group at same time

*P < .05 versus control values

**P < .025 versus control values

pressures and blood gas tensions. Induction of anesthesia caused a significant reduction in ICP in both groups of patients, whereas mean arterial pressure was unchanged. Laryngsocopy and endotracheal intubation resulted in a significant increase in both ICP and arterial pressure in the patients who received only saline pre-treatment. This was apparent immediatley after intubation (30 seconds after laryngoscopy) and persisted for over a minute thereafter (Fig 1).

In contrast, ICP did not increase after intubation in the group pre-treated with lidocaine, and the mean increase in arterial pressure was not significant.

Discussion

Several possible mechanisms may explain the effect of lidocaine in preventing raised ICP after endotracheal intubation. Lidocaine blunts the arterial hypertensive and tachycardic response to intubation (1), and there is evidence that it acts as a specific depressant of the cough reflex (5). Prevention of arterial hypertension could reduce blood flow through a mass lesion with impaired auto-regulation and thus might prevent intracranial hypertension.

Intravenous lidocaine also acts as a general anesthetic at sub-seizure blood levels such as those obtained in this study. In dogs a single IV bolus of 15 mg/kg slows the EEG and significantly reduces CBF and $CMRO_2$(3). It is possible, then, that the effect of lidocaine on ICP may be mediated by an anesthetic function similar to that observed with barbiturate anesthesia. We find that a bolus injection of lidocaine in the dose range of 1½ - 2 mg/kg IV often controls raised ICP in patients with head trauma. In this setting, lidocaine is particularly advantageous because, unlike ultra-short acting barbiturates, it produces minimal cardiovascular and respiratory depression.

Summary

The efficacy of intravenous lidocaine for prevention of raised ICP following endotracheal intubation was studied in 20 patients with intracranial neoplasms. Using a double-blind, random sequence protocol we observed that addition of lidocaine, 1.5 mg/kg IV, to a thiopental-nitrous oxide anesthetic technique prevented increased ICP after intubation. The same anesthetic technique resulted in significant intracranial hypertension after intubation when saline placebo was given instead of lidocaine. We believed lidocaine should be used for prevention and control of increased ICP under these conditions.

References

1. Abou-Madi MN, Keszler H, Yacoub JM(1977) Cardiovascular reactions to laryngoscopy and tracheal intubation following small and large intravenous doses of lidocaine. Canad Anesth Soc J 24:12-19

2. Burney RG, Winn HR (1975) Increased cerebrospinal fluid pressure during laryngoscopy and intubation for induction of anesthesia. Anesth and Analg 54:687-690

3. Skabe T, Maekawa T, Ishkawa T, Takeshita H(1974) The effects of lidocaine on canine cerebral metabolism and circulation related to the electroencephalogram. Anesthes 40:433-441

4. Shaprio HN, Whyte SR, Harris AB, Galindo A(1972) Acute intraoperative intracranial hypertension in neurosurgical patients. Mechanical and pharmacologic factors. Anesthes 37:399-405

5. Steinhaus JE, Gaskin L (1963) A study of intravenous lidocaine as a suppressant of cough reflex. Anesthesiol 24:285-290

6. Winn HR, Dacey RG, Jane JA (1977) Intracranial subarachnoid pressure recording: experience with 650 patients. Surg Neurol 8:41-46

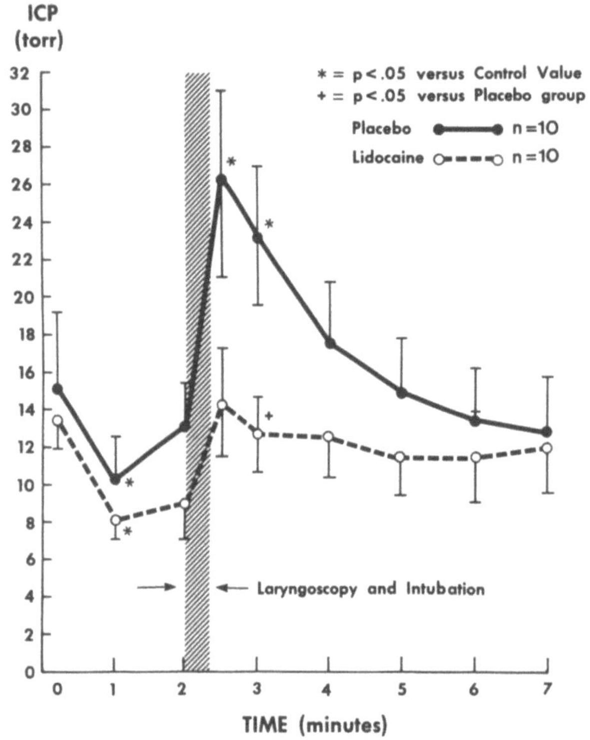

Fig. 1. ICP response to laryngoscopy and endotracheal intubation in anesthetized patients pretreated with either lidocaine or saline placebo. Lidocaine prevented the significant intracranial hypertension associated with endotracheal intubation in patients who received placebo at the time of anesthetic induction.

INCOMPATIBILITY OF HALOGENATED ANESTHETICS WITH BRAIN SURGERY

A. SCHETTINI

Introduction

Most neurosurgeons are reluctant to accept the use of volatile halogenated anesthetics in brain surgery, even when intracranial pressure (ICP) is normal. The reasons for these are twofold: 1) volatile halogenated anesthetics may increase cerebral vascular volume; and 2) even with hyperventilation, they cause a tight brain. The second reason means that brain elastance increases and suggests that mechanisms other than vasodilation might be responsible for this increase.

In our laboratory, brain elastance is obtained by measuring the Pressure-Depth Ratio (G_o) of the subpial region. The parameter G_o is closely related to the elastic modulus of the brain (7).

In this paper we have summarized our studies on the effects of halogenated volatile anesthetics on intracranial fluid dynamics in dogs with normal intracranial tension. These studies provide clear evidence that, as observed by the neurosurgeon, these volatile anesthetics increase brain elastance, which, at least for halothane, may be due to increased cerebral vascular volume and/or metabolic brain edema.

Material and methods

Three series of experiments were performed on 51 dogs (18-30 kg). In the first series, 23 dogs were chronically implanted for measurement of both surface brain pressure epidurally and low frequency (1kHz) brain electrical impedance (4). Fourteen out of the 23 dogs were studied at 0.8, 1.0, 1.5 and 2.0% inspired concentrations of halothane. Ten of these 14 dogs were studied, in random fashion, at 1.2% halothane following thiopental-hyperventilation induction. Six of the 14, also chosen at random, were studied during thiopental narcosis. The other nine implanted dogs were induced with thiopental (30 mg/kg), hyperventilated ($PaCO_2$:26-28 mmHg) and then exposed, at random, for one hour, to decreasing inspired concentrations of halothane(1.5-0.8%), enflurane (4-2%) or isoflurane (2.5-1.5%) (3).

In the second series, 16 dogs were implanted for measurement of both ICP and brain mechanical response properties, epidurally (7). The elastic parameters derived from these tests were: <u>Initial Tangent</u> (G_o) and the (equilibrium) <u>Secant Modulus</u> (G_s) (8). Control measurements were made during light thiopental narcosis (20 mg/kg). Following additional thiopental (100-150 mg) the mechanical tests were repeated during halothane (1 MAC[1] and 1.5 MAC) in random order. We also monitored alveolar anesthetic concentration, CO_2 and arterial blood pressure which was pharmacologically maintained near control values. Arterial blood gas tensions, pH and acid-base balance were measured frequently.

1. MAC=Minimal alveolar anesthetic concentration that prevents any movement with skin incision in 50% of cases.

The third series of experiments in 12 dogs was acute. In Group I (6 dogs) we measured plasma and cerebrospinal fluid (CSF) osmolality and electrolytes (Na,K,Cl), water and electrolyte (Na,K,Cl) content for the gray and white matter and total brain osmolality during pentobarbital narcosis (30 mg/kg) and normocarbia. In Group II (6 dogs) we repeated the same measurements during 1% (alveolar) haolthane under normocarbia and normotensive blood pressure (5).

Results

I. Surface Brain Pressure and Brain Electrical Impedance: 1. At normocarbia: 0.8 to 2% halothane increased both surface brain pressure and brain electrical impedance ($P<.05$, analysis of variance). The rise in brain pressure was dose related ($P<.05$) but the rise in impedance was not. 2. Thiopental-Hyperventilation Induction. This did not prevent a small (2-3 mmHg) increase in surface brain pressure and a moderate impedance rise with the subsequent haolthane (1.2%) inhalation. The same findings were observed with enflurane and, to a lesser degree, with isoflurane (Fig 1). 3. Thiopental Narcosis. As opposed to the above anesthetics, thiopental caused a significant decrease in both surface brain pressure and brain impedance ($P<.05$) (4).

II. Brain Elastance: under thiopental, control values for G_o and G_s were within the range of our normal values (6). With halothane and enflurane both G_o and G_s increased ($P<.05$, paired T tests) despite thiopental-hyperventilation induction (Fig 2). A dose-related response could not be established.

III. Brain Water and Electrolytes: With pentobarbital narcosis, brain concentration of Na,K,Cl, water content and total brain osmolality were within the range of values reported as normal (1). In dogs exposed to 1% halothane (alveolar) we found a net increase ($P<.05$, analysis of variance) of Na, Cl and H_2O content, but no change in K for the gray matter; in the white matter only Cl increased ($P<.05$). The computed brain swelling was 3.7%. These findings were associated with a decrease in total brain osmolality in the face of normal plasma and CSF osmolality (Table I).

Discussion

In the normocarbic dog, the increase in surface brain pressure with haolgenated anesthetics may be attributed to cerebral vascular expansion. The impedance rise, however, suggested that a second mechanism was also responsible for the increased brain bulk. The increase in brain elastance which behaved like brain electrical impedance, adds further support to the impedance findings.

A rise in brain electrical impedance is mainly (43-45%) due to water and ion shifts intracellularly and in part (20%) to a reduction in brain extracellular space (ECS) because of loss in highly conductive ions (e.g. Na) from brain ECS (4). Direct measurements of brain water and electrolyte distribution during halothane confirmed the impedance findings, since there was an increase in Na, Cl and H_2O content limited to the gray matter. Similar findings, including the impedance rise, have been reported by BAETHMANN and VAN HARREVELD in rats pretreated with the metabolic inhibitor 6 aminonicontinamide(2). In their experiments, the increase in brain water uptake was 13%. With halothane it was 3.7% (5).

TABLE I. WATER AND ELECTROLYTE DISTRIBUTION OF THE CORTICAL GRAY AND SUBCORTICAL WHITE MATTER OF DOGS BRAIN DURING HALOTHANE ANAESTHESIA. (FROM THE Br. J. Anaesth., 1979, in press).

	CORTICAL GRAY MATTER									
	Na+ (mEq/Kg OF WET WT.)	K+ (mEq/Kg OF WET WT.)	Cl- (mEq/Kg OF WET WT.)	Na+ (mEg/Kg OF DRY WT.)	K+ (mEg/Kg OF DRY WT.)	Cl- (mEg/Kg OF DRY WT.)	H_2O g/100g OF WET WT.	H_2O g/100g OF DRY WT.	H_2O g/100g FROZEN WT.[A]	OSMOLALITY[B] mOsm/Kg OF H_2O
CONTROL GROUP N=6 DOGS										
MEAN	51.37	93.36	38.45	237.51	435.86	175.43	78.32	361.96	75.55	306.4
S.D.	3.04	6.95	3.79	20.83	54.65	19.52	1.66	29.83	1.44	17.7
S.E.M.	0.72	1.69	0.89	4.91	13.25	4.61	0.39	7.03	0.36	6.4
HALOTHANE GROUP N=6 DOGS										
MEAN	54.21	94.87	42.42	258.92	454.67	201.56	79.07	378.54	75.47	272.1
S.D.	3.14	2.87	2.70	11.47	33.83	11.15	1.13	25.06	1.73	23.0
S.E.M.	0.74*	0.68	0.64*	2.70*	7.97	2.63*	0.26*	5.90*	0.42	6.9*

	SUBCORTICAL WHITE MATTER							
	Na+ (mEq/Kg OF WET WT.)	K+ (mEq/Kg OF WET WT.)	Cl- (mEq/Kg OF WET WT.)	Na+ (mEg/Kg OF DRY WT.)	K+ (mEg/Kg OF DRY WT.)	Cl- (mEg/Kg OF DRY WT.)	H_2O g/100g H_2O	H_2O g/100g OF DRY WT.
CONTROL GROUP N=6 DOGS								
MEAN	53.45	81.58	39.45	178.52	274.26	131.60	69.92	234.04
S.D.	5.70	8.79	4.82	20.21	35.65	15.53	1.00	13.97
S.E.M.	1.34	2.13	1.11	4.76	8.65	3.66	0.23	3.29
HALOTHANE GROUP N=6 DOGS								
MEAN	57.87	84.32	43.80	194.43	287.24	147.53	70.16	237.08
S.D.	4.19	4.85	2.68	14.92	31.53	14.58	1.88	22.58
S.E.M.	0.99	1.20	0.63*	3.52	7.65	3.44*	0.44	5.47

A. WHOLE BRAIN SAMPLE

B. OSMOLALITY FOR WHOLE BRAIN

*$p < .05$ DIFFERENCE FROM CONTROL

Supported by our data, and the evidence above mentioned, we postulate that halothane, and presumably halogenated volatile anesthetics, in addition to being a cerebral vasodilator also causes some degree of matabolic brain edema. It is metabolic because the edema is restricted to the gray matter which is unable to pump out the excess intracellular Na, due to decreased active transport (2).

Summary

The present studies show that even with hyperventilation, volatile halogenated anesthetics make the brain stiffer and raise the low frequency brain electrical impedance. Measurement of brain water and electrolyte content show that halothane inhalation induces metabolic brain edema.

References

1. Arieff AI, Kleeman CR, Keushkerian A, Bagdoyan A (1972) Brain tissue osmolality: Method of determination and variation in hyper- and hypo-osmolar states. J Lab Clin Med 29:334-343

2. Baethmann I, Van Harreveld A (1973) Water and electrolyte distribution in gray matter rendered edematous with a metabolic inhibitor. J Neuropath Exp. Neurol 32:408-423

3. Schettini A (1975) Intracranial ionic imbalance induced by halogenated anesthetics. Excerpta Medica International Congress Series #347. Excerpta Medica, Amsterdam, p 807

4. Shcettini A, Morsehead G (1978) Effects of halothane and sodium thiopentone on surface brain pressure and brain electrical impedance in dogs with normal intracranial tension. Br J Anesth 50: 1003-1012

5. Schettini A, Furniss WW (to be published) Brain water and electrolyte distribution during halothane. Br J Anesth

6. Schettini A, Walsh EK (1979) Influence of large doses of steroids on brain compression, epidurally. In this symposium.

7. Walsh EK, Schettini A (1976) Elastic behavior of brain tissue in vivo. Am J Physiol 230:1058-1062

8. Walsh EK, Schettini A (1979) Parameters for identifying brain response properties in vivo. In this symposium.

Supported by V.A. Medical Research.

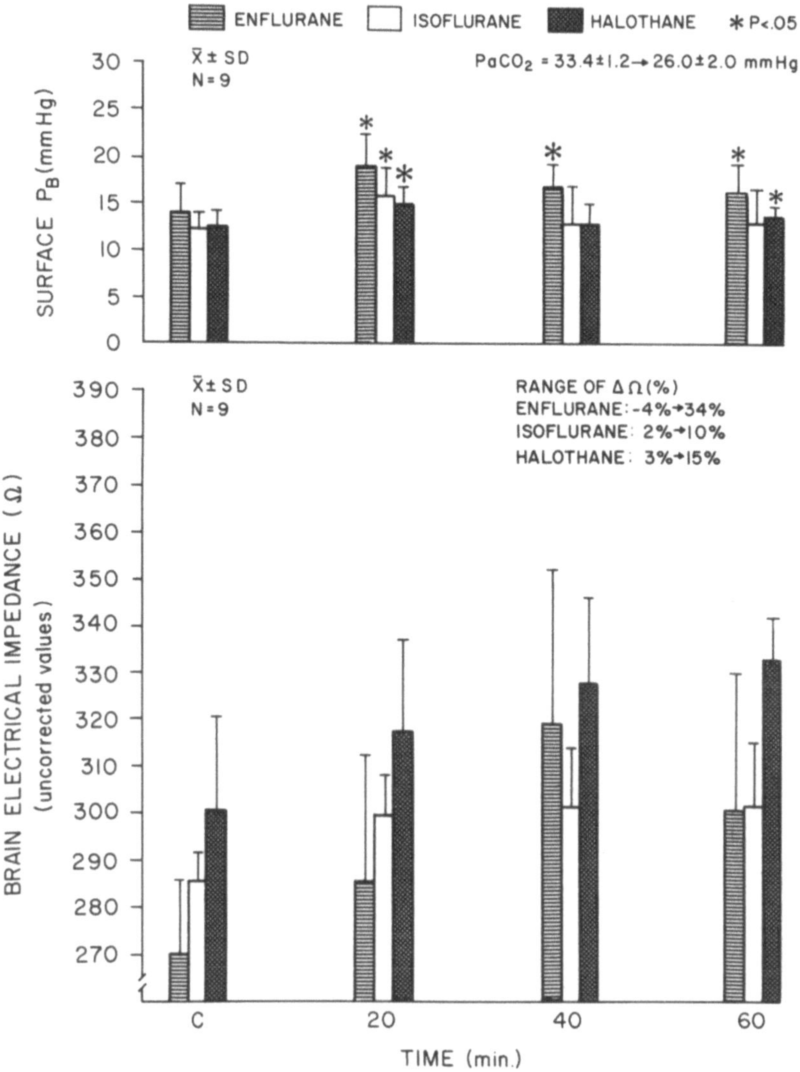

Fig. 1. The upper half of the figure is surface brain pressure (mmHg); the lower half is brain electrical impedance (ohms). Control (C) values were obtained under light sedation. Measurements during inhalational anesthesia were made after thiopental-hyperventilation induction. Arterial anesthetic concentrations (Vol%; X±SD) were 1.1±.2 for halothane, 2.0±.3 for isoflurane and 2.4±.3 for enflurane. Significant difference from control is not given for the impedance, in view of its wide range with enflurane (diphasic behaior).
(Reproduced from Ref 3 with permission).

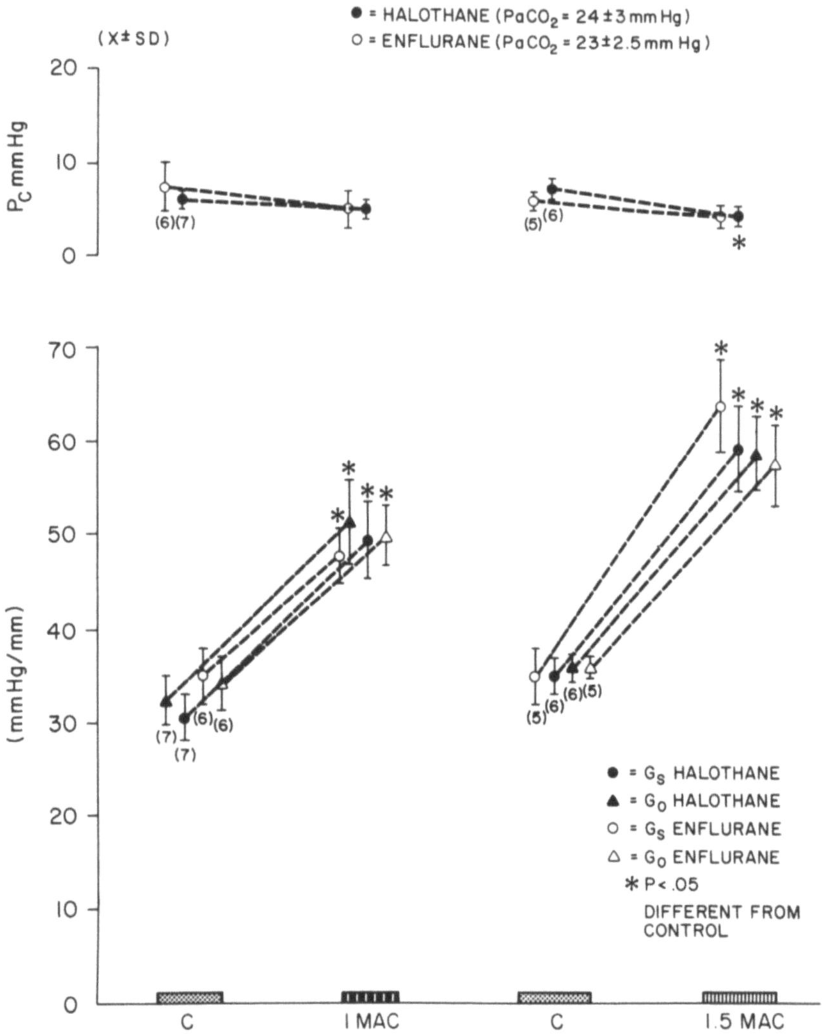

Fig. 2. The upper tracings are CSF pressure values (P_c) derived from the Pressure Tests. The ordinate of the lower tracings is the Pressure-Depth Ratio (mmHg/mm) of the elastic parameters measured: Secant (G_s, equilibrium), and Initial Tangent (G_o). Figures in parenthesis are the number of dogs for each experimental series. The abcissa is the alveolar anesthetic concentration. The control (C) measurements were made under thiopental and normocarbia. Those during inhalational anesthesia were made after thiopental-hyperventilation induction.

THE EFFECTS OF NITROUS OXIDE, ALTHESIN AND THIOPENTONE ON INTRACRANIAL PRESSURE DURING CHEST PHYSIOTHERAPY IN PATIENTS WITH SEVERE HEAD INJURIES

E. MOSS, J.S. GIBSON, AND D.G. MCDOWALL

Introduction

Chest physiotherapy causes intracranial pressure (ICP) increases in patients with severe head injury (2), increases which are partially due to noxious stimulation. The analgesic property of nitrous oxide might help to reduce these ICP increases. Thiopentone and Althesin both reduce ICP (5,13) and would be expected to reduce ICP increases during chest physiotherapy. This paper describes the effects of nitrous oxide, Althesin and thiopentone on ICP during chest physiotherapy in head injuries, and also the effect of nitrous oxide on ICP in head injured patients in the absence of chest physiotherapy.

Method

These patients had severe head injuries and were being hyperventilated ($PaCO_2$ 3.3 - 4.0 kPa), receiving non-depolarizing muscle relaxants. During chest physiotherapy, the lungs were hyperinflated by anesthetists. Before any study was performed the patient received further muscle relaxant. ICP was recorded from a subdural catheter or device or an extradural device (1), using a transducer, amplifier and chart recorder. The maximum rise in mean ICP during the period of chest physiotherapy was read from the chart recordings.

The initial study was to compare the effects of chest physiotherapy on ICP in the presence of 100% oxygen or 50% nitrous oxide in 50% oxygen (Entonox). This study was stopped when Entonox had been given 12 times to 3 patients. In a second study 100% oxygen, thiopentone (3 mg/kg) and 100% oxygen, or Althesin (0.03 ml/kg) and 100% oxygen were given at random to 6 patients for chest physiotherapy. The thiopentone or Althesin was given to the patient over 30 sec, and 30 sec later the systolic arterial pressure was measured. Chest physiotherapy was then performed for 5 minutes.

In the third study, the effect of Entonox on ICP in a further nine patients was investigated when they were not receiving chest physiotherapy. Mechanical ventilation had been established for at least six hours and the inspired oxygen concentration was less than 50%. The maximum change in mean ICP during the administration of Entonox was measured. During the last six administrations of Entonox, end tidal carbon dioxide concentration was measured by mass spectrometry.

Results

There was a greater increase in ICP when Entonox was used during chest physiotherapy than when 100% oxygen alone was used ($0.02 > P > 0.01$) (Table 1). In 2 patients A-waves (7) occurred during physiotherapy with Entonox, but an A-wave also occurred in one patient given physiotherapy with 100% oxygen. There was a small, but not statistically

Table 1. Increases in ICP (mmHg) produced by chest physiotherapy during 100% oxygen or Entonox administration. Controls are the values of mean ICP before physiotherapy. *0.02 > P > 0.01

	OXYGEN		ENTONOX	
	Control	Change from Control	Control	Change from Control
n	11		12	
$\bar{x}$	12.8	+10.5*	12.2	+22.7*
S.D.	5.6	10.4	3.5	10.6

significant, reduction in the ICP increase associated with chest physiotherapy when thiopentone and Althesin were used, compared with 100% oxygen alone (Table 2). In all three study groups the mean ICP prior to chest physiotherapy was not significantly different. In no patient did the systolic arterial pressure drop below 110 mmHg at 30 sec after the administration of thiopentone or Althesin. Without physiotherapy, Entonox caused an increase in ICP and its withdrawal caused a decrease (Table 3). The end tidal carbon dioxide concentration did not change significantly during Entonox adminstration.

Discussion

Increases in ICP have been reported during induction of anesthesia with nitrous oxide in patients with intracranial tumors and aneurysms (12,6,4,3,9) and during established anesthesia with hypocapnia in patients with cerebral tumors when nitrous oxide was added. The effect of nitrous oxide on ICP in patients with severe head injuries has not been reported, although it has been suggested that ICP may increase(4). Rises in ICP during chest physiotherapy have been reported in patients with severe head injuries (2). These could be due to noxious stimulation causing systemic hypertension and cerebral activation. As Entonox is analgesic, it might be expected to reduce ICP increases during chest physiotherapy. However, when Entonox had been given on twelve occasions during chest physiotherapy, it was clear that it exacerbated the ICP increases. This can be explained by the subsequent work showing that Entonox alone increases ICP in severe head injuries (Table 3). This ICP increase is almost certainly due to a cerebral vasodilating action of the drug, as end tidal carbon dioxide concentration remained unchanged during the Entonox administration.

Table 2. Increases in ICP (mmHg) produced by chest physiotherapy during 100% oxygen, or thiopentone and 100% oxygen, or Althesin and 100% oxygen administration. Controls are the values of mean ICP before physiotherapy

	OXYGEN		THIOPENTONE + OXYGEN		ALTHESIN + OXYGEN	
	Control	Change from Control	Control	Change from Control	Control	Change from Control
n	12		11		11	
$\bar{x}$	13.9	+7.2	11.5	+4.1	12.6	+5
S.D.	7.0	4.9	8.5	3.1	7.7	5.3

Table 3. ICP (mmHg) before, during and after Entonox (16 administrations)

	Control	max. change during Entonox administration	max. change after Entonox withdrawal
$\bar{x}$	10.6	$\bar{d}$ = + 3.8 (o – + 8.5)	$\bar{d}$ = - 4.6
S.D.	8.53	2.40	2.83
		P < 0.001	P < 0.001

Thiopentone and Althesin reduce ICP (5,13) and cerebral blood flow (10,11); thus they would be expected to reduce the ICP increases associated with chest physiotherapy in severe head injuries. The ICP increases were smaller in both the thiopentone and Althesin groups than in the group receiving oxygen alone, but these differences failed to reach statistical significance. From our results we conclude that, in patients with severe head injrues, 50% nitrous oxide in oxygen increases ICP and exacerbates the ICP increases associated with chest physiotherapy. Thiopentone and Althesin may help to control the ICP increases associated with chest physiotherapy, but the numbers to date are small and we are unable to draw any conclusions about the efficacy of these agents.

Summary

In patients with severe head injuries, 50% nitrous oxide in oxygen (Entonox) exacerbated the increase in intracranial pressure (ICP) mean 22.7 mmHg) during chest physiotherapy (3 patients, 12 administrations) in comparison with oxygen (mean 10.5 mmHg) ($P < 0.02$)(11 administrations). Without chest physiotherapy, Entonox caused a mean increase in ICP of 3.8 mmHg (S.D.2.4) ($P < 0.001$) and a mean fall of ICP of 4.6 mmHg(S.D. 2.8) ($P < 0.001$) (9 patients, 16 administrations). In 6 patients, the addition of thiopentone or Althesin to physiotherapy with oxygen reduced the increase in ICP, but these results were not statistically significant.

References

1. Coroneos NJ, McDowall DG, Gibson RM, Pickerodt, VWA, Keaney NP (1973) Measurement of extradural pressure and its relationship to other intracranial pressures. J Neurol Neurosurg Psychiat 36: 514-522

2. Gibson RM, McDowall DG, Turner JM, Nahhas MF (1975) Clinical experience of a method of continuous intracranial pressure recording in 50 neurosurgical patients. In: Lundberg N, Ponten U, Brock M (eds) Intracranial Pressure III. Springer, Berlin Heidelberg New York, p 496

3. Greenbaum R, Cooper R, Hulme A, Mackintosh IP (1975) The effect of induction of anesthesia on intracranial pressure. In: Arias A (ed) Recent Progress in Anesthesiology and Resuscitation. International Congress Series no. 347. Excerpta Medica, Amsterdam,p 794

4. Henriksen HT, Jorgensen PB (1973) The effect of nitrous oxide on intracranial pressure in patients with intracranial disorders. Br J. Anesth 45:486-491

5. Horsley JS (1937) The intracranial pressure during barbital narcosis. Lancet 1:141-143

6. Hulme A, Cooper R (1972) Changes in intracranial pressure and other variables during the induction of general anesthesia. Proc roy Soc Med 65:883-884

7. Lundberg N (1960)Continuous recording and control of ventricular fluid pressure in neurosurgical practice. Acta psychiat scand 36 (Suppl 149)

8. Misfeldt BB, Jorgensen PB, Rishoj M (1974) The effect of nitrous oxide and halothane upon the intracranial pressure in hypocapnic patients with intracranial disorders. Br J Anesth 46:853-858

9. Phirman JR, Shapiro HM (1977) Modification of nitrous oxide-induced intracranial hypertension by prior induction of anesthesia. Anesthesiol 46:150-151

10. Pierce EC, Lambertsen CJ, Deutsch S, Chase PE, Linde HW, Dripps RD, Price HL (1962) Cerebral circulation and metabolism during thiopental anesthesia and hyperventilation in man. J Clin Invest 41:1664-1671

11. Sari A, Maekawa T, Tohjo M. Okuda Y, Takeshita H (1976) Effects of Althesin on cerebral blood flow and oxygen consumption in man. Br J Anesth 48:545-549

12. Sondergard W (1961) Intracranial pressure during general anesthesia. Dan med Bull 8:18-25

13. Turner JM, Coroneos NJ, Gibson RM, Powell D, Ness MA, McDowell DG (1973) The effect of Althesin on intracranial pressure in man. Br J Anesth 45:168-171

EFFECT OF ALTHESIN ON INTRACRANIAL HYPERTENSION IN PATIENTS WITH SEVERE HEAD INJURY

P.VERSARI, G.VECCHI, M.AROSIO, M.COLLICE, AND M.ROSANDA

Alphaxalone - alphadolone (Althesin) causes a marked reduction of intracranial pressure (ICP, cerebral blood flow and metabolism (1,2). Thiopentone has a similar effect and has been successfully used against severe intracranial hypertension (HICP) in man (3).

This report describes the results of repeated i.v. bolus injections of Althesin (1-2 ml) in 8 cases of severe head injury, subjected to continuous ventricular fluid pressure (CVFP) monitoring. These patients developed severe HICP in spite of hyperventilation, dexamethasone, osmotic diuretics and standard sedation with phenobarbital, diazepam, opiates:

Case No.	Years	Midbrain Dysfunc.	HICP duration (days)	Highest Value mmHg	Althesin Adm. Total	Effective(%)	Outcome
1	4	+	10	100	72	72 (69)	alive
2	8	+	8	56	15	12 (80)	dead
3	10	-	5	50	10	9 (90)	alive
4	13	-	6	50	13	13(100)	alive
5	14	-	7	30	5	5(100)	alive
6	15	+	10	40	8	2 (25)	dead
7	19	+	3	40	10	5 (50)	dead
8	25	+	7	40	10	9 (90)	alive

The number of bolus injections given to a single patient ranged from 5 to 15 over 2 to 8 days. One child of 4 with multiple injuries, who developed ICP peaks as high as 100 mmHg in spite of heavy analgesia was given 72 doses over 8 days. He made a full recovery. Althesin bolus proved effective in most cases, with one exception (case No.6).

VFP dropped immediately after the injection. Following 15 injections of 1 ml bolus and 17 of 2 ml bolus, the VFP could be recorded for at least 1 hour without any interference caused by either stimuli or further medication. VFP increased slowly but did not reach the initial level (Fig 1). The hypotensive effect of 2 ml bolus looks more marked and persistent. Following Althesin injection, ICP remained acceptably low for several hours in only one-third of the instances, when its course could be observed, and in the absence of interfering artifacts. However, in most cases the effect subsided within 1 to 2 hours.

The duration of the ICP reduction following Althesin bolus cannot be related to persistent cerebral depression, due to the quick removal of the drug from the brain; also in this group of patients the anesthetic effect was not prolonged. Moreover, a few attempts to maintain Althesin anesthesia by continuous i.v. injection was not always effective in preventing further ICP elevations. Therefore, the bolus administration is still being tested, with the limited purpose of achieving a quick ICP reduction when it begins to rise to a dangerous level.

This scheme does not afford the continuous brain depression that has been advocated for cerebral protection (3). On the contrary, the patient's reactivity can be checked between the administrations of Althesin. In such a program the single bolus injections of anesthetic drugs (either Althesin or thiopentone) can be usefully combined with osmotics and CSF drainage, thus avoiding overdosage when it is not absolutely required.

References

1. Pickerodt VWA, McDowall DG, Coroneos NJ, Deaney NP (1972) Effect of Althesin on cerebral perfusion, cerebral metabolism and intracranial pressure in the anesthetized baboon. Brit J Anesth 44: 751-758

2. Rasmussen JJ, Rosendal T, Overgaard J (1978) Althesin in neurosurgical patients: Effect on cerebral hemodynamics and metabolism. Acta Anesth Scand 22:257-269

3. Shapiro HM, Wyte SR, Loeser J (1974) Barbiturate augmented hypothermia for reduction of persistent intracranial hypertension. J Neurosurg 40:90-100

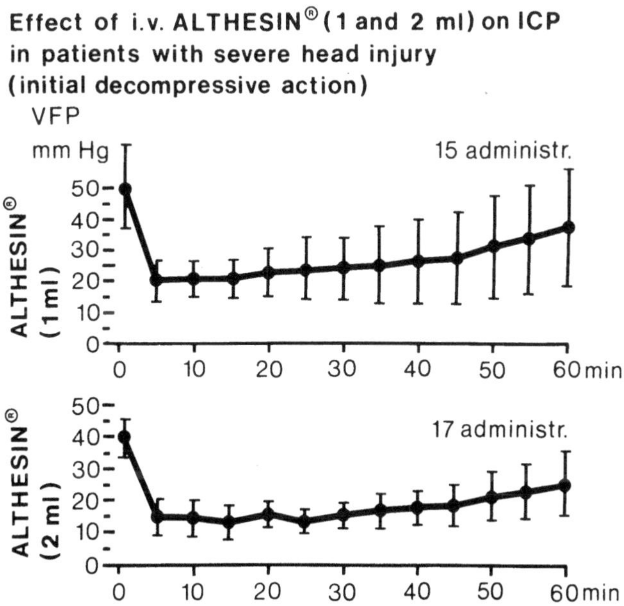

Fig.1. Mean values and S.E. of VFP following bolus injections of either 1 or 2 ml of Althesin.

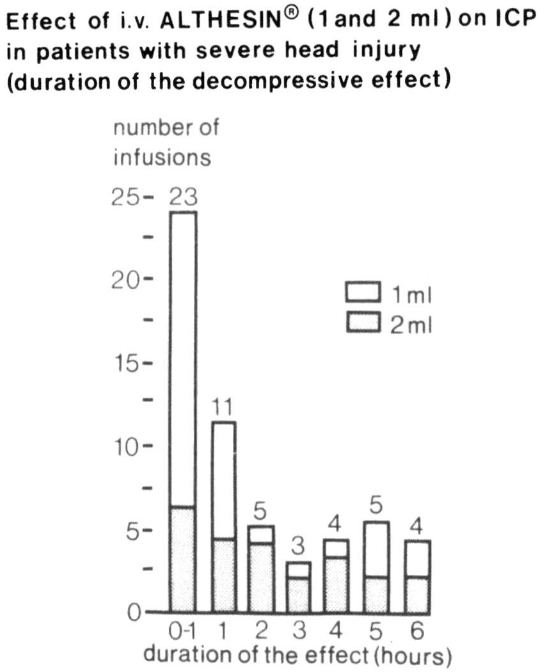

Fig. 2. Duration of VFP decrease following bolus injections of Althesin.

NITROPRUSSIDE AND NITROGLYCERIN INDUCED INTRACRANIAL PRESSURE CHANGES

B. GUPTA AND J.E. COTTRELL

Introduction

Induced hypotension is frequently used in neurosurgical patients for clipping of aneurysm, to reduce blood loss and to provide a relatively bloodless field to decrease operative time. Previous methods to induce hypotension were inadequate due to lack of easy controllability, toxic metabolites or increase in intracranial pressure (ICP). Recently, sodium nitroprusside's (SNP) popularity in neurosurgical patients has been threatened because of reports of increased ICP(3,5). Nitroglycerin (NTG) has been suggested as an alternate because of reported lack of ICP effects (2). We conducted the present study with NTG and compared it with our previous study.

Material and methods

Patients scheduled for neurosurgical procedures were divided into groups A and B. Ten patients received SNP (A) and five patients received NTG (B). All patients in group A and four patients in group B had intracranial tumor, and one patient had an A-V malformation.

All patients were selected for the study based on the potential need to induce hypotension for the control of bleeding during surgery. A subarachnoid screw was placed under local anesthesia. General anesthesia consisted of a standardized thiopental, nitrous oxide, oxygen, narcotic and muscle relaxant sequence. Patients were monitored for arterial blood gases, direct intraarterial pressure recording, airway pressure (AWP), ICP, central venous pressure (CVP), urinary output and body temperature. Four of five patients in group B had balloon tipped flow directed pulmonary artery catheters. Ventilation was controlled to maintain $PaCO_2$ at 25-30 torr.

After ICP, MAP, CFP, AWP and pulmonary artery diastolic pressures(PAD), were stable, SNP (0.01%) or NTG (0.015%) was given until MAP reduced to two thirds control pressure. Cerebral perfusion pressure (CPP) was calculated, (MAP-ICP) when the desired hypotensive response was achieved. Statistical analysis was performed utilizing the Student's t test for paired data.

Results (Table I)

Group A (SNP): As MAP decreased from 104 ± 2.55 to 70.90 ± 3.61 torr, ICP increased from 14.58 ± 1.76 to 27.61 ± 3.16 torr ($p < 0.0005$). CPP decreased significantly from 89.32 ± 3.57 to 43.23 ± 4.60 torr ($p < 0.005$).

Group B (NTG): As MAP decreased from 104.40 ± 3.91 to 69.0 ± 1.82 torr, ICP increased from 14.20 ± 0.66 to 30.80 ± 1.06 torr ($p < 0.005$). CPP decreased from 90.20 ± 3.59 to 38.20 ± 2.28 ($p < 0.005$).

Table 1. MAP, ICP & CPP After SNP and NTG-Induced Hypotension

Measurement* (torr)	Pre SNP	Post SNP	Pre NTG	Post NTG
MAP	104 ± 2.55	70.9 ± 3.61	104.40 ± 3.91	69.0 ± 1.82
ICP	14.58 ± 1.76	27.61 ± 3.16	14.20 ± 0.66	30.8 ± 1.06
CPP	89.32 ± 3.57	43.23 ± 4.60	90.20 ± 3.59	38.2 ± 2.28

* Mean ± S.E.M.

Discussion

SNP is widely used in neurosurgery because of its ability to maintain cerebral blood flow despite CPP's of 50 torr or less (8). This is due to direct dilatation without significant myocardial depression or decrease in cardiac output (1). Cerebral vessels therefore dilate and if intracranial compliance is compromised, ICP will increase in a linear relationship to increase in cerebral blood flow (CBF). In our study, intracranial pressure increased significantly as MAP decreased with SNP infusion. CPP decreased from 89.32 ± 3.57 to 43.23 ± 4.60 torr in group A when the desired hypotensive effect occurred. One patient developed a calculated CPP of 28.8 torr, but did not exhibit signs of cerebral hypoxia postoperatively, presumably because of suppression of cerebral oxygen requirements by anesthetics (barbiturate and narcotics) used (7). In the unanesthetized brain, a CPP of 30 to 40 torr is necessary to prevent hypoxic encephalopathy (5).

Intravenous NTG dilates venous capacitance vessels without significant reduction in cardiac output or increase in CBF (4) and theoretically is less likely to increase ICP. Recently, no change in ICP was reported in animals with normal or raised ICP after epidural balloon inflation, whereas others (GONZALEZ-ABOLA) demonstrated an increase in ICP in dogs with normal intracranial dynamics, but no change with experimentally produced mass lesions (2). In our study ICP increase was found to be greater after NTG than after SNP (Fig 1). as MAP reduced by one third. Decrease in CPP therefore, was also greater with NTG than with SNP but signs of postoperative cerebral hypoxia were not seen.

NTG dilates capacitance vessels within the relatively non-compliant cranial cavity and increases cerebral blood volume (CBV). Intracranial venous outflow tracts and CSF displacement cannot rapidly accommodate for this change and ICP increases. NTG is presently not approved by the Food and Drug Administration for intravenous use.

References

1. Adams AP, Clarke TNS, Edmonds-Seal J. et al (1974) The effects of sodium nitroprusside on myocardial contractability and hemodynamics. Brit J Anesth 46:807-817

2. Chestnut SJ, Albin MS, Gonzalez-Abola E et al (1978) Clinical evaluation of intravenous nitroglycerin for neurosurgery. J Neurosurg 48:704-711

3. Cottrell JE, Patel K, Turndorf H et al (1978) Intracranial pressure changes induced by sodium nitroprusside in patients with intracranial mass lesions. J Neurosurg 48:329-331

4. Ferrer MI, Bradley SE, et al(1975) Some effects of nitroglycerin upon the splanchnic, pulmonary and systemic circulations. Circulation 51:132-139

5. Kaasik AE, Nilsson L. Siesjo BK (1970) The effects of arterial hypotention upon lactate, pyruvate and bicarbonate concentrations of brain tissue and cisternal CSF, and upon the tissue concentrations of phosphocreatine and adenine nucleotides in anesthetized rats. Acta Physiol Scand 78:448-458

6. Keykkah MM, Shapiro HM, Van Horn et al (1976) ICP response to nitroprusside during progressive intracranial hypotension. ASA Annual Meeting (Abstract)

7. Smith AL, Wollman H (1972) Cerebral blood flow and metabolism. Effects of anesthetic drugs and techniques. Anesthes 36:378-400

8. Stoyka WW, Schutz H (1975) The cerebral response to sodium nitroprusside and trimethapan controlled hypotension. Can Anesthes Soc J 22:275-283

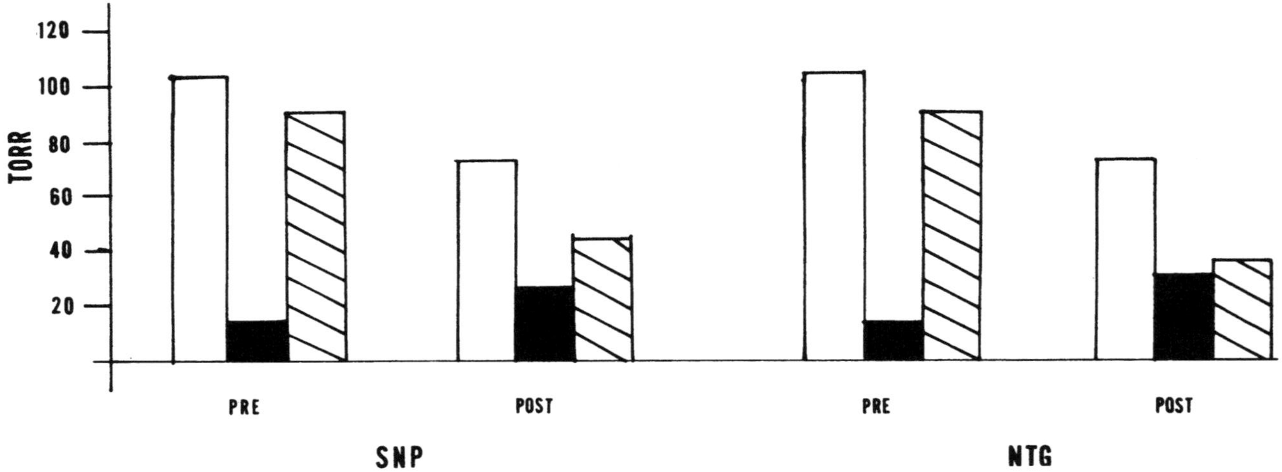

Fig I. Relation between MAP, ICP and CPP after SNP and NTG induced hypotension.

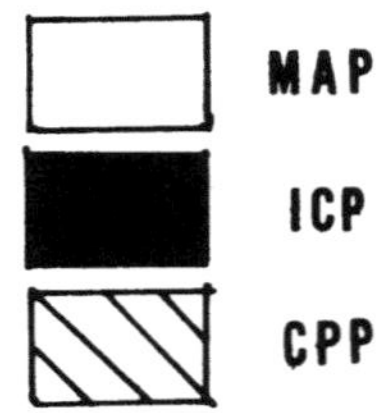

EFFECTS OF ENFLURANE AND HALOTHANE ON ICP IN DOGS

A. STEVENAERT, P. HANS, AND D. GODIN

Introduction

It is admitted that the halogenated volatile anesthetics induce cerebral vasodilatation with a resulting increase of intracranial pressure. The purpose of this study is to control the effects of enflurane and halothane on ICP, blood pressure (SAP) and cerebral perfusion pressure (CPP).

Material and methods

Eleven dogs were anesthetized using intraperitoneal injection of pentobarbital, ventilated with a Harvard respirator giving a constant volume of a gas mixture containing 70% H_2O and 30% O_2; the dogs were maintained in normocapnia and normoxia, except for one which was hypercapnic. One hour after the induction, enflurane (0.5%, 1% and 2%) was introduced for 15 minutes in the anesthetic circuit by an Enfluratec Vaporizer; after return to control values, halothane (0.5% and 1%) was sprayed for 15 minutes by a Draeger Vapor. This procedure was again used in four dogs who received an intracarotid injection of sodium laurylsulfate.

The surgical procedures included the cannulation of the inferior vena cava and the thoracic aorta via a femoral artery and vein. The cisterna magna was punctured with an 18-g needle. All catheters and needles were connected to a Statham P23Db transducer; pressures were recorded on a magnetic recorder (Ampex SP 700).

Results

In all dogs, neither central venous pressure nor temperature changed. In dogs with normocapnia and normal ICP, enflurane 1% and 2% raised ICP and decreased SAP while there was no significant change with enflurane 0.5%. Halothane had similar significant effects at 0.5%, 1% and 2%. With both anesthetics, the effects were dose-dependent, and potentiated by hypercapnia. In dogs who received an intracarotid injection of laurylsulfate, the control ICP level was raised but it failed in two thirds of the experiments during anesthetics vaporization, while SAP decreased as expected.

Discussion

The results confirmed that halogenated anesthetics bring about SAP decrease, ICP increase and consequently CPP decrease. ICP increase is probably due to the cerebral vasodilatator effect of the anesthetics and is enhanced by hypercapnia, which adds a supplementary cause of vasodilatation.

The variations in ICP and SAP are dose-dependent; the sequence of effects can be expressed as follows:

ICP : E 0.5% < E 1% < H 0.5% < E 2% < H 1%
SAP : E 0.5% < H 0.5% < E 1% < E 2% < H 1%

In these sequences, there is an inversion of the effects of enflurane 1% and halothane 0.5%; this could be due to the difference of their mechanisms of arterial hypotension. The changes in CPP are similar to that in SAP.

Intracarotid injection of sodium laurylsulfate induces brain edema with vasogenic component and temporary loss of cerebral autoregulation. In this particular situation, halogenated anesthetics decrease ICP. This "paradoxical" effect could be explained by the systemic arterial hypotension and the resulting decrease in the hydrostatic pressure in the arterial cerebral vessels, which plays a role in the genesis and the maintenance of vasogenic edema.

Summary

Experiments in dogs demonstrate that enflurane and halothane increase ICP, decrease SAP and consequently CPP; the effects are dose-dependent, potentiated by hypercapnia, and halothane is more effective than enflurane. In vasogenic brain edema, the anesthetics induce an ICP decrease, in relation with their arterial hypotensive effect.

1. Adams RW, Gronert GA, Sundt TM, Mickenfelder JD (1972) Halothane, hypocapnia and cerebrospinal fluid pressure in neurosurgery. Anesthesiol 37:510

2. Boop WC, Knight R (1978) Enflurane anesthesia and changes of intracranial pressure. J Neurosurg 48:228-231

3. Christensen MS, Hoedt Rasmussen K, Lassen NA (1967) Cerebral vasodilatation by halothane anesthesia in man and its potentiation by hypotension and hypercapnia. Brit J Anesth 39:927

4. Dobkin AB, Nishioka K, Gengade DB, Ducksook K, Evers W, Israel JS (1969) Ethrane (compound 347) anesthesia, a clinical and laboratory review of 700 cases. Anesth Anal Res 43:477

5. Jennett WB, McDowall DG, Barker J (1967) The effect of halothane on intracranial pressure in cerebral tumors. J Neurosurg 26:270

6. McDowall DG (1967) The effects of linical concentrations of halothane on the blood flow and oxygen uptake of the cerebral cortex. Crit J Anesthes 39:186

7. McDowall DG, Barker J, Jennet WB (1966) Cerebrospinal fluid pressure measurements during anesthesia. Anesth 21:189

8. Wilkinson HA, Wepsic JG, Austin G (1971) Diuretic synergy in the treatment of acute experimental edema. J Neurosurg 34:203

Work supported by the Fonds National de la Recherche Scientifique.

EFFECT OF SOME ANALGESICS, SEDATIVES AND I.V. ANESTHETICS ON ICP IN MAN

G. CUNITZ AND M. GAAB

Introduction

Analgesics and sedatives are widely used in neurosurgical anesthesia and in the intensive care unit. Intravenous anesthetics may be given to rapidly lower an elevated ICP. In the following study the effect of some of these drugs on ICP is described.

Methods

The following drugs were investigated in neurosurgery patients who were either awaiting an elective operation or were being treated in the intensive care unit: 1. Fentanyl (Sublimaze[R]), 2. Pentazocine (Talwin[R]), 3. Diazepam (Valium[R]), 4 Etomidat, 5. Methohexital (Brietal[R]), 6. Thiopental (Pentothal[R]) and 7. Droperidol (Inapsine[R]). Drugs 1-6 were used during a neuroleptanalgesia (NLA) and during a phenobarbital-diazepam sedation. These patients were artificially ventilated. Drugs 4-7 were used for the induction of a general anesthesia in patients who were breathing spontaneously. Further details are listed in the table. Predominant disorders were: Hydrocephalus, tumors and head injuries. ICP was continuously recorded by use of an external Statham pressure transducer (puncture of a Hakim-shunt or a Rickham reservoir or via an epidural miniature transducer (Gaeltec). In most cases blood pressure (BP) was also recorded. Cerebral perfusion pressure (CPP) was calculated. For statistical analysis the paired t-test was used

Results (See table and figure)

The analgesics fentanyl and pentazocine did not change the ICP level, provided care was taken (by artificial ventilation) that respiratory depression did not occur. The sedative diazepam, clearly lowered ICP. Droperidol also dropped ICP. The higher the pre-existing ICP value, the greater was the drop after this neuroleptic drug was used.

The true i.v. anesthetics etomidat, methohexital and thiopental all promptly lowered ICP. This occurred during the maintenance of general anesthesia. BP (where it was recorded) and CPP reached their lowest levels after the use of the barbiturates methohexital and thiopental.

Discussion

Because of their depressive effect on respiration, it was necessary to investigate some of the drugs under ventilatory control. Consequently, two groups, one with and one without artificial respiration were established. When comparing the absolute ICP changes after drug injections, one must keep in mind that drug interaction may have taken

Table 1. Results - effect of the listed drugs.

mg/kg	ICP from	ICP to	CPP from	CPP to	BP from	BP to	n	PCO_2
1. During artificial ventilation, basic anesthesia and sedation								
Fentanyl (0.003)	11.8± 1.7	11.7± 1.7+	72.4± 4.1	68.6± 4.4*	83.7± 5.0	79.8± 5.2*	12	36
Pentazocine (0.78)	7.8± 1.9	7.9± 1.9+	66.8± 9.6	69.0± 9.1+	79.4± 7.3	81.2± 7.0+	8	32
Diazepam (0.26)	15.1± 3.6	13.1± 3.4*	66.0± 5.4	64.9± 5.9+	83.6± 5.0	81.1± 4.9+	12	32
Etomidat (0.24)	11.7± 6.8	9.2± 6.8**	72.3±16.6	68.6±16.8*	84.3±19.0	78.1±18.6**	10	33
Methohexital (1.1)	14.7± 7.7	11.6± 7.8**	67.0±18.4	60.3±16.7*	82.3±20.9	72.5±19.0**	7	32
Thiopental (3.1)	11.7± 4.1	8.9± 4.8**	59.0±15.8	55.1±15.0*	70.7±17.5	64.0±16.8**	7	31
2. For induction								
Droperidol (0.26)	8.0± 2.4	6.8± 2.5*	80.7± 5.4	71.3± 6.6*	88.7± 4.5	78.2± 6.0*	6	
(0.22)	51.5	38.5					2	
Etomidat (0.20)	15.6± 2.5	10.7± 1.5**				** P< 0,01	12	
Methohexital (1.0)	14.1± 2.9	11.1± 2.1*				* < 0.05	8	
Thiopental (3.0)	12.3± 3.3	6.8± 2.2**				+ n.s.	8	

place between the underlying anesthetics or sedatives and the newly injected test drug. However, the general trends are more important than the absolute values. The results show that fentanyl and pentazocine did not have an adverse effect on ICP. Diazepam, Droperidol and the i.v. anesthetics used, on the other hand, had a favorable effect on ICP. Previous studies have shown (4,5) that ICP remained unchanged after fentanyl. However, MILLER et al (3) noted a pressure increase. BARKER et al (1) described an ICP-drop after injection of pentazocine. However, our study showed that ICP remained unchanged after pentazocine. The combination of fentanyl with droperidol (Innovar[R] or Thalamonal[R]), mainly used in NLA is known to slightly lower ICP, an effect probably related to droperidol. Since diazepam lowers cerebral blood flow (2), and ICP drop could be expected. Etomidat, methohexital and thiopental all seem suitable for rapidly lowering ICP as proposed by SHAPIRO et al (6) for thiopental. Finally, this study showed that the new anesthetic, etomidat, which has relatively favorable effects on the cardiovascular system, possesses ICP lowering properties similar to those of thiopental.

Summary

In neurosurgical patients diazepam, droperidol and the i.v. anesthetic etomidat, methohexital and thiopental caused an ICP drop. The analgesics fentanyl and pentazocine left ICP unchanged. It was necessary to investigate some drugs under ventilatory control. BP was also measured and CPP calculated.

References

1. Barker J, Miller JD, Johnston IH (1972) The effect of pentazocine on pupillary size and intracranial pressure. Brit J Anesth 44:202

2. Cotev S, Shalit MN (1975) Effects of diazepam on cerebral blood flow and oxygen uptake after head injury. Anesth 43:117-122

3. Miller R, Tausk HC, Stark DCC (1975) Effect of innovar fentanyl and droperidol on the cerebrospinal fluid pressure in neurosurgical patients. Canad Anesth Soc J 22:502-508

4. Misfeldt BB, Jorgensen PB, Spotoft H, Ronde F (1976) The effects of droperidol and fentanyl on intracranial pressure and cerebral perfusion pressure in neurosurgical patients. Brit J Anesth 48: 963-968

5. Moss E, Powell D. Gibson RM, McDowall DG (1978) Effects of fentanyl on intracranial pressure and cerebral perfusion pressure during hypocapnia. Brit J Anesth 50:779-784

6. Shapiro HM, Galindo A, Wyte SR, Harris AB (1973) Rapid intraoperative reduction of intracranial pressure with thiopentone. Br J Anesth 45:1057-1062

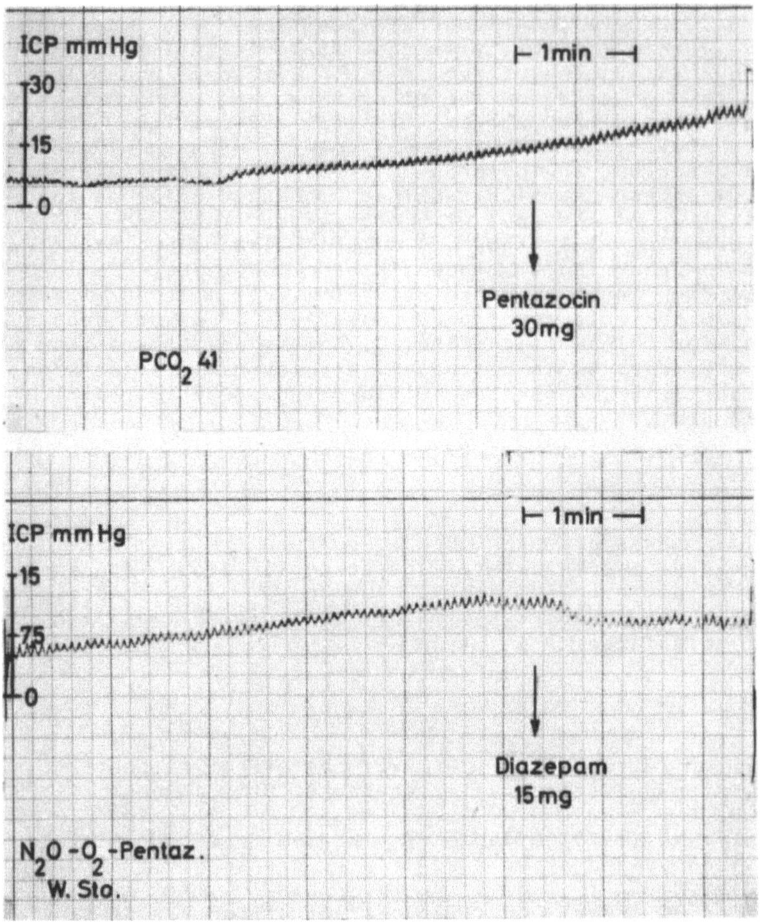

Fig.1. Effect of i.v. pentazocine and diazepam on rising ICP. The 51 year old man has a basic anesthesia. Diagnosis: cerebellar metastasis.

Session XII

BARBITURATE, STEROID, AND OSMOTHERAPY

Chairman: J.T.Hoff
Co-chairman: W.Gobiet

SUMMARY

The collection of papers from Session XII outlines recent advances in our understanding of barbiturate, steroid, and osmotherapy in animals and man with raised intracranial pressure from brain swelling.

Barbiturates appear to be most effective in man with increased ICP from severe head injury or Reye's syndrome, particularly in children and young adults. Intracranial hypertension greater than 20mmHg which is refractory to standard treatment, including osmotherapy and hyperventilation, can be reduced to near-normal levels by intravenous pentobarbital. Careful monitoring of ICP, EEG, pulmonary function, EKG, blood pressure, fluid-electrolyte balance, and blood barbiturate levels (optimal = 3-4mg%) in an intensive care unit is essential. The San Diego and Philadelphia groups both show significant improvement in outcome from severe head injury, complicated by raised ICP, with this adjunctive therapy. DRS. MCGRAW and HOWARD confirmed the ICP reduction effect of pentobarbital in patients with brain swelling, but found no significant change in the effect of Mannitol on ICP when barbiturates were given in addition.

The beneficial effect of barbiturates on focal and global ischemia remains unconfirmed. DR. KASSEL and his colleagues administered pentobarbital to patients with severe cerebral ischemia-hypoxia from vasospasm caused by subarachnoid hemorrhage and were unable to confirm previous anecdotal reports of barbiturate protection from ischemia in man. DRS. BRUCE and MARSHALL also noted no significant improvement in outcome in patients with severe global cerebral ischemia-hypoxia even though ICP could be consistently controlled by barbiturates.

Steroids in traditional or high doses were shown to have no significant effect on increased ICP in patients with severe head injury. Independent, randomized, and blinded studies with dexamethasone recently reported from two head injury centers (Pitts, San Francisco; Cooper, Dallas) were discussed. While the effect of steroids on outcome from severe head injury remains uncertain, the drug appears to have no role in the reduction of ICP in trauma victims. Animal studies by SCHETTINI and WALSH confirmed the limited role of steroids in reducing brain stiffness caused by epidural brain compression.

Doses, duration, and distribution of the effect of Mannitol on brain water and raised ICP were reported by groups from Barcelona and Kansas City. Mannitol in excess of 1.0gm/kg given over 5-10 minutes did not reduce ICP more in patients with brain swelling. Furthermore, rebound ICP elevation and water intoxication occurred when that dose was exceeded. In rats, Mannitol has a greater effect when it is given rapidly, dehydrating regions of the brain non-uniformly.

Furosemide and THAM have important therapeutic effects on raised ICP, by different mechanisms. SKLAR and his colleagues demonstrated reduced ICP in patients with pseudotumor, presumably by reduced CSF formation, particularly during periods of elevated ICP. THAM, on the other hand, may control brain water by reducing intracellular acidosis caused by trauma in patients and by cold injury in cats.

Papers in this session indicate a growing interest in the pharmacologic approach to control of raised ICP. More work, particularly with drugs which have a barbiturate-like effect on ICP without the inherent risks of "iatrogenic coma", is required to improve outcome from severe brain swelling further. Non-sedative agents such as furosemide, Mannitol, and THAM may provide that future therapeutic direction.

BARBITURATES FOR INTRACRANIAL HYPERTENSION: A TEN YEAR PERSPECTIVE

L.F.Marshall and H.M.Shapiro

Introduction

There has been much recent interest in the utilization of high-dose barbiturates in the treatment of a variety of acute brain injuries. We have previously demonstrated that barbiturates can rapidly lower intracranial pressure, and we have described our experience in patients with severe head injury and in Reye's syndrome (1,2,3). It appeared from our initial studies that the reduction of intracranial pressure (ICP) accomplished in these early patients may have prevented potential secondary cerebral ischemic insults.

Materials and Methods

In an attempt to assess the effectiveness of high-dose barbiturate therapy in a more rigorous fashion, we have utilized intravenous pentobarbital in 45 consecutive patients suffering from acute severe head injury in whom the intracranial pressure exceeded 40mmHg for at least 15 minutes and/or a reduction in the mean cerebral perfusion pressure to less than 50mmHg occurred.

Intra-arterial and intracranial pressures were monitored in all patients. Emergency computerized axial tomographic scanning was carried out in each patient. Extraparenchymal hematomas were evacuated when indicated. In all instances, high doses of barbiturates were administered only after standard therapy to control ICP had failed. This included control of hyperventilation, intravenous mannitol, blood pressure reduction, maintenance of normothermia, and a standardized regimen of high-dose dexamethasone (80mg/day). Pentobarbital was initially administered intravenously in a dose of 5mg/kg followed by 1-2mg/kg/hr supplements to maintain a blood pressure of above a mean of 60mmHg, and an ICP of less than 15mmHg. A serum barbiturate level of 3-4mg% usually gave adequate control of ICP; levels of greater than 5mg% did not appear to have any beneficial clinical effect. The initial criteria for the slow withdrawal of barbiturates in the head-injured patients included normalization of the ICP for 36 hours or more, a normal ventricular volume-pressure response, and a systolic arterial blood pressure of less than 160mmHg in an adult without vasodilator therapy. If there was no initial response to barbiburates a second dose was administered. If there was still no reduction in ICP, the drug was discontinued.

In addition, eight children with uncontrolled intracranial hypertension following the development of a post-infectious encephalitis were also treated. Criteria for treatment in these children varied slightly in that if the ICP remained above 30mmHg for at least 30 minutes, barbiturate therapy was begun. The rest of their management did not differ.

Table 1

Glasgow coma score	No.of patients[a]	Good recovery	Moderate disability	Vegetative	Dead
INITIAL RESPONDERS[b]					
3	7	4	1	0	2
4	9	4	1	1	3
5	5	3	1	0	1
6	11	6	2	1	2
7	4	3	1	0	0
Total	36	20	6	2	8
INITIAL NONRESPONDERS					
3	4	0	0	0	4
4	2	0	0	0	2
5	2	0	0	1	1
6	1	0	0	0	1
7	0	0	0	0	0
Total	9	0	0	1	8

[a] All patients treated with barbiturates had an ICP > 40 mm Hg for least 15 min.

[b] Initial responders (N=36) are defined as having reduction in ICP > 10 mm Hg (29 of these had normalization of ICP < 15 mm Hg). See text for discussion.

Results

Head Injury: The Glasgow Coma Scale (GCS) scores of the patients with head injury described below are shown in Table I. This series includes no patients with GCS scores of greater than 7 when barbiturates were begun, although four of the 45 patients subsequently deteriorated from higher admitting scores. ICP was reduced by more than 10mmHg in 36 of the 45 patients within 10 minutes of the initial barbiturate dose. Rapid normalization of ICP was accomplished in 29 of these initial responders; however, of these patients six developed "late escape" from barbiturate-augmented ICP control, and four subsequently died of uncontrolled intracranial hypertension. Of the nine patients who had no ICP response to barbiturate therapy, eight died and one is vegetative. Non-responsiveness could be predicted by a lack of response to manipulation of pCO_2

Encephalitis: In the children with Reye's syndrome (n=7) and in herpes encephalitis, the results were uniformly good. Only one child was significantly brain damaged following therapy, and the rest are normal on sophisticated psychometric examination, where such testing was possible.

Discussion

In patients suffering severe head injury, control of ICP is often a major determinant of survival and quality of outcome. Prior to our initiation of high-dose barbiturate therapy, 17 patients with persistent ICP's of greater than 40mmHg had been treated in our institution using identical management without barbiturates by our neurosurigcal intensive care unit team. Fifteen of 17 expired and two are vegetative survivors.

Thus, the mortality of 36% in the present group of head-injured patients with high ICP's strongly implies that barbiturates do influence both survival and the qualtiy of outcome. The inability to reduce elevated ICP with barbiturates is a grave prognostic sign, in our hands. We believe that the GCS score does provide a comparative common reference for assessing severity of injury. This data indicates that the outcome in these severely brain-injured patients has been altered favorably.

Our experience in post-infectious encephalitis is also favorable. The nil mortality demonstrated in this group is in sharp contrast to the mortality rate in patients reported with neurologic states similar to our patients.

How barbiturates act to reduce ICP remains unclear. The rapidity of response in most instances leads one to conclude that the major initial effect is cerebral vasoconstriction with an immediate reduction in brain-blood volume. Supporting this conclusion is the fact that the response to high-dose barbiturate administration appears to be an age-related phenomenon with younger patients having an almost uniformly good response to high-dose barbiturate therapy. In view of the fact that BRUCE and his colleagues have demonstrated that head injury in children is most often associated with vascular engorgement of the brain, this conclusion appears logical. The reduction in brain-blood volume and cerebral blood flow, which one sees with barbiturates, is better tolerated because the cerebral metabolic rate is depressed on a long-term basis by high serum barbiturate levels. Whether other mechanisms such as depression of free radical formation, alteration in short-chain fatty acid metabolisms, or suppression of abnormal catecholamine release or reuptake play any role in explaining the reduction in ICP we have observed is unknown. It appears unnecessary to invoke these hypothesis.

In disease processes where ischemia is secondary to intracranial hypertension, high-dose barbiturate therapy is a useful adjunct in the treatment of such brain-injured patients. Our dismal experience in treating patients with primary ischemia, either focal or global in nature, despite the fact that intracranial hypertension was well controlled as long as these patients were maintained on high doses of barbiturates, leads us to believe that the use of barbiturates following global ischemia is unwarranted in efforts to protect the brain following clinical stroke or cerebral circulatory arrest in 1979.

References

1. Marshall LF, Shapiro HM, Rauscher A, Kaufman NM (1978) Pentobarbital therapy for intracranial hypertension in metabolic coma. Reye's syndrome. Crit Care Med 6:1-5

2. Marshall LF, Smith RW, Shapiro HM (1979) The outcome with agressive treatment in severe head injuries. Part I: The significance of intracranial pressure monitoring. J Neurosurg 50:20-25

3. Marshall LF, Smith RW, Shapiro HM (1979) The outcome with aggressive treatment in severe head injuries. Part II: Acute and chronic barbiturate administration in the management of head injury. J Neurosurg 50:26-30

THE EFFECTIVENESS OF IATROGENIC BARBITURATE COMA IN CONTROLLING INCREASED ICP IN 61 CHILDREN

D.A.BRUCE, R.A.RAPHAELY, D.SWEDLOW, AND L.SCHUT

Introduction

Shapiro et al (1) in 1974 recorded that intravenous barbiturates were effective in lowering intracranial pressure (ICP). Since then little evidence has accrued as to which barbiturate is most effective, which disease processes respond to this therapy and what the end points of therapy should be. Further, there is little information as to the relative complications of this therapy. We have had the opportunity to monitor the ICP in 180 children between 1975 and 1979. Of this group, 61 patients have received barbiturates in large doses as an ancillary measure to control elevated ICP. This report concerns our observations in this group of children.

Methods

61 children aged 8 months to 17 years have received barbiturates as therapy to control or maintain an ICP of less than 20 torr. Table 1 shows the diseases for which treatment was required. The barbiturates used were either Sodium Pentothal (Pentothal - Abbott) or Pentobarbital Sodium (Nembutal - Abbott) alone or in combination. Only 2 children received Pentothal alone, 20 others had intermittent boluses of Pentothal superimposed on the continuous infusion of Pentobarbital. In 50 patients, Pentobarbital was used when other methods (i.e. hyperventilation, mannitol and hypothermia) had failed to effectively maintain the ICP below 20 torr. In 9 patients with Reye's Syndrome, Pentobarbital was administered early in the course of the disease as the first therapy in an effort to prevent an increase in ICP. In the 50 patients, 5-10mg/Kg of Pentobarbital were administered by bolus i.v. injection and a continuous infusion of 1-3mg/Kg/hr begun. If this dosage was adequate to control the ICP, no increase in dosage was required immaterial of blood levels of Pentobarbital. If the ICP was not controlled, the blood levels of barbiturates were increased by further bolus injections of 5-10mg/Kg. The end points for barbiturate administration were: control of the ICP below 20 torr, a flat EEG, or evidence of a dropping cardiac output. The barbiturate levels required for adequate ICP control range from 2.5mg% to 7mg%.

Barbiturates were discontinued when the ICP had remained below 20 torr for 48 hours. If the ICP rose again as the barbiturate level decreased, the barbiturate therapy was begun again. During the course of barbiturate therapy, episodic increases in ICP were treated with bolus injections of Pentothal or mannitol, if necessary; the $PaCO_2$ was maintained in the low 20's and hypothermia from 32-34° was present.

Results

Head Injuries: In 20 of 23 head-injured patients the addition of barbiturates to the treatment regimen was effective in lowering the ICP and maintaining it around 20 torr or less. In 5 of these patients, further doses of mannitol or Lasix were necessary to maintain the ICP below 20 torr despite barbiturate therapy. Although 3 patients in this group died, none died from elevated ICP. In the remaining 3 patients the barbiturates were ineffective in lowering or controlling the ICP and all 3 patients died with ICP equal to arterial pressure. One of these patients had no cerebral perfusion pressure when therapy was begun and 1 other, a perfusion pressure of only 16 torr. The third developed an increasing ICP despite adequate barbiturate therapy and died an intracranial death. One patient out of the 23 died after developing progressive arterial hypotension while on barbiturate therapy. This did not seem to be due to the barbiturates since the Swan Ganz catheter showed initially a high cardiac output with an extremely low peripheral resistance and peripheral vasculature that was unresponsive to catecholamines. Fifteen of the survivors made a good recovery or were moderately disabled and 2 patients were left in a vegetative or severely disabled state.

Reye's Syndrome: Fifteen stage III-V and 1 stage II patients with Reye's Syndrome were treated with Pentobarbital. Seven patients were given the barbiturates because other methods of ICP control (i.e. hyperventilation, mannitol, hypothermia and/or exchange transfusion) had failed to maintain an ICP below 20 torr. The addition of this therapy controlled the ICP in 5, 2 already had no perfusion when the drug was begun and in 1 a sudden drop in blood pressure occurred and the arterial and intracranial pressures became equal. Nine patients were immediately placed into deep barbiturate coma with blood levels of 3-5mg% and either a flat or burst surpressed EEG. One of these 9 patients died of uncontrollable intracranial hypertension and the pressure was well controlled in the other 8. One patient in this group also died with a hypotensive episode. This was also associated with a lack of peripheral response to catecholamines and initially a high output cardiac state.

Anoxia: Barbiturates were effective in lowering the ICP in 7 of 9 patients who had suffered severe anoxic or ischemic insults to the brain. Despite good ICP control, however, 3 of these patients died and the remaining 4 were left in a severely vegetative state. In the 2 patients in whom barbiturates were ineffective in controlling ICP, death occurred due to intracranial hypertension.

In the other disease states shown in Table I the addition of barbiturates in large doses was effective in maintaining ICP control in 9 of 13 patients. Three of the total 61 patients died of progressive arterial hypotension. This may be related to the high barbiturate therapy and cardiovascular monitoring with a Swan Ganz catheter, which is a necessary part of monitoring in these children.

Conclusions

Large doses of intravenous Pentobarbital or Sodium Pentothal are an effective way of controlling the ICP in children when other, more standard methods have failed. A positive response to barbiturate therapy can be expected in approximately 80% of patients. In patients with severe anoxic brain damage, however, the use of barbiturates failed to effect a useful functional outcome in any of the survivors. To be effective, barbiturates should be used before the CPP is reduced below 30 torr. Other than in Reye's Syndrome, there is no evidence to suggest that barbiturates should replace more standard therapy or should be the first drug of choice in intracranial hypertension. Alterations in cardiovascular function are common in these very sick children and adequate monitoring of ICP, systemic arterial pressure (SAP) and usually of cardiovascular function with Swan Ganz catheter are necessary if this therapy is to be

Table 1. Number of patients in whom barbiturates failed to maintain ICP below SAP

	Number Patients	Number Deaths	Deaths due to ↑ ICP
Head Injury	23	6	3
Reye's Syndrome	16	5	1(2)
Anoxia & drowning	9	5	2
Tumors	5	2	2
Encephalitis	6	2	2
Miscellaneous	2	1	1
	61	21	11

used. Individualization of dose is necessary to balance the least amount of drug to an adequate ICP. Finally, no comment can be made on any protective effect of barbiturates nor can any inferences of mechanism be made.

Reference

1. Shapiro HM, Wyte SR, Loeser JD (1974) Barbiturate-augmented hypothermia for reduction of persistent intracranial hypertension. J Neurosurg 40:90-100

EFFECTS OF BARBITURATES ON INTRACRANIAL PRESSURE AND THE AMOUNT OF MANNITOL REQUIRED TO CONTROL THE INTRACRANIAL PRESSURE

C.P.McGRAW AND G.HOWARD

Introduction

Benefits have been described for barbiturates administered following severe cerebral injury (4,5); decreases in intracranial pressure (ICP) also have been observed (3,2). Therefore, ICP data from ICP-monitored patients were gathered to delineate the ICP response to phenobarbital, pentobarbital and thiopental given by bolus administration or on a regimen.

Because of the clinical nature of these observations, the data were not collected in the most desirable planned study for statistical analysis. However, the response of ICP to administrations of barbiturates was delineated.

Methods

We gathered data on three types of barbiturate administrations in 30 patients with elevated ICP (19 with head injuries, 8 with hemorrhages, 2 with inflammations, 1 with infarction) (Table 1).

Bolus Administration: Information on bolus administrations consisted of: 1) the amount of drug administered, and 2) the ICP at fixed periods before and after the bolus administration (-6, -4, -2, 0, 0.5, 1.5, 3, 6, and 10 minutes for pentobarbital and thiopental, plus 15 and 30 minutes for pentobarbital). A "repeated measures analysis of variance" and a "2-factor mixed design analysis of variance" (1) were used to examine the response of ICP with respect to time following administration of the bolus doses.

Barbiturate Regimens: Data collected on each barbiturate regimen change were: 1) phenobarbital and thiopental regimens both before and after any change in dosage; 2) average ICP over the pre- and post-change periods; 3) the average hourly amount of mannitol given during the pre- and post-change periods; 4) the length of time the patient had been monitored up to the change in dosage; and 5) the number of hours the patient was maintained at the new dosage. Analysis was aimed at establishing the ICP response and the amount of mannitol required with respect to the change in barbiturate dosage. In order to remove the influence of ICP and mannitol, regression analysis was used to demonstrate the effects of barbiturates on ICP, change in ICP, amount of mannitol required, and the change in the amount of mannitol required.

Results

1) Pentobarbital caused a change ($p<0.001$) in mean ICP from 25 to 19mmHg in the first 10 minutes after administration. The ICP had not returned to the postadministration levels by 30 minutes, which was as long as data could be collected before artifacts interfered. 2) Thiopental so-

Table 1. Dosage and observations

DRUG	BOLUSES	REGIMEN
Phenobarbital		15 to 160 mg/8 hr, IM
.2-2.3 mg/kg		73 observations (74%*)
Pentobarbital	150 mg, IV	
2.5 mg/kg	32 observations (56%*)	
Thiopental sodium	10 to 500 mg, IV	50 to 500 mg/hr, IV
.1-7.5 mg/kg	260 observations (19%*)	92 observations (67%*)

* Percentage of administrations selected for analysis; the other administrations were rejected because of simultaneous manual hyperventilation, suctioning, mannitol administrations, and other artifactual interferences. IM = intramuscular; IV = intravenous.

dium caused a change with respect to time ($p<0.001$), suggesting that different doses have different effects at different times. 3) By regression analysis, when variations in ICP and mannitol were taken into consideration, phenobarbital caused a significant ($p<0.05$) decrease in ICP. No relationship ($p>0.05$) could be established between phenobarbital and the amount of mannitol required to maintain the ICP below 25mm Hg. 4) By regression analysis, no relationship was found ($p>0.05$) to the change in dosage of thiopental when administered on a continuous basis.

Discussion

Boluses of pentobarbital decreased ICP and sustained that decrease for an average of at least 30 minutes, while boluses of thiopental decreased ICP for less than 10 minutes. No relationship could be found for continuous administrations of thiopental. This could reflect the fact that the ICP response to thiopental boluses lasted for less than 10 minutes or that tachyphylaxis was occurring. These findings suggest that thiopental doses do not have a lasting effect on ICP while phenobarbital and pentobarbital doses do. These findings are statistically significant, but should be verified in a planned prospective study.

Summary

The effects on ICP of boluses of pentobarbital or thiopental and of continuous administrations of phenobarbital or thiopental were delineated. All except continuous thiopental had a significant effect on ICP. Bolus pentobarbital had an effect on ICP that lasted longer than that of bolus theopental.

References

1. Bruning JL, Kintz BL (1977) In: Computational Handbook of Statistics, 2nd edition. Scott, Foresmen and Co, Glenview, Illinois, p 44

2. Marshall LF, Shaprio HM, Rauscher A, Kaufman NM (1978) Pentobarbital therapy for intracranial hypertension in metabolic coma. Reye's syndrome. Crit Care Med 6:1-5

3. Marshall LF, Smith RW, Shaprio HM (1979) The outcome with aggressive treatment in severe head injuries. Part II: Acute and chronic barbiturate administration in the management of head injury. J Neurosurg 50:26-30

4. McGraw CP (1977) Experimental cerebral infarction effects of pentobarbital in Mongolian gerbils. Arch Neurol 34:334-336

5. Smith AL, Wollman H (1972) Cerebral blood flow and metabolism: Effects of anesthesia drugs and techniques. Anesthesiol 36:378-400

CEREBRAL VASOSPASM, ICP AND BARBITURATE COMA

N.F.KASSELL, S.J.PEERLESS, AND C.G.DRAKE

Introduction

Many patients with subarachnoid hemorrhage (SAH) from ruptured aneurysms develop vasospasm and ischemic neurological deficits which progress relentlessly despite agressive measures to improve cerebral perfusion. In such situations barbiturate coma may prevent infarction from occurring by decreasing the metabolic needs of the brain to approximate the availability of substrates provided by the compromised circulation. Furthermore, intracranial hypertension is common in these patients (1) and the decrease in ICP which results from barbiturate therapy should improve cerebral blood flow (2,3).

Materials and Methods

Pentobarbital coma was employed in 11 patients with life-threatening neurological deterioration from vasospasm refractory to more conventional measures. Seven patients were treated pre-operatively and four post-operatively. Barbiturate coma was induced between four and 16 days after subarachnoid hemorrhage (mean of nine). Within three hours after the patients became unresponsive the coma was induced with pentobarbital sodium 15 to 30mg/kg, and maintained with an infusion of 2mg/kg/hr resulting in a blood level between 2 and 4mg.% and electrocerebral silence or burst suppression in the EEG of between 30 and 60 seconds. Barbiturates were discontinued when vasospasm was significantly reduced angiographically and intracranial pressure was less than 25 torr.

Results

Immediately prior to induction of barbiturate coma five patients had normal ICP. In two ICP remained normal throughout their course, except when one patient rebled. In the other three the ICP increased to equal the systemic arterial pressure (SAP). Six patients had elevated ICP ranging from 20 to 70 torr before administration of barbiturates. In five a prompt reduction of ICP occurred after pentobarbital infusion and in one the ICP remained elevated.

Five patients died during barbiturate therapy, three from uncontrollable intracranial hypertension presumably related to massive infarction, one from aneurysmal rebleeding and one from inadvertent puncture of the subclavian artery. The six survivors were emerged from barbiturate coma after five to 13 days. One showed no improvement three days after discontinuation of therapy and died from hydrocephalus when her ventriculostomy malfunctioned. One patient improved slightly and died suddenly from cardiac arrhythmia ten days after the barbiturates were stopped. Another died from unknown causes after 18 hours.

Three patients were significantly improved. All awakened and were responsive to verbal commands. These three patients were treated postoperatively and, in addition to the barbiturate coma, had arterial hypertension induced. One perished from meningitis, another from an intracerebral hematoma. The third survived but is disabled.

In three patients where hypothermia to core temperatures of 30-32°C was used in conjunction with barbiturate coma profound metabolic alterations resulted characterized by massive third space losses, pulmonary insufficiency and renal failure.

Discussion

The prognosis in patients with vasospasm who deteriorate on an ischemic basis to the point of being unresponsive with no purposeful motor response is uniformly unfavorable. In only seven of the 11 patients studied in this series could the effectiveness of the barbiturate therapy be evaluated. Two patients died during treatment, one from rebleeding and one from exsanguination. Two patients died after being emerged from the coma but too soon to be able to determine the results of therapy. One perished from a malfunctioning ventriculostomy and the other from an unknown cause.

Of the seven patients in whom a judgement could be made, therapy failed in four. Three of these died from massive infarction and uncontrollable intracranial hypertension while in barbiturate coma and one died ten days after being emerged but was improved only minimally. Dramatic improvement was seen in three patients. While this improvement was encouraging, all three were treated post-operatively and the improvement may have been related to factors other than the barbiturate therapy, such as induced arterial hypertension.

Summary

Hypothermia seems contra-indicated in conjunction with barbiturate coma. Barbiturate coma therapy is of assistance in decreasing intracranial hypertension in patients with vasospasm after SAH. This modality may be effective in preventing infarction in patients with a severe degree of vasospasm but therapy must be initiated before irreversible changes in the brain have occurred. A further trial of barbiturate coma in severely ill patients with vasospasm is warranted, but therapy should commence at an earlier stage than in this series.

References

1. Kassell NF, Peerless SJ, Reilly PL (1976) ICP, aneurysms and subarachnoid hemorrhage. In: Beks JWF, Bosch DA, Brock M (eds) Intracranial Pressure III. Springer, Berlin Heidelberg New York p. 147

2. Marshall LF, Bruce DA, Bruno L et al (1977) The role of intracranial pressure monitoring and barbiturate therapy in malignant intracranial hypertension. Case report. J Neurosurg 47:481-485

3. Shapiro HM, Galindo A, Wyte SR et al (1973) Rapid intra-operative reduction of intracranial pressure with thiopentone. Br J Anaesthesiol 45:1057-1062

EFFECT OF MEGADOSE STEROIDS ON ICP IN TRAUMATIC COMA

L.H.PITTS AND J.V.KAKTIS

Introduction

There is general agreement that corticosteroids diminish cerebral edema in a variety of central nervous system pathological states, including malignant brain tumors and brain abscesses. In the hope that such edema reduction also occurs in head injured patients, corticosteroids are widely used in patients with craniocerebral trauma, although no well-controlled clinical trials have been conducted to demonstrate unequivocally the benefit of steroids in this setting.

If corticosteroid administration were to improve outcome after head injury, steroids might accomplish this by reducing the formation of edema fluid or enhancing its resolution and, secondarily, lowering intracranial pressure (ICP). In this study, we have examined this possible effect of steroids on ICP.

Materials and Methods

Head injured adults admitted to San Francisco General Hospital, who were comatose on admission or who lapsed into coma for 6 or more hours, were prospectively randomized into one of 3 steroid regimens: placebo, low-dose (16mg of dexamethasone/day), or megadose (24mg of dexamethasone/day). Steroids were given for a maximum of 7 days with a 5 day taper, or until patients were awake and oriented. Comatose patients did not follow commands or open their eyes in response to pain, and made no verbal response. Daily neurological examinations were recorded as well as any complications that arose. ICP was monitored after placement of a subdural or intraventricular catheter shortly following admission. Patients were studied by CT scan or angiogram, and surgical decompression of mass lesions was performed when clinically indicated. Management in an intensive care unit included osmotherapy and intubation with controlled ventilation to maintain ICP below 25 torr. An estimated mean ICP was recorded hourly. Subsequently these values were grouped in 6 hour blocks starting from the time of admission, and mean values calculated for each time period. Subjects who were monitored for less than 12 hours were excluded from analysis. Values after 72 hours were not analyzed because only a small portion of our patient population required continued monitoring after that time.

Results

Mean ICP values were analyzed for 76 patients admitted between February, 1977, and March, 1979. The study groups were remarkably similar in age distribution, physical exam findings, and frequency of mass lesions (Figure 1).

There were no differences among the groups when 6 hour ICP averages at any time during the first 72 hours after head injury were compared (Figure 2). The mean value among the groups ranged from 13 to 25 torr, but were within 7 torr during most intervals. Analysis of variance by ranks (KRUSKAL-WALLIS test) showed no statistically significant difference between the groups (α = 0.05).

Steroid administration did not increase the complication rate (Figure 3), except to produce hyperglycemia in approximately 20% of patients in both groups. Diabetes insipidus or inappropriate antidiuretic hormone secretion was more frequent in the low-dose group, although this increase was not statistically significant (x^2 = 4.0597, p>0.10). Central nervous system infections occurred in 3 patients receiving magadose steroids, which was not a significant increase by a log-likelihood test (G = 4.159, p>0.10).

Discussion

It has been hypothesized that glucocorticoids affect the course of head injury by reducing associated cerebral edema and subsequent secondary injury. Previous work has indicated that administration of steroids produces lower ICP values and decreases the frequency of plateau waves within the first 48 hours of use.

KULLBERG (4) examined the effects of corticosteroids on ICP in a small number of patients including 2 with head injury. Using early pretreatment levels as the control with which to compare her observations, she found a modest reduction of mean pressure values as well as a reduction in the pattern of plateau waves that she felt resulted from steroid administration. BROCK (1) attempted to quantify changes in ICP distribution induced by dexamethasone in a series of 12 patients with supratentorial mass lesions. Again, comparisons made between the pretreatment and post-treatment values in the same subject showed a significant reduction in the range of ICP fluctuation and a shift toward lower pressure values in the entire series after corticosteroids were administered. Neither of these studies excluded the possibility that this improvement in ICP was a function of time only and unrelated to steroid use.

In a study that varied steroid therapy by year (i.e., no dexamethasone the first year, 16mg of dexamethasone per day the second year, 96mg per day on Days 1 and 3, and 48mg per day on Days 2 and 4 the third year), GOBIET (3) investigated the effects of dexamethasone on the number of high (50 torr or more) pressures in the respective study groups. He found minimal differences between placebo and low dose groups, with significantly fewer ICP increases in the high dose dexamethasone group. This information is difficult to interpret because of the study design and high level of ICP that he chose to examine.

MILLER and LEECH (4) examined ventricular fluid pressure (VFP) and volume-pressure response (VPR) in 7 patients with elevated ICP from a variety of conditions who received beta-methasone for a 24 hour period. Using each patient as his or her own control, they found a significant reduction in the VPR, but no difference in the VFP after 24 hours of therapy. This study seems to indicate that corticosteroids may reduce ICP elevations, although the study's small patient population and choice of controls makes it difficult to interpret.

In our investigation, mean ICP values in all groups decreased over time, in agreement with the findings of previous investigators (1,2,3,4). In patients not receiving steroids, mean ICP values decreased from 27 to 14 torr over 48 hours. This same pattern was observed in both steroid groups (from 26 to 19 torr in "low dose" patients and from 17 to 13 torr in "megadose" patients), and was not significantly different from the placebo group. The minor differences among the study groups represent random variation during repeated testing under steady state conditions.

Summary

Intracranial hypertension in head injured patients falls toward normal values in the first 72 hours after injury if no steroids have been used or if megadose or conventional dose steroids have been used. Improvement in intracranial hypertension previously attributed to steroids is probably the result of improving brain function or intracranial volume adjustments in response to brain trauma, which occurs in the first few days after injury.

The question of efficacy of steroids in the treatment of craniocerebral trauma remains under investigation. Glucocorticoids may improve outcome in head injured patients, but such a benefit is not a result of improved ICP control in patients with traumatic coma.

References

1. Brock M, Wiegand H, Zillig C, Zywietz C, Mock P, Dietz H (1976) The effect of dexamethasone on intracranial pressure in patients with supratentorial tumors. In: Pappius HM, Feindel W. (eds) Dynamics of Brain Edema. Springer, Berlin Heidelberg New York, p. 330

2. Gobiet W (1976) The influence of various doses of dexamethasone on intracranial pressure in patients with severe head injury. In: Pappius HM, Feindel W (eds) Dynamics of Brain Edema. Springer, Berlin Heidelberg New York, p. 351

3. Gobiet W, Bock WJ, Liesegang J, Grote W (1976) Treatment of acute cerebral edema with a high dose of dexamethasone. In: Beks JWF, Bosch DA, Brock M (eds) Intracranial Pressure III. Springer, Berlin Heidelberg New York, p. 231

4. KULLBERG G (1976) Clinical studies on the effect of corticosteroids on the ventricular fluid pressure. In: Reulen HJ, Schurman K (eds) Steroids and Brain Edema. Springer, Berlin Heidelberg New York p. 253

5. Miller JD, Leech P (1975) Effects of mannitol and steroid therapy on intracranial volume-pressure relationships in patients. J Neurosurg 42:274-281

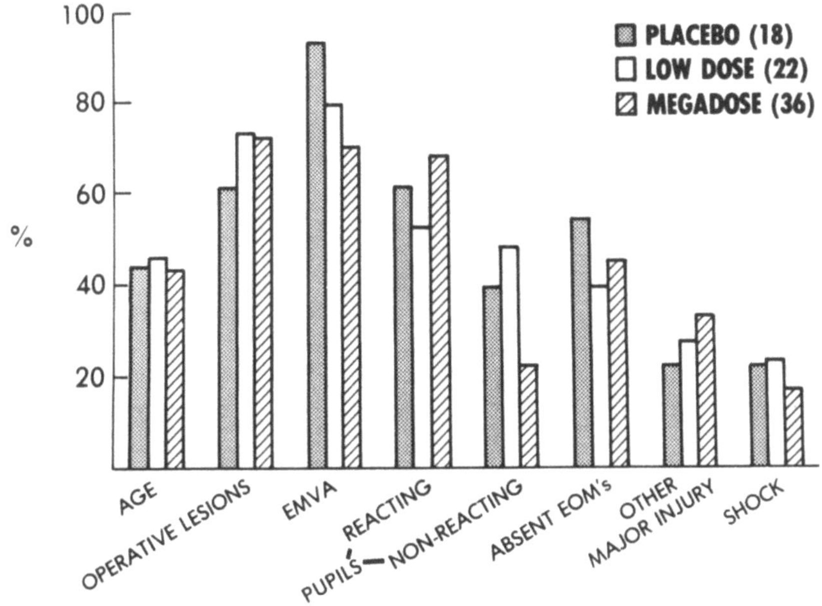

Figure 1.
Characteristics of the study population by steroid group showing comparable study groups.

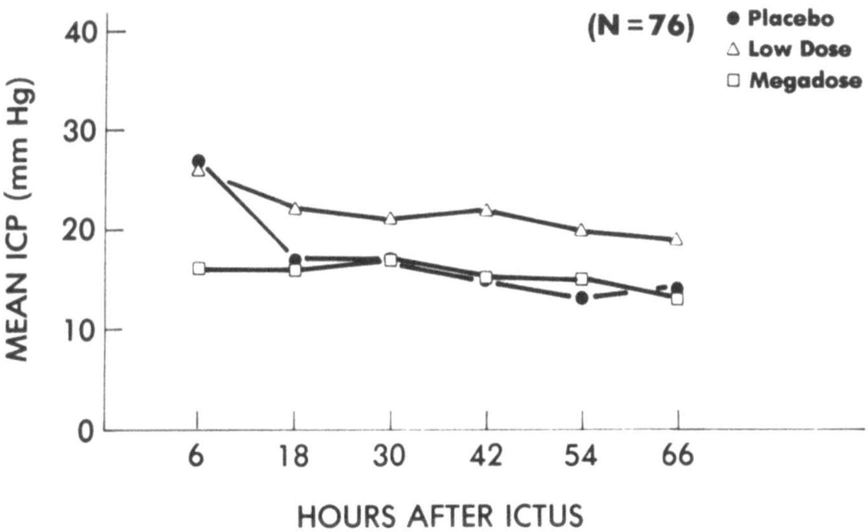

Figure 2.
Plot of 6 hour mean ICP values at 12 hour intervals for each steroid group. The trend for ICP to decrease over time is not limited to those patients who received dexamethasone.

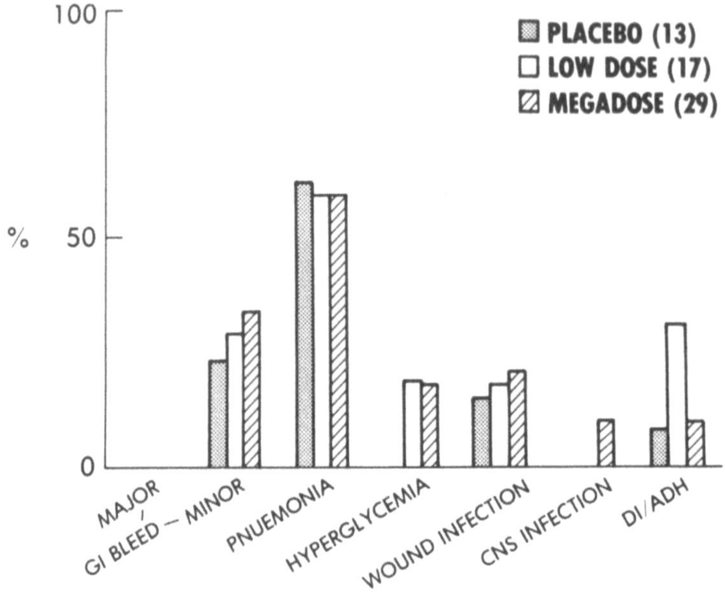

Figure 3.
Distribution of complications in the study groups. There is no significant increase in the complication rate in patients receiving steroids.

INFLUENCE OF LARGE DOSES OF STEROIDS ON BRAIN COMPRESSION, EPIDURALLY

A. SCHETTINI AND E. K. WALSH

Introduction

This study was designed to investigate the efficacy of large doses of glucocorticosteroids (Dexamethasone) in reversing the stiffening of the intracranial system as induced by a prolonged mechanical loading.

Materials and Methods

The procedure to quantitate the influence of Dexamethasone on brain mechanical properties, in particular, the elastic response properties (brain stiffness) was: 1) to measure the response properties of each animal under normal conditions; 2) to then cause a change in the stiffness of the brain tissue and administer the steroid; and 3) to reevaluate the response properties. The study required three days of testing for each animal. Twenty-four dogs were chronically implanted for measurement of intracranial pressure (ICP) and brain mechanical properties, epidurally (1). The first day of testing, the third day after implant, we measured the normal mechanical response properties. These included the 1) pressure test; 2) elastic response test; and 3) pressure relaxation test. The pressure test served to identify the positions of the subpial region (2). The elastic response test provided a quantitative measure of the subpial brain tissue response properties (3). The pressure relaxation test gave a qualitative evaluation of the anelastic behavior of the response. Following this the subpial region was subjected to an extended creep response test to cause an increase in the stiffness of the brain tissue beneath the transducer. A weight of approximately 300gms was applied to the region through the transducer core shaft for 45-50 minutes while cerebral perfusion pressure was kept at or below 45mmHg. On the second day of testing, the change in stiffness was measured by the pressure test and elastic response tests (3). After these tests, the Control Group dogs received no treatment, while the Experimental Group dogs were randomly placed on Dexamethasone, 4mg/kg, given I.m. in three equally divided doses, i.e. q8h. On the following day, the tests were repeated to quantify the effects of steroids and the progression of stiffening. Of 24 implants, 8 Control and 5 Experimental dogs succumbed during the three day tests, as a result of coma and major neurological deficits, including brain herniation. The present study includes 4 control and 7 experimental dogs.

Results

1. Effects of the extended compression: This caused, 1) inconsistent cerebrospinal fluid (CSF) pressure response, epidurally; 2) anomalous response behavior in the mechanical response tests, for example, a lowering of pressure during the insertion phase of an elastic response test, and changes in the anelastic behavior; and 3) measured increase in the parameters identifying brain stiffness (Figure 1).

II. Effects of 24 hours of Dexamethasone treatment: 1) a recovery of the earlier anomalous response noted in the mechanical response test; 2) a normalization of brain viscoelastic behavior in several, but not all, of the animals tested (Figure 2); 3) the elastic response parameters indicated a continued increase (above normal) of the brain stiffness. This correlated with the post mortem findings of swollen congested brain.

Discussion

The anomalous response behavior reflected the brain deformation which affected the transducer coplanarity. The changes in viscoelastic properties (pressure relaxation) and the increase in the elastic parameters (stiff brain) suggested a swollen congested brain and was confirmed at the autopsy. The first 24 hours of large dose steroid therapy abolished the anomalous response but was ineffective in reversing the increased brain stiffness. This may be interpreted to mean that: 1) either steroids are ineffective against a traumatized congested brain; or 2) normalization of the mechanical response properties occurs in two phases. The first, qualitative is followed by a second phase of slow normalization of the quantitative changes in the mechanical parameters. The tendency of brain viscoelastic behavior (pressure relaxation) to normalize in the majority of dogs, strongly supports the second hypothesis.

Summary

Creep compression consistently produced a stiffening of the brain and anomalous response behavior. The 24 hours of a large dose of Dexamethasone normalized the response but failed to reverse the increased brain stiffness.

References

1. Walsh EK, Schettini A (1977) On measurement of brain elastic response in vivo. Am J Physiol 232:R27-30

2. Schettini A, Walsh EK (1974) Experimental identification of the subarachnoid and subpial compartments by intracranial pressure measurements. J Neurosurg 40:609-616

3. Walsh EK, Schettini A, Parameters for identifying brain response properties in vivo. (In ICP IV)

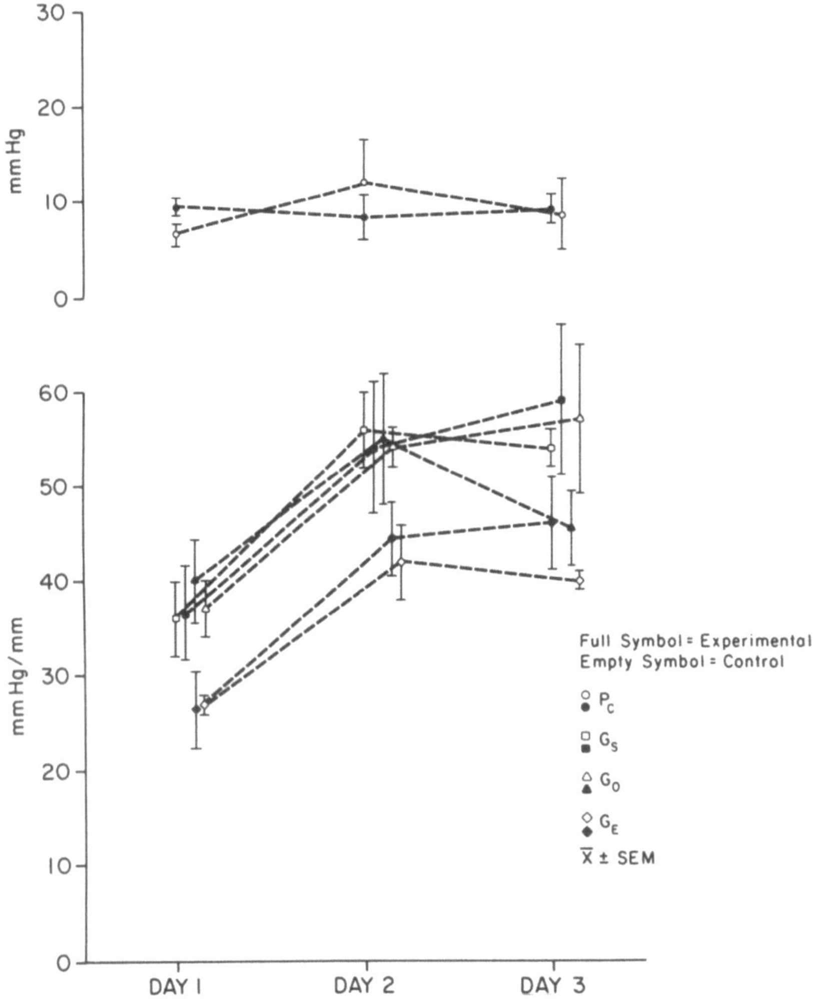

Figure 1.
The upper part of the figure is the subarachnoid CSF pressure (mmHg) at the vault. It was derived from the Pressure Test done on that day. The lower parts of the figure are the measured elastic parameters in the controls and in the steroid treated dogs. The ordinate here is the Pressure-Depth Ratio (mmHg/mm). The abscissa is the day of measurement.

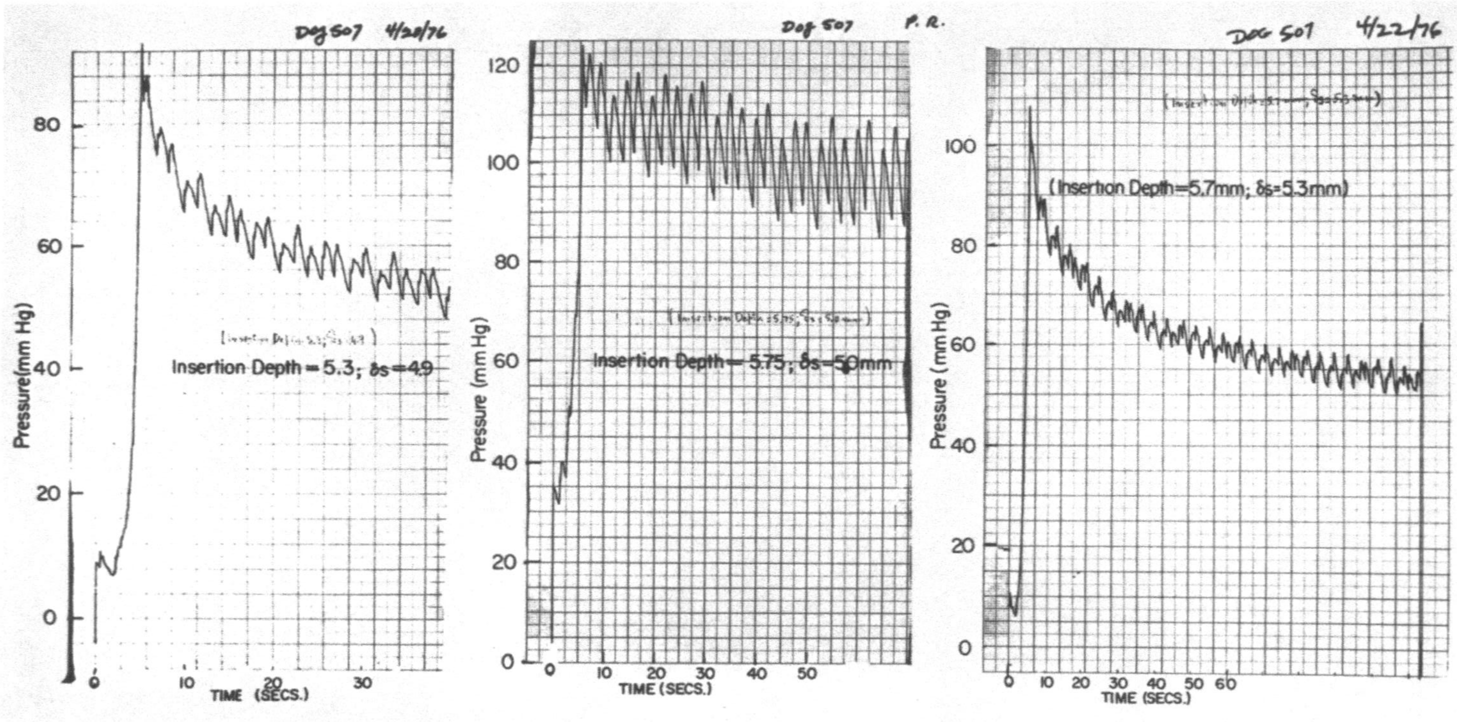

Figure 2.
Retrieved data of pressure relaxation response (left to right), under normal condition, after creep compression and 24 hours after Dexamethasone (4mg/kg) treatment. Note the amplitude of pulsations and lack of relaxation after creep compression.

MANNITOL RESPONSE AND HISTOGRAM ANALYSIS IN RAISED ICP

E. FERRER, F. VILA, AND F. ISAMAAT

Introduction

For many years, drugs producing a rapid decrease of the intracranial pressure (ICP), have been the standard management and indeed an important step forward in neurosurgical patients' therapy. The effects of osmotic diuretics are well known. Mannitol is, no doubt, the one that has attracted most attention.

WISE, in 1961, proved its convenience over other osmotic diuretics like urea; thereafter a number of papers have ascertained this fact (5,7). The purpose of this work is to analyze the ICP response to Mannitol given to 22 of our patients.

Materials and Methods

We have measured the epidural ICP in 22 patients after placing a fiber optic sensor through a frontal burrhole. Simultaneously, in all of them, a histogram was drawn using a frequency analyzer. After an initial recording for one or two hours, a single dose of Mannitol 20% was given intravenously in 5 to 10 minutes. Dosage ranged from 0.25 to 2gm/kg. 1gm/kg was given to 15 of our patients. 4 patients received 0.5gm/kg and 2 received 0.25gm/kg. One last patient received 2gm/kg.

Histograms were made each hour, during the next 4 or 5 hours. Relevant data was: Initial pressure (P_o), Minimal pressure (P_{min}), Total time of effectiveness and Rebound effect. Special emphases were placed in mode, median and range and hourly translation of these histogram parameters. The different patients' pathologies were: 10 malignant gliomas, 3 meningiomas, 4 metastases and other malignant tumors, and 5 with severe head injuries (focal or diffuse brain contusion).

Results

The different results obtained are summarized in Table 1.

Discussion

In accordance with previous observations (2,5,7), we found that the minimal pressure was reached 25 to 35 minutes after Mannitol infusion. ICP was below the initial level during the first two hours. All our cases showed an ascendent ICP line during the third hour. A rebound effect was found in 31.8% of patients. During the fourth and fifth hours the ICP tended to reach the initial levels once again. Regarding the range of the histograms, during the first two hours, we saw a range decrease in 17 of our patients, that is to say, stabilization of the recording due, we presume, to the effect of Mannitol on the patients' elastance. The range was altered again during the third hour, occasionally being

Table 1

NUMBER OF CASES TOTAL NUMBER: 22	MALIGNANT GLIOMAS 10	MENINGIOMAS 3	OTHER MALIGNANT TUMOURS 4	SEVERE BRAIN CONTUSION 5
PREVIOUS MEAN ICP: Po (mmHg)	33,5	22,5	38,6	44,8
MEAN TIME OF MINIMAL PRESSURE	34,4'	26,6'	35'	35,6'
MINIMAL PRESSURE Pm (mmHg)	18,8	16,3	20,6	24,7
DECREASE ICP AVERAGE: Po-Pm	43.88%	27.56%	53.37%	55.13%
REBOUND NUMBER OF CASES	4	0	1	2
MEAN EFFECTIVENESS TIME (minutes)	133'	118'	120'	145'

superior to initial level. Obviously, the stabilizing pressure effect was more pronounced in patients with unstable initial tracing. The ICP pattern was different with the diverse lesions: a marked reduction of ICP was seen in severe head injuries and in metastasis; on the other hand, only a slight decrease of ICP followed meningioma. The rebound effect, however, did not depend on the dosage, where as the initial pressure reduction was closely related to the amount of drug given. Despite our reduced number of cases, and after taking into account the minimal pressure reached, total time of effectiveness and the apparition of rebound effect, we believe that optimal dosage would be 1gm/kg.

Summary

The ICP response to a single dose of Mannitol 20% was studied in 22 patients. For 4 or 5 hours we registered the ICP line and we made hourly histograms after the initiation of Mannitol treatment. The minimal pressure was reached in 25 to 35 minutes after Mannitol infusion, unrelated to the dosage of Mannitol used. The mean total time of effectiveness was 130 minutes. A rebound effect was seen in 31.8% of the cases. The histograms showed stabilizing recordings for the first two hours, followed by a return to the initial level. Finally, the third hour is decisive due to the instabilizaton of the tracing and the possibility of rebound effect.

References

1. Kullberg G, Sundbarg G (1976) Reduction of raised ICP following infusion of Mannitol. A Review of clinical recordings. In: Beks JWF, Bosch DA, Brock M (eds) Intracranial Pressure III. Springer, Berlin Heidelberg New York, p. 224

2. Lundberg N (1960) Continuous recording and control of ventricular fluid pressure in neurosurgical practice. Acta Neurol Scand 36: Suppl 149:1-193

3. Marshall LF, Smith RW, Rauscher LA, Shaprio HM (1978) Mannitol dose requirements in brain injured patients. J Neurosurg 48:169-172

4. Miller JD, Leech P (1975) Effects of Mannitol and steroid therapy on intracranial volume-pressure relationships in patients. J Neurosurg 42:274-281

5. Shenkin HA, Goluboff B, Haft H (1962) The use of Mannitol for the reduction of intracranial pressure in intracranial surgery. J Neurosurg 19:897-901

6. Szewczykowski J, Slivka S, et al (1975) Computer-assisted analysis of intraventricular pressure after mannitol administration. J Neurosurg 43:136-141

7. Wise BL, Chater N (1962) The value of hypertonic mannitol solution in decreasing brain mass and lowering cerebrospinal fluid pressure. J Neurosurg 19:1038-1043

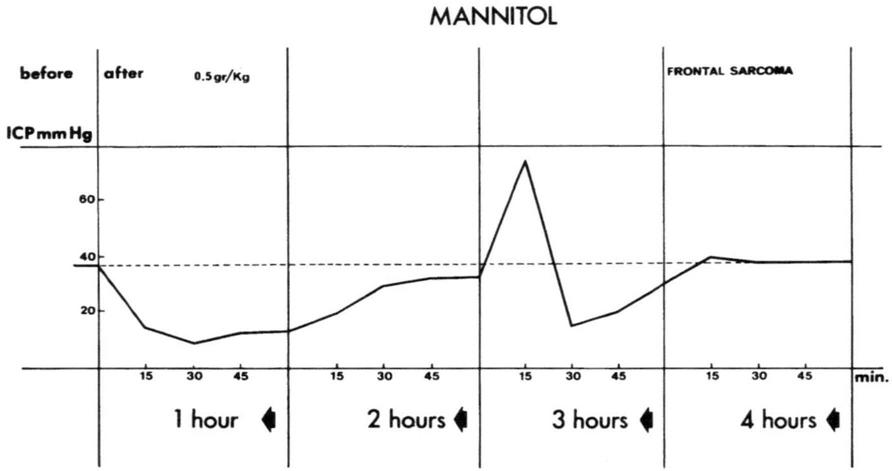

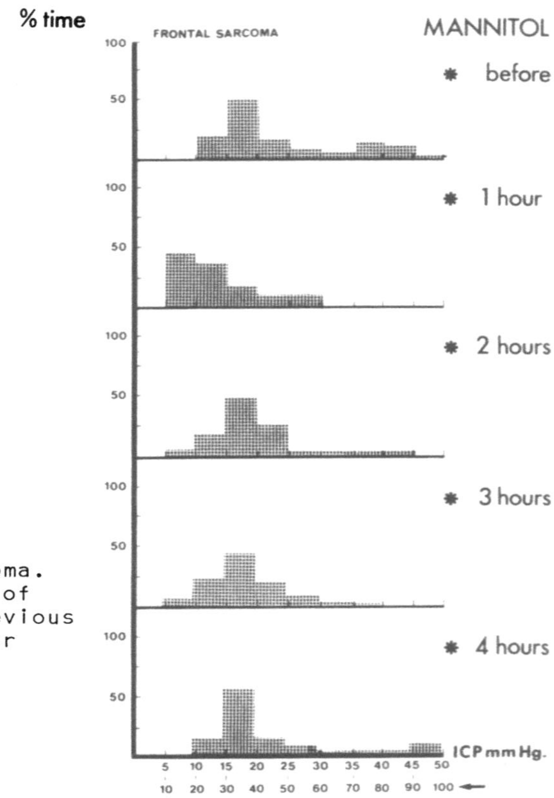

Figure I.
Theoretical mean pressure from a patient suffering a frontal sarcoma. Notice the rebound effect appeared in the third hour. Total time of effectiveness was two hours. Histogram series: Wide range in previous histogram and left translation of mode and median during first hour after treatment.

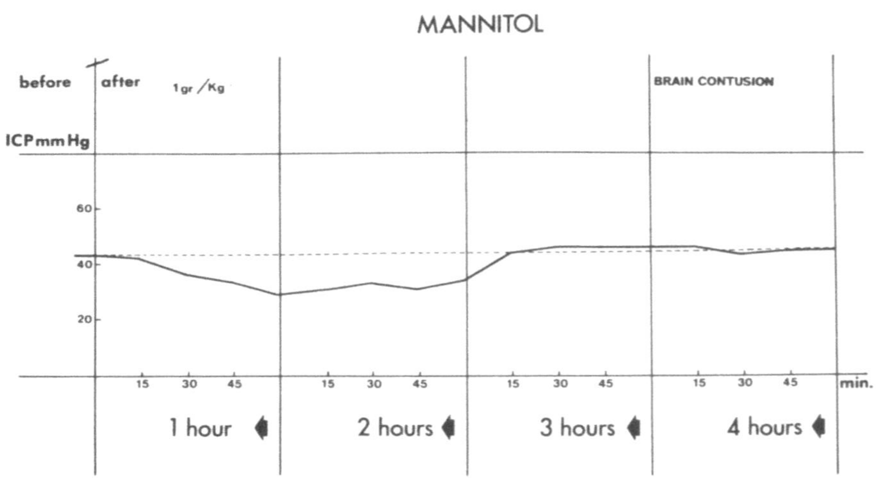

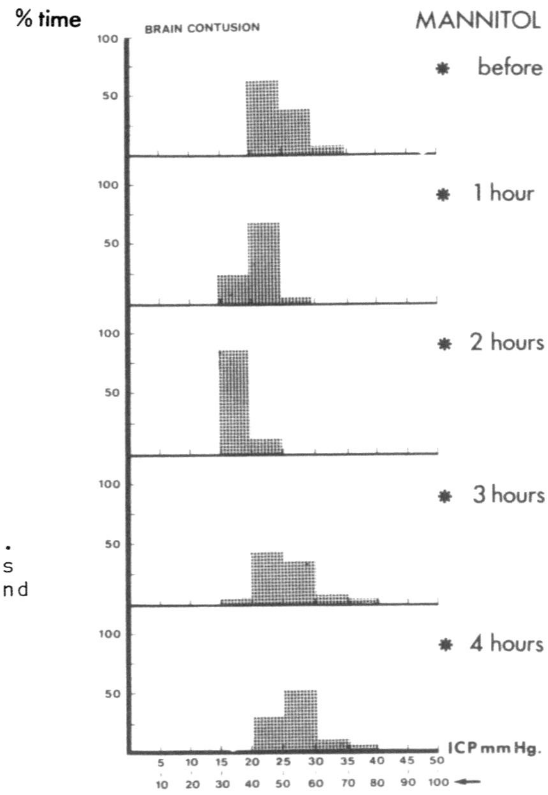

Figure 2.
Focal brain contusion. Total time of effectiveness of 135 minutes. Slight rebound effect occurred in the third hour. Histogram series shows a reduction of range during the second hour, and clear rebound effect since third hour.

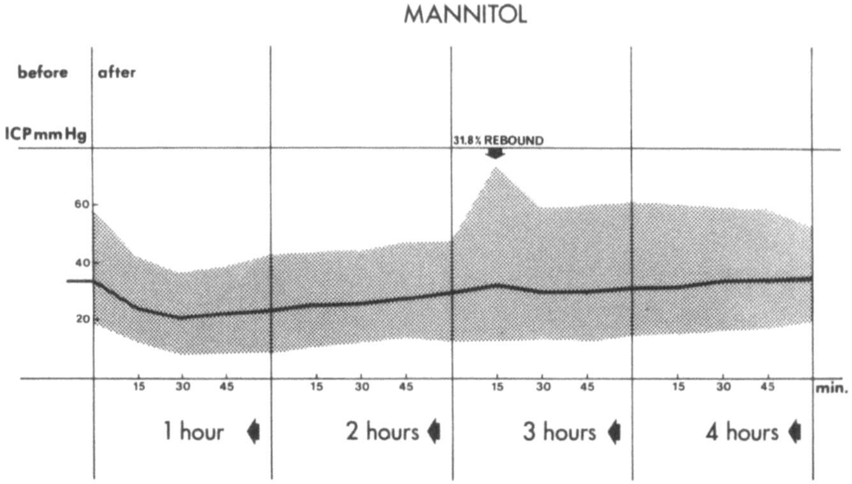

Figure 3.
Chart summarized all the responses observed. Continuous line represents mean values of mean pressures. The shadowed area includes all the values from the different responses. It is the dispersion area. Upper and lower limits of this zone are the most extreme responses.

METHODOLOGY FOR THE CONTROL OF INTRACRANIAL PRESSURE WITH HYPERTONIC MANNITOL

H.E.JAMES

Introduction

Hypertonic agents have been successfully employed in the management of intracranial pressure (ICP) for many years (2). There is in the literature information regarding the administration of the agent via intravenous infusions (4) rather than by bolus administrations (5). Arguments have been put forth in favor of small frequent dosages (3) over large less frequent bolus administrations. The objective of this presentation is to demonstrate several methods that are available to administer hypertonic mannitol to control ICP.

Materials and Methods

Sixty patients whose ages range from 1 to 73 years with elevated ICP (25 torr or more for 3 minutes or longer) form part of this study. All had ICP continuously monitored by a subarachnoid screw or an intraventricular cannula (1). All patients received a bolus administration of 20% mannitol (dosage 0.18-2.5 gm/kg/dose). Eighteen of these patients who had subsequent elevations of ICP (>25 torr for 3 or more minutes) then underwent a continuous infusion of a 20% solution of mannitol to control ICP (2-20gm/kg/total, 6 to 100 hour period), and the infusion discontinued when ICP was persistently low. A response to hypertonic mannitol is defined as a reduction in ICP of more than 10% of control values.

Results

Of the 120 bolus administrations of mannitol in 60 patients, there was a reduction of ICP in 113 administrations, with a maximum low 44 minutes (range 18 to 120 minutes), from the initiation of the bolus. In the 14 bolus administrations with a dosage under 1gm/kg/dose, there was a failure to reduce ICP in 6. In 106 bolus administrations with a dosage of 1 gm/kg or more, there was a reduction of ICP in all but one trial (Table 1). In 18 patients there was a return to pretreatment ICP levels or higher within two hours following the bolus administration of mannitol, and in these a continuous infusion of mannitol controlled pressure waves and maintained ICP below 25 torr in 16. The total dosage required was 2-20gm/kg. Serum osmolality levels ranged from 276-354 mosm/liter in 28 patients who received bolus mannitol, and 276-301 mosm/liter in the patients with continuous infusions.

We conclude that a hypertonic mannitol bolus will reduce ICP when administered in a dosage ranging from 1.0 to 2.5gm/kg. If careful assessment and judicious replacement of fluids is maintained, continuous mannitol infusion has a definite role in patient management.

Table 1. Dosage and response in 120 administrations of hypertonic mannitol (*)

Dose (Gm/Kg)	No. of Administrations	Responded (**)	Did Not Respond	Percent Response
0.18	1	0	1	0
0.25	4	1	3	25.0
0.5	9	7	2	77.7
1.0	86	85	1	98.8
1.5	5	5	0	100.0
2.0	12	12	0	100.0
2.5	3	3	0	100.0

(*) in 60 patients.

(**) reduction in ICP of more than 10% of control value.

References

1. James HE, Bruno L, Shapiro HM, Levitt JD, Aidinis S, Langfitt TW (1976) Methodology for intraventricular and subarachnoid continuous recording of intracranial pressure in clinical practice. Acta Neurochir 33:45-51

2. James HE, Langfitt TW, Kumar VS, Ghostine SY (1977) Treatment of intracranial hypertension. Acta Neurochir 36:189-200

3. Marshall LF, Smith RW, Rauscher LA, Shapiro HM (1978) Mannitol dose requirements in brain-injured patients. J Neurosurg 48:169-172

4. Scewczykowski J, Slivka S, Kunicki A, Korsach-Slivka J, Dziduszko J, Dytko P, Augustyniak B (1975) Computer-assisted analyses of intraventricular pressure after mannitol administration. J Neurosurg 43:136-141

5. Troupp H, Valtonen S, Vapalahti M (1971) Intraventricular pressure after administration of dehydrating agents to severely brain injured patients: Is there a rebound phenomenon? Acta Neuroshir 24:89-95

EFFECT OF INFUSION RATE OF GLYCEROL, MANNITOL AND UREA ON REGIONAL BRAIN DEHYDRATION IN THE RAT

S.R.NELSON AND C.A.CONRY

Introduction

Hyperosmotic diuretics continue to be used in patients where rapid, predictable brain dehydration is essential; however, short duration of action and side effects limit their use. Optimal infusion rates of these agents may extend the duration of action of these agents. In this report the results of studies correlating infusion rate and brain dehydration are presented. Normal rats were used because, in injured brain, osmotic diuretics appear to dehydrate those areas with normal capillary permeability (1).

Materials and Methods

Female Wistar rats were anesthetized with pentobarbital and after the insertion of a venous catheter, osmotic diuretics were infused into the animal with an infusion pump. Glycerol and urea were given at both 33 and 16 mmole/kg doses while mannitol was given at 16mmole/kg. The rats were decapitated at intervals after the drug infusion and the brain was removed and divided into 4 coronal sections. The sections (3 mm thick) were placed under kerosene to prevent drying while samples were dissected for density measurement. The specific gravity (sp gr) of six brain areas was determined using a continuous gradient column made with bromobenzene and kerosene (3).

Results

Regional differences in brain dehydration: The study in Figure 1 shows the decrease in tissue volume in 6 areas of rat brain after drug infusions for 30 min and decapitation 30 min later. High doses of urea and glycerol (33 mmole/kg) caused the greatest dehydration in all 6 areas of brain (5 to 9% volume decrease). At a lower dose, 16 mmole/kg, urea appeared more effective than glycerol in removing H_2O from cortex, thalamus, hippocampus and caudate, but in cerebellum and brainstem the drugs were equally effective (Figure 1). For all three agents used, thalamus and caudate showed the greatest dehydration when the infusion period was 30 min and decapitation occurred 30 min later (Figure 1). This regional selectivity was much less when mannitol was used; mannitol produced a uniform dehydration with a percent volume decrease of about 1.5 to 2% for the six areas studied.

While caudate and thalamus showed greatest dehydration with a 30 min infusion, this was not the case at different infusion rates. When urea (33 mmole/kg) was given over a 5 min period, brainstem had the most rapid and largest volume decrease (Figure 2).

Infusion rate and brain dehydration: Different infusion periods were used to determine how infusion rate affects brain dehydration. When urea(33 mmole/kg) was infused for 5, 30 and 60 min, the maximum percent volume decrease was about 6% (Figure 2). For these three infusion rates, the density of the samples from all four areas of brain had returned to near control levels by 180 min (Figure 2). Similar results occurred when glycerol and mannitol were used (data not shown).

The rehydrationof tissue occurred in spite of a sustained elevation in serum osmolality. When urea (33 mmole/kg) was infused for 30 min, the serum osmolality increased 37 mosmoles/l, from 292 to 329, at 30 min and remained at near this level for 6 hours.

Discussion

Although greater dehydration occurred in caudate and thalamus than in other areas after a 30 min urea infusion, this regional selectivity varied with infusion rate. At infusion rates of 5 and 30 min, brainstem dehydrated more rapidly than the other tissues and tended to remain high in the animals infused for 5 min. Since brainstem has a relatively large amount of white matter, it may be that there is less resistance to H_2O movement in the intercellular spaces, along fiber tracts, as has been described for the spread of edema fluid through white matter (2).

For infusion periods from 5 through 60 min, there was no indication of altered duration of tissue dehydration. In all cases rehydration had occurred at 180 min. With a 180 min infusion (urea, 33 mmole/kg), the dehydration response was delayed and of marginal effectiveness. This longer infusion period represents an infusion of 0.18 mmole/kg per min. Increasing the infusion to 0.28 mmole/kg per min caused progressive dehydration of all brain regions; brainstem volume decrease was 4% at the end of 3 hrs (data not shown). If the dose is further increased to 0.56 mmole/kg per min, brainstem dehydration reached 10% volume decrease in 3 hrs. These findings indicate that brain dehydration can be extended with continuous infusions, limited only by the side effects of the accumulated drugs.

Summary

Thirty min. infusions of glycerol and urea were associated with greater dehydration of caudate and thalamus than cortex, brainstem, cerebellum and hippocampus. The duration of infusion (5, 30 or 60 min) did not influence the duration of dehydration; rehydration occurred in 3 hrs. An infusion of urea (33 mmole/kg) for 180 min resulted in minimal brain dehydration which was slow in onset. For effective and rapid brain dehydration in the rat, the minimum dose for urea is about 0.28 mmole/kg per min.

References

1. Clasen RA, Cooke PM, Pandolfe S, Carnecki G, Bryar G (1965) Hypertonic urea in experimental cerebral edema. Arch Neurol 12:424-434

2. Klatzo I (1968) Aspects of the blood-brain barrier in brain edema. Clin Neurosurg 16:472-473

3. Nelson SR, Mantz ML, Maxwell JS (1971) Use of specific gravity in the measurement of cerebral edema. J Appl Physiol 30:268-271

Work supported by NIH Grant NS 14390.

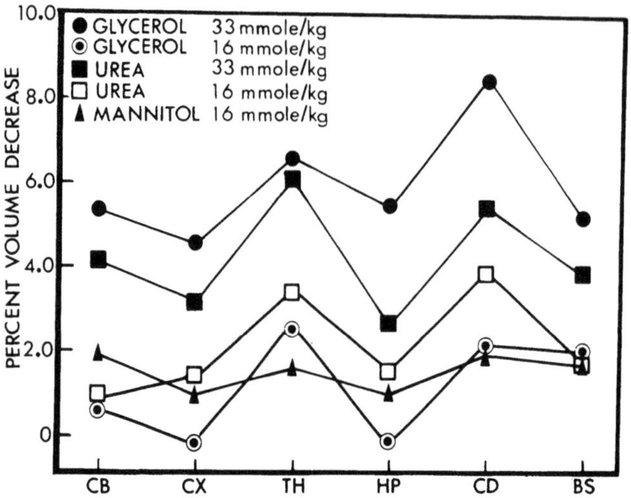

Figure 1.
Rats were infused for 30 min with glycerol, urea and mannitol and decapitated 60 min after the infusion was started. The brains were removed and the density of the following regions was determined: cerebellum (CB), cortex (CX), thalamus (TH), hippocampus (HP), caudate (CD) and brainstem (BS). Each point is the mean percent volume decrease for samples from 3 to 5 rats.

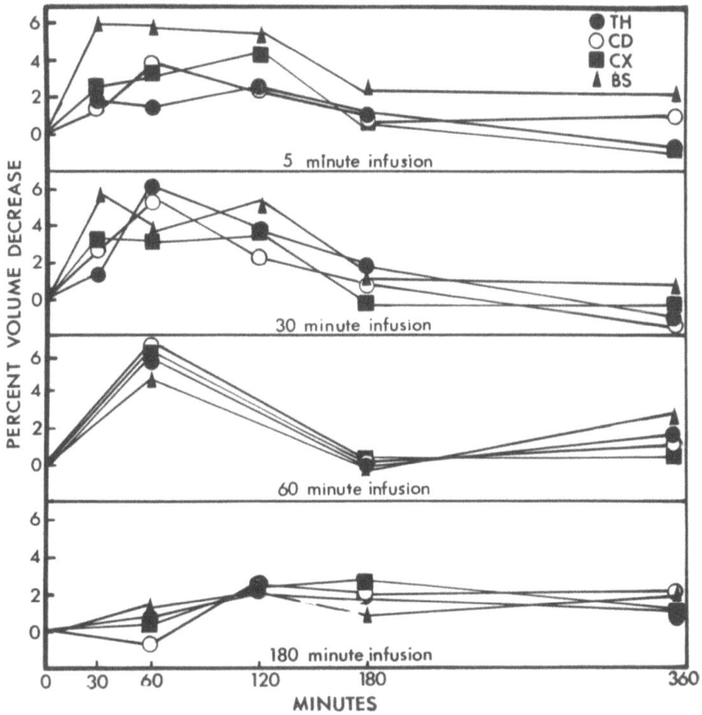

Figure 2.
Rats were infused with urea (33 mmole/kg) for periods of 5, 30, 60 and 180 min. The rats were decapitated at intervals after the infusions and the density of samples from thalamus (TH), caudate (CD), cortex (CX) and brainstem (BS) was determined. The volume decrease for these areas was calculated from the difference in density between experimental and control samples. Each point is the mean percent volume decrease for samples from 3 to 5 rats.

THE EFFECTS OF FUROSEMIDE ON CSF DYNAMICS IN PATIENTS WITH PSEUDOTUMOR CEREBRI

F.H.SKLAR, C.W.BEYER,JR., M.RAMANATHAN, AND W.K.CLARK

Introduction

Clinical studies suggest that the potent sulfonamid diuretic furosemide is a useful drug in the management of intracranial hypertension. Parenternal furosemide (1 mg/kg) decreases intracranial pressure (ICP) in patients undergoing neurological surgery (1). Oral furosemide (120 mg/day) in combination with dexamethasone appears to be more effective in reducing peritumoral water content than dexamethasone alone (4). Animal studies indicate the diuretic to be of therapeutic benefit in the treatment of vasogenic cerebral edema related to cortical cold lesions(3) and head trauma(10). Furosemide induced inhibition of cerebrospinal fluid (CSF) production with a concurrent reduction of intraventricular pressure is thought to enhance the clearance of vasogenic edema fluid(7).

A quantitative study of the effects of fuorsemide on CSF dynamics in man has not been reported previously. The present work examines these drug effects in patients with pseudotumor cerebri.

Methods

Net CSF absorptive capacity and resting pressure were determined in four patients with pseudotumor cerebri with the servo-controlled lumbar infusion technique (8). The test determines the arithmetic difference between CSF absorption and formation (A-F) as a linear function of ICP. The slope of the resulting (A-F) versus ICP curve is a measure of the net CSF absorptive capacity measured in cc/min/mmHg. The pressure axis intercept corresponds to the resting pressure.

Eight infusions were done in four patients. Two patients were first studied when symptomatic with headache and papilledema and were re-studied when asymptomatic on oral furosemide. One patient(R.W.) was begun on furosemide 160 mg/day and re-studied after 40 days on the medication. The second patient(S.E.) was re-studied 10 days after the furosemide dose was increased from 160 mg to 320 mg/day. Intravenous furosemide 40mg was administered during four infusion studies in three patients. CSF dynamics were measured before and 30-60 min.after the drug was given.

Results

All of the patients showed a linear relationship between (A-F)and ICP. As reported elsewhere (9),all but one of these patients had abnormally low CSF absorptive capacities with measurements under 0.13cc/min/mmHg.

In the two patients re-studied after treatment with oral furosemide, there were no significant changes in the calculated slope relating(A-F) to ICP.,i.e.,net CSF absorptive capacity. However, in both patients, the curve was shifted to the left on the pressure axis, decreasing the resting pressure P_O. These data are summarized in Table I.

Table 1. Effects of Oral Furosemide on CSF Dynamics

Patient (age, sex)	CSF absorptive capacity (cc/min/mm Hg) Before	After	Probability 2 slopes different*	P_0 (mm Hg) Before	After
S.E. (21 y, F)	0.165 ($p < 0.005$)[+]	0.178 ($p < 0.001$)[+]	$p > 0.5$ (NS[†])	22.7	13.6
R.W. (16 y, M)	0.0778 ($p < 0.001$)	0.0725 ($p < 0.01$)	$p > 0.5$ (NS)	14.9	8.4

* Determined from Student's t test for comparing two slopes.

[+] Significance level of regression slope calculation.

[†] NS, not significant.

Table 2. Effects of Parenteral Furosemide 40 mg on CSF Dynamics

Patient (age, sex)	CSF absorptive capacity (cc/min/mm Hg) Before	After	Probability 2 slopes different*	P_0 (mm Hg) Before	After
W.A. (45 y, F)	0.0992 ($p < 0.001$)[+]	0.124 ($p < 0.005$)[+]	$p > 0.5$ (NS[†])	9.5	-0.4
W.A. (45 y, F)	0.0610 ($p < 0.002$)	0.110 ($p < 0.001$)	$p < 0.05$	10.0	9.0
J.P. (17 y, F)	0.0609 ($p < 0.001$)	0.0810 ($p < 0.001$)	$p \approx 0.35$ (NS)	7.9	10.2
S.E. (21 y, F)	0.125 ($p < 0.001$)	0.184 ($p < 0.001$)	$p < 0.2$ (NS)	14.4	15.8

* Determined from Student's t test for comparing two slopes.

[+] Significance level of regression slope calculation.

[†] NS, not significant.

On the other hand, the administration of intravenous furosemide in each of four infusion studies resulted in an increased slope value (net CSF absorptive capacity). The magnitude of the slope increases reaches statistical significance in only one of four observations. In three of the four studies, there was little change in P_O, although an impressive reduction of resting pressure was noted in one instance. These results are summarized in Table 2.

In addition, the data from the parenteral furosemide studies were examined with multiple linear regression techniques as to whether the observed changes in CSF dynamics could have been related to drug induced alterations of mean arterial blood pressure or cerebral perfusion pressure. The inclusion of either parameters in the analysis did not improve the multiple correlation coefficients.

Discussion

It is unclear in the literature as to what effect furosemide has on CSF dynamics. From traditional ventriculocisternal perfusion studies,DOMER reported that large doses of intravenous furosemide (20mg/kg) had no effect on CSF production in cats (2).In his experimental protocol, indicator concentrations were measured during three 30-minute sampling periods after administration of the drug, and these results were averaged. Because of the strict requirement of steady state conditions with the ventriculocisternal perfusion technique, it is likely that his experimental design could have missed furosemide induced changes in CSF dynamics. Certainly,the ventriculocisternal perfusion technique is insensitive to rapid or subtle changes in CSF formation.With ventriculocisternal perfusion techniques, McCARTHY and REED showed a reduction of CSF production to 50% control values with intravenous furosemide(4). Similarly, REED noted 50% reductions of cisternal drainage with intravenous furosemide50mg/kg but only small changes in CSF drainage with 10mg/kg(6).

The results of the present study are consistent with a furosemide induced reduction of CSF formation in patients, since a constant inhibitory effect on CSF production would shift the (A-F) versus ICP curve to the left on the pressure axis,not changing the slope. The two patients treated with oral furosemide showed a reduction in resting pressure P_O, with no change in the net CSF absorptive capacity. These findings suggest a drug-related reduction of CSF formation.

On the other hand,the observed slope increased with parenteral furosemide possibly indicate a drug induced pressure-sensitive inhibition of CSF formation with greater inhibition occurring at higher pressures. Slope increases were observed in all four infusion studies, although these changes reach statistical significance in only one case. In a single patient,the resting pressure showed an impressive reduction(9.5 mmHg to 0.4mmHg). Parenteral furosemide appeared to alter favorably CSF dynamics in these studies, but only one with statistical significance. Again,these findings are consistent with furosemide induced reduction of CSF production. Moreover, the mechanisms for action of parenteral furosemide may be more complicated than simple inhibition of the choroid plexus active transport system.

Summary

On the basis of servo-controlled lumbar infusion studies in patients with pseudotumor cerebri, oral furosemide favorably effects CSF dynamics to reduce resting pressure.The infusion data are consistent with a constant inhibitory effect on the CSF formation rate. On the other hand, parenteral furosemide does not consistently reduce resting pressure but appears to increase the net CSF absorptive capacity. A pressure sensitive inhibition of CSF formation could explain these results.

References

1. Cottrell JE, Robustelli A, Post K, Turndorf H (1977) Furosemide- and mannitol-induced changes in intracranial pressure and serum osmolaltiy and electrolytes. Anesthesiol 47:28-30

2. Domer FR (1969) Effects of diuretics on cerebrospinal fluid formation and potassium movement. Exp Neurol 24:54-64

3. Long DM, Maxwell R, Choi KS (1976) A new therapy regimen for brain edema. In: Pappius HM, Feindel W (eds) Dynamics of Brain Edema. Springer, Berlin Heidelberg New York, p. 293

4. McCarthy KD, Reed DJ (1974) The effect of acetazolamide and furosemide on cerebrospinal fluid production and choroid plexus carbonic anhydrase activity. J Pharmacol Exp Therapeutics 189:194-201

5. Meinig G, Aulich A, Wende S, Reulen HJ (1976) The effect of dexamethasone and diuretics on peritumor brain edema: Comparative study of tissue water content and CT. In: Pappius HM, Feindel W (eds) Dynamics of Brain Edema. Springer, Berlin Heidelberg New York, p 301

6. Reed DJ (1969) The effect of furosemide on cerebrospinal fluid flow in rabbits. Arch Int Pharmacodyn 178:324-330

7. Reulen HJ, Graham R, Spatz M, Klatzo I (1977) Role of pressure gradients and bulk flow in dynamics of vasogenic brain edema. J Neurosurg 46:24-35

8. Sklar FH, Beyer CW Jr, Ramanathan M, Elashvili I, Cooper PR, Clark WK (1978) Servo-controlled lumbar infusions: A clinical tool for the determination of CSF dynamics as a function of pressure. Neurosurg 3:170-175

9. Sklar FH, Beyer CW Jr, Ramanathan M, Clark WK (in press) Cerebrospinal fluid dynamics in patients with pseudotumor cerebri. Neurosurg

10. Tornheim PA, McLaurin RL, Sawaya R (1979) Effect of furosemide on experimental traumatic cerebral edema. Neurosurg 4:48-52

EFFECT OF THAM ON ICP, EEG AND TISSUE EDEMA PARAMETERS IN EXPERIMENTAL AND CLINICAL BRAIN EDEMA

M. GAAB, O.E. KNOBLICH, A. SPOHR, H. BONEKE, AND U. FUHRMEISTER

Introduction

In the treatment of brain swelling, it is not only necessary to reduce the elevated intracranial pressure (ICP), which is a symptom, but also to counteract the causal pathogenetic factors, one of which is the lactacidotic local metabolism (1,8). This acidotic disturbance of metabolism and vasoregulation intensifies, ending in fatal elevation of ICP, by penetration of arterial pressure into vasoparalyzed edema (1,8). As THAM (tromethamine, "Tris-buffer"), in contrast to Na-bicarbonate, crosses plasmatic membranes and directly influences intracellular acidosis (7,9), we tested its action in experimental and clinical brain edema.

Materials and Methods

In 25 cats we induced a right hemispheric cold brain injury by applying a cooling stamp (maintained at -73°C) for 4 minutes to the intact dura, following parietal trepanation. The latter was then dosed by a Palacos^R graft. Miniaturized force transducers continuously recorded the epidural pressures (rEP, lEP) over both hemispheres and the cerebellum (posterior brain fossa, pEP) (5). The ventricular (VP, left lateral ventricle), systemic arterial (aP, aorta) and central venous (cvP) pressures were also registered. The bipolar fronto-occipital EEG was continuously evaluated over both hemispheres by FFT (Power spectra, Intertechnique Plurimat S). Total power (1-25 Hz, arbitrary units), power % of α, ϑ, δ-ranges and dominant frequencies (Figure 1b) were calculated. Arterio-venous metabolite differences (AVD) were measured after catheterization of the superior sagittal sinus. On attaining significantly elevated ICP (VP 30mmHg, 1-2.5 hrs after injury), 5 cats were treated with THAM i.v. (app. 5 mmol/kg b.wt.), 5 were infused with 40% sorbitol (5), and 15 untreated cats served as controls.

In rats (12 per group) brain tissue water and electrolyte contents were analyzed 6 hrs (artificially respirated rats) or 24 hrs (those breathing spontaneously) after a cold brain trauma had been induced by a 3 minute application of a stamp at -73°C on right parietal skull. These values, and the survival rates of untreated controls, were compared with those after i.v. therapy with THAM (3.9 mmol/6 hrs), Na-bicarbonate (1.8 mmol/6 hrs), dexamethasone (2mg/6 hrs) or Phenobarbitol (3mg/6 hrs).

Clinically, we investigated the action of THAM (2mmol/kg per dose), in 14 patients with severe head injury, by continuous recording of the ICP with extradurally implanted miniature transducers (4), and evaluation of the EEG by FFT. All patients were respirated.

Results

In the cats, the ICP increased progressively after cold brain injury with marked pressure gradients (Figure 1a). The rEP over the lesion rose more sharply than the lEP and VP. The pED increased slowly. The EEG (Figure

1b) rapidly deteriorated after cooling, especially on the right, then recovered significantly on the left although finally deteriorating with increasing ICP. THAM rapidly, but only transiently, and to varying degrees from cat to cat, lowered the ICP (Figure 1a) without affecting blood osmolality. In contrast to osmotherapy (5), the decrease was more pronounced on the right hemisphere. The EEG progressively improved after THAM (frequency acceleration, increasing α- and decreasing δ-power), even on the right. This improvement outlasted the ICP decrease, unlike osmotherapy (5). The survival time (until isoelectric EEG) was significantly prolonged (234 ± 49 min) compared with controls (160 ± 57 min) and osmotic infusion (205 ± 33 min). The AVD values however, showed no differences to controls, in contrast to operative edema resection (6).

In the rats, THAM improved the water and electrolyte contents of the hemispheres in respirated animals, but in those breathing spontaneously, survival rates were lower (68% controls, 50% after THAM).

Clinically, in collating results from several patients with brain edema, THAM appeared to reduce the ICP (Figure 2a). This effect however, (lower THAM dosage), was not as consistent as in the standardized animal experiment and the decrease not as steep, although longer-lasting. Initially there was a concommitant slight decrease in aP but the ICP remained low despite a subsequent re-increase in aP. The EEG also improved (Figure 2b). During and after infusion, the dominant frequency accelerated, and after the slow frequency decrease following infusion, the Σ-power remained elevated.

Discussion

Since the reports of DOS et al in 1962 (2), which indicated a rapid correction of intracranial hypertension in hypercapnia with THAM, and EWERBECK et al in 1966 (3), which described beneficial effects of THAM in preventing brain damage after severe burns, little attention has been paid to this buffering drug in intracranial hypertension. However, at the last ICP Symposium, AKIOKA et al (1) reported the effect of THAM on decreasing ICP in acute hyperemia after balloon inflation in dogs. Our experiments confirm the efficacy of THAM also in cases of proven clinical and experimental brain edema. The decrease in ICP appears to be due to counteraction of vasoparalysis by rapid buffering of the acidosis in the vessel wall, which results in a vasoconstriction. This would explain the more marked effect of THAM on the injured side in the cats, where the vasoparalysis was more pronounced. It has also been suggested that there is a direct interaction with the catecholamine sensitive vascular receptors (1). Due to subsequent THAM diffusion into the extra-vascular space, the concentration remaining in the vessel walls is reduced, therefore explaining the temporary effect on ICP. However, the long-lasting EEG improvement and the effect on tissue edema parameters, observed in the rat experiments, suggests an additional metabolic effect, which may well be due to increasing the tissue pH as seen in glial cells (1), which results in the re-establishment of the aerobic metabolism and interruption of anaerobic acidosis-edema.

These observations clearly indicate the need for further studies on THAM in brain edema and congestion. The breath-depressing effect of THAM, which resulted in reduced survival rates in the rats, does however limit its use to patients receiving artificial respiration. But higher dosages may well give more profound effects.

Summary

In cats with cold brain injury edema, THAM rapidly but transiently lowers the ICP. The EEG, evaluated by computer, is markedly improved, outlasting the ICP decrease and the survival time is significantly prolonged. In respirated rats with similar cold brain trauma, water and electrolyte contents are improved by THAM. However, the breath-depressing effect reduces survival rates in animals breathing spontaneously. In patients with traumatic brain edema, a corresponding lowering of ICP and long-lasting improvement in EEG are seen. The results indicate an effect of THAM on vasoparalysis and acidotic disturbed metabolism in edema, but its breath-depressing effect limits its use to patients receiving artificial respiration.

References

1. Akioka T, Ota K, Matsumoto A, Iwatsuki K, Doi A, Akao S, Ninomya K, Nishimoto A (1976) The effect of Tham on acute intracranial hypertension. In: Beks JWF, Bosch DA, Brock M (eds) Intracranial Pressure III. Springer, Berlin Heidelberg New York, p. 219-233

2. Dos SJ, Nahas GG, Pappen EM (1962) Experimental correction of hypercapnic intracranial hypertension. Anesthesiology 23:46-50

3. Ewerbeck H, Hager J, Welte W (1966) Tris-Pufferbehandlung schwerer Verbrennungen bei Kindern zur Vermeidung von Hirndauerschäden. Dtsch med Wschr 91:1333-1338

4. Gaab M, Knoblich OE, Dietrich K, Gruss P (1978) Miniaturized methods of monitoring intracranial pressure in craniocerebral trauma before and after operation. In: Frowein RA, Wilcke O, Karimi-Nejad A, Brock M, Klinger M (eds) Advances in Neurosurgery 5. Springer, Berlin Heidelberg New York, p. 5-11

5. Gaab M, Knoblich OE, Schupp J, Dietrich K, Fuhrmeister U (1978) Wirkung unterschiedlicher Osmo- and Onkotherapie auf Hirndruck und elektrische Hirnaktivität beim experimentellen Hirnödem. Acta Neurochir 40:203-221

6. Gaab M, Knoblich OE, Pflughaupt KW, Fuhrmeister U (1979) Surgical decompression and resection of local edema in the therapy of experimental brain trauma. Investigation on metabolism, ICP and EEG. Acta Neurol Scand Suppl (in Press)

7. Henschler D (1963) Trispuffer (Tham) als Therapeutikum. Dtsch med Wschr 88:1328-1331

8. Meinig G, Reulen JH, Magawly C, Zöllner EJ (1978) Brain energy metabolism in global brain oedema. Acta Neurochir 41:273-286

9. Nahas GG (1966) The clinical pharmacology of THAM. Clin Pharm Ther 4:784-803

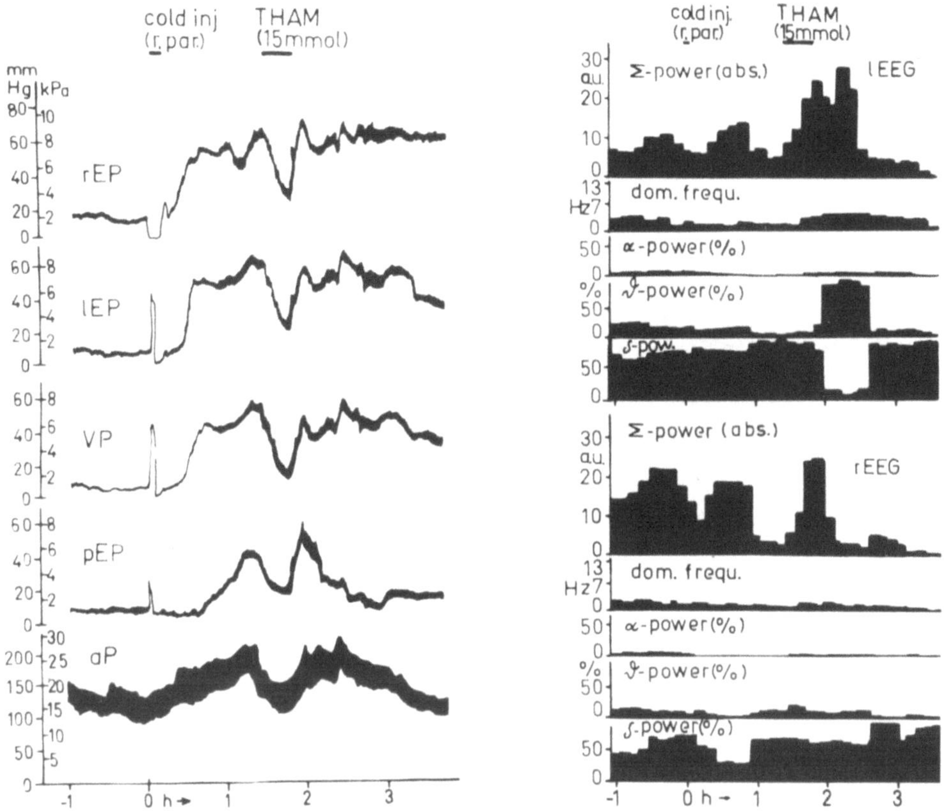

Figure la and b.
Effect of THAM on ICP (a) and EEG (b) in cat after cold brain injury. THAM rapidly but transiently lowers ICP, and markedly improves EEG power and frequency (pronounced on left, uninjured hemisphere). Note considerable pressure gradients after trauma (rEP right-, lEP left epidural press.; VP ventricular press., pEP epidural press. over cerebellum. aP arterial-, cvP central venous press.).

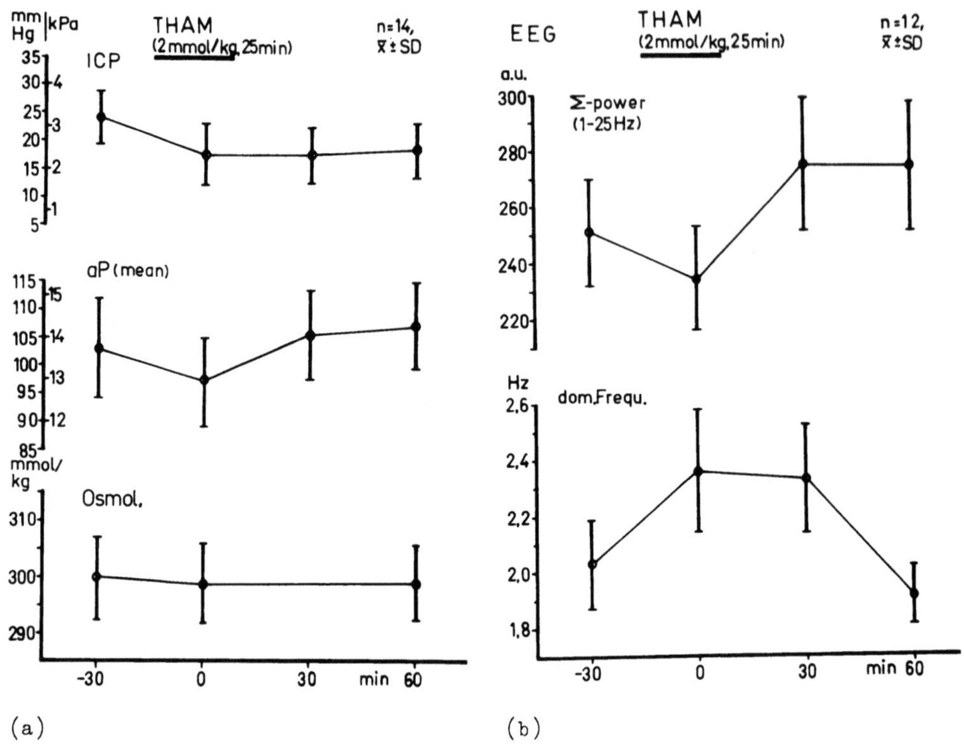

Figure 2a and b.
Effect of THAM on ICP (a) and EEG (b) in patients with severe head injuries (summarized values). THAM lowers ICP (measured epidurally without affecting blood osmolality; EEG frequency is increased, and also, after slow drop in frequency, EEG power remains elevated.

CLOSING DISCUSSION: "WHERE HAVE WE BEEN, WHERE ARE WE NOW, AND WHERE DO WE GO FROM HERE?"

T.W. LANGFITT

The title assigned to me for this summary is both challenging and appropriate. I will not spend much time on where we have been, because most of you are well aware of the modern history of ICP investigations. I will say that twenty years ago we were nowhere. JANNY had published an important paper on continuous recording of ICP in man, and LUNDBERG'S first paper on ICP recordings was published in 1959. Ten years ago only a handful of neurosurgeons were recording ICP routinely in an attempt to unravel the pathophysiology of intracranial hypertension and better manage their patients. It is probably true that at the moment, as we conclude this symposium, several hundred patients are having their ICP monitored throughout the world, a demonstration that the usefulness of ICP recording has now been established in the minds of a large number of neurosurgeons.

I will address the questions--where are we now and where do we go from here?--within three categories that, in my opinion, are the three principal goals of the study of intracranial pressure in the years ahead. The goals follow one upon the other. The first one is to continue to better understand the pathophysiology of increased intracranial pressure, in order to develop more effective methods of diagnosis and treatment, which is the second goal, so as to improve outcome in patients with a variety of intracranial pathologies, the third goal. In this summary, the essayists of a number of papers presented at the symposium will be cited by name. I hesitate to do so because many important contributions will be left out. Since there have been 150 communications during the course of the symposium, however, it would not be feasible to mention all of them even briefly.

Pathophysiology:
In one form or another the pathophysiology of increased intracranial pressure has occupied much of our time at this conference. Three subjects under that heading have received the most attention: volume/pressure relationships, edema and CSF dynamics.

Volume/Pressure Relationships: I believe the greatest advances in our understanding of the pathophysiology of increased intracranial pressure in the past few years have been made in the general area of the biomechanical properties of the craniospinal space and its contents in normal and pathological conditions. There have been many contributors. Most noteworthy have been LOFGREN and ZWETNOW, MILLER and LEACH, MARMAROU and SHULMAN, SCHETTINI and WALSH, and more recently SKLAR, BENABID, SULLIVAN and others. The relationship of pressure and of the compliance or the elastance of the intracranial space and its contents to volume perturbations has proved to be complex. Some of the problems in understanding these relationships relate to the manner in which the system is perturbed. Three principal methods have been used. The first method, the one that was employed to derive the first volume/pressure curves, consists of expansion of an intracranial, extracerebral balloon either in increments or by slow infusion of water into the balloon. The second method is infusion of mock CSF into the ventricles or subarachnoid space at various rates, and the third method is a bolus injection of saline through an intraventricular cannula. The engineers and mathematicians among us have developed models of the craniospinal space and its contents and have demonstrated quite elegantly the validity of these models in a variety of experimental circumstances. However, there are still a number of areas of disagreement in the interpretation of the results and some confusion among those in the field of ICP who have not done specific research in volume/pressure relationships.

In my opinion some of that confusion relates to the fact that often a proper distinction is not made between the brain and spinal cord on the one hand and the CSF spaces on the other when the mechanical properties of the system are described. They respond very differently to a stress applied to the system, and they also respond differently according to the precise nature of that stress. Although there is a reciprocal relationship between compliance and elastance, and therefore both brain and CSF possess both elastance and compliance, I find it more convenient to think of the CSF spaces as the primarily compliant part of the system and the brain as being an essentially elastic substance, although it has significant viscous (compliant) properties.

Looking now at the volume/pressure curve in response to constant rate infusion of an intracranial balloon over a period of many hours, a situation that roughly simulates the most common volume/pressure relationship encountered in clinical neurosurgery, the initial, nearly horizontal portion of the curve is largely a function of the compliance of the intracranial space. Two principal physical events occur during this time. CSF is expressed from the intracranial space, largely into the spinal theca, in order to accommodate the balloon, and the brain is distorted and molded to the expanding mass. The rate at which the molding takes place, and the consequent alterations in brain substance, are a function of the elastance of the brain. It is probably true that even with the slowest rates of infusion there is a pressure gradient across the underlying brain, and the height of the pressure gradient is a function of the rate of expansion of the balloon. However, shortly after cessation of expansion of the mass, irrespective of the level of intracranial pressure at that time, the pressure gradient is dissipated, probably within a few minutes, by viscous or plastic creep of the brain away from the balloon. When pressures are equalized throughout the brain the creep ceases. On the rapidly ascending portion of the volume/pressure curve much of the CSF has been expelled, and each increment added to the balloon is now "testing" the elastance of the brain more than the compliance of the CSF pathways.

The volume/pressure relationship responds somewhat differently to infusion of mock CSF compared to expansion of a balloon. The infusate is absorbed by increased conductance through the arachnoid villi, a pressure dependent phenomenon. When the rate of infusion exceeds the maximum rate of absorption, ICP rises at a rapid rate in much the same way that it rises on the rapidly ascending portion of the volume/pressure curve during expansion of a balloon. At very high pressures during infusion the curve tends to flatten giving it the sigmoid shape that has been described in the literature so frequently in recent years. The flattening of the curve means that a decrease in resistance must have occurred somewhere within the system, and the observations presented by LOVE during the symposium show that during prolonged infusion outflow resistance does decrease in the cat. In discussion, EKSTEDT presented evidence that a late decrease in resistance does not occur in man, and I suspect that flattening of the volume/pressure curve in experimental animals occurs only with infusion, not with expansion of a balloon.

The bolus method for testing the compliance/elastance of the intracranial space is quite different from the other two methods. Because a small amount of fluid is injected into the intracranial space very rapidly, both the CSF spaces and the brain behave in a highly elastic fashion in contrast to balloon expansion and infusion where there is time for the compliance of the system to come into play, mainly through displacement of CSF but also by plastic creep of the brain. This issue was addressed in a presentation by SULLIVAN who compared outflow resistance during infusion and bolus injection and attributed the large differences at high outflow resistance to tissue relaxation with the infusion method but not with bolus injections.

As a final comment on the volume/pressure relationships I believe that at all times they are multiexponential. The two principal exponents relate to the CSF and the brain, but surely the brain itself does not react homogeneously to expansion of an extracerebral mass, for example. Probably cerebral blood volume decreases in a heterogeneous, multiexponential pattern in response to the expanding mass, and the elastic properties of the brain tissue itself must be very complex.

The principal interest in volume/pressure relationships derives from the importance of assessing the compliance/elastance of the intracranial space in clinical management. It is well recognized that a patient with a slightly elevated ICP who has a large compliance is at less risk to develop a rapid, dangerous increase in ICP in response to changes in respiration or physical movements, for example, than is a patient with the same resting level of ICP but reduced compliance. The bolus method that is used to assess compliance clinically carries small but significant risks. The bolus can set off a pressure wave, and any time fluid is injected into the intracranial space through a ventricular cannula the risk of infection is increased. Therefore, a non-invasive method for assessing compliance is badly needed. EIJNDHOVEN and AVEZAAT and PORTNOY addressed this issue. The former authors postulated that the amplitude of the CSF pulse is principally a function of the amount of increase in cerebral blood volume with each cycle and the slope of the craniospinal volume/pressure curve. Thus, if the increase in cerebral blood volume that occurs with each systole can be assumed to be constant the amplitude of the pulse wave becomes an estimate of compliance/elastance. PORTNOY described an increase in the amplitude of the second wave of the pulse which he attributed to a decrease in resistance within the resistance vessels of the brain, and, therefore, an increase in brain volume and a decrease in intracranial compliance.

Edema: Two persistent questions about edema recur in the ICP symposia and in the recent conferences on brain edema. They are the incidence and significance of brain edema in acute head injury, and the contribution of edema to brain damage and neurologic dysfunction in any pathological condition. GENNARELLI demonstrated large increases in ICP in a model of acceleration head injury in the monkey and concluded that the rapid time course of the pressure changes was much more compatible with cerebral vasodilatation and an increase in cerebral blood volume than with the formation and absorption of edema. In a model of percussion injury of the cat, CORALES showed increases in ICP but no increase in the water content of the brain. Although it is clear that edema does develop in the brain surrounding contusions and traumatic intracerebral hematomas, and the time course of the formation and absorption of that edema has now been studied by CT scanning, the papers presented at this symposium provided additional evidence that diffuse, traumatic cerebral edema does not exist.

A cold lesion of the cerebral cortex simulates reasonably well a severe cortical contusion. Edema fluid seeps from the broken blood vessels through the white matter of the ipsilateral cerebral hemisphere. If the lesion is large enough, and particularly if the systemic blood pressure is elevated during the course of edema formation, swelling of the hemisphere may be sufficient to raise intracranial pressure so high that the animal dies. Cerebral blood flow is reduced adjacent to the injury, secondary to the mass effects of the lesion, and blood flow is reduced throughout the brain if ICP increases to high enough levels. However, there is not a good correlation between the amount of edema and regional flow as demonstrated in the paper presented by DICK. MARMAROU showed that even a very marked increase in water content in the white matter produced by a slow infusion of fluid does not reduce blood flow. Therefore, there continues to be compelling evidence that edema per se does not disturb brain function. Brain function appears to be impaired only when the volume of edema is sufficient to reduce focal blood flow, by an increase in tissue pressure, or the volume of edema fluid is large enough to cause a marked, generalized rise in ICP and a reduction of blood flow throughout the brain to ischemic levels.

CSF Dynamics: It has been known for a long time that cerebral vessels are liberally supplied with nerve endings of autonomic origin. However, extensive effort was required to demonstrate that this neural system was important in the control of the cerebral circulation in normal and pathological conditions. At this symposium, for the first time, a very important contribution of the autonomic system to the formation of CSF by the choroid plexus was demonstrated by EDVINSSON and LINDVALL. Sympathetic stimulation decreased CSF formation one third and sympathectomy resulted in a one third increase in CSF production. Norepinephrine administered both intravenously and through the ventricles had a significant effect on CSF production.

The valves within the arachnoid villi that provide the principal resistance to CSF absorption have become more and more important in our understanding of a number of pathological conditions. For a number of years, blockage of the villi by red blood cells following subarachnoid hemorrhage and by exudate in the course of intracranial infections has been well recognized. The result is hydrocephalus which may require shunting or may resolve spontaneously with resolution of the clogging of the villi. KASARSKIS demonstrated that vitamin A deficiency results in a reversible structural alteration of arachnoid villi in rats resulting in a syndrome similar to pseudotumor cerebri, rather than hydrocephalus, and also presented a clinical case where there were good reasons to believe that the patient had the same disorder produced experimentally in the rats. These observations and others during the course of the symposium emphasized two important issues. First, increases in the resistance to CSF absorption might occur in response to a variety of systemic "toxins" and not only from physical obstruction of the arachnoid villi, and second, there is still little understanding of the reasons why an increase in outflow resistance either at the arachnoid villi or within the dural sinuses results in hydrocephalus in some patients and benign intracranial hypertension due to brain swelling in other patients.

The communications in this symposium have demonstrated more than ever before that changes in CSF production cannot be neglected in the interpretation of clinical or experimental data related to the CSF system. MANN found a marked increase in outflow resistance with Enflurane and Ketamine compared to pentobarbital, and estimates of CSF production indicated a doubling with Enflurane compared to the other agents. One can only imagine the magnitude of the alterations in CSF production that occur in a patient with a severe head injury in whom there are marked fluctuations in sympathetic activity and in the catecholamine content of the blood in response to the severe stresses to which the body is subjected, and in a head injured patient who undergoes anesthesia and is treated with barbiturates.

The Diagnosis and Management of Patients with Intracranial Pathology--The Second Goal

Hydrocephalus: Two of the most pressing issues in the field of hydrocephalus are the diagnosis of normal pressure hydrocephalus, that is, making the differential diagnosis between NPH and cerebral atrophy, and second, the diagnosis of arrested hydrocephalus, defined as persistent hydrocephalus that does no harm to the patient.

The CSF infusion test shows great promise in distinguishing between NPH and atrophy. The observations of GJERRIS were particularly striking. When the value for CSF conductance (C_{out}) was less than .075, shunting resulted in clinical improvement in 28 of the 29 patients in that category. In contrast, among 11 patients with a value for C_{out} between .075 and .125, none improved with shunting. In discussion, GJERRIS stated that among the 28 patients who improved with shunts, none had a CT picture compatible with the diagnosis of atrophy. TEASDALE was not quite so optimistic about the value of the infusion test, and FIRTH had a small number of patients with a diagnosis of atrophy who did improve with the shunt. CROCKARD reminded the group that the postoperative evaluation of these patients must be extremely rigorous. In particular, he noted that many of the standard psychometric tests are useless in these patients.

The presence of pressure waves was also a good indication for shunting in the view of LAMAS. GJERRIS also noted that B waves were present in the large majority of patients who benefitted from the shunt. EKSTEDT made the interesting observation that if conductance is always reduced in NPH then ICP must always be increased. In the beginning the condition was called low pressure hydrocephalus. Then came recognition of the fact that intracranial pressure was not below normal, and the term normal pressure hydrocephalus was substituted. If EKSTEDT is correct, another substitution might be necessary, perhaps moderate pressure hydrocephalus (MPH).

Where do we go from here in further studies of hydrocephalus? I believe mainly toward acquisition of more clinical data, particularly on the infusion test, the incidence and the nature of pressure waves in patients who respond well to shunting, and very careful analysis of resting or mean overall ICP in order to determine if pressure is, in fact, normal or increased in these patients. Three points appear to be important with regard to the infusion test. First, all investigators should agree on the methodology. It would be unfortunate to have disagreements at our next symposium based on different techniques. Second, the methodology must be applied meticulously. Leaks around the needle and other technical problems can lead to artifacts. Finally, the preoperative and postoperative status of each patient must be examined rigorously, and in particular, the social and mental status of the patients must be tested adequately.

Head Injury: ICP continues to be measured more commonly in severely head injured patients than in any other clinical condition. The purposes are to determine if ICP is increased, if it is increased then treat the intracranial hypertension with whatever means are necessary, and finally correlate the clinical outcome with the level of ICP during the patients' illness in order to assess the significance of intracranial hypertension in the morbidity and mortality of head injury.

It has been difficult to establish the overall incidence of intracranial hypertension in head injured patients because a definition of increased ICP has not been clearly established and because most patients have therapy of varying degrees of intensity before the first recording of ICP is obtained. From a number of observations made at this symposium, and from a variety of other contributions in recent years, it now seems reasonable to divide severely head injured patients into three categories based on the neurological examination, the CT scan, continuous recording of ICP, and measurements of cerebral blood flow.

The first category of patients are those who have diffuse impact injury or its synonym, diffuse white matter shearing injury. They are immediately comatose and on admission to the hospital are in profound coma with decerebration or decortication and other brainstem signs. The CT scan is normal except for the frequent occurrence of small hemorrhages in the corpus callosum and other midline structures. The patients do not have extracerebral hematomas, and ICP is normal. The cerebral metabolic rate of O_2 utilization ($CMRO_2$) is greatly reduced, often below 1.0 ml/100gm/min, and CBF is reduced proportionately. It appears that these patients have massive, irreversible brain injury from the moment of impact, ICP is not a problem, and current therapy is of no avail.

The second group of patients are those in whom the cerebral hemispheres bear the brunt of the injury in the form of contusions, especially large contusions of the temporal and frontal lobes, intracerebral hematomas, and subdural hematomas. The level of ICP in these patients is a function of the volume of extracerebral blood, and, subsequently, the volume of edema fluid that develops around the contusions and hematomas. Generalized CBF in these patients correlates well with the level of consciousness, but focal changes in the form of either decreased CBF or hyperemia are common in brain adjacent to hematomas and contusions. In many of these patients--the incidence has not been clearly established--successful treatment of intracranial hypertension produced by the hematomas, contusions and edema can be life-saving.

The third category of patients are those with diffuse cerebral swelling as described by BRUCE. Most of the patients are children and diffuse cerebral swelling over the age of 30 appears to be quite rare. Some of the children with moderate injuries have a lucid interval followed by loss of consciousness whereas those with more severe injuries remain unconscious from the time of the accident. There are many cases in the latter group who have very severe injuries manifested by deep coma and brainstem signs. The diagnosis of diffuse swelling is made by CT scan which shows small to absent ventricles and CSF spaces. ICP may be normal or only slightly elevated even when the CT scan shows severe swelling. In the more severely injured group of patients, however, ICP is nearly always elevated and very often is the principal factor related to outcome. If ICP can be controlled in these patients, the mortality is quite low and the quality of survival is good. CBF is increased either absolutely or relative to $CMRO_2$, and the density of the brain on CT scan is also increased, demonstrating that much if not all of the brain swelling is due to increased cerebral blood volume, not edema. Further categorization of severe head injuries, based on ICP and other criteria is a major challenge for the future.

Papers on therapy for intracranial hypertension dealt primarily with steroids, hypertonic mannitol and barbiturates. In recent years, improved outcome in patients treated with large doses of steroids has been reported. A number of investigators have found it difficult to accept these results because of the great difficulty in adequately comparing two groups of severely head injured patients under any circumstances. JAMES described a greater variability in the response of ICP to mannitol than did FERRER, and the latter essayist also observed a much higher incidence of rebound with mannitol than has been described in the literature.

The largest part of the discussion on therapy was devoted to barbiturates. MARSHALL described a significant improvement in outcome in head injured patients treated with barbiturates and confirmed previous observations by his group and by others that barbiturates not only produce a prompt decrease in ICP in most head injured patients but often will reduce ICP when all other agents have failed. BRUCE provided confirmation of these observations in children and provided evidence that the decrease in morbidity and mortality in his series of patients was due in significant part to control of marked intracranial hypertension with barbiturates. KASSELL described a reduction in ICP in a number of patients with severe vasospasm secondary to subarachnoid hemorrhage. MCGRAW presented evidence that pentobarbital is more effective in the control of ICP than is thiopental.

It was clear during the course of the symposium that at the present time the principal thrust in the treatment of intracranial hypertension is in the direction of better understanding of barbiturate therapy and its interaction with other forms of treatment. There are a number of areas for investigation: --How do barbiturates work? Are the beneficial effects due entirely to a reduction in ICP? Does pentobarbital further reduce metabolism in a patient with a severe head injury who already has a marked reduction in metabolic rate, and if so, is this beneficial? --Under what circumstances should barbiturate therapy be used? This is a corollary of the first question and related to its mechanisms of action and the reasons why the therapy is beneficial. --When should it be started? Thus far, barbiturates have been used mainly when other methods of treatment have failed. Might they be even more beneficial if started earlier? --How long should barbiturate therapy be continued? If reduction in ICP is the principal beneficial effect, then it follows that the therapy should be discontinued when it is no longer necessary to control ICP. If there are other beneficial effects, such as a reduction in metabolism, the end point for therapy could be quite different. --What is the incidence and significance of complications of the therapy related to the beneficial effects? The therapy if often difficult to control, and a number of systemic problems have been described. Therefore, in some patients the risk of complications could outweigh the chances of benefit. This is particularly so in patients who do not have increased ICP, which at the moment is the only clearly delineated indication for barbiturate therapy.

ICP and Clinical Outcome

The final test of any field of research that deals ultimately with clinical problems is the contribution that the research makes toward improving the morbidity and mortality from those clinical disorders. Studies of the influence of ICP measurements on outcome have been mainly in head injured patients. The amount of information available in patients with intracranial hemorrhage and other acute brain insults is insufficient to make any comment on the value of ICP measurements. ICP measurements will become very important in the outcome of normal pressure hydrocephalus if further studies confirm the importance of the pressure waves in differentiating NPH from brain atrophy.

Since VAPALAHTI'S original publication on the correlation of ICP and outcome demonstrating that nearly all patients with an ICP over 60 torr died, there has been much discussion about the level of ICP that is significant in terms of brain function and therefore should be significant in terms of outcome. In this symposium, PITTS and RICHARD described a good correlation between high ICP and outcome, and the latter investigators noted that high ICP was related to both neurological status and advancing age in predicting a bad outcome. No patients survived who were unconscious more than three days and had an ICP of more than 20 torr. ROSSANDA, who presented the paper by COLLICE and colleagues, did not find a difference in outcome in patients who had their ICP monitored and patients who were not monitored.

Clearly this is an area that needs to be pursued vigorously. The fact that many neurosurgeons throughout the world monitor ICP in severely head injured patients is not proof that the monitoring is beneficial either in managing the patients or especially in improving the results of management. One can think of a great many diagnostic methods and therapeutic regimens in the field of medicine that are of questionable effectiveness. The task is staggering in its dimensions because of the complexity of head injury, which means that no two patients are completely alike, and because the patients are so severely ill that true randomization of management is difficult if not impossible.

Both the organization and the scientific quality of this Fourth International Symposium on Intracranial Pressure were superb. It has been an honor and a pleasure to summarize briefly the proceedings.

LIST OF SENIOR AUTHORS

AKIOKA, T.
Division of Neurosurgery, Mizushima Central Hospital, 4-5, Aoba-cho, Mizushima, Kurashiki-shi 712 (Japan)

ALBIN, M.S.
Department of Anesthesiology, University of Texas Health Science Center, 7703 Floyd Curl Drive, San Antonio, TX 78284 (USA)

ALEXANDER, C.
Department of Anesthesiology, University of Wisconsin School of Medicine, Madison, WI 53706 (USA)

ARNOLD, H.
Abteilung für Neurochirurgie, Neurologische Universitätsklinik Hamburg, Martinistrasse 52, D-2000 Hamburg 20 (FRG)

ARTRU, F.
Département d'Anesthésie-Réanimation, Hôpital Neurologique, Unité 800, F-69394 Lyon Cedex 3 (France)

AUER, L.
Universitätsklinik für Neurochirurgie, Auenbruggerplatz, A-8036 Graz (Austria)

AVEZAAT, C.J.J.
Department of Neurosurgery, Dijkzigt-Hospital, Dr. Molewaterplein 40, Rotterdam-3002 (The Netherlands)

BAETHMANN, A.
Neurochirurgische Klinik, Klinikum Grosshadern, Ludwig-Maximilians-Universität München, Marchioninistrasse 15, D-8000 München 70 (FRG)

BECKER, D.P.
Virginia Commonwealth University, Medical College of Virginia, Division of Neurological Surgery, 1200 East Broad Street, Richmond, VA 23298 (USA)

BEDFORD, R.F.
Department of Anesthesiology, University of Virginia Medical Center, P.O.Box 238, Charlottesville, VA 22908 (USA)

BEKS, J.W.F.
Kliniek voor Neuro-Chirurgie, Akademisch Ziekenhuis, Oostersingel 59, Groningen (The Netherlands)

BENABID, A.L.
Service de Neurochirurgie, C.H.U. de Grenoble, F-38700 La Tronche (France)

BLASBERG, R.
National Institutes of Health, Building 37 5A-13, Bethesda, MD 20205 (USA)

BLESSER, M.
Royal Alexandra Hospital for Children, Pyrmont Bridge Road, Camperdown, NSW 2050 (Australia)

BONGARTZ, E.B.
Neurochirurgische Klinik der Universität Essen, Hufelandstrasse 55, D-4300 Essen 1 (FRG)

BROCK, M.
Universitätsklinikum Steglitz, Neurochirurgische Klinik und Poliklinik, Freie Universität Berlin, Hindenburgdamm 30, D-1000 Berlin 45 (FRG)

BROCKLEHURST, G.
Hull Royal Infirmary, Anlaby Road, Kingston Upon Hull, Humberside (U.K.)

BRUCE, D.A.
Division of Neurosurgery, University of Pennsylvania, 3400 Sprace Street, Philadelphia, PA 19104 (USA)

BUTLER, A.B.
Department of Neurological Surgery, University of Virginia Hospital, P.O.Box 212, Charlottesville, VA 22908 (USA)

BYRNES, D.P.
Maryland Institute for Emergency Medical Services Systems, University of Maryland, Baltimore, MD 21202 (USA)

CALBUCCI, F.
Divisione di Neurochirurgica, Ospedale Bellaria, Via Altura, I-65020 Bologna (Italy)

CASTEL, J.-P.
Service de Neurochirurgie A, Hôpital Pellegrin, F-33076 Bordeaux (France)

CHAPMAN, P.H.
Neurosurgical Service, Massachusetts General Hospital, Boston, MA 02114 (USA)

CLUBB, R.J.
Department of Neurosurgery, National Naval Medical Center, Bethesda, MD 20014 (USA)

COLLICE, M.
Divisione di Neurochirurgica, Ospedale Ca'Granda, Piazza Ospedale Maggiore 3, I-20162 Milano-Niquarda (Italy)

COOPER, P.R.
450 Clarkson Avenue, P.O.Box 1189, Brooklyn, NY 11203 (USA)

CORALES, R.L.
Division of Neurological Surgery, Medical College of Virginia, Richmond, VA 23298 (USA)

CORBIN, S.D.
Cardiovascular Surgery, Stanford University School of Medicine, Medical Center, 300 Pasteur Dr., Stanford, CA 94305 (USA)

CROCKARD, H.A.
Department of Neurosurgical Studies, National Hospital for Nervous Diseases, Queen Square, London WCI (U.K.)

CUNITZ, G.
Knappschaftskrankenhaus-Bochum-Langendreer, Universitätsklinik der Ruhr Universität, In der Schornau 23-25, D-4630 Bochum-Langendreer (FRG)

CZERNICKI, Z.
Department of Neurosurgery, Medical Research Centre, Polish Academy of Sciences, Bialobrzeska 58, 02-325 Warsaw (Poland)

DACEY, R.G.
Department of Neurosurgery, University of Virginia Hospital, P.O.Box 212, Charlottesville, VA 22908 (USA)

DICK, A.R.
Department of Neurology, University of Kansas Medical Center, Room 101-B, Kansas City, KS 66103 (USA)

DUNKER, R.O.
Division of Neurosurgery, West Virginia University, Morgantown, West VA 26506 (USA)

EIJNDHOVEN, VAN, J.H.M.
Department of Electro-Neurology (EE 2238), Erasmus University, P.O. Box 1738, Rotterdam-3002 (The Netherlands)

EKSTEDT, J.
Department of Neurology, University Hospital of Umeå, S-90185 Umeå (Sweden)

ERDMANN, W.
Departments of Anesthesiology, Neurosurgery and Pharmacology, Rijksuniversiteit, Groningen (The Netherlands)

ESPARZA, J.
Servicio de Neurocirurgia, Ciudad Sanitaria "I° de Octubre", Carretera de Andalucia, Km. 5.400, Madrid-16 (Spain)

FASOL, P.
II. Universitätsklinik für Unfallchirurgie, Spitalgasse 23, A-1090 Wien (Austria)

FERRER, E.
Servicio de Neurocirurgia, C.S. Principes de España, Hospitalet de Llobregat, Barcelona (Spain)

FRIDÉN, H.
Department of Neurology, University Hospital of Umeå, S-90185 Umeå (Sweden)

FUHRMEISTER, U.
Neurologische Universitätsklinik, Kopfklinik, Josef-Schneider-Strasse 11, D-8700 Würzburg (FRG)

FUJIMOTO, S.
Department of Neurological Surgery, Okayama University Medical School, 2-5-1 Shikata-cho, Okayama 700 (Japan)

FURUSE, M.
Department of Neurosurgery, Nagoya University School of Medicine, 65 Tsuruma-cho, Showa-ku, Nagoya 466 (Japan)

GAAB, M.
Neurochirurgische Universitätsklinik, Kopfklinikum, Josef-Schneider-Strasse 11, D-8700 Würzburg (FRG)

GARCIA, J.H.
Department of Pathology, University of Alabama Medical Center, Birmingham, AL 35294 (USA)

GARCIA DE SOLA, R.
Servicio de Neurocirurgía, Clínica Puerta de Hierro. San Martín de Porres 4, Madrid-35 (Spain)

GAZENDAM, J.
National Institutes of Health, Building 37 5A-13, Bethesda, MD 20205 (USA)

GEGA, A.
Department of Neurosurgery, Nara Medical University, Kashihara, Nara 634 (Japan)

GENNARELLI, T.A.
Division of Neurosurgery, University of Pennsylvania, 3400 Sprace Street, Philadelphia, PA 19104 (USA)

GESSEY, G.
Department of Cardio-thoracic Measurement, Derbyshire Royal Infirmary, Derby DE1 2QY (U.K.)

GJERRIS, F.
University Clinic of Neurosurgery, Rikshospitalet, DK-2100 Copenhagen (Denmark)

GOBIET, W.
Universitätsklinikum der Gesamthochschule Essen, Neurochirurgische Klinik, Hufelandstrasse 55, D-4300 Essen 1 (FRG)

GODIN, D.
Clinique Neurochirurgicale, Hôpital de Bavière, 66 Boulevard de la Constitution, B-4020 Liège (Belgium)

GRAHAM, D.I.
Department of Neuropathology, Institute of Neurological Sciences, Southern General Hospital, Glasgow G51 4TF (U.K.)

GRAHAM, S.I.
Division of Neurosurgery, University of Texas Medical School at Houston, Health Science Center, 6431 Fannin Street, Houston, TX 77030 (USA)

GRIFFITH, R.L.
Virginia Commonwealth University, Medical College of Virginia, Division of Neurological Surgery, 1200 East Broad Street, Richmond, VA 23298 (USA)

GUCER, G.
Division of Neurosurgery, Baltimore City Hospitals, 4940 Eastern Avenue, Baltimore, MD 21224 (USA)

GUPTA, B.
Department of Anesthesiology, New York University Medical Center, 560 First Avenue, New York, NY 10016 (USA)

HAAR, F.L.
Division of Neurosurgery, University of Texas Medical School at Houston, Health Science Center, 6431 Fannin Street, Houston, TX 77030 (USA)

HARTMANN, A.
Neurologische Universitätsklinik, Vosstrasse 2, D-6900 Heidelberg (FRG)

HAYASHI, M.
Department of Neurosurgery, University of Kanazawa School of Medicine, 13-1 Takaramachi, Kanazawa 920 (Japan)

HOCHWALD, G.M.
Department of Neurology, New York University Medical Center, 550 First Avenue, New York, NY 10016 (USA)

HOFF, J.T.
Department of Neurosurgery, University of California Medical Center, San Francisco, CA 94143 (USA)

IKAYAMA, A.
Department of Neurosurgery, Nagoya University School of Medicine, 65 Tsuruma-cho, Showa-ku, Nagoya 446 (Japan)

JAMES, H.E.
Division of Neurosurgery (H-893), University Hospital, 225 W.Dickinson Street, San Diego, CA 92103 (USA)

JANE, J.A.
Department of Neurosurgery, University of Virginia School of Medicine, Charlottesville, VA 22901 (USA)

JANNY, P.
Hôpital Fontmaure, F-63400 Chamalières (France)

JENNETT, S.
Institute of Physiology, University of Glasgow, Glasgow G12 8QQ (U.K.)

KASARSKIS, E.J.
Department of Neurology, University of Virginia Hospital, P.O.Box 212, Charlottesville, VA 22908 (USA)

KASSELL, N.F.
Division of Neurosurgery, University of Iowa Hospitals and Clinics, Iowa City, IA 52242 (USA)

KINDT, G.W.
Division of Neurosurgery, University of Michigan Medical Center, Ann Arbor, MI 48109 (USA)

KNOBLICH, O.E.
Psychiatrische Klinik und Poliklinik, Universität München, Nussbaumstrasse 7, D-8000 München 2 (FRG)

KOSTER, W.G.
Philips Medical Systems Division, QM45, Eindhoven (The Netherlands)

KRISHNAN, K.L.M.
Institute of Neurology, Madras Medical College and Government General Hospital, Plot 64, "F" Block, Anna Nagar, Madras-600 040 (India)

KUCHIWAKI, H.
3-12-6 Minamigaoka, Nisshincho, Aichi-gun, Aichi 471-01 (Japan)

KUYAMA, H.
Department of Neurological Surgery, Okayama University Medical School, 2-5-1 Shikata-cho, Okayama 700 (Japan)

LAMAS, E.
Servicio de Neurocirurgia, Ciudad Sanitaria "1º de Octubre", Carretera de Andalucia, Km. 5.400, Madrid-16 (Spain)

LANGFITT, T.W.
Division of Neurosurgery, University of Pennsylvania, 3400 Sprace Street, Philadelphia, PA 19104 (USA)

LINDVALL, M.
Department of Histology, University of Lund, Biskopsgatan 5, S-223 62 Lund (Sweden)

LOBATO, R.D.
Servicio de Neurocirurgia, Ciudad Sanitaria "1º de Octubre", Carretera de Andalucia, Km. 5.400, Madrid-16 (Spain)

LOVE, J.A.
Department of Physiology and Biophysics, CH. Tupper Building, Faculty of Medicine, Dalhousie University, Halifax, Nova Scotia, B 3H 4H7 (Canada)

LUNDBERG, N.
Department of Neurosurgery B, University Hospital, S-223 62 Lund (Sweden)

MANN, J.D.
751 Burnett-Womack Clinical Sciences Building 229H, University of North Carolina, Chapel Hill, NC 27514 (USA)

MARMAROU, A.
Leo M. Davidoff Department of Neurological Surgery, Albert Einstein College of Medicine, Yeshiva University, 1300 Morris Park Avenue, Bronx, NY 10461 (USA)

MARSHALL, L.F.
Division of Neurosurgery (H-893), University Hospital, 225 W.Dickinson Street, San Diego, CA 92103 (USA)

MASON, J.
Department of Medical Physics, Pinderfields General Hospital, Wakefield, West Yorkshire WF1 4DG (U.K.)

McGRAW, C.P.
Department of Neurology, The Bowman Gray School of Medicine, Wake Forest University, 300 S. Hawthorne Road, Winston-Salem, NC 27103 (USA)

MENEZES, A.
Division of Neurosurgery, University of Iowa Hospitals and Clinics, Iowa City, IA 52242 (USA)

MESANGEAU, D.
Laboratoire d'Innothera, 10 Avenue P.V. Couturier, F-94110 Arcueil (France)

MEYER, G.A.
Department of Neurosurgery, Room 1034, The Medical College of Wisconsin, 8700 West Wisconsin Avenue, Milwaukee, WI 53226 (USA)

MILLER, J.D.
Virginia Commonwealth University, Medical College of Virginia, Division of Neurological Surgery, 1200 East Broad Street, Richmond, VA 23298 (USA)

MINGRINO, S.
Istituto Neurochirurgica, Via Giustiniani 5, I-84034 Padova (Italy)

MITCHELL, P.H.
Department of Physiological Nursing, SM-28, University of Washington, Seattle, WA 98195 (USA)

MOHR, P.
Abteilung für Neurochirurgie der Justus Liebig-Universität Giessen, Klinikstrasse 29, D-6300 Giessen (FRG)

MORAWETZ, R.B.
Division of Neurosurgery, University Station, Birmingham, AL 35294 (USA)

MOSS, E.
Leeds General Infirmary, Great George Street, Leeds LS1 3EX, West Yorkshire (U.K.)

MOSZYNISKI, K.
Balladyny 16/36, 2061 Lublin (Poland)

NAGAI, H.
Department of Neurosurgery, Nagoya University School of Medicine, 65 Tsuruma-cho, Showa-ku, Nagoya 466 (Japan)

NAKAGAWA, Y.
Department of Neurosurgery, Hokkaido University School of Medicine, North 14 West 5, Sapporo, Hokkaido (Japan)

NAKATANI, S.
Department of Neurosurgery, Osaka University Medical School, 1-1-50, Fukushima, Osaka 553 (Japan)

NELSON, S.R.
Departments of Pharmacology and Surgery, University of Kansas Medical Center, 39th and Rainbow Boulevard, Kansas City, KS 66103 (USA)

NEMOTO, E.M.
Anesthesia Research Laboratories, Department of Anesthesiology and Critical Care Medicine, University of Pittsburgh School of Medicine, Pittsburgh, PA 15261 (USA)

NISHIMURA, M.C.
Department of Neurological Surgery, M784, University of California Medical Center, San Francisco, CA 94143 (USA)

NYARY, I.
National Institute of Neurosurgery, Budapest (Hungary)

OBERBAUER, R.W.
Universitätsklinik für Neurochirurgie, Auenbruggerplatz, A-8036 Graz (Austria)

PALTSEV, E.I.
Laboratory for Biophysical Aspects of Complex Biological Systems, Institute for Problems of Information Transmission, Academy of Sciences USSR, 19 Ermolovoy Street, Moscow 103051 (USSR)

PAPO, I.
Divisione die Neurochirurgica, Ospedale Generale Regionale, Via Panoramica 34, I-60100 Ancona (Italy)

PICKARD, J.D.
Department of Neurosurgery, Institute of Neurological Sciences, Southern General Hospital, Glasgow G51 4TF (U.K.)

PITTS, L.H.
Department of Neurological Surgery, University of California Medical Center, San Francisco, CA 94143 (USA)

PORTNOY, H.D.
Oakland Neurological Clinic, P.C., 1431 Woodward, Bloomfield Hill, MI 48013 (USA)

PRICE, D.J.
Department of Neurosurgery, Pinderfields General Hospital, Wakefield, West Yorkshire WF1 4DG (U.K.)

RAJU, T.N.K.
Department of Pediatrics, University of Illinois Hospital, 840 South Wood Street, Chicago, IL 60612 (USA)

RAP, Z.M.
Department of Neuropathology, Medical Research Centre, Polish Academy of Sciences, 3, Dworkowa Str., 00-784 Warsaw (Poland)

RICHARD, K.E.
Neurochirurgische Universitätsklinik, Joseph-Stelzmann-Strasse 9, D-5000 Köln 41 (FRG)

ROTTENBERG, D.A.
Department of Neurology, Memorial Hospital, 1275 York Avenue, New York, NY 10021 (USA)

ROWAN, J.O.
Division of Clinical Physics, Institute of Neurological Sciences, Southern General Hospital, Gowan Road, Glasgow G51 4TF (U.K.)

SCHETTINI, A.
Anesthesiology Section (112), Medical College of Virginia, McGuire V.A. Hospital, Richmond, VA 23235 (USA)

SHAPIRO, K.
Leo M. Davidoff Department of Neurological Surgery, Albert Einstein College of Medicine, Yeshiva University, 1300 Morris Park Avenue, Bronx, NY 10461 (USA)

SHIGENO, T.
Department of Neurosurgery, University of Tokyo, 7-3-1 Hongo, Bunkyo-ku, Tokyo 160 (Japan)

SHULMAN, K.
Leo M. Davidoff Department of Neurological Surgery, Albert Einstein College of Medicine, Yeshiva University, 1300 Morris Park Avenue, Bronx, NY 10461 (USA)

SILVERBERG, G.D.
Division of Neurosurgery, Stanford University School of Medicine, Medical Center, 300 Pasteur Dr., Stanford, CA 94305 (USA)

SKLAR, F.H.
Division of Neurosurgery, University of Texas Health Science Center at Dallas, 5323 Harry Hines Boulevard, Dallas, TX 75235 (USA)

SØRENSEN, S.C.
University Clinic of Anaesthesiology, Rikshospitalet, DK-2100 Copenhagen (Denmark)

STÅHLHAMMAR, D.
Department of Neurosurgery, Sahlgrens Hospital, S-413 45 Göteborg (Sweden)

STEVENAERT, A.
Clinique Neurochirurgicale, Hôpital de Bavière, 66 Boulevard de la Constitution, B-4020 Liège (Belgium)

SULLIVAN, H.G.
Virginia Commonwealth University, Medical College of Virginia, Division of Neurological Surgery, 1200 East Broad Street, Richmond, VA 23298 (USA)

SZWECZYKOWSKI, J.
Department of Neurosurgery, Medical Research Centre, Polish Academy of Sciences, Bialobrzezeska 58, 02-325 Warsaw (Poland)

TABADDOR, K.
Leo M. Davidoff Department of Neurological Surgery, Albert Einstein College of Medicine, Yeshiva University, 1300 Morris Park Avenue, Bronx, NY 10461 (USA)

TAKAGI, H.
Department of Neurosurgery, Kitasato University School of Medicine, 1, Asamizodai, Sagamihara-shi, Kanagawa 228 (Japan)

TAKIZAWA, H.
Department of Neurosurgery, Tokyo Rosai Hospital, Ota-ku, Omori-minami 4-13-21, Tokyo 160 (Japan)

TEASDALE, G.
Department of Neurosurgery, Institute of Neurological Sciences, Southern General Hospital, Glasgow G51 4TF (U.K.)

TSEMENTZIS, S.A.
Department of Surgical Neurology, Western General Hospital, Crewe Road, Edinburgh EH4 2XU (U.K.)

VAJDA, J.
National Institute of Neurosurgery, Budapest (Hungary)

VERSARI, P.
Divisione di Neurochirurgica, Ospedale Ca'Granda, Piazza Ospedale Maggiore 3, I-20162 Milano-Niquarda (Italy)

VILA, F.
Servicio de Neurocirurgica, C.S. Príncipes de España, Hospitalet de Llobregat, Barcelona (Spain)

VOLBY, B.
Neurokirurgisk afdeling, Kommunehospitalet, DK-8000 Aarhus C (Denmark)

WALLENFANG, Th.
Neurochirurgische Universitätsklinik, Langenbeckstrasse 1, D-6500 Mainz (FRG)

WALSH, E.K.
College of Engineering, University of Florida, Gainesville, FL 32611 (USA)

WALSTRA, G.
Department of Neurology, University Hospital, Groningen (The Netherlands)

WOOD, D.H.
Department of Neurology, Howard University Hospital, Washington, DC 20046 (USA)

YAMAMOTO, M.
Cerebral Blood Flow Laboratory, Houstan VA Medical Center, Houston, TX 77025 (USA)

YONEDA, S.
Department of Neurosurgery, Kyoto University Medical School, 54 Kawahara-cho, Shogoin, Sakyo-ku, Kyoto 606 (Japan)

ZERVAS, N.T.
Neurosurgical Service, Massachusetts General Hospital, Boston, MA 02114 (USA)

ZIERSKI, J.
Neurochirurgische Universitätsklinik, Klinikstrasse 29, D-6300 Giessen (FRG)

ZWETNOW, N.N.
Department of Neurosurgery, Karolinska Sjukhuset, S-10401 Stockholm (Sweden)

AUTHOR INDEX

SUBJECT INDEX

MIX
Papier aus verantwortungsvollen Quellen
Paper from responsible sources
FSC® C105338
www.fsc.org

If you have any concerns about our products,
you can contact us on
ProductSafety@springernature.com

In case Publisher is established outside the EU,
the EU authorized representative is:
Springer Nature Customer Service Center GmbH
Europaplatz 3, 69115 Heidelberg, Germany

Printed by Libri Plureos GmbH
in Hamburg, Germany